PROSTHETICS
AND
ORTHOTICS

Lower Limb and Spinal

PROSTHETICS AND ORTHOTICS

Lower Limb and Spinal

RON SEYMOUR, PT, PHD

Associate Professor
Department of Physical Therapy Education
College of Health Professions
SUNY Upstate Medical University
Syracuse, New York

with contributors

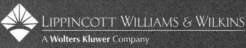

LIPPINCOTT WILLIAMS & WILKINS
A **Wolters Kluwer** Company

Philadelphia · Baltimore · New York · London
Buenos Aires · Hong Kong · Sydney · Tokyo

Senior Acquiring Editor: Tim Julet
Managing Editor: Ulita Lushnycky
Development Editor: Nancy Peterson
Senior Marketing Manager: Debby Hartman
Production Editor: Jennifer Ajello

Printed in the United States of America

Library of Congress Cataloging-in-Publication Data

Seymour, Ron, PhD.
    Prosthetics and orthotics : lower limb and spinal / Ron Seymour.
        p. cm.
    Includes index.
    ISBN-13: 978-0-7817-2854-6
    ISBN-10: 0-7817-2854-1
        1. Prosthesis. 2. Orthopedic apparatus. 3. Artificial limbs. 4. Artificial legs. 5. Amputees—Rehabilitation. I. Title.

RD756.4 .S49 2002
617.5'803—dc21

                                                                2001050351

The publishers have made every effort to trace the copyright holders for borrowed material. If they have inadvertently overlooked any, they will be pleased to make the necessary arrangements at the first opportunity.

To purchase additional copies of this book call our customer service department at **(800) 638-3030** or fax orders to **(301) 824-7390**. International customers should call **(301) 714-2324.**

06
4 5 6 7 8 9 10

To Nora and Sid, for an excellent beginning

To Rachel and Jamie, the joys of my life

To Mary, for her love and support

CONTRIBUTORS

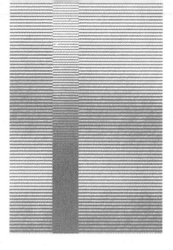

Mary Evans, PT
Physical Therapy
Children's Hospital
Buffalo, New York

Carol Gambell, MSM, ATC, BOC
Director of Orthotics
The Training Room
Syracuse, New York

Karen Kott, PT, PhD
Department of Physical Therapy Education
Upstate Medical University
Syracuse, New York

Kendra Miller, PT
Physical Therapy
Burke Rehabilitation Center
White Plains, New York

Susan D. Miller, PT, MS
Department of Physical Therapy Education
Upstate Medical University
Syracuse, New York

Gabriel Yankowitz, PT
VanBeveren and Yankowitz Physical Therapy
Syracuse, New York

PREFACE

As an instructor of prosthetics and orthotics for over 25 years and as a clinician working with patients requiring a prosthesis or orthosis, I saw a need for an updated combined text in prosthetics and orthotics. In addition, information using the *Guide to Physical Therapist* terminology was needed. Much of the material in this text was expanded from class notes used in teaching prosthetics and orthotics at two physical therapy academic institutions.

The fields of prosthetics and orthotics have undergone tremendous strides in the past several years. Development of materials, examination and casting procedures, and fabrication have made enormous advances. One of the aims of this text is to familiarize the physical therapy and physical therapist assistant student, as well as the practitioner, with these advances. This text also provides a systematic method of examination, evaluation, and implementation of various interventions in the management of the patient requiring a prosthesis or orthosis. The team approach to assist in maximizing potential for successful recovery is emphasized in this text.

The number of prosthetic and orthotic components is varied and overwhelming. It would be impossible to include all these components. In this text, some of the most commonly used components are presented. Regional differences may affect the use of specific components for a particular patient.

An attempt has been made throughout this extensively illustrated text to provide the student or practicing clinician with clinical decision-making cases that would parallel patient examples. Other features include

- Chapter objectives and summary key points
- Case studies involving prescription of a prosthesis or orthosis
- An in-depth analysis of gait deviations and ways to correct these deviations
- Critical thinking questions or laboratory activities at the end of each chapter
- Practical application boxes
- Pediatric and geriatric perspectives
- Pros and cons boxes
- Detailed case studies in *Guide to Physical Therapist* format

This text is divided into four parts. Part I consists of Chapters 1–5, which provide introductory information regarding conditions that may require use of a prosthesis or orthosis, examination, team approach, psychosocial issues, and biomechanics. Part II contains Chapters 6–13, which provide information regarding transtibial, transfemoral, bilateral, hip disarticulation, and transpelvic prostheses. Prostheses for pediatric and sports populations are also included. Part III includes Chapters 14–17 regarding the orthopedic or neurologic patient and spinal orthotics. Part

IV is the Appendix, which contains three detailed case studies in Guide to Physical Therapist format. Bolded terms throughout the text are defined in the glossary beginning on page 464.

Many hours of research and preparation were spent in the publishing of this text. The reader is encouraged to provide feedback so that subsequent editions of this text may meet the changing needs of the practitioner and ultimately the needs of the patient requiring a prosthesis or orthosis.

ACKNOWLEDGMENTS

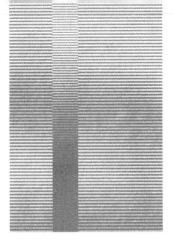

Many people have spent numerous hours in the preparation and review of this text. I would like to thank the contributors for sharing their expertise. Thank you to my colleagues at the Department of Physical Therapy Education, College of Health Professions, SUNY Upstate Medical University for allowing me to undertake this project and for their review of the manuscript. I am appreciative of Richard V McDougall (Mac) of the University of Kentucky for getting me started in prosthetics and orthotics. Special thanks to Mike Hall, CPO; Tony Marschall, CPO; Karen Hughes, PT; Karen Kemmis, PT; Pamela Lamb, PTA; Tim Damron, MD; Terry Hall; and Pamela Gramet, PhD, PT, for their suggestions. Thank you to Pamela Hitchcock, Deborah Rexine, and Rich Whelsky of the Upstate Medical University Photography staff. Thank you to the individuals who agreed to be photographed, including Harold Foyer, Erin Dolan, Patty Cannella, and Chantelle Hollenbeck. I would also like to thank the excellent staff at Lippincott Williams & Wilkins for their expertise and patience; Ulita Lushnycky, Managing Editor, who was always available when I needed her advice, Nancy J. Peterson, Developmental Editor; V. Helm, artist; and Amy Amico, Editorial Assistant. A special thank you to Margaret M. Biblis for her support of this undertaking. Also, thank you to my constant editorial assistant, my wife, Mary.

CONTENTS

Introduction

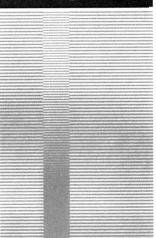

Chapter 1

INTRODUCTION TO PROSTHETICS AND ORTHOTICS

Objectives

1. Describe briefly the history of amputation, prosthetics, and orthotics
2. Portray the demographics associated with the use of a prosthesis or orthosis
3. Describe the causes and levels of amputations
4. Differentiate between two assessments of blood flow
5. Distinguish between wound-staging methods
6. Define different levels of amputation
7. Examine conditions that may require use of an orthosis

This chapter is divided into the following sections:

An appreciation of the history of amputations, prosthetics, and orthotics provides an understanding of how far technology has advanced in these fields. Knowledge of the causes and levels of amputation and conditions that may require an orthosis will result in better practitioners.

In 1970, the International Society for Prosthetics and Orthotics was founded to improve communication between researchers and clinicians. To make international communication more efficient, a standard nomenclature was adopted to refer to the level of amputation and related prostheses. The term *trans* is used when an amputation extends across the axis of a long bone such as the tibia. When two bones are involved together, such as the tibia and fibula, the primary bone is identified, such as *transtibial* for a below-the-knee amputation. Amputations between long bones or through a joint are referred to as *disarticulations*, such as a hip or knee disarticulation.

♦♦♦

History

A historical perspective of amputation, prosthetics, and orthotics makes one appreciate the advances of present-day technology. This perspective also makes us realize the progress made in surgical techniques and in improving prosthetic and orthotic design. A historical timeline of amputations, prosthetics, and orthotics is presented in Figure 1-1.

Amputation

Therapeutic, ritualistic, and punitive amputation was practiced thousands of years ago. Neolithic man is known to have survived amputation. The remains of Neanderthal man show evidence of survival after amputation.[1] Hippocrates, whose moral and ethical principles form the basis of medical practice, advocated amputation in cases of gangrene to control pain and hemorrhage. Evidence has been found that 43,000 years before the Christian era, amputation was done with primitive tools such as knives, saws, and axes. Peruvians used stone knives and saws constructed by setting flint into wood or jawbone.[2] The discovery of gunpowder led to the use of cannon balls and shot, resulting in the need for battlefield amputation. In the early 1800s, Baron Larrey, surgeon to Napoleon Bonaparte, performed 200 amputations on the battlefield in 1 day. He advocated operating on wounds within the first 24 hours of injury. Larrey is also known for introducing the flying horse ambulance used in the evacuation of wounded soldiers from the battlefield.[3]

One of the most famous surgeons was Lisfranc (1790–1847), who could amputate a foot in less than 1 minute and had a foot amputation procedure named after him. In these early times, surgical bleeding was controlled by pressure, crow's beak forceps, cautery, and plant and animal products. Sutures were made of cotton or human hair, thorns, and ant jaws.[3]

Before antiseptic technique, mortality rates were extremely high. At the Battle of Waterloo,

there was a 70% mortality rate for thigh amputations. In London in the 1860s, the mortality rates due to sepsis for transtibial and transfemoral amputations were 50 and 80%, respectively.[3] Surgical antisepsis, started in 1865 by Lord Lister, helped to decrease these high mortality rates.[4]

After World War I, centers to treat patients with amputation were established to coordinate surgical and prosthetic care.[5] Common reasons for amputation during this time were explosive and gunshot wounds as well as frostbite and sepsis.[6] The methods of amputation have greatly advanced from these early days. Limb salvage, prosthetic implantation in cases of malignancy, and reattachment of severed limbs have recently been described. Today, multidisciplinary rehabilitation team care exists in many health-care facilities. A coordinated team approach is often used in these centers, which is discussed in more detail in Chapter 3.

Prosthetics

It is not known exactly when the first prosthesis was fabricated. Indian literature describes artificial legs as early as 1500 BC.[5] Following this era, the earliest historical record of a prosthesis comes from Herodotus (485–425 BC), who described an individual imprisoned by Sparta who obtained a knife and performed an amputation of his foot. He thus was able to escape from the stocks. Ultimately he supplied himself with a wooden foot.[5]

A prosthesis unearthed in the ruins of Pompeii that dated to 300 BC is thought to be the first prosthesis. This prosthesis was made of thin pieces of bronze fixed to a central wooden core and secured to the residual limb with a leather skirt.[2] During this time, prostheses were made of fiber, wood, bone, and metals and were often lined with rags.[3] Designs for prostheses were made by a number of influential figures including Ambroise Paré, a military surgeon of the 16th century, and Leonardo da Vinci[2]

43,000 BC	Evidence found that amputation was done with primitive tools.
2730–2625 BC	A device to stabilize the knee joint was found.
1500 BC	Indian literature describes artificial legs.
370 BC	Hippocrates used splints on the legs.
485–425 BC	Herodotus described an individual imprisoned by Sparta who supplied himself with a wooden foot.
300 BC	A prosthesis unearthed in the ruins of Pompeii is thought to be the first prosthesis.
131–201	Galen used dynamic orthoses for scoliosis and kyphosis.
476–1453	During the Middle ages, knights wore elaborate armor to conceal prostheses.
1200	Medical school at Bologna considers orthotics as an important part of medical knowledge.
1509–1590	Ambroise Pare' established technical standards for surgical amputations and described spinal corsets and shoe modifications.
1690	Verduin constructed a transtibial prosthesis with copper socket, leather thigh corset, and a wooden foot.
1790–1847	Lisfranc, a famous surgeon, amputates a foot in less than 1 minute.
1800	Baron Larrey, surgeon to Napoleon Bonaparte performs 200 amputations on the battlefield in 1 day. He advocates wounds being operated on within the first 24 hours.
1860	Mortality rate due to sepsis in London for transtibial and transfemoral amputations were 50 and 80% respectively.
1865	Lord Lister starts surgical antisepsis to decrease high mortality rates.
1865	J.E. Hangar, sustains an amputation while serving in the Confederate Army, places rubber bumpers in solid feet, and produces the first articulated prosthetic foot.
1918	After World War I, The Limb Fitting Centre at Queen Mary's Hospital, Roehampton becomes a primary development and supply center to military veterans.
1945	The U.S. Veterans Administration supports the development of the patellar tendon bearing and the quadrilateral sockets. Canada develops a prosthetic research program at Sunnybrook Hospital in Toronto.
1970	The U.S. Veterans Administration develops the endoskeletal prosthesis.
2000	A microprocessor controlled knee with hydraulic swing and stance phase control is developed.

Figure 1-1. Historical timeline of amputations, prosthetics, and orthotics.

(Fig. 1-2). Early prosthetists were blacksmiths, armor makers, and often the patients themselves. During the Middle Ages, the privileged classes of knights attempted to conceal their battle disabilities by wearing elaborate armor for protection. In contrast, the common person used a peg or wooden leg as a makeshift substitute. Many of these individuals with an amputation were ostracized from society, unable to earn a living, and often lived as beggars.[5] This society is depicted in the 16th-century painting by Pieter Breughel. *The Cripples* portrays a street scene that may have been common during the 16th century (Fig. 1-3).

Ambroise Paré established technical standards for surgical amputation in the late 1500s. He was responsible for the design used by the French armor industry using concepts similar to those of modern day prosthetics. These concepts included harnesses, knee and ankle joints, and sockets.[6] Verduin, a Dutch surgeon in 1690, constructed a transtibial prosthesis with a copper socket, a leather thigh corset to bear weight through hinged side bars, and a wooden foot.[7] This prosthesis was a precursor to the thigh corset suspension used for transtibial amputation.

In the early 19th century, with the advent of general anesthesia and the increasing number of civilian industrial accidents, the limbmaker was no longer a skilled carpenter or blacksmith but a trained prosthetist.[5] Early limbs manufactured in Europe and in North America used metal, wood, and leather. In the mid-1800s, J. E. Hangar, who sustained an amputation while serving in the Confederate army, placed rubber bumpers in solid feet and thus produced the first articulated prosthetic foot.

War continued to provide the major impetus for research and development in prosthetics. After World War I, in the United Kingdom, the Limb Fitting Centre at Queen Mary's Hospital, Roehampton, became a primary development and supply center to military veterans. Following World War II, the National Academy of Sciences, under the direction of the U.S. government, started a prosthetic research program. The Armed Forces, the Veterans Administration (VA), the National Institutes of Health, the Vocational Rehabilitation Administration, universities, and private industry were recruited to assist in prosthetic research and development.[5] Soon after, fiscal responsibility for this research and development was gradually transferred to the VA.[8]

Following World War II, the VA supported the development of the patellar tendon bearing socket used for transtibial amputations and the quadrilateral socket used for transfemoral amputations. Suction suspension for transfemoral prostheses was introduced in 1949.[7] Up until the 1950s, prostheses used a 'plug fit' design in which the body weight was supported by the proximal end of the prosthetic socket rather

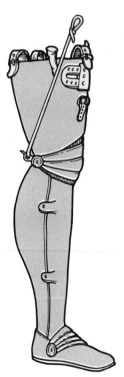

Figure 1-2. Artificial limb designed by Ambroise Paré from the middle of the 16th century. (Adapted from a painting in the Royal College of Surgeons Museum.)

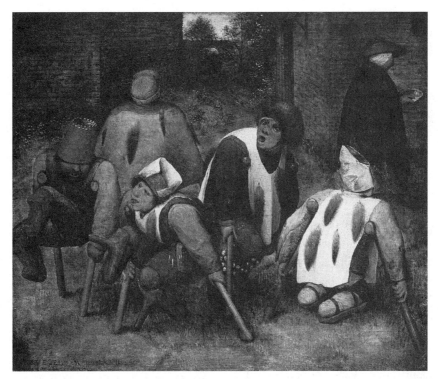

Figure 1-3. *The Cripples* by Pieter Breughel hangs in the Louvre. (Permission received from the Louvre.)

than a total-contact weight-bearing socket. The 'plug fit' socket created large pressures on the distal end of the residual limb and increased skin shearing forces.[7]

After World War II, Canada developed a prosthetic research program at Sunnybrook Hospital in Toronto. Much of this prosthetic and orthotic research is conducted today at the Ontario Crippled Children's Center in Toronto. This program produced the Canadian hip disarticulation and Syme prostheses.[8] During and after the Vietnam War, renewed funding by the VA led to further refinements in prostheses, including the endoskeletal or modular prostheses.[9] Additional refinements are continually being made as evidenced by a recently developed microprocessor-controlled knee with hydraulic swing and stance control. Each of these prostheses is described in more detail in Chapters 8 and 9.

Orthotics

Orthotics has a much longer history than the field of prosthetics. The word *orthosis* is derived from the Greek *ortho,* meaning straight, upright, or correct. *Orthosis* refers to a static or dynamic device and is preferable to *splint* or *brace,* which refers only to a static device. Perhaps the oldest of all devices to stabilize the knee joint was known as early as the Fifth Dynasty (2730–2625 BC). Mummies were found with intact orthoses, used for fracture bracing. Hippocrates, around 370 BC, used splints on the leg, avoiding placement of pressure points over bony prominences. Galen (AD 131–201) used dynamic orthoses for scoliosis and kyphosis. In the 12th century, the medical school at Bologna considered orthotics an important part of medical knowledge. They standardized, simplified, and lightened orthoses by

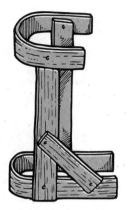

Figure 1-4. Early ankle–foot orthosis designed by Arcaeo (1574). (Adapted from a diagram in Murdoch, G. (Ed.) (1976). *The advance in orthotics (p. 8)*. Baltimore: Williams & Wilkins.)

using wood and metal. Figure 1-4 illustrates an early orthosis.

Ambroise Paré (1509–1590), known for his pioneering work in prosthetics, also contributed to orthosis fabrication. Paré's book described spinal corsets, fracture orthoses, weight-relieving orthoses for hip disease, and shoe modifications. He commissioned armor makers who became proficient in the use of metal, leather, and wood to produce orthoses.[9] The craft of orthosis making was often handed down from father to son, as masters to apprentices.[10]

The use of orthoses in the management of spinal deformity dates back to the 1500s. In the 1800s, an orthosis maker was part of every orthopedic office.[10] Until 1915, when surgical treatment of scoliosis became possible, orthoses were used extensively.[11] Present-day orthoses are discussed in Chapters 14–17.

Demographics

The National Center for Health statistics estimates more than 300,000 persons with lower extremity amputation are currently living in the United States.[12] From 1988 to 1992 there were an estimated 130,000 amputations performed yearly in the United States, including 65,000 individuals with diabetes.[13] Worldwide, however, the number of individuals with amputations is not currently traced by any organization.[14] The number of lower extremity amputations performed in nonfederal and federal hospitals as well as the total number in the United States in 1997 are shown in Table 1-1.[15,16] In the United States, 173,000 prosthetic lower limbs or feet were used in 1994, contrasted with 21,000 prosthetic upper limb or hand devices.[17] It is estimated that the worldwide annual demand is over 2 million prostheses per year.[7] The number of land mines in foreign countries has dramatically increased the number of amputations, particularly in children[18–20]

Factors that increase amputation rates include having a chronic disease, being male, increasing age, and being a member of a racial or ethnic minority.[21–25] Over 70% of amputations in the United States are performed for vascular disease, including diabetic complications, arteriosclerosis, and thromboembolism. The remaining 30% includes 22% due to trauma, 4% due to malignancies, and 4% due to congenital deformities.[14] A study of hospital patient dis-

Table 1.1. Lower Extremity Amputations in the United States in 1997			
Involved Area	**Incidence**		
	Nonfederal	*Federal*	*Total*
Toe	51,000	2,010	53,010
Foot	12,000	504	12,504
Transtibial	38,000	1,479	39,479
Transfemoral	35,000	1,478	36,478
			141,471

Data from Detailed diagnoses and procedures, National Hospital Discharge Survey. (1997). *Vital and Health Statistics Series 13, 145,* 138, and *Lower extremity complications in Veterens Health Administration. FY 89-99 Part 1: Lower extremity amputation rates, progression and utilization.* January 2000, p. 67.)

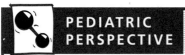

PEDIATRIC PERSPECTIVE

Land Mines and Children

Between 60 and 70 million land mines are currently in place in over 70 countries. Land mines injure an estimated 1200 persons and kill another 800 every week; many of these victims are children. Victims of land mines often face repeated operations because of widespread infection. The fight against infection is further hampered by the large number of blood transfusions that are needed. During the 1991–1992 war in Croatia, antipersonnel mines were mostly laid without a plan. As a result, at least 10 years of intensive work by 2000 to 3000 trained experts will be required to clear some 2 million mines laid all over the area. The devastating effect of land mines can only be resolved by preventing the further placement of these mines and by removing those already in place.

charges from the United States Veterans Health Administration facilities from 1989 to 1998 found 60,234 discharges with a diagnosis of amputation.[26] Major indications for amputation were diabetes (62.9%) and peripheral vascular disease alone (23.6%). Similar reasons for amputation have been found in southern Finland.[27]

Complications of diabetes (discussed in more detail later in this chapter) are associated with vascular changes, **neuropathy**, insensitivity, skin ulcers, and amputation. Although persons with diabetes represent only 3% of the total United States population, 51% of the discharge diagnoses for amputation also listed the diagnosis of diabetes.[13] Chronic skin ulcers were present in 2.7% of all hospital diagnoses that listed diabetes, and the average hospital stay was 59% longer for those with ulcer conditions.[28]

The development of preoperative objective measurements, such as the use of the Doppler ultrasound blood pressure examination and impedance plethysmography, allowed more-distal amputations. As an example, the ratio of transfemoral to transtibial amputation in the United States between 1965 and 1975 was almost reversed from 70:30 to 30:70. The use of a long posterior myofasciocutaneous flap, with its increased blood supply, improved the success rate in transtibial amputations.[29]

The number and percentages of lower extremity amputations by amputation level and the presence or absence of diabetes for 1989–1992 in the United States are depicted in Table 1-2.[15] Overall, toe amputations made up the largest category, followed by transfemoral and transtibial amputations. Individuals with diabetes had a greater frequency of toe, foot, ankle, and transtibial amputations than nondiabetics.

Individuals with diabetes compose only 2–5% of the population. Yet this group includes 40 to 45% of those with amputation.[30] Data show that 9–20% of individuals with diabetes experience a second leg (contralateral) amputation during a separate hospitalization within 12 months after amputation. Five years following an initial amputation, 28–51% of patients with diabetes undergo a second leg amputation.[28] It is estimated that the 5-year survival rate for patients with an amputation with diabetes is 40%.[31] Advances in diabetes management with newer medications and more rigid control of elevated blood glucose levels may reduce this incidence of amputations.

Health-care professionals have an important role to play in preventing complications that may lead to amputation. A number of amputation prevention programs have reported marked pre- and postintervention differences in amputation frequency as a result of comprehensive, multidisciplinary foot-care programs.[28] However, despite education regarding diabetes, smoking cessation, and limb-saving techniques, the number of vascular amputa-

**Table 1-2. Lower Extremity Amputations by Level
and the Presence of Diabetes 1989–1992**

Level	Diabetes		No Diabetes		Total	
	Number	*%*	*Number*	*%*	*Number*	*%*
Toe	21,671	40	12,427	24	34,098	32
Foot or ankle	7,773	14	2,967	6	10,740	10
Transtibial	13,484	25	11,048	21	24,527	23
Knee disarticulation	704	1	778	1	1,482	1
Transfemoral	8,612	16	20,028	39	28,640	27
Hip or pelvis	87	0.2	386	0.7	473	0.5
Not specified	1,378	2.6	3,971	7.7	5,349	5.1
Total	53,709	100	51,605	100	105,309	100

Data from Detailed diagnoses and procedures, National Hospital Discharge Survey. (1997). *Vital and Health Statistics Series 13, 145.*

tions in the civilian sector of the United States has not declined significantly over the past decade. The incidence and complications of peripheral vascular disease unfortunately continue to be an unresolved major public health concern in the United States.[32]

The numbers and percentages of individuals using orthoses in the United States in 1994 are depicted in Table 1-3. [17] Lumbar orthoses constitute the largest category, possibly because of the high incidence of low back pain in the United States. Knee orthoses are the second largest group, perhaps because of the number of sports injuries and the incidence of osteoarthritis.

Causes of Amputations

Causes of amputations are divided into six categories:

1. Peripheral vascular disease
2. Diabetes

**Table 1-3. Number of Persons Using Orthoses
by Age of Person and Type of Orthosis**

Orthosis	All Ages	44 Years and younger	45–64 Years	65 Years and older
Lumbar	1,688,000	795,000	614,000	279,000
Cervical	168,000	76,000	78,000	13,000
Hand	332,000	171,000	119,000	42,000
Arm	320,000	209,000	86,000	25,000
Leg	596,000	266,000	138,000	192,000
Foot	282,000	191,000	59,000	31,000
Knee	989,000	694,000	199,000	96,000
Other	399,000	239,000	104,000	56,000

Data from Russell, J. N., Hendershot, G. E., LeClere, F., Howie, L. J., & Adler, M. (1997). Trends and differential use of assistive technology devices: United States 1994. *Advance Data, 292, 3.*

3. Trauma
4. Infections
5. Tumors
6. Limb deficiencies

Each of these causes of amputation is discussed in detail below.

Peripheral Vascular Disease

Most amputations today, in adults, are performed because of **peripheral vascular disease (PVD)**. PVD is any abnormal condition affecting blood vessels peripheral to the heart. PVD can be caused by embolism, thrombosis, trauma, vasospasm, inflammation, or arteriosclerosis leading to deficits in the arterial, venous, and lymphatic circulatory systems. PVD is uncommon in the pediatric age group.

Clinical manifestations of chronic arterial occlusion due to PVD may not be readily apparent and may appear as late as 20–40 years after onset.[33] The lower limbs are far more susceptible to arterial and venous occlusive disorders and atherosclerosis than are the upper limbs. Common symptoms of chronic arterial occlusive disease include intermittent claudication due to ischemia. **Intermittent claudication** occurs when the arterial diameter decreases, resulting in insufficient blood flow. As the disease progresses, the individual is able to walk less and less before claudication occurs. The individual with claudication often reports a dull, aching tightness deep in the muscle. Severe ischemia may lead to foot ulcers. Only relaxation of the affected limb will reduce muscle cramping and permit increased blood flow, thus relieving the symptoms. Interventions may include energy conservation techniques, frequent rests, and avoidance of prolonged standing.

Arteriosclerosis, a type of PVD, is the most common occlusive arterial disease. It is characterized by thickening, hardening, and narrowing of the arterial walls. Fibrous plaques narrow the vessels, eventually leading to ischemia of the lower extremities. This condition is most often seen in elderly patients but can appear in younger individuals.[34] Arteriosclerosis occurs in about 5% of men over age 50 and women over age 60. About 25% of individuals with arteriosclerosis eventually require reconstructive surgery, and about 5% eventually require major amputation.[35]

The number of arteriosclerosis cases increases when associated with diabetes. Approximately 15% of individuals with diabetes have arteriosclerosis after onset of diabetes, while 45% have arteriosclerosis 20 years after onset of diabetes.[34,36]

Risk factors in arteriosclerosis are diabetes, elevated serum cholesterol concentrations and low-density lipid (LDL) levels in the blood, smoking, hypertension, obesity, and a sedentary lifestyle.[34,36]

Arteriosclerosis interventions consist of smoking cessation, daily walking exercise, dietary management, pain control, and pharmacologic management. Associated pharmacologic management for hypertension that is frequently associated with arteriosclerosis includes the use of β-blockers, calcium channel blockers, angiotensin-converting enzyme (ACE) inhibitors, and angiotensin-receptor blockers (ARBs).[37]

Chronic Venous Insufficiency

Chronic venous insufficiency (CVI) is an abnormal circulatory condition characterized by decreased return of the venous blood from the legs to the trunk. CVI may involve both superficial and deep veins, leading to skin ulcers and eventual amputation. Common findings associated with CVI include edema, dilated veins, and dermatitis that does not respond well to topical preparations.

The incidence of CVI increases with age and obesity. CVI may be associated with conditions such as sickle cell anemia, systemic lupus erythematosus, and hemolytic anemia. The etiology of CVI may involve the loss of the valvular mechanism in the deep venous system. As a re-

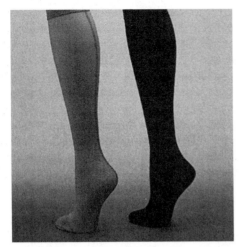

Figure 1-5. Compression stockings to aid in venous return in cases of CVI. (Photo courtesy of Beiersdorf-Jobst Inc.)

sult, venous and capillary pressures increase, leading to edema, subcutaneous fibrosis, and lymphatic obstruction. Edema is often worse at the end of the day, and stasis skin ulcers fre-

quently result. Cutaneous pigmentation often results from the deposition of proteins in the skin. These ulcers are frequently found above the superior medial malleolus or on the lower leg, and pain is often relieved by elevation.[38] Interventions may include elevation of the lower extremities, compression stockings (Fig. 1-5), and the use of an intermittent compression pump (Fig. 1-6) to reduce hydrostatic pressure. If ulcers are present, cleansing and wound-care preparations are indicated. An interdisciplinary approach to wound care is given at specialty wound care centers.

Diabetes

An estimated 15.7 million people, or 5.9% of the population in the United States, have diabetes.[39] While an estimated 10.3 million have been diagnosed, 5.4 million are not aware they have the disease. Each day, approximately 2200 people are diagnosed with diabetes. Diabetes is an incurable but manageable chronic disease

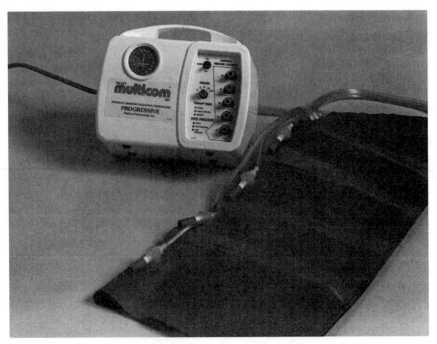

Figure 1-6. Use of an intermittent compression pump to reduce hydrostatic pressure.

and is the seventh leading cause of death in the United States. The cost of health care as well as lost productivity for individuals with diabetes in 1997 was estimated to be $98 billion.[39]

Diabetes mellitus is defined as a group of metabolic diseases characterized by **hyperglycemia** resulting from defects in insulin secretion, insulin action, or both. Impaired insulin secretion and defects in insulin action frequently coexist in the same patient. It is often unclear which abnormality causes hyperglycemia.[40] The body needs insulin to convert glucose into energy. The main goal of diabetes intervention is to bring glucose levels down to normal. Suggested glucose level goals are less than 140 milligrams per deciliter (mg/dL) before meals and less than 160 mg/dL at bedtime.[41]

Classification

The classification of diabetes has moved from a system based on pharmacologic intervention toward a system based on disease etiology. As a result, terms such as insulin-dependent diabetes mellitus (IDDM) or non–insulin-dependent diabetes mellitus (NIDDM) are no longer used. In addition, the use of arabic numerals (types 1 and 2) rather than roman numerals (I and II) has been adopted to avoid confusion. The roman numeral II can be confused by the public with the number 11.[40]

The incidence of diabetes increases with advancing age. Approximately 10% of individuals with diabetes have type 1 (formerly called IDDM).[41] Type 1 is characterized by insulin deficiency due to an autoimmune process that destroys the beta cells of the pancreas. Type 1 usually presents in childhood or early adulthood, with symptoms such as polyuria, polydipsia, and weight loss. Type 2 (formerly called NIDDM) is present in approximately 90% of diabetics, usually presents in middle-to-older age, and increases with age. For those in high-risk populations (African American, Hispanic, Asian or Native American heritage), the onset of type 2 diabetes can be very early in life. Type 2 diabetes is characterized by insulin resistance

and an insulin secretory deficit. Type 2 diabetes can go undiagnosed for many years because the hyperglycemia develops insidiously, and the patient often fails to notice any of the classic symptoms of diabetes. The number of individuals with type 2 diabetes is expected to double within the next decade.[42] Factors such as obesity and inactivity in a patient with a genetic predisposition to diabetes contribute to the incidence of type 2 diabetes. Some insulin resistance is simply caused by obesity.[40]

Complications

Duration is directly related to morbidity, i.e., the longer one has diabetes, the greater the risk of developing long-term complications. These complications may include microvascular, macrovascular, and neurologic disorders. Macrovascular disorders include PVD, coronary artery disease, and cerebrovascular accidents. Many studies have demonstrated that the combination of insulin resistance and hyperinsulinemia is a major risk factor for coronary artery disease.[43] Microvascular disorders include nephropathy leading to renal failure, retinopathy with potential loss of vision, and neuropathy including peripheral sensory deficits that could lead to foot ulcers, Charcot joints, and amputation.[40,44] Sensory loss, weakness, abnormal sensations (paresthesias), and degeneration of the peripheral nerves (neuropathy), develop in most diabetic patients. Minor traumatic events in the insensitive limb can result in limb-threatening ulcers. In addition, the altered metabolic state in uncontrolled diabetes can decrease granulocyte function and collagen synthesis and result in an increased susceptibility to infection and delayed wound healing.[45]

Interventions

All individuals with type 1 diabetes and some with type 2 diabetes require insulin injection for optimal blood glucose control. The insulin dosage schedule depends on several factors including the activity level and severity of diabetes. The individual who is administering insulin several times a day is less likely to develop hypoglycemia during exercise or activity. Individuals with type 2 diabetes generally do not need insulin injections and may be treated successfully with diet, exercise, and oral pharmacologic agents.[37] Commonly used pharmaceutic classifications for the management of type 2 diabetes include

Sulfonylureas
Biguanides
Meglitinides
Thiazolidinediones
α-Glucosidase inhibitors[46]

Signs and symptoms the patient with diabetic neuropathy should be made aware of are depicted in Resource Box 1-1[34,47] Specific foot care guidelines are discussed in Chapter 16, "Orthoses for Patients with Neurologic Disorders—Clinical Decision Making."

A study of patients with diabetes showed that a multidisciplinary approach played an

important role in reducing and maintaining a low incidence of major amputation in patients with diabetes.[48] The Diabetes Control and Complications Trial (DCCT) demonstrated that in patients with type 1 diabetes, the risk of development or progression of retinopathy, nephropathy, and neuropathy is 50–75% lower with intensive intervention regimens than with conventional intervention.[49] Morbidity, mortality, and costs of care were substantial in a study of patients with diabetes and foot ulcers compared with those of patients without diabetes. This study supported the value of foot ulcer–prevention programs for patients with diabetes.[50]

Interventions for skin ulcers may include bed rest; limb protection; tobacco avoidance; protection of pressure areas (particularly between toes); dietary balance of protein, carbohydrate, and fat; and control of blood glucose levels. Pre- and postoperative nutritional screening is recommended to allow a diet conducive to optimal wound healing. Those with arteriosclerosis and diabetes may also benefit from extra-depth shoes or a total-contact cast and an assistive device such as a cane to decrease pressure. Since neuropathic ulcers frequently affect the metatarsal heads, a rocker sole may be indicated to decrease pressures over this area. An extra-depth shoe with rocker sole is depicted in Figure 1-7. A study of lower-

RESOURCE BOX 1-1

Signs and Symptoms of Neuropathy That May Be Caused by Diabetes

1. Lowered temperature in the feet
2. Decreased sensation, including vibratory and position sense in the feet or hand
3. Loss of deep tendon reflexes
4. Dry, scaly skin due to decreased foot perspiration
5. Callus and blister formation, which can ulcerate, providing a good medium for bacterial and fungal infections
6. Weakness of foot musculature, which can lead to structural changes

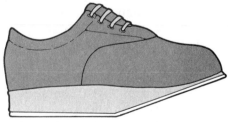

Figure 1-7. Extra-depth shoe with rocker sole. (Adapted from Laing, P. W., Cogley, D. I., & Klenerman, L. (1992). Neuropathic foot ulceration treated by total contact casts. *Journal of Bone & Joint Surgery, 74B,* 133–136.)

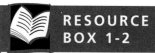

RESOURCE BOX 1-2

Diabetes Resources

The National Diabetes Information Clearinghouse
  1 Information Way
  Bethesda, MD 20892-3560
  301-654-3327
  http://ndep.nih.gov/health/diabetes
The American Diabetes Association
  1660 Duke Street
  Alexandria, VA 22314
  703-549-1500
  http://www.diabetes.org
Centers for Disease Control and Prevention
  1600 Clifton Road
  Atlanta, GA 30333
  404-639-3311
  http://www.cdc.gov/diabetes
Canadian Diabetes Association
  15 Toronto Street Suite 800
  Toronto On M5C2E3
  416-363-3373
  http://www.diabetes.ca

limb amputation by the United States Veterans Administration Healthcare System found that the prescription of protective footwear has the potential to reduce the incidence of shoe-related ulcers and amputations.[51]

Excellent resources for individuals with diabetes, which provide free information, are listed in Resource Box 1-2.

Trauma

Common accidental causes of traumatic amputation include automobile accidents, freezing, burns, nonunion fractures, and farm machinery and power tool accidents. Damage to the nervous system, such as a brachial plexus in-

jury, may result in such debilitating paralysis to the limb that amputation is required.

Trauma or infection increases energy requirements 30–55% above basal values. Protein malnutrition, a common complication of trauma, has an adverse affect on morbidity and mortality in hospitalized patients. Malnourished patients have a 40–50% risk for wound failure or infection. Patients with corrected wound-healing environments average 90% healing.[52] In one study, malnutrition was present in 90% of patients who underwent transtibial amputation secondary to occlusive arterial disease.[53] Surgery in these malnourished patients may need to be delayed until nutritional deficiencies are corrected and protein balance is improved. In cases of trauma, adequate protein and albumin levels promote healing and help prevent secondary complications such as infection, atrophy, and neuropathy.

Normal electrolyte values are presented in Table 1-4.[38] Any electrolyte disturbance aris-

Table 1-4. Normal Electrolyte Values	
Electrolytes	*Values*
Albumin	3.5–5.5 g/dL
Bicarbonate	21–28 meq/L
BUN (blood, urea, nitrogen)	3.6–7.1 mmol/L
Calcium	9.0–10.5 mg/dL
Chloride	98–106 meq/L
Creatinine	Less than 1.5 mg/dL
Glucose	75–115 mg/dL
Magnesium	1.3–2.1 meq/L
Phosphorus	3.0–14.5 mg/dL
Potassium	3.5–5.0 meq/L
Protein (total)	5.5–8.0 g/dL
Sodium	136–145 meq/L

Data adapted from Braunwald, E., Isselbacher, K. J., Petersdorf, R. G., Wilson, J. D., Martin, J. B., & Fauci, A. S. (1994). *Harrison's principles of internal medicine* (13th ed., pp. 1045–1046). New York: McGraw Hill.

ing from trauma, burns, or chronic disease can have deleterious effects on multiple organ systems. To prevent these systemic problems, oral hyperalimentation or parenteral (intravenous) nutritional supplements may be administered via a peripheral or central line. These supplements contain essential nutrients such as amino acids, calories, electrolytes, and vitamins, which provide energy for healing. The average adult needs a minimum of 1600 calories per day to meet basic energy needs. However, the metabolic need in response to stress for injured patients is frequently much greater.

In cases of severe trauma resulting in bone shortening or in cases of congenital abnormalities, limb-lengthening procedures have been used. Limb lengthening may be indicated when more than 60% of predicted femoral length is present.[54] Limb-lengthening procedures typically consist of the Wagner (diaphyseal lengthening) or the Ilizarov (circular frame)[55] (Fig. 1-8). Both of these procedures allow elongation of approximately 1–1.5 mm per day.

Whether to attempt limb salvage or amputate in the case of trauma is one of the most difficult decisions a surgeon and patient must make. Factors such as the extent of injury, overall health and activity of the patient, and the patient's support system enter into the decision-making process. The timing of an amputation is important. Immediate amputation is often viewed by the patient and family as a result of the injury. On the other hand, delayed amputation may be viewed as an intervention failure. If feasible, a shared decision-making approach among the patient, family, and surgeon is critical.

Many investigators have identified a number of factors that predict failure of limb-salvage management. A mangled extremity severity score (MESS) has been used to determine the success probability of limb salvage in the case of trauma. The MESS considers 10 factors: injury severity score; injury to integument, nerve, and bone; arterial and venous injury;

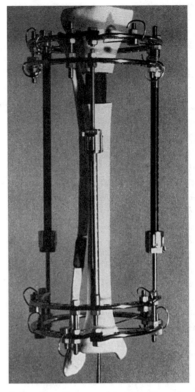

Figure 1-8. The Ilizarov (circular frame) used for limb lengthening. (Photo courtesy of Dr. Christopher Geel, Department of Orthopedics, Upstate Medical University, Syracuse, NY.)

delay of more than 6 hours in treatment; patient age; preexisting disease; and shock. In one study of severe lower-extremity fractures, 94% of the patients with MESS values of 5–7 were able to achieve functional recovery.[56]

Another scale of limb-salvage prediction following trauma is called the limb salvage index (LSI). This index rates seven factors including arterial injury; injury to nerve, bone, skin, and muscle; deep vein injury; and warm ischemia time. Those with an LSI below 6 had successful limb salvage. Conversely, those with an LSI of 6 or above underwent an amputation.[57]

Due to the improvement in surgical techniques, even patients with severely traumatized limbs and vascular or nerve injuries may be candidates for limb salvage. Disrupted major vessels must be repaired to bring oxygenated blood necessary for wound healing to ischemic and traumatized limbs. Options available to the vascular surgeon include balloon angioplasty, laser surgery, and bypass grafts using autologous veins or synthetic graft material. Multiple surgeries to salvage a limb may result in functional limitations and disability. A limb-sparing procedure is more complex than amputation and is often associated with longer hospitalizations and greater complications.[58] In some cases, early amputation may lessen the disability. Therefore, the cost/benefit ratio is also a factor in the decision to attempt to salvage a limb or amputate.[59]

Physical therapy procedures for patients with severe trauma consist of prevention of contractures, use of the extremity, and partial to eventually full weight-bearing activities using an assistive device such as crutches. Weight bearing allows compression of the new bone and promotes osteogenesis.[60,61] Pain, pin site infection, and the bulkiness of the limb-lengthening device produce difficulties with activities of daily living such as transfers and dressing.

Infections

Infections are often a complication of PVD or diabetes or are acquired in a hospital setting. **Osteomyelitis** is an infection spread by numerous pathogens including *Staphylococcus aureus* that commonly affects the long bones such as the femur or tibia. Common symptoms reported by the patient with an infection include fever, malaise, and pain. However, the perception of pain may be altered in cases of decreased skin sensitivity. Hyperglycemia, commonly seen in patients with diabetes, impairs resistance to infection.[37]

The prevention of major lower-limb amputation by the salvage of all or most of the foot in patients with diabetic foot infections has become more common. Success depends on

timely presentation of the patient and control of infection and hyperglycemia with a combination of early debridement and appropriate antibiotics and insulin.[29]

Infection can occur following placement of a prosthetic implant, as in a total hip procedure. Rheumatoid arthritis, corticosteroid therapy, poor nutritional status, and advanced age are also contributing factors. The most common pathogens associated with a prosthetic implant are staphylococci. Regardless of placement with or without cement, organisms often become attached to the prosthetic implant. Most implant infections must be treated with temporary implant removal and antibiotics given for several weeks. Treatment of infection has been further compromised by the emergence of drug-resistant organisms. Amputation may result.[37]

Tumors

Amputations may be done as an intervention for bone sarcomas, soft tissue tumors, and metastatic disease. Although amputations may be done for primary tumor control of extremity sarcomas, these procedures may also be done for complications following limb-sparing surgery. The goals of limb-sparing surgery are total eradication of the tumor and preservation of a functional limb. The decision to spare a limb is made after ensuring that the neurovascular structures are not compromised by tumor and that the expected function following reconstruction would be superior to that with amputation.

The most common bony sarcoma is **osteosarcoma (osteogenic sarcoma)**, which has a peak occurrence between the ages of 10 and 25 years and is slightly more common in boys. Osteosarcomas are most commonly primary but may also occur as secondary tumors in Paget's disease and as a result of irradiation of other tumors. Osteosarcoma may involve any bone in the body; however the usual sites for this tumor are the metaphyses of the long bones, particularly the lower end of the femur, upper end of the tibia, and upper end of the humerus. Osteosarcoma presents with pain surrounding the knee in patients with femoral or tibial involvement. The pain may initially be mild and intermittent but often becomes progressively more severe, worse during the night or with extended periods of rest, and constant over time. Another relatively common bone sarcoma, **Ewing's sarcoma**, is most common between the ages of 5 and 30 and is also slightly more common in boys. Ewing's sarcoma is typically a rapidly growing tumor that aggressively erodes the bone cortex to produce a tender, palpable mass.

There has been a dramatic improvement in the survival rate of patients with osteosarcoma and Ewing's sarcoma over the last 30 years. Multiagent neoadjuvant chemotherapy has dramatically increased the overall survival rate from less than 5% to 20% in the 1960s to 55 to 80% in the 1990s.[62] Although amputation was used frequently in the past for surgical treatment of bone sarcomas, limb-sparing surgery has become the standard of care for most malignant and aggressive benign bone tumors. An example of this limb-sparing surgery is shown in Figure 1-9. In large part because of the improved survival with chemotherapy and improved imaging techniques, the percentage of amputations has decreased from 80–90% to 10–20%.[63]

Limb Deficiencies

Limb deficiencies are malformations of the limb bud, occurring near day 28 in utero. Medications (e.g., thalidomide taken by the mother to alleviate nausea), virus infections, rubella, diabetes, or abortion attempts have resulted in limb deficiencies.[64] The International Society for Prosthetics and Orthotics (ISPO) classified

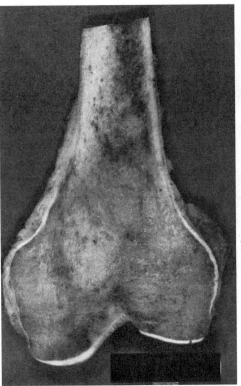
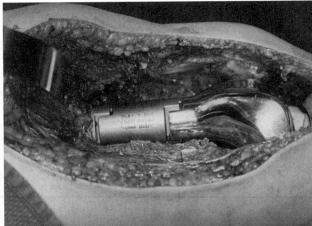

Figure 1-9. **A.** Coronal thin slice of resected distal femur following neoadjuvant chemotherapy with osteosarcoma in medial metaphysis and femoral condyle. **B.** Endoprosthetic total knee replacement. (Photo courtesy of Dr. Timothy Damron, Department of Orthopedics, Upstate Medical University, Syracuse, NY.)

congenital limb deficiencies as longitudinal or transverse.[65] A *transverse deficiency* is one in which no distal structures exist. Therefore, the limb ends at the location of the deficit. A *longitudinal deficiency* is a total or partial absence of a structure along the long axis of a segment, beyond which normal skeletal elements may exist. An example is the congenital absence of a tibia with an essentially normal foot. Other longitudinal anomalies include partial or complete absence of the femur (**proximal femoral focal deficiency, or PFFD**) and absence of the fibula.[64] PFFD is described further in Chapter 12, "Pediatric Patients with Lower Extremity Amputations—Clinical Decision Making."

Limb deficiencies have also been described as follows:

- Amelia—absence of a whole limb
- Apodia—absence of a hand or foot
- Adactylia—absence of one or more fingers or toes and associated metacarpals or metatarsals
- Aphalangia—absence of one or more fingers or toes
- Phocomelia—flipper limb due to absence of a limb segment[64]

Children with limb deficiencies often require many surgeries to facilitate maximal function. These may include tendon transfers, osteotomies, fusion, amputation, and limb lengthening.[66] Additional information concerning limb deficiencies is found in Chapter 12, "Pediatric Patients with Lower Extremity Amputations—Clinical Decision Making."

Assessment of Blood Flow

Assessment of blood flow is critical in a variety of these causes of amputation. There are many ways to assess blood flow including auscultation through a stethoscope, palpation, Doppler ultrasound blood-pressure, and impedance plethysmography. Doppler ultrasound blood-pressure examination is the most readily available objective measurement of limb blood flow and perfusion.[13] This method can detect even minimal blood flow and pulses that are inaudible. The ultrasound transducer or probe beams waves into the limb. Each tissue interface of different density reflects a portion of the wave. The reflected waves are changed in frequency in proportion to the velocity of the moving surface.[67] When evaluating blood flow, the Doppler signal increases or decreases as a result of the motion of red blood cells, which have different velocities depending on their location in the blood vessel. In a straight vessel with uniform walls, the blood flow has a consistent smooth velocity called *laminar flow*. In a diseased vessel with plaque formation or stenosis, the blood-flow pattern is disturbed and has a higher velocity through the stenotic area. A turbulent flow results distal to the stenosis.[68] The Doppler ultrasound blood-pressure unit is shown in Figure 1-10.

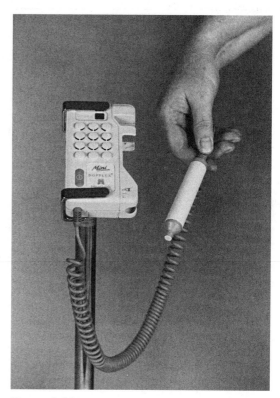

Figure 1-10. Use of the Doppler ultrasound blood pressure unit.

The procedure using the Doppler ultrasound blood-pressure unit and the ankle brachial index (ABI) is described in the Geriatric Perspective Box.[45,52,69,70]

Blood flow may be assessed by palpating various lower extremity arteries such as the dorsalis pedis and posterior tibial. The dorsal pedis artery, a continuation of the anterior tibial artery, lies between the anterior tibialis and extensor digitorum longus tendons. The posterior tibial artery lies behind the medial malleolus and the posterior tibialis and flexor digitorum longus tendons, respectively. The location of these arteries is shown in Figure 1-11. Surgical procedures, such as arterial and/or venous bypass, may be done to restore blood flow and decrease the need for amputation.

GERIATRIC PERSPECTIVE

Doppler Ultrasound Procedure and the Ankle Brachial Index

To assess compromised blood flow, which is often present in the geriatric population, a Doppler probe is placed over a blood vessel distal to a blood pressure cuff. The cuff is inflated to a pressure above systolic pressure and then slowly deflated. The systolic blood pressure is signaled by the onset of blood flow, detected either acoustically or by a graph recorder. Arterial systolic pressure determinations can be used to make an ankle brachial index (ABI). The ABI is calculated as the foot systolic pressure (using the posterior tibial or dorsal pedis artery) divided by the brachial artery systolic pressure. The ABI is normally 1.1. An ABI of 0.75–0.95 shows arterial insufficiency, although the patient may be asymptomatic. An ABI between 0.50 and 0.75 indicates significant arterial symptomatology, including lower extremity pain with walking and rest pain. However, blood pressures can be falsely elevated in cases of noncompressible, noncompliant, calcified, atherosclerotic peripheral arteries.

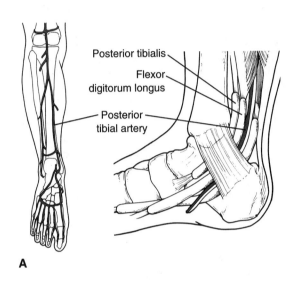

A

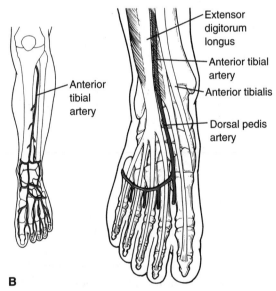

B

Figure 1-11. Location of the dorsalis pedis and posterior tibial arteries.

Table 1-5. Wound Staging for Pressure Ulcers (Agency for Health Care Policy and Research, AHCPR)	
Stage 1	Nonblanchable erythema of intact skin. Erythema does not resolve within 30 minutes of pressure relief. Epidermis remains intact. In individuals with darker skin, skin discoloration, warmth, edema, and hardness also may be indicators.
Stage 2	Partial-thickness loss of skin layers involving epidermis and possibly the dermis. The ulcer is superficial and presents clinically as an abrasion, blister, or shallow crater. The wound base is moist, pink, and painful, but free of necrotic tissue.
Stage 3	Full-thickness skin loss involving damage to, or necrosis of, subcutaneous tissue that may extend down to, but not through, underlying fascia. The wound may include necrotic tissue, sinus tract formation, exudate, and/or infection. The wound base is usually not painful.
Stage 4	Full-thickness skin loss with extensive tissue necrosis or damage to muscle, bone, tendon, and/or joint capsule. This wound presents as a deep crater, and the wound base is usually not painful.

Data adapted from Smyth, K., & Maguire, D. P. (1999). Wound Care Management. *Nursing Clinics of North America, 34,* 816.

Impedance plethysmography is another method of assessing blood flow. Like Doppler ultrasound, impedance plethysmography is noninvasive. Impedance plethysmography is often used to detect deep-vein thrombosis. In contrast, Doppler ultrasound is used to detect both arterial and venous blood flow.[70] Four electrodes are placed on the skin, and a small current is passed between electrodes. The changes in electrical impedance between electrodes is measured as the limb volume changes. For example, volume increases as arterial blood flows into an insufficient venous system.[69–71] Therefore, measurement of the voltage change allows indirect assessment of limb flow volume.

Wound Staging

Decreased blood flow may result in dermal wounds that may necessitate physical therapy and multidisciplinary intervention. There are numerous systems used to classify or stage a wound. One of the most common staging systems has been recommended by the Agency for Health Care Policy and Research (AHCPR) (Table 1-5).[72] This system was designed only for wounds due to pressure ulcers. Another staging method applicable to extremity vascular wounds is shown in Table 1-6.[73,74] Use of wound classification systems, such as those in Tables 1-5 or 1-6, can serve as an objective measure for initially establishing a baseline as well as evidence of wound improvement or progression.

Table 1-6. Wagner's Grading System for Extremity Vascular Wounds	
Grade	*Wound Description*
0	Preulcerative lesion, healed ulcers, presence of bony deformity
1	Superficial ulcer without involvement of subcutaneous tissue
2	Wound penetrates through the subcutaneous tissue (may expose bone, tendon, ligament, or joint capsule)
3	Osteitis, abscess, or osteomyelitis are present
4	Gangrene of a digit
5	Gangrene of the foot, requiring disarticulation

Adapted from Wagner, F. W., Jr. (1981). The dysvascular foot: A system for diagnosis and treatment. *Foot & Ankle, 2,* 64–122, and Bryant, R. A. (2000). *Acute and chronic wounds.* Nursing management (2nd ed.). St Louis: Mosby.

Amputation Levels

The terms *myoplasty, myofascial flap,* and *myodesis* are used when describing an amputation surgical procedure. They are defined as follows: **myoplasty** is the attachment of muscle to muscle; **myofascial flap** is the attachment of muscle to fascia; and **myodesis** is the attachment of muscle to periosteal bone. An example of the use of these terms is a description of a transtibial amputation. A well-padded, cylindrical transtibial limb is best achieved with fascia (myofascial flap) and muscle stabilization (myoplasty) over the anterior tibia and securing this to the periosteum (myodesis).[13]

Amputation Levels

Amputation levels above the knee are shown in Figure 1-12. These levels include the following:

- **Hemipelvectomy** is the loss of any part of the ilium, ischium, and pubis.
- **Hip disarticulation** is the loss of all of the femur. The hemipelvectomy and hip disarticulation procedures are usually done in cases of malignant tumors, extensive gangrene, massive trauma, or advanced infection.
- Short transfemoral amputations occur when less than 35% of femoral length is present. A larger weight-bearing surface can be created if femoral transection can be done at the level of the lesser trochanter. This level retains the femoral head and neck and the greater trochanter, resulting in improved prosthetic fit.[75] The number of transfemoral amputations has declined since the 1980s.[76] This decline is due to improved surgical techniques and better preoperative assessment of vascular status.[77]
- Medium transfemoral amputations occur when between 35 and 60% of femoral length is present. Ideally, transfemoral limbs should be at least 4 inches or 10 cm above the lower end of the femur to allow room for

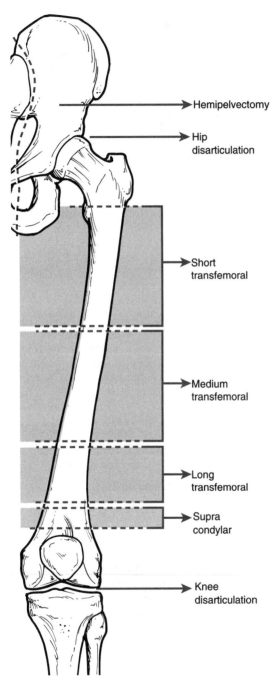

Figure 1-12. Amputation levels above the knee.

Hemipelvectomy

Hip disarticulation

Short transfemoral

Medium transfemoral

Long transfemoral

Supra condylar

Knee disarticulation

the prosthetic knee.[78] In a transfemoral amputation, both anterior and posterior muscular surfaces are well vascularized; therefore, equal flaps are fashioned.

- A **rotationplasty** is applicable to patients who have a malignant tumor in the middle or distal femur. It is also done in cases of PFFD. A rotationplasty involves an osteotomy in the proximal third of the femur, distal to the lesser trochanter, and in the proximal part of the tibia, distal to the tibial tuberosity. The foot is rotated 180° and the tibia reattached to the remaining femur. The foot is fit into the prosthesis and acts as a knee joint. Prosthetically, this amputation has the advantage of preserving the anatomic ankle joint, which acts as a knee joint, and a long lever arm for better prosthesis control.[79] The rotationplasty procedure is illustrated in Figure 1-13.

- Long transfemoral amputations occur when more than 60% of femoral length is present but not capable of end bearing. A transfemoral amputation is depicted in Figure 1-14.

- In a **supracondylar** amputation, the patella may be left for better end bearing. However, the area created between the end of the femur and the patella may delay healing.

- A **knee disarticulation** amputation offers good weight distribution and retains a long, powerful, muscle-stabilized femoral lever arm. In addition, the thigh muscles are completely preserved, thereby ensuring good muscular balance. This amputation maintains the femoral length in growing children by preserving the growth potential of the distal femoral epiphysis. However, the knee disarticulation amputation yields a noncosmetic socket because of the need for an external joint mechanism and resulting difficulty with swing-phase control. Knee disarticulation amputation is often performed on the patient who will not become a prosthetic walker. This amputation avoids the possibility of knee flexion contractures

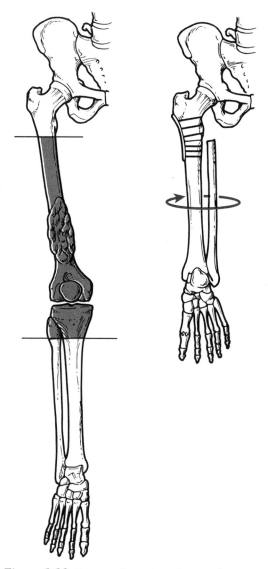

Figure 1-13. Rotationplasty procedure used in cases of a tumor in the middle or distal femur. *Diagram on the left* shows intact leg with tumor. *Diagram on right* shows that the foot has been rotated 180° and the tibia attached to the shortened femur. (Adapted from Hillmann, A., Rosenbaum, D., Schroter, J., Gosheger, G., Hoffmann, C., & Winkelmann, W. (2000). Electromyographic and gait analysis of forty-three patients after rotationplasty. *Journal of Bone & Joint Surgery, 82A,* 187–196.)

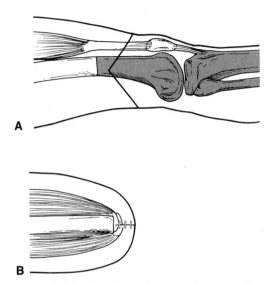

Figure 1-14. Transfemoral amputation procedure. **A.** Equal anterior and posterior soft tissue sections extending longer than the transected femur. **B.** A myodesis (attachment of muscle to periosteal bone) and a myoplasty (attachment of muscle to muscle) have been done. (Adapted from Shea, J. D. (1972). Surgical techniques for lower extremity amputation. *Orthopedic Clinics of North America, 3,* 287–301.)

and provides an excellent platform for sitting and transfers.[52,75] A knee disarticulation procedure is depicted in Figure 1-15.

Transtibial amputation levels are depicted in Figure 1-16.These include the following:

- A very short transtibial amputation occurs when less than 20% of tibial length is present. This amputation may result from trauma and is usually not done as an elective procedure. A very short transtibial amputation results in a small-moment arm, making knee extension difficult. Moment arms are further described in Chapter 5, "Biomechanic Implications of Prosthetics and Orthosis."
- A standard transtibial amputation occurs when between 20 and 50% of tibial length is present. An elective amputation in the middle third of the tibia, regardless of measured

length, provides a well-padded and biomechanically sufficient lever arm.[75] At least 8 cm of tibia is required below the knee joint for optimal fitting of a prosthesis.[80]

- A long transtibial amputation occurs when more than 50% of tibial length is present. This amputation is not advised because of poor blood supply in the distal leg.

The level of tibial transection should be as long as possible between the tibial tubercle and the junction of the middle and distal thirds of the tibia. A long posterior flap for transtibial amputations is advantageous because it is well vascularized and provides an excellent weight-bearing surface. In addition, the scar is on the anterior border, an area that is subject to less weight bearing. The deep calf musculature is often thinned to reduce the bulk of the posterior flap.[81]

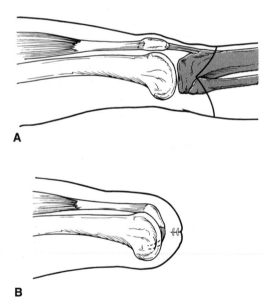

Figure 1-15. Knee disarticulation amputation. **A.** Equal anterior and posterior flaps are used. **B.** The patella and patellar ligament are wrapped around the distal femur. The patellar ligament and hamstrings are attached to the cruciate ligaments. (Adapted from Shea, J. D. (1972). Surgical techniques for lower extremity amputation. *Orthopedic Clinics of North America, 3,* 287–301.)

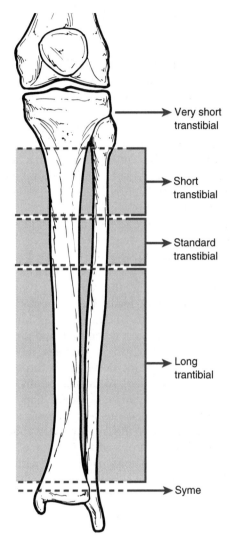

Figure 1-16. Transtibial amputation levels.

In a transtibial amputation, the fibula is transected 1 to 2 cm shorter than the tibia to avoid distal fibula pain. If the fibula is transected at the same length as the tibia, the patient senses that the fibula is too long, which may cause pain over the distal fibula. If the fibula is cut too short, a more conical shape, rather than the desired cylindrical-shape residual limb results. The cylindrical shape is better suited for total-contact prosthetic fitting techniques. A bevel is

placed on the anterior distal tibia to minimize tibial pain on weight bearing. The surgical technique for a transtibial amputation is depicted in Figure 1-17. To avoid a painful **neuroma**, a collection of axons and fibrous tissue, nerves should be identified, drawn down, severed, and allowed to retract at least 3 to 5 cm away from the areas of weight-bearing pressure.[13]

A **Syme amputation** was named for James Syme, a noted University of Edinburgh surgeon, in the mid-1800s. This amputation is an ankle disarticulation in which the heel pad is kept for good weight bearing. The Syme amputation results in a residual limb that possesses good function due to the long lever arm to control the prosthesis and the ability to ambulate without the prosthesis.

Associated problems with the Syme amputation include an unstable heel flap, development of neuromas of the posterior tibial nerve, and poor cosmesis. Performed properly, the residual limb is ideally suited for weight bearing and lasts virtually the life of the patient.

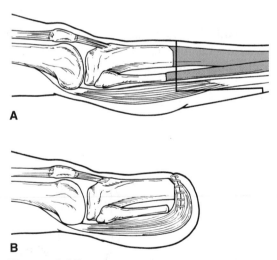

Figure 1-17. Transtibial amputation procedure A. Long posterior flap is used. B. Fibula is cut higher than the tibia and the anterior surface of the tibia is beveled (Adapted from Shea, J. D. (1972). Surgical techniques for lower extremity amputation. *Orthopedic Clinics of North America, 3,* 287–301.)

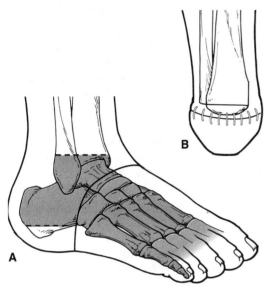

Figure 1-18. Syme amputation. **A.** The tibia and fibula may be shaved, creating a narrowed end. A thin layer of calcaneous with the intact heel pad is fixed to the distal tibia. **B.** The completed amputation with an anterior incision.(Adapted from Shea, J. D. (1972). Surgical techniques for lower extremity amputation. *Orthopedic Clinics of North America, 3,* 287–301.)

The bulky residual limb that results from a Syme amputation may be streamlined by trimming the remaining metaphyseal flares of the tibia and fibula. The Syme surgical technique is depicted in Figure 1-18.

Foot amputations levels are depicted in Figure 1-19. These include the following:

- A transmetatarsal amputation (TMA) may be performed for deformities resulting from trauma to the toes, infection or gangrene due to frostbite, diabetes, arteriosclerosis, or autoimmune circulatory connective tissue disorders.[82] There are approximately 10,000 TMAs a year in the United States, with a failure rate of about 30%.[82] Of all the amputations done in the United Kingdom, this amputation has the highest failure rate.[80] This high failure rate is due to a combination of substantial loss of weight-bearing areas on the neuropathic foot and the decreased foot length available to generate a plantarflexor moment. As a result, the remaining tissues bear an increased load. This amputation should be limited to patients with an intact posterior tibial pulse, a warm foot, and localization of osteomyelitis or gangrene to the phalanges. A dorsal incision is made through the mid- to proximal metatarsal shafts. A long, thick, myocutaneous plantar flap including the flexor tendons is used, with closure of this flap onto the dorsum of the foot[75] The transmetatarsal procedure is depicted in Figure 1-20. A custom-made shoe with a rigid rocker-bottom sole and a polypropylene ankle–foot orthosis (AFO) has been advo-

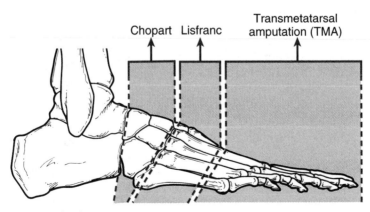

Figure 1-19. Foot amputation levels

cated for some patients with a TMA. This orthosis adaptation is depicted in Figure 1-21. This shoe with an AFO results in a longer ankle moment-arm resulting in a greater ankle plantarflexor moment and overall stability.[83] Conversely, a subsequent study found that use of the AFO generated many complaints about cosmesis and restriction at the ankle. These investigators recommended only a rigid rocker sole and not an AFO for most patients with diabetes mellitus and a TMA.[84]

- The **Lisfranc amputation** is done at the tarsometatarsal joint and involves a disarticulation of all five metatarsals and digits.
- The **Chopart amputation**, at the talonavicular and calcaneocuboid joints, involves a disartic-

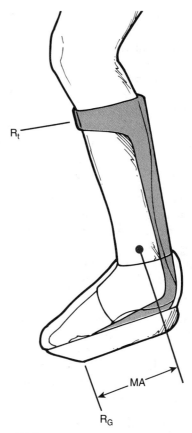

Figure 1-21. A regular shoe and ankle–foot orthosis (AFO) generate a long ankle moment-arm (ma) and more stability than a shortened shoe. (*Rg*, ground reaction force; *Rt*, reaction force of orthosis on tibial or leg) (Adapted from Mueller, M. J., & Sinacore, D. R. (1994). Rehabilitation factors following transmetatarsal amputation. *Physical Therapy, 74*, 1027–1033.)

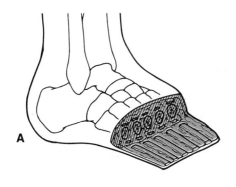

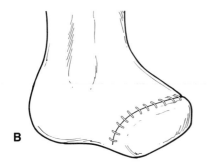

Figure 1-20. Transmetatarsal amputation. **A.** A long posterior flap extending to the toe crease results in an incision on the top of the foot. **B.** The completed amputation. (Adapted from Shea, J. D. (1972). Surgical techniques for lower extremity amputation. *Orthopedic Clinics of North America, 3*, 287–301.)

ulation through the midtarsal joint leaving only the calcaneus and talus. Both the Lisfranc and Chopart amputations were introduced before blood transfusions and antibiotics were available. They were planned as disarticulations to be performed as rapidly as possible. These amputations often result in an equinus and varus deformity due to the pull of the plantarflexors and loss of dorsiflexor and peroneal muscles. In addition, a distal sensitive end often leads to skin breakdown. There is much less indication for their use today.[85]

- A transphalangeal (toe disarticulation) amputation is done at the metatarsophalangeal joint. Toe disarticulations result in biomechanical deficiencies. Amputation of the great toe affects push-off during fast walking and running; as a result, patients with PVD often have a nonpropulsive gait pattern. If the base of the proximal phalanx with the insertion of the flexor hallucis brevis is saved, stability is enhanced.[52] Second-digit amputation results in severe hallux valgus.

Note: For the Lisfranc, Chopart, and transphalangeal amputations, shoe fillers or shoe modifications such as a spring-steel shank extending to the metatarsal heads, and a rocker sole or padding of the tongue of the shoe to assist in holding the hindfoot firmly in the shoe may be used.

- Phalangeal or partial toe amputation involves excision of any part of one or more toes. The lesser toes serve little function in patients with ischemic PVD. As a result, gait is not markedly affected with amputation of the lesser toes.[52] A prosthesis is usually not necessary for toe amputations.

Conditions Associated with the Need for an Orthosis

The following descriptions offer a brief background of the conditions that may necessitate use of an orthosis. Orthoses that may be used for these conditions and their implications are explained in more detail in Chapters 15 and 16.

Cerebral Palsy

Cerebral palsy (CP) is a nonprogressive, nonhereditary lesion of the cerebral cortex resulting in postural and motion disturbances. Children with CP may exhibit inaccurate sequencing and timing of muscle activation, abnormalities between agonist–antagonist muscle control, insufficient balance, and insufficient production of muscular force.[86] CP may be associated with speech, vision, hearing, and perceptual difficulties; hydrocephalus; microcephalus; or mental retardation. CP is often classified by the type of muscle tone and predominant limb involvement. The patterns of motor involvement are listed in Table 1-7. The reported incidence of CP ranges from 2.5 to 4.2 cases per 1000 births in

Table 1-7. Classification of Cerebral Palsy

Type by Muscle Tone and Body Part	Description
Spastic (75% incidence)	Increased reflexes; rapid alternating muscle contraction and relaxation; scissors gait common
Diplegia	Primarily involves trunk and lower limbs
Hemiplegia	Primarily one side involved, usually upper more than lower extremity
Quadriplegia (tetraplegia)	Involvement of all four limbs, trunk, head
Ataxia (15% incidence)	Irregularity of total body muscular action; fine movements impossible; decreased reflexes
Dyskinesia (5% incidence)	Impairment of total body voluntary movement; rapid, ceaseless, involuntary movements (chorea) alternating with repetitive, slow, writhing movements (athetosis); arms usually more affected than legs; movements may interfere with speech
Hypotonia (less than 1% incidence)	Reduced reflexes and muscle tone

Adapted from Goodman, C. C., & Boissonnault W. G. (1998). *Pathology: Implications for the physical therapist* (pp. 292–293). Philadelphia: W. B. Saunders.

the United States, with 7,000–12,000 children affected per year.[37] Low birth weight, premature birth, poor prenatal care, and anoxia are commonly associated with CP. Musculoskeletal problems of altered muscle tone, weakness, and joint contractures are common. Most of these children have some type of spasticity and hypertonicity. About 70% of these children become ambulatory in spite of delayed motor development. The gait pattern is affected by hypertonicity, which often produces a toe-walking pattern with sustained equinus, excessive knee and hip flexion, early heel rise, foot drop, excessive limb flexion during swing, and decreased step length.[87] Individuals with CP may benefit from various orthoses used to support a joint, such as a dynamic ankle–foot orthosis (DAFO). Likewise, a floor-reaction orthosis (FRO) may assist muscle action during ambulation in cases of a crouched stance.

Spina Bifida

The term *spina bifida* is often used to describe embryonic neural tube deficits. The three most common deficits include

1. **Spina bifida occulta**—incomplete fusion of the vertebral lamina, often asymptomatic. This is the most common type of spina bifida and the least likely to result in lower extremity paralysis.
2. **Meningocele**—external protrusion of the meninges. Depending on the severity of the protrusion, there may not be any paralysis of the lower extremities.
3. **Myelomeningocele**—protrusion of the meninges and spinal cord. There is paralysis of the lower extremity, possibly infection (meningitis), and hydrocephalus. These spina bifida deficits are most commonly found in the lumbosacral area. These deficits occur in 1–2 cases per 1000 live births. There are 6000–10,000 children with some form of spina bifida born each year in the United States.[37] The prognosis for ambulation by children with spina bifida is related to the

level of motor function. The higher the level of defect, the smaller the percentage of the group who are ambulatory. Other factors that may influence ambulation are mental retardation, muscle strength within the level of defect, orthopedic deformities, and hydrocephalus.[88] A variety of orthopedic interventions may be necessary as the child with spina bifida grows older. These include hip dislocation repair, scoliosis fusion, tendon transfers, and muscle releases. Individuals with spina bifida may benefit from standing frames and orthoses, such as a parapodium to achieve ambulation.

Arthritis

The most common forms of **arthritis** are osteoarthritis (OA) and rheumatoid arthritis (RA). OA, or degenerative joint disease, is a slow, progressive process leading to the breakdown of joint articular cartilage with subsequent pain and stiffness. The primary cause of osteoarthritis is unknown. The articular cartilage breaks down because of an imbalance between the mechanical stresses and the ability of the joint structures to absorb weight-bearing forces. It is estimated that 60–85% of those over 60 years of age have some type of joint articular cartilage changes.[37] RA is a chronic systemic autoimmune disorder, usually involving bilateral joints. RA is characterized by the inflammation of the cartilage and lining of the joints, which may cause redness, warmth, pain, and swelling. The cardiovascular, gastrointestinal, hematologic, and pulmonary systems may also be involved. Approximately 1–2% of the adult population has RA, with a two to three times higher incidence in women than in men.[37] The differences between OA and RA are shown in Table 1-8.

Individuals with either form of arthritis may benefit from orthoses used to unload, support, or protect a joint. These individuals may also benefit from shoe modifications such as rocker soles, soft heels, and metatarsal bars to de-

Table 1-8. Differences between Osteoarthritis and Rheumatoid Arthritis

Osteoarthritis	Rheumatoid Arthritis
Usually begins after age 40	Usually begins between ages 25 and 50
Usually develops slowly, over many years	Often develops suddenly
Often affects joints on one side of the body	Usually affects same joint on both sides of body (e.g., knees)
Usually doesn't cause redness, warmth, or inflammation of a joint	Causes redness, warmth, and joint effusion
Affects weight-bearing joints primarily; rarely affects elbows or shoulders	Affects multiple joints including elbows and shoulders

crease weight bearing on various aspects of the foot. These shoe modifications are discussed in Chapter 16, "Orthoses for Clients with Neurologic Disorders—Clinical Decision Making."

Diabetes Mellitus

Diabetes was described earlier in this chapter as a predisposing factor for amputation. An individual who has diabetes may also need an orthosis. Diabetes can result in vascular complications and neuropathies. Individuals with diabetes may benefit from shoe modifications such as an extra-depth shoe with molded inserts.

Spinal Cord Injury

Spinal cord injury can be caused by trauma such as a motor vehicle accident, a fall, or a tumor or may be due to congenital defects such as spina bifida. The damage to the spinal cord may be caused by laceration, compression, or blood in the spinal canal. Recent advances, especially in the area of neuron preservation, have resulted in fewer complete spinal cord injuries.[37] The use of high-dose steroid therapy during the first few days after injury has dramatically decreased the spinal shock and edema leading to neurologic deficits. Transplantation of nerve cells may soon negate the effects of spinal cord injury. A complete spinal cord injury often results in excessive muscle tone. An incomplete spinal

cord injury may result in joint contractures due to muscle imbalance. Individuals with paralysis secondary to a spinal cord injury may benefit from various orthoses to assist with ambulation, such as AFOs, knee–ankle–foot orthoses (KAFOs), or reciprocating-gait orthoses (RGOs). Those in the more acute phases may benefit from spinal orthoses such as a molded thoracolumbosacral orthosis (TLSO), hyperextension brace, or a halo cervical orthosis. These orthoses are described in more detail in Chapters 16 and 17.

Cerebrovascular Accident (CVA)

A CVA is a primary cause of disability in adults.[37] Factors that increase the risk of CVA include atherosclerosis, hypertension, cardiac dysrhythmias, diabetes, high serum triglyceride levels, lack of exercise, use of oral contraceptives, and cigarette smoking.[89] A CVA may be caused by a thrombus, embolus, or aneurysm resulting in loss of proprioception, sensation, motor power, and cognition. The average incidence of first CVA is 114 per 100,000 persons.[37] Some deficits due to a CVA have been limited as a result of infusional clot-dissolving agents. However, the infusion must be given within the first 2 hours after symptoms develop. New research in this area may limit the extent of disability.[89]

As a result of the CVA, gross limb synergies often result. A **synergy** occurs when specific movements of various joints occur together. A flexion synergy in the upper extremity usually predominates, characterized by scapular retraction; shoulder depression, internal rotation, and adduction; elbow flexion; forearm pronation; and wrist/finger flexion. Conversely, an extension synergy often predominates in the lower extremity. Pelvic retraction; hip extension, internal rotation, and adduction; knee extension; and ankle plantarflexion/inversion are often noted. As part of this extension synergy, the knee frequently goes into recurvatum or rigid knee extension from initial contact to the end of stance phase. In addition, flexion of the knee is difficult. Instead of a normal heel-to-toe gait, the foot often contacts the ground on the ball and lateral border. As a result, the patient may adopt a number of gait deviations to compensate for excessive lower-extremity extensor tone. These gait deviations are discussed in subsequent chapters. Patients with a CVA may benefit from an AFO with limited plantarflexion to assist with toe clearance in swing phase and to prevent recurvatum.

Traumatic Brain Injury (TBI)

A **traumatic brain injury (TBI)** occurs when the brain comes into forced contact with the harder skull, resulting in significant bruising and bleeding within the brain. There are about 2 million cases of head injury per year, with about 90,000 persons left with lifelong disabilities.[37] Head injury may result in damage to several structures including the brain, brainstem, blood vessels, and cranial nerves. As a result of this damage, excessive extensor tone often results in the lower extremity, which interferes with normal ambulation. Individuals with a TBI may benefit from an orthosis such as an AFO to assist in safe ambulation.

Peripheral Nerve Injuries

A peripheral nerve injury may occur from a nerve root compression due to, for example, a spinal disk protrusion or laceration of the peripheral nerve itself. A common peroneal nerve injury will affect the strength of the ankle dorsiflexors and evertors, resulting in a plantarflexed or inverted (**equinovarus**) foot position. Individuals with weakness of these muscles may benefit from an AFO with a dorsiflexion assist.

Ligamentous or Tendon Injuries

Ligaments or tendons may be sprained or torn, which necessitates some type of orthotic support. Sprains are classified as first, second, or third degree. First-degree sprains involve some discomfort, microtearing of collagen fibers, local tenderness, mild swelling, and ecchymosis but no loss of ligamentous integrity. Second-degree sprains result in increased pain, detectable joint instability, and muscle weakness. Third-degree sprains are characterized by severe pain and complete loss of structural or biomechanical integrity.[90]

Ligamentous or tendon injuries may be treated with orthosis supports ranging from a functional knee brace in the case of an anterior cruciate ligament sprain to a simple heel cup in cases of Achilles tendinitis.

KEY POINTS

- Care of the patient with an amputation has evolved from the primitive setting with no postoperative rehabilitation to a coordinated team approach involving many disciplines.
- The development of new materials and knowledge of biomechanical approaches has led to an ever-expanding improvement in prosthetic and orthotic components.
- Most amputations in the United States are performed in individuals more than 65 years of age for vascular disease. Those with diabetes make up a large segment of those with vascular disease.
- A patient's level of function is determined by the level of amputation as well as the presence of comorbidities.

• Common conditions associated with the need for an orthosis include cerebral palsy, spina bifida, arthritis, diabetes, spinal cord injury, cerebral vascular accident, traumatic brain injury, peripheral nerve injuries, and various ligamentous or tendon injuries.

CRITICAL THINKING QUESTIONS

1. Differentiate among the six causes of amputation. Which are the most common causes? Which risk factors are associated with each cause?

2. Compare and contrast type 1 and type 2 diabetes as to cause, possible complications, pharmaceutic interventions, and other interventions.

3. Define the different types of limb deficiencies.

4. Contrast the methods of assessing blood flow.

5. Discuss the different levels of amputation and, if appropriate, the advantages and disadvantages of each.

6. Assess various conditions that may necessitate use of an orthosis.

REFERENCES

1. Datta, D. (1998). Rehabilitation of amputees: Clinical management in the brave new world. *Journal of Tissue Viability, 8,* 14–16.
2. Magee, R. (1998). Amputation through the ages: The oldest major surgical operation. *Australian & New Zealand Journal of Surgery, 69,* 675–678.
3. Padula, P. A., & Friedmann, L. W. (1987). Acquired amputation and prostheses before the sixteenth century. *Angiology, 38,* 133–141.
4. Gordon, R. (1996). *The Literary Companion to Medicine (p. 1).* New York: St. Martin's Press.
5. Fliegel, O., & Feuer, S. F. (1966). Historical development of lower extremity prostheses. *Archives of Physical Medicine and Rehabilitation, 47,* 275–285.
6. Mustapha, N. M. (1985). Artificial limbs, past, present and future. *National News, 22,* 18–20.
7. Orr, J. F., James, W. V., & Bahrani, A. S. (1982). The history and development of artificial limbs. *Engineering in Medicine, 11,* 155–161.

8. Wilson, A. B. (1972). The modern history of amputation surgery and artificial limbs. *Orthopedic Clinics of North America, 3,* 267–285.
9. Shurr, D. G., & Cook, T. M. (1990). *Prosthetics & orthotics.* Norwalk, CT: Appleton & Lange.
10. Bunch, W. H., & Keagy, R. D. (1976). *Principles of orthotic treatment (pp. 1–2).* Baltimore: Williams & Wilkins.
11. Winter, R. B. (1994). The pendulum has swung too far. *Orthopedic Clinics of North America, 25,* 195–204.
12. Pandian, G., & Kowalske, K. (1999). Daily functioning of patients with an amputated lower extremity. *Clinical Orthopaedics and Related Research, 361,* 91–97.
13. Smith, D. G., & Fergason, J. R. (1999). Transtibial amputations. *Clinical Orthopaedics and Related Research, 361,* 108–115.
14. *Causes of amputation.* Albert Einstein Healthcare Network. Available at: http://www.einstein.edu/mossrehab/show.asp?durki=8214. Accessed December 29, 2000.
15. Detailed diagnoses and procedures, National Hospital Discharge Survey. (1997). *Vital and Health Statistics Series 13, 145.*
16. *Lower extremity complications in Veterans Health Administration. FY 89–99 Part 1: Lower extremity amputation rates, progression and utilization.* January 2000, p. 67.
17. Russell, J. N., Hendershot, G. E., LeClere, F., Howie, L. J., & Adler, M. (1997). Trends and differential use of assistive technology devices: United States 1994. *Advance Data, 292, 3.*
18. Soldo, S., Puntaric, D., Petrovicki, Z., & Prgomet, D. (1999). Injuries caused by antipersonnel mines in Croatian Army soldiers on the East Slavonia front during the 1991–1992 war in Croatia. *Military Medicine, 164,* 141–144.
19. Newman, R. D., & Mercer, M. A. (2000). Environmental health consequences of land mines. *International Journal of Occupational and Environmental Health, 6,* 243–248.
20. Atesalp, A. S., Erler, K., Gur, E., & Solakoglu, C. (1999). Below-knee amputations as a result of land-mine injuries: Comparison of primary closure versus delayed primary closure. *Journal of Trauma-Injury Infection and Critical Care, 47,* 724–727.
21. Group, T. G. (2000). Epidemiology of lower extremity amputation in centres in Europe, North America, and East Asia. *British Journal of Surgery, 87,* 328–337.

22. Resnick, H. E., Valsania, P., & Phillips, C. L. (1999). Diabetes mellitus and nontraumatic lower extremity amputation in black and white Americans: The National Health and Nutrition Examination Survey Epidemiologic Follow-up Study 1971–1992. *Archives of Internal Medicine, 159,* 2470–2475.

23. Moss, S. E., Klein, R., & Klein, B. E. (1999). The 14 year incidence of lower extremity amputations in a diabetic population. The Wisconsin Epidemiologic Study of Diabetic Retinopathy. *Diabetes Care, 22,* 951–959.

24. Lavery, L. A., VanHoutum, W. H., Ashry, H. R, Armstrong, D. G, & Pugh, J. A. (1999). Diabetes related lower extremity amputations disproportionately affect blacks and Mexican Americans. *Southern Medical Journal, 92,* 593–599.

25. Eggers, P. W., Gohdes, D., & Pugh, J. (1999). Nontraumatic lower extremity amputations in the Medicare end-stage renal disease population. *Kidney International, 56,* 1524–1533.

26. Mayfield, J. A., Reiber, G. E., Maynard, C., Czerniecki, J. M., Caps, M. T., & Sangeorzan, B. J. (2000). Trends in lower limb amputation in the Veterans Health Administration 1989–1998. *Journal of Rehabilitation Research and Development, 37,* 23–30.

27. Pohjolainen, T., & Alaranta, H. (1999). Epidemiology of lower limb amputees in southern Finland in 1995 and trends since 1984. *Prosthetics and Orthotics International, 23,* 88–92.

28. Reiber, G. E., Boyko, E. J., & Smith, D. G. (1995). Lower extremity foot ulcers and amputation in diabetes. In M. I. Harris, C. C. Cowie, M. P. Stern et al. (Eds.) *Diabetes in America* (2nd ed., pp. 409–428). (NIH Publication No. 95-1468). Washington, DC: National Institutes of Health.

29. Bowker, J. H., & Michael, J. W. (1992). *Atlas of limb prosthetics.* St Louis: Mosby Year Book.

30. Dormandy, J., Heeck, L., & Vig, S. (1999). Major amputations: Clinical patterns and predictors. *Seminars in Vascular Surgery, 12,* 154–161.

31. Slovik, D. M. (1997). Diabetes and rehab: Treating, managing, and rehabilitating diabetic patients. *Rehab Management,* 46–54.

32. Stern, P. H. (1991). The epidemiology of amputations. *Physical Medicine and Rehabilitation Clinics of North America, 2,* 253–261.

33. Dennison, P. D., Black, J. M. (1993). Nursing care of clients with peripheral vascular disorders. In J. M. Black & E. Matassarin-Jacobs (Eds.). (1993). *Luckmann and Sorrensen's medical surgical nursing* (4th ed., pp. 1253–1314). Philadelphia: WB Saunders.

34. Goodman, C. C., & Snyder, T. K. (2000). *Differential diagnosis in physical therapy* (3rd ed., p. 118). Philadelphia: WB Saunders.

35. Krajewski, L. P., & Olin, J. W. (1991). Atherosclerosis of the aorta and lower extremities arteries. In J. R. Young, R. A. Graor, J. W. Olin, & J. R. Bartholomew (Eds.) (1991). *Peripheral vascular diseases (pp. 179-200).* St. Louis: Mosby-Year Book.

36. Price, J. F., Mowbray, P. I., Lee, A. J., Rumley, A., Lowe, G. D., & Fowkes, F. G. (1999). Relationship between smoking and cardiovascular risk factors in the development of peripheral arterial disease and coronary artery disease: Edinburgh Artery Study. *European Heart Journal, 20,* 344–353.

37. Goodman, C. C., & Boissonnault, W. G. (1998). *Pathology: Implications for the physical therapist* (pp. 292–293). Philadelphia: W. B. Saunders.

38. Braunwald, E., Isselbacher, K. J., Petersdorf, R. G., Wilson, J. D., Martin, J. B., & Fauci, A. S. (1994). *Harrison's principles of internal medicine* (13th ed., pp. 1045–1046). New York: McGraw Hill.

39. Diabetes Facts and Figures 1999. Available at: http://www.diabetes.org/ada/facts.asp. Accessed December 29, 2000.

40. Report of the Expert Committee on the Diagnosis and Classification of Diabetes Mellitus. (1998). *Diabetes Care, 21,* S5–19.

41. Standards of Care. American Diabetes Association, 1660 Duke Street, Alexandria, VA 22314,1994.

42. American Diabetes Association. *The dangerous toll of diabetes.* Available at: (http://www.diabetes.org/ada/facts.asp. Accessed December 29, 2000.

43. DeFronazo, R. A. (1999). Pathophysiology of type 2 diabetes: The role of insulin resistance. *Consultations in Primary Care Consultant, 39,* S8–16.

44. Nathan, D. M. (1993). Long-term complications of diabetes mellitus. *New England Journal of Medicine, 328,* 1676–1685.

45. Falanga, V. (2000). *Text atlas of wound management* (p. 133). London: Martin Dunitz.

46. Anon. (Winter 2000–2001). *Nurse Practitioners Prescribing Reference (p. 108).* New York: Prescribing Reference.

47. Rijken, P. M., Dekker, J., Dekker, E., Lankhorst, G. J., Bakker, K., Dooren, J., & Rauwerda, J. A. (1998). Clinical and functional correlates of foot pain in diabetic patients. *Disability & Rehabilitation, 20,* 330–336.

48. Larsson, J., Apelqvist, J., Agardh, C. D., & Stenstrom. (1995). A decreasing incidence of major amputation in diabetic patients: A consequence of a multidisciplinary foot care team approach. *Diabetic Medicine, 12,* 770–776.

49. Position Statement. (1998). Standards of medical care for patients with diabetes mellitus. *Diabetes Care, 21,* S23–31.

50. Ramsey, S. D., Newton, K., Blough, D., McCulloch, D. K., Sandhu, N., Reiber, G. E., & Wagner, E. H. (1999). Incidence, outcomes and cost of foot ulcers in patients with diabetes. *Diabetes Care, 22,* 382–387.

51. Fotieo, G. G., Reiber, G. E., Carter, J. S., & Smith, D. G. (1999). Diabetic amputations in the Veterans Administration: Are there opportunities for interventions? *Journal of Rehabilitation Research and Development, 36,* 55–59.

52. Pinzur, M. S. (1997). Current concepts: Amputation surgery in peripheral vascular disease. *Instructional Course Lectures, 46,* 501–509.

53. Eneroth, M., Apelqvist, J., Larsson, J., & Persson, B. M. (1997). Improved wound healing in transtibial amputees receiving supplementary nutrition. *International Orthopaedics, 21,* 104–108.

54. Gillespie, R. (1990). Principles of amputation surgery in children with longitudinal limb deficiencies of the femur. *Clinical Orthopedics & Related Research, 256,* 29–38.

55. Tachdjian, M. O. (1997). *Clinical pediatric orthopedics (pp. 244–246).* Stamford, CT: Appleton & Lange.

56. Lin C. H., Wei, F. C., Levein, L. S., Su, J. I., & Yeh, W. L. (1997). The functional outcome of lower extremity fractures with vascular injury. *Journal of Trauma-Injury Infection & Critical Care, 43,* 480–485.

57. Russell W. L., Sailors, D. M., Whittle, T. B., et al. (1991). Limb salvage versus traumatic amputation: A decision based on a seven-part predictive index. *Annals of Surgery, 213,* 473–481.

58. Hudson, M. M., Tyc, V. L., Cremer, L. K., Luo, X., Li, H., Rao, B. N., & Meyer, W. H. (1998). Patient satisfaction after limb-sparing surgery for pediatric malignant bone tumors. *Journal of Pediatric Oncology Nursing, 15,* 60-69.

59. Tornetta, P., & Olson, S. A. (1997). Amputation versus limb salvage. *Instructional Course Lectures, 46,* 511–518.

60. Moseley, C. F. (1991). Leg lengthening: The historical perspective. *Orthopedic Clinics of North America, 22,* 555–561.

61. Green, S. A. (1997). Patient management during limb lengthening. *Instructional Course Lectures, 46,* 547–554.

62. Craft, A. W. (1997). Challenges in the management of bone tumors. *Annals of the New York Academy of Sciences, 824,* 167–179.

63. Picci, P. (1992). Osteosarcoma and other cancers of bone. *Current Opinion in Oncology, 4,* 676–680.

64. Sharrard, W. J. W. (1993). *Paediatric orthopaedics and fractures* (3rd ed.). London: Blackwell Scientific Publications.

65. Day, H. B. (1991). The ISO/ISPO classification of congenital limb deficiency. *Prosthetics Orthotics International, 15,* 67–69.

66. Tecklin, J. S. (1999). Pediatric physical therapy (3rd ed., p.391). Philadelphia: J. B. Lippincott.

67. Loscalzo, J. L, Creager, M. A., & Dzau, V. J. (1996). *Vascular medicine. A textbook of vascular biology and disease* (2nd Ed., pp. 418–422). Boston: Little, Brown & Co.

68. Aburahma, A. F., & Bergan, J. T. (Eds.) (2000). *Noninvasive vascular diagnosis.* London: Springer-Verlag.

69. Krebs, C. A., Giyanani, V. L., & Eisenberg, R. L. (1999). *Ultrasound atlas of vascular diseases (pp. 4–5).* Stamford, CT: Appleton & Lange.

70. McCulloch, J. M., Kloth, L. C., & Feedar, J. A. (1995). *Wound healing: Alternatives in management* (2nd ed.). Philadelphia: F. A. Davis.

71. Irwin S., & Tecklin, J. S. (1995). *Cardiopulmonary physical therapy* (3rd ed., p. 225). St. Louis: Mosby-Yearbook.

72. Smyth, K., & Maguire, D. P. (1999). Wound care management. *Nursing Clinics of North America, 34,* 816.

73. Wagner, F. W., Jr. (1981). The dysvascular foot: A system for diagnosis and treatment. *Foot & Ankle, 2,* 64–122.

74. Bryant, R. A. (2000). *Acute and chronic wounds. Nursing management* (2nd ed.). St Louis: Mosby.

75. Rutherford, R. B. (2000). *Vascular surgery* (5th ed.). Philadelphia: W. B. Saunders.

76. Pernot, H. F., deWitte, L. P., Lindeman, E., & Cluitmas, J. (1997). Daily functioning of the lower extremity amputee: An overview of the literature. *Clinical Rehabilitation, 11,* 93–106.

77. Cutson, T. M. & Bongiorni, D. R. (1996). Rehabilitation of the older lower limb amputee: A brief review. *Journal American Geriatric Society, 44,* 1388–1393.

78. Coletta, E. M. (2000). Care of the elderly patient with lower extremity amputation. *Journal of the American Board of Family Practice, 123,* 23–34.

79. Hillmann, A., Rosenbaum, D., Schroter, J., Gosheger, G., Hoffmann, C., & Winkelmann, W. (2000). Electromyographic and gait analysis of forty-three patients after rotationplasty. *Journal of Bone and Joint Surgery, 82A,* 187–196.

80. Spark, I., Vowden, K., & Vowden, P. (1998). Lower-limb amputation: Wound care and rehabilitation. *Journal of Wound Care, 7,* 137–140.

81. Gottschalk, F. (1999). Transfemoral amputation. Biomechanics and surgery. *Clinical Orthopaedics & Related Research, 361,* 15–22.

82. Hodge, M. J., Peters, P. G., Efird, W. G. (1989). Amputations of the distal portion of the foot. *Southern Medical Journal, 82,* 1138–1142.

83. Mueller, M. J., & Sinacore, D. R. (1994). Rehabilitation factors following transmetatarsal amputation. *Physical Therapy, 74,* 1027–1033.

84. Mueller, M. J., & Strube, M. J. (1997). Therapeutic footwear: Enhanced function in people with diabetes and transmetatarsal amputation. *Archives of Physical Medicine & Rehabilitation, 78,* 952–956.

85. Roach, J. J., Deutsch, A., & McFarland, D. S. (1987). Resurrection of the amputations of Lisfranc and Chopart for diabetic gangrene. *Archives of Surgery, 122,* 931–934.

86. Dormans, J., & Pellegrino, L. (1998). *Caring for children with cerebral palsy: A team approach (p. 393).* Baltimore: Paul H. Brookes.

87. Fish, D. J., & Kosta, C. S. (1997, September). Neuromuscular characteristic gait patterns influence therapy. *Biomechanics/O&P,* 7–15.

88. Hinderer, K., Hinderer, S., & Shurtleff, D. (2000). Myelodysplasia. In S. K. Campbell, D. W. Van der Linden, & R. J. Palisano (Eds.) *Physical therapy for children* (2nd ed.). Philadelphia: W. B. Saunders.

89. Benson, R. T., & Sacco, R. L. (2000). Stroke prevention: hypertension, diabetes, tobacco, and lipids. *Neurologic Clinics, 18,* 309–319.

90. Anderson, M. K., & Hall, S. J. (1995). *Sports Injury Management (pp. 41–42).* Baltimore: Williams & Wilkins.

Chapter 2

EXAMINATION OF THE PATIENT WITH AN AMPUTATION AND THE PATIENT REQUIRING AN ORTHOSIS

Objectives

1. Correctly evaluate an individual with an amputation or an individual requiring an orthosis by use of either a generic examination form or the *Guide to Physical Therapist Practice*
2. Depict conditions associated with the need for an orthosis
3. Compare and contrast skin complications that may be encountered by a patient with a prosthesis or orthosis
4. Differentiate intrinsic and extrinsic phantom pain and phantom limb sensation

This chapter is divided into the following sections:

This chapter uses the *Guide to Physical Therapist Practice* terminology.[1] Physical therapists examine, evaluate, diagnose, determine prognoses, use intervention techniques, and establish outcomes to interact more effectively with patients with an amputation or requiring an orthosis. We, as physical therapists, perform these activities at various levels of the disablement process, including impairment, functional limitation, and disability.

♦ ♦ ♦

Evaluation of Patients with Amputations

A patient with an amputation may be evaluated in various ways. Two methods are presented that may serve as mechanisms to evaluate the patient effectively. One method is the *Guide to Physical Therapist Practice*, which is described later in this chapter.[1] Another method uses the examination for patients with an amputation, depicted in Figure 2-1.

Demographic and Health Information Section:
1. Date
2. Name
3. Address
4. Age
5. Height
6. Weight
7. Living Arrangements:
    ____ with family ____ alone ____ facility
8. Occupation (past/future plans)
9. Recreational Activities
10. Vocational Rehabilitation Potential
    ____ yes ____ perhaps ____ no
11. Date of amputation/site/reason
12. Date and Reason for Revision, if any
13. Past Medical History
14. Medications
15. Current Problems
16. Purpose/goal for prosthesis

Functional Assessment Section:
1. Ambulation
    ____ non ambulatory
    ____ community (independent indoors and outdoors on all surfaces)
    ____ household (independent mainly indoors and some outdoors if flat, smooth surfaces)
    ____ therapeutic (indoors under assistance or supervision or chairbound)
    ____ type of assistive device used
2. Transfers
    ____ independent
    ____ requires assistance (describe)
3. Bandaging
    ____ independent ____ with assistance
    ____ properly ____ needs improvement
    ____ not bandaging

Tests and Measures Residual Limb Condition Section:
1. Length from:
    ____ tibial tubercle (transtibial) to end of bone
    ____ tibial tubercle (transtibial) to end of soft tissue
    ____ ischial tuberosity (transfemoral) to end of bone
    ____ ischial tuberosity (transfemoral) to end of soft tissue
2. Circumference Measurements at:
    0cm ____ 4cm ____ 8cm ____
    12cm____ 16cm____ 20cm____
    24cm____ 28cm____ 32cm____

3. Shape of Residual limb
    ____ conical ____ cylindrical ____ bulbous
4. Distal view: Note areas of Tenderness (t) Adherence (a) Invagination (i) Callus (c) Discoloration (d) Non-healing (nh)

ANTERIOR
CENTER
POSTERIOR

5. Condition of hip:

Abduction		Flexion		Extension		Adduction	
Strength	ROM	Strength	ROM	Strength	ROM	Strength	ROM

6. Condition of knee:

Flexion		Extension	
Strength	ROM	Strength	ROM

7. Stability:
    ____ anterior/posterior ____ medial/lateral
    ____ crepitus ____ recurvatum
8. Skin condition
    ____ warm ____ abnormally warm
    ____ adherent scar ____ cool ____ impaired sensitivity ____ smallest Semmes-Weinstein Monofilament perceived (Inability to feel the touch of 5.07 or smaller indicates loss of protection)
9. Phantom pain/limb (describe)
10. Areas of possible complications (neuroma, redundant tissue)

Remaining Extremity Section
1. Strength
    ____ normal ____ decreased (describe)
2. ROM
    ____ normal ____ decreased (describe)
3. Vascular pulses:

Pulse	0 (absent)	1+ (diminished)	2+ (normal)	3+ (increased)
Femoral				
Tibial				
Posterior tibial				
Doral Pedis				

4. Refill time after blanching toenails ____ seconds. (Normal refill time is 3 seconds)
5. Temperature
    ____ abnormally warm ____ cool
6. Skin condition
    ____ warm ____ abnormally warm
    ____ cool ____ impaired sensitivity
    ____ smallest Semmes-Weinstein Monofilament perceived (Inability to feel the touch of 5.07 or smaller indicates loss of protective extension)
7. Extent of distal hair growth
    Assessment
Outcomes
Signature   Date

Figure 2-1. Examination of patients with an amputation.

Examination of Patients with an Amputation

Description of each section of this form as depicted in Figure 2-1 is as follows:

Demographic and Health Information

The demographic and health information section includes the patient's personal information such as living arrangements, occupation, and health information. A clear understanding of this information will assist in discharge planning. Current medications may affect the individual's ability to participate in an aggressive rehabilitation program. For example, anticoagulants may result in bruising easily. Diuretics, to control hypertension, may cause residual limb volume changes and frequent urination. Antihypertensive medications may limit exercise tolerance because of dizziness and weakness.

Functional Assessment

The functional assessment section includes ambulation, transfers, and residual limb bandaging. A patient may need further instruction to bandage the residual limb independently.

Residual Limb Condition

In the tests and measures area, the residual limb condition section contains information regarding the dimensions, skin condition, flexibility, and strength of the residual limb. Length from the tibial tubercle for a transtibial amputation or from the ischial tuberosity for a transfemoral amputation can be determined. Length measurements are taken to the end of the bone and to the end of the soft tissue. If these measurements differ markedly, redundant tissue is the likely cause. This redundant tissue may be decreased with proper residual limb wrapping, exercise, and weight-bearing activities. Circumferential measurements are then taken. The 0 cm point corresponds to the tibial tubercle for a transtibial amputation or

the proximal thigh/ischial tuberosity level for a transfemoral amputation. Circumferential measurements can be taken at each 4 cm of length. A conical residual limb has a smaller circumference at the distal end of the residual limb than at the proximal area. A cylindrical residual limb would have approximately equal circumferences at the proximal and distal ends, while a bulbous residual limb would have a greater circumference at the distal end. The cylindrical shape is better suited for total-contact prosthetic fitting techniques. These residual limbs are illustrated in Figure 2-2.

Areas on the anterior, posterior, and center aspects of the residual limb may be noted for various conditions. The center is the bottom of the residual limb, and notations are tenderness (t), adherence (a), invagination (i), callus (c), discoloration (d), and nonhealing (nh).

The condition of the residual limb hip and knee (in cases of a transtibial amputation) may be assessed in terms of strength and range of motion (ROM). The affected knee is assessed for anterior and posterior drawer, medial and lateral (valgus and varus) stability, crepitus, and recurvatum. The skin is assessed for scar adherence, coolness (possibly indicating arterial insufficiency), abnormal warmth (possibly indicating infection), and impaired sensitivity.

Skin sensitivity may be assessed using Semmes-Weinstein Monofilaments.[2] Semmes-Weinstein Monofilaments are calibrated nylon monofilaments that generate a reproducible buckling stress. The manufacturer has assigned numbers to the monofilaments that range from 1.65 to 6.65.[3] If a patient cannot consistently feel the touch of a 5.07 Semmes-Weinstein Monofilament, protective sensation has been lost.[4] Research has shown that the Semmes-Weinstein Monofilament is an inexpensive, reliable, valid, and easy-to-use clinical indicator for identifying patients at risk for developing foot ulcers and subsequent amputations.[3] The Semmes-Weinstein Monofilament is shown in Figure 2-3.

Phantom limb and pain (described later in this chapter) may be described as well as areas

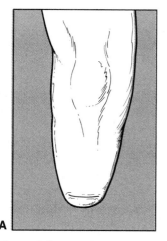 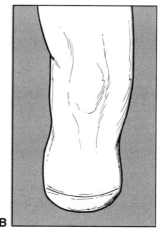 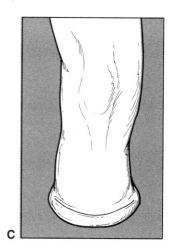

Figure 2-2. Residual limb shapes: A. conical; B. cylindrical; C. bulbous.

of possible complications such as the presence of a neuroma (also described later) or redundant tissue.

Remaining Extremity

Strength and ROM of the remaining extremity as well as vascular pulses (femoral, tibial, dorsal pedis, and posterior tibial) may also be evaluated. The femoral pulse is found in the groin area, and the tibial pulse in the popliteal area. The dorsal pedis pulse is found between the extensor hallucis longus and anterior tibialis tendons; the posterior tibial pulse is found behind the medial malleolus. Locations of these pulses are shown in Figure 1-11. Palpation of the femoral, popliteal, posterior tibial, and dorsalis pedis pulses can indicate diminished circulation. Inadequate circulation may also lead to dependent rubor. Pulses are graded as follows:

0, absent
1+, diminished
2+, normal
3+, increased

Arterial blood flow may be determined by blanching the toenails of the remaining extremity with one's fingertips and counting the time needed for return of normal toenail color.

Normal refill time is 3 seconds. If this time is delayed, arterial blood flow may be compromised. Another test to determine vascular status is to elevate the limb at an angle of about 60° for 1 minute. The limb is then placed in a

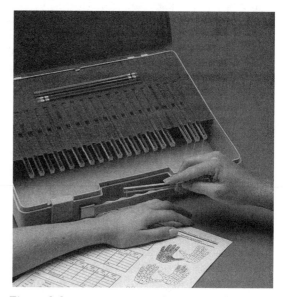

Figure 2-3. Semmes-Weinstein Monofilament. (Photo courtesy of the Rehabilitation Division of Smith & Nephew, Inc.)

dependent position. If the limb turns red, this is a rebound from the period of hypoxia and an indication of dysvascularity.[5] Blood flow may also be assessed by Doppler ultrasound or impedance plethysmography as described in Chapter 1.

Temperature of the remaining extremity may be rated warm (normal), abnormally warm, or cool (indicating possible vascular problems). Skin sensitivity may be assessed similarly to that of the residual limb. The extent of distal hair growth is checked to determine if arterial problems are present. A gross determination may be made; if someone has hair on the dorsal surface of the fingers, it is likely to be present on the dorsum of the foot and toes as well.

This form also contains areas to document the assessment and outcomes and provides space for signatures and date.

Guide to Physical Therapist Practice

Another system of managing the patient with an amputation uses the American Physical Therapy Association's *Guide to Physical Therapist Practice* (the *Guide*).[1] The *Guide*, using a disablement model, describes the sequelae of an injury or disease process.[6] Physical therapy interventions should not focus on pathology or disease but rather on functional loss and disability of the patient.

Terminology

The disablement model uses the terms *impairments, functional limitations,* and *disability.* These are defined, with examples specific to a patient with an amputation, as follows.

Impairments are losses or abnormalities of anatomic, physiologic, psychologic, or mental structure or function. Loss of full knee extension or loss of strength of the hip extensors are examples of impairments.

Functional limitations are restrictions of the ability to perform at the level of a whole person a physical action, activity, or task in an efficient, typically expected, or competent manner. Inability to bandage the residual limb is an example of a functional limitation.

Disability is the inability to perform, or limitation in the performance of, actions, tasks, and activities usually expected in social roles that are customary for the individual in a specific sociocultural context and physical environment. In the *Guide,* required roles may involve self-care, home management, and work that may involve job, school, play, and community and leisure categories.[1] Inability to return to one's prior employment is an example of a disability.

The *Guide* advocates the following terms or elements be used in communication and documentation.

Examination is the process of history taking, systems review, and selecting and administering specific tests and measures. Examination leads to a diagnostic classification or, as appropriate, to referral to other practitioners. The *Guide* states that the examination includes the patient's history, systems review, and tests and measures. Types of data that may be generated from a patient/client history are shown in Figure 2-4. The systems review may include

- Cardiovascular/pulmonary (blood pressure, edema, heart, and respiratory rates)
- Integumentary (presence of scar formation, skin color, and integrity)
- Musculoskeletal (gross ROM, strength, and symmetry, height, and weight)
- Neuromuscular (gross coordinated movements)

Tests and measures that may be done with a patient with an amputation or one requiring an orthosis are listed in Resource Box 2-1.

Evaluation is a dynamic process in which the therapist makes a clinical judgment based on the examination. The term *evaluation* should be used instead of *assessment.*

Diagnosis is the process and the end result of evaluation information obtained from the

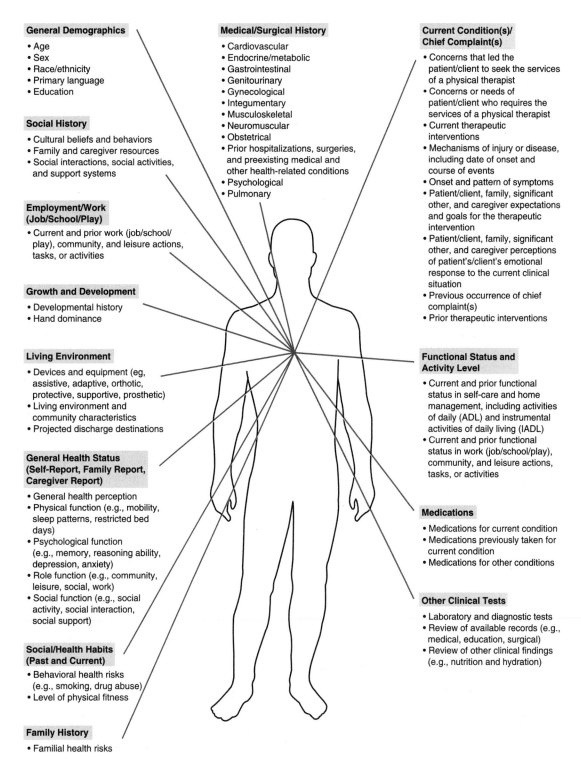

General Demographics

- Age
- Sex
- Race/ethnicity
- Primary language
- Education

Social History

- Cultural beliefs and behaviors
- Family and caregiver resources
- Social interactions, social activities, and support systems

Employment/Work (Job/School/Play)

- Current and prior work (job/school/play), community, and leisure actions, tasks, or activities

Growth and Development

- Developmental history
- Hand dominance

Living Environment

- Devices and equipment (eg, assistive, adaptive, orthotic, protective, supportive, prosthetic)
- Living environment and community characteristics
- Projected discharge destinations

General Health Status (Self-Report, Family Report, Caregiver Report)

- General health perception
- Physical function (e.g., mobility, sleep patterns, restricted bed days)
- Psychological function (e.g., memory, reasoning ability, depression, anxiety)
- Role function (e.g., community, leisure, social, work)
- Social function (e.g., social activity, social interaction, social support)

Social/Health Habits (Past and Current)

- Behavioral health risks (e.g., smoking, drug abuse)
- Level of physical fitness

Family History

- Familial health risks

Medical/Surgical History

- Cardiovascular
- Endocrine/metabolic
- Gastrointestinal
- Genitourinary
- Gynecological
- Integumentary
- Musculoskeletal
- Neuromuscular
- Obstetrical
- Prior hospitalizations, surgeries, and preexisting medical and other health-related conditions
- Psychological
- Pulmonary

Current Condition(s)/Chief Complaint(s)

- Concerns that led the patient/client to seek the services of a physical therapist
- Concerns or needs of patient/client who requires the services of a physical therapist
- Current therapeutic interventions
- Mechanisms of injury or disease, including date of onset and course of events
- Onset and pattern of symptoms
- Patient/client, family, significant other, and caregiver expectations and goals for the therapeutic intervention
- Patient/client, family, significant other, and caregiver perceptions of patient's/client's emotional response to the current clinical situation
- Previous occurrence of chief complaint(s)
- Prior therapeutic interventions

Functional Status and Activity Level

- Current and prior functional status in self-care and home management, including activities of daily (ADL) and instrumental activities of daily living (IADL)
- Current and prior functional status in work (job/school/play), community, and leisure actions, tasks, or activities

Medications

- Medications for current condition
- Medications previously taken for current condition
- Medications for other conditions

Other Clinical Tests

- Laboratory and diagnostic tests
- Review of available records (e.g., medical, education, surgical)
- Review of other clinical findings (e.g., nutrition and hydration)

Figure 2-4. Types of data that may be generated from a patient/client history. (Adapted from American Physical Therapy Association. (2001). A guide to physical therapist practice. *Physical Therapy, 81.*)

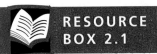

RESOURCE BOX 2.1

Tests and Measures

Aerobic Capacity and Endurance
Anthropometric Characteristics
Arousal, Attention, and Cognition
Assistive and Adaptive Devices
Circulation (Arterial, Venous, and Lymphatic)
Cranial and Peripheral Nerve Integrity
Environmental, Home, and Work (Job/School/Play) Barriers
Ergonomics and Body Mechanics
Gait, Locomotion, and Balance
Integumentary Integrity
Joint Integrity and Mobility
Motor Function (Motor Control and Motor Learning)
Muscle Performance
Orthotic, Protective, and Supportive Devices
Pain
Posture
Prosthetic Requirements
Range of Motion including Muscle Length
Self-care and Home Management
Sensory Integrity
Work (Job/School/Play), Community, and Leisure Integration or Reintegration (Including Independent Activities of Daily Living)

Reprinted with permission from American Physical Therapy Association. (2001). A guide to physical therapist practice. *Physical Therapy, 81.*

examination. This information is organized into defined categories to help determine the prognosis, the plan of care, and the most appropriate interventions.

Prognosis is a determination of the level of optimal improvement that may be attained and the amount of time to reach that level.

Intervention is a purposeful and skilled interaction of the therapist with the patient and, when appropriate, with other individuals involved in the care of the patient, to produce changes consistent with examination findings, the evaluation, the diagnosis, and the prognosis. The term *intervention* should be used instead of *treatment.* Intervention has three major components:

1. Communication, coordination, and documentation
2. Patient-related instruction
3. Procedural interventions; examples of interventions are illustrated in Figure 2-5.

Outcomes are the expected results of patient management. Outcomes should be measurable and involve a specified period needed to meet them. The term *outcomes* should be used instead of *goals.*[6]

The relationship of these various elements of patient/client management is shown in Figure 2-6.

Episode of care encompasses all patient activities that are provided, directed, or supervised by the physical therapist from initial contact through discharge, in an unbroken sequence. A range of number of visits is established for an episode of care. The episode of care may involve the patient in a variety of settings such as acute, subacute, home health, or outpatient care. It also includes reclassification of the patient among practice patterns.

Treatment is the total of all interventions provided by the physical therapist during an episode of care.

Practice Patterns

Decisions about which diagnostic pattern to use with a particular patient are based on information from the evaluation. Selection of the correct diagnostic pattern is confirmed by the examination results, an effective intervention and prognosis, and communication with other members of the patient's health-care team. A patient may have more than two patterns (e.g., a patient with diabetes and skin breakdown

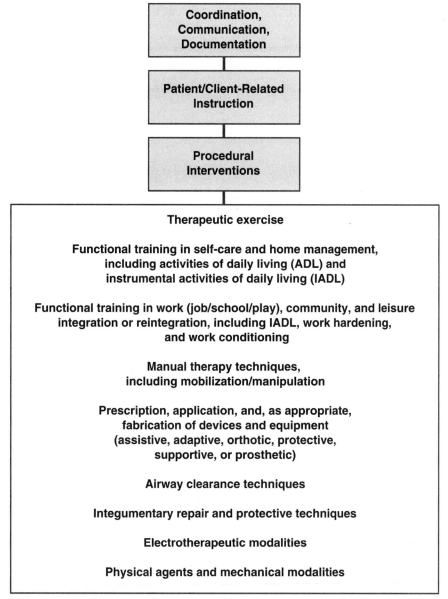

Figure 2-5. Examples of physical therapist interventions. (Adapted from American Physical Therapy Association. (2001). A guide to physical therapist practice. *Physical Therapy, 81.*)

due to neuropathy that resulted in an amputation). This patient would have both an integumentary pattern and a musculoskeletal pattern.

The *Guide* describes a practice pattern for dealing with lower extremity amputation in a pattern called "Impaired Gait, Locomotion, and Balance and Impaired Motor Function Secondary to Lower Extremity Amputation" (pattern 4J).[1] According to this practice pattern, the expected range of visits during a single

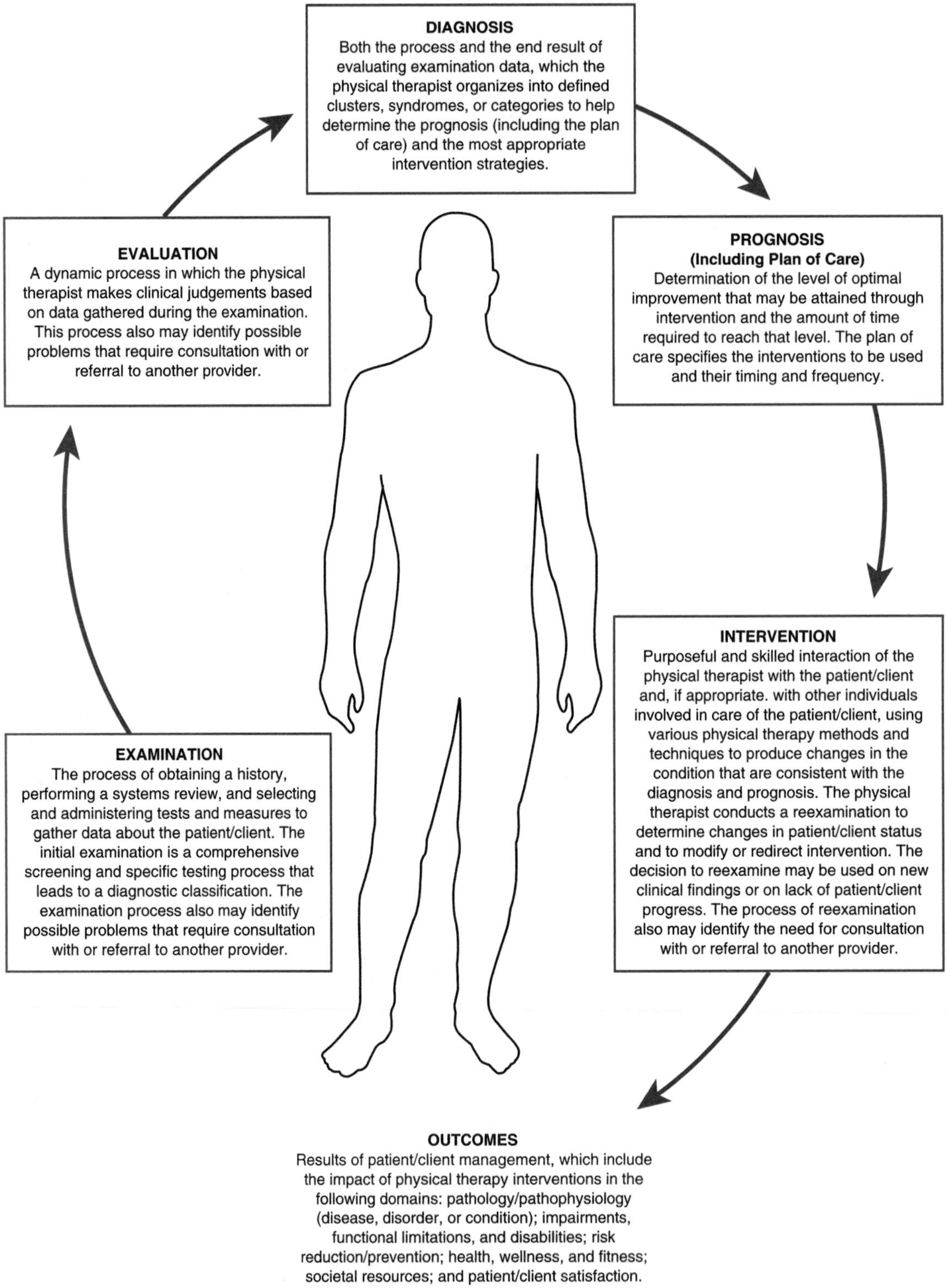

DIAGNOSIS
Both the process and the end result of evaluating examination data, which the physical therapist organizes into defined clusters, syndromes, or categories to help determine the prognosis (including the plan of care) and the most appropriate intervention strategies.

EVALUATION
A dynamic process in which the physical therapist makes clinical judgements based on data gathered during the examination. This process also may identify possible problems that require consultation with or referral to another provider.

PROGNOSIS
(Including Plan of Care)
Determination of the level of optimal improvement that may be attained through intervention and the amount of time required to reach that level. The plan of care specifies the interventions to be used and their timing and frequency.

EXAMINATION
The process of obtaining a history, performing a systems review, and selecting and administering tests and measures to gather data about the patient/client. The initial examination is a comprehensive screening and specific testing process that leads to a diagnostic classification. The examination process also may identify possible problems that require consultation with or referral to another provider.

INTERVENTION
Purposeful and skilled interaction of the physical therapist with the patient/client and, if appropriate. with other individuals involved in care of the patient/client, using various physical therapy methods and techniques to produce changes in the condition that are consistent with the diagnosis and prognosis. The physical therapist conducts a reexamination to determine changes in patient/client status and to modify or redirect intervention. The decision to reexamine may be used on new clinical findings or on lack of patient/client progress. The process of reexamination also may identify the need for consultation with or referral to another provider.

OUTCOMES
Results of patient/client management, which include the impact of physical therapy interventions in the following domains: pathology/pathophysiology (disease, disorder, or condition); impairments, functional limitations, and disabilities; risk reduction/prevention; health, wellness, and fitness; societal resources; and patient/client satisfaction.

Figure 2-6. Relationship of elements of patient/client management leading to optimal outcomes. (Adapted from American Physical Therapy Association. (2001). A guide to physical therapist practice. *Physical Therapy, 81.*)

episode of care is 15 to 45. This range represents the lower and upper limits of the number of physical therapist visits required to achieve anticipated and desired outcomes. It is anticipated that 80% of patients with an amputation in this diagnostic group will achieve the outcomes within 15 to 45 visits during a single continuous episode of care.[1]

Other practice patterns for patients with an amputation include:

- Impaired motor function and sensory integrity associated with acute or chronic polyneuropathies (5G)
- Primary prevention/risk reduction for integumentary disorders (7A)
- Impaired integumentary integrity associated with partial- or full-thickness skin involvement and scar formation (7C and 7D)

Impaired integumentary integrity associated with skin involvement extending into fascia, muscle, or bone and scar formation (7E)

Either of these, the examination for patients with an amputation form or the *Guide* may serve as a valuable tool to examine and evaluate the patient with an amputation effectively.

Evaluation of Patients Needing Orthoses

There are a number of methods for the evaluation of a patient needing an orthosis. Many generic patient examination forms may effectively evaluate a patient who needs an orthosis. One form that may be used is shown in Figure 2-7. The functional assessment section defines ambulation ability in community, household, and therapeutic terminology. Many of the categories in this form were described for the examination form for patients with an amputation. In the tests and measures section, proprioception, response to tactile input, and extremity shortening may be present with orthopedic or neurologic conditions.

The *Guide* contains many practice patterns that apply to a patient with an orthosis. These include the following patterns:

- Impaired posture including scoliosis (4B)
- Impaired muscle performance (4C)
- Impaired joint mobility, motor function, muscle performance, and ROM associated with connective tissue dysfunction (4D)
- Impaired joint mobility, motor function, muscle performance, and ROM associated with localized inflammation (4E)
- Impaired motor function and sensory integrity associated with nonprogressive disorders of the central nervous system—congenital or acquired in infancy or childhood (5C)
- Motor function and sensory integrity associated with nonprogressive disorders of the central nervous system—acquired in adolescence or adulthood (5D)
- Impaired motor function, peripheral nerve integrity, and sensory integrity associated with nonprogressive disorders of the spinal cord (5H)
- Primary prevention/risk factor reduction for integumentary disorders (7A)[1]

Common Skin Complications

Problems with skin integrity may be noted in the systems review of the examination. Common skin complications that may be encountered by patients wearing a prosthesis or orthosis include abrasions, blisters, contact dermatitis, and distal edema.

Abrasion

Abrasions or areas of skin breakdown often develop if the patient does not have sufficient sensation to judge the amount of weight bearing to the limb. To reduce this complication, the fit of the prosthetic socket or orthosis or the amount of time the patient is using the prosthesis or orthosis needs to be assessed. Initially, a prosthesis or orthosis may be worn for

Demographic and Health Information Section:
1. Date
2. Name
3. Address
4. Age
5. Height
6. Weight
7. Living Arrangements:
   ____ with family ____ alone ____ facility
8. Occupation (past/future plans)
9. Recreational Activities
10. Date of surgery(ies)/site/reason
11. Past Medical/Surgical History
12. Medications
13. Orthoses used
14. Assistive Devices used
15. Current Problems
14. Purpose/goal for Orthoses

Functional Assessment Section:
1. Ambulation
   ____ non ambulatory
   ____ community (independent indoors and outdoors on all surfaces)
   ____ household (independent mainly indoors and some outdoors if flat, smooth surfaces)
   ____ therapeutic (indoors under assistance or supervision or chairbound)
   ____ type of assistive device used
2. Tranfers
   ____ type of transfer
   ____ independent
   ____ requires assistance (describe)
3. Balance
   ____ position assessed (sitting, standing, walking)
   ____ normal
   ____ impaired (describe)
4. Postural Analysis
   ____ normal
   ____ asymmetry (describe)
5. Gait Analysis
   ____ normal
   ____ impaired (describe)

Tests and Measures Section:
1. Condition of hip:

Abduction		Flexion		Extension		Adduction	
Strength	ROM	Strength	ROM	Strength	ROM	Strength	ROM

2. Condition of knee:

Flexion		Extension	
Strength	ROM	Strength	ROM

3. Condition of ankle:

Dorsiflexion		Plantarflexion		Inversion		Eversion	
Strength	ROM	Strength	ROM	Strength	ROM	Strength	ROM

4. Knee Stability:
   ____ anterior/posterior
   ____ medial/lateral
   ____ crepitus
   ____ recurvatum
5. Ankle Stability:
   ____ anterior/posterior
   ____ medial/lateral
6. Skin condition:
   ____ warm
   ____ abnormally warm
   ____ cool
   ____ impaired sensitivity
   ____ smallest Semmes-Weinstein Monofilament perceived
7. Proprioception:
   ____ normal
   ____ impaired (describe)
   ____ absent
8. Response to Tactile Input:
   ____ normal
   ____ impaired (describe)
   ____ absent
9. Extremity shortening:
   ____ none
   ____ right
   ____ left
Measured from:

Assessment

Outcomes

Signature

Date

Figure 2-7. Examination of patients needing an orthosis.

only 10 minutes between skin checks. An abrasion in a patient with poor skin sensitivity may delay prosthetic or orthotic gait training.

Blisters

Blisters may be caused by friction between the limb and the prosthetic socket or orthosis. For the patient with a prosthesis, a solution might be the use of a nylon sheath to decrease this friction or a better prosthetic fit such as increasing the ply of socks. The patient with an orthosis should wear a sock on the limb and put on the orthosis over the sock. The orthosis may need to be reevaluated for correct fit. Abrasions and blisters must be treated aggressively to avoid more serious complications such as skin infections, ulcers, and gangrene. In cases of insensitive skin, weight should be kept off the blistered area until healing occurs. The risk of further skin trauma outweighs the benefits of continued ambulation.

Contact Dermatitis

Contact dermatitis is an inflammatory response to an irritant. A burning sensation, blistering, itching, rash, and peeling may occur. Once the integrity of the skin is breached, the area may become a site for infection and development of an ulcer. Contact dermatitis is often a reaction to either the inner coating of the prosthetic socket or orthosis, prosthetic socks, or detergents. One must determine the source of the irritant and eliminate this irritating source.

Distal Edema

Distal edema occurs when swelling is noted at the distal aspect of a limb. This edema may be related to cardiac, lymphatic, or renal insufficiency. It may also be caused by the lack of total contact between the limb and the prosthesis

or orthosis, prosthetic socks of insufficient ply, improper wrapping of the residual limb or constriction of the orthosis.[7] Management of distal edema may need the intervention of a physician to adjust medication, a prosthetist or orthotist to ensure total contact, or physical therapy personnel to correct residual limb wrapping or decrease constriction of the prosthesis or orthosis.

Pain

Patients with a prosthesis or orthosis may experience complex types of pain such as intrinsic pain (within the limb) or extrinsic pain (caused outside the limb). In addition, those with an amputation may experience phantom limb pain.

Intrinsic Pain

There are many causes of intrinsic pain including ambulating on a bone with minimal soft tissue covering or vascular spasm, which can be described as throbbing or pulsating. Vascular pain results from muscle tissues being deprived of adequate blood supply when plaque formation decreases the arterial patency. Intermittent claudication may be present if leg pain occurs with activities such as ambulating or stationary bicycle riding and disappears with rest. Intermittent claudication is common in a patient with peripheral vascular disease (PVD) or diabetes. In a patient with an amputation, localized nerve pain can be caused by a neuroma. The development of a neuroma is a natural repair process that occurs after peripheral nerve transection. During the repair phase, the axons combine with the fibrous repair tissue to form a small enlargement at the distal end of the nerve.[8] If the neuroma is superficial, it can cause sharp, shooting, and localized pain when irritated by weight bearing or touch. Reliefs built into the prosthetic socket often alleviate pain due to a neuroma. Patients with arthritis often have joint pain due to inflammation. Referred pain can occur in the residual limb from, for example, the lumbar spine or the sacroiliac joint. Low back pain may be aggravated by prolonged sitting in a wheelchair. Sympathetic involvement such as **reflex sympathetic dystrophy (RSD)** or **complex regional pain syndrome (CRPS)** may also cause pain in the residual limb.

Extrinsic Pain

Examples of pain caused by extrinsic factors include overly constrictive prosthetic shrinkers or inadequate prosthetic or orthotic fitting. Common causes include excessive end bearing; uneven skin pressure due to increased muscle hypertrophy, weight gain, or edema; and increased skin friction. Areas of prosthetic pain in the patient with a transfemoral amputation include excessive pressure on the ischial tuberosity with a quadrilateral socket, groin pain from an adductor roll, and excessive end bearing. Common areas of pain due to excessive pressure in an individual wearing an orthosis include

- Navicular tuberosity
- Malleoli
- Crest of the tibia
- Fibular head

Phantom Pain and Phantom Limb Sensation

Patients with an amputation frequently experience phantom pain. **Phantom pain** is characterized by a perception of pain in the absent distal extremity. Phantom pain is often described as shooting, burning, cramping, or crushing. Phantom pain can interfere with vocational activities. In contrast, **phantom limb sensation** is a perception of the absent distal extremity. Phantom limb sensations are universal with acquired amputations and occur to a lesser extent with congenital limb deficiency.[9] This sensation may be described as numbness, pressure, position, temperature, or pins-and-needles feeling in the amputated part. Phantom limb sensation is projected to areas of the body from areas previously serving the amputated limb. Investigators have concluded that phantom limb sensation is caused by cortical plasticity with reorganization involving sprouting into adjacent laminae in the somatotopically organized dorsal horn.[10,11]

A survey of 590 British veterans with amputation found a strong correlation between phantom pain and phantom limb sensation. The intensity of phantom limb sensation was a significant predictor for the duration of phantom pain. In this study, phantom pain became worse over time in only 3% of the respondents.[12]

Results of studies reporting the incidence of phantom pain are conflicting. In a study of 5000 veterans with an amputation, 33% of respondents who were employed reported phantom pain interfered with work. In addition, 82% stated that phantom pain interfered with sleep.[13] Conversely, one study of 92 patients with an amputation found that back pain was rated more bothersome than phantom pain.[14] The different results in these two studies may reflect the large difference in the number of subjects between studies.

Patients with an amputation should be informed that phantom pain is an expected sequela after surgery. Phantom pain is thought to occur because the surgical amputation destroys a large number of sensory fibers to the reticular formation, thus diminishing the inhibitory influence. As a result, self-sustaining neural activity can be initiated by the remaining fibers, often resulting in pain.[15] The rehabilitation team must determine if this pain has a physical origin or is, in fact, phantom pain. Pain differentiation involves a thorough inspection of the residual limb, involving neuroma location, areas of skin adherence, vascular insufficiency, or infection. Persistent pain in the affected limb prior to amputation may contribute to phantom pain. Infection and emotional distress may also trigger episodes of phantom pain.[16]

Intervention measures that increase peripheral input may provide at least temporary, partial relief of phantom pain. These include use of the prosthesis, massage, wrapping, or application of heat to the residual limb.[8] Techniques include a variety of sensory inputs, such as tapping or rubbing the residual limb for 20–60 minutes. The resultant neurosensory overload may be effective in decreasing phantom pain.[17] Like other chronic pain syndromes, chronic phantom pain is affected by stress, anxiety, and depression.[18] Some patients have obtained relief from phantom pain with repeated injections of local anesthetics and steroid preparations in trigger areas or neuromas.[19] One study found that 75% of patients had no phantom limb pain after 10 days of intravenous treatment with salmon calcitonin. Follow-up examinations at 3-, 6-, and 12-month intervals showed long-term success.[20] The combined use of transcutaneous electrical nerve stimulation (TENS) and appropriate psychotherapy may also be a beneficial approach to the management of phantom pain.[8] Multiple interventions have been proposed for the control of phantom pain; no one method works in every case, and each case should be considered individually. Pain management centers may be helpful in providing pharmacologic agents, nerve blocks, or injections and counseling. In summary, phantom pain appears to be common, yet unpredictable, in etiology, severity, frequency or duration. Symptom stability generally occurs after a few months.

KEY POINTS

- Examination and evaluation of patients with an amputation or those requiring an orthosis may be done using a generic form or the *Guide to Physical Therapist Practice.*[1]

- Common skin complications include abrasions, blistering, contact dermatitis, distal edema, and skin ulcerations.

- Patients with a prosthesis or orthosis often develop intrinsic or extrinsic pain. Those with an amputation may experience phantom limb or phantom pain.

LABORATORY ACTIVITIES

1. Using the generic form in Figure 2-1, perform an examination on a simulated patient with an amputation.
  a. Discuss possible impairments, functional limitations, and disability that this patient may possess.
  b. Integrate appropriate interventions to the problems encountered with this patient.

2. Using the *Guide to Physical Therapist Practice*, review the practice patterns that pertain to patients with an amputation or needing an orthosis.

3. Using the generic form in Figure 2-7, perform an examination on a simulated patient needing an orthosis.
  a. Discuss possible impairments, functional limitations, and disability that this patient may possess.
  b. Integrate appropriate interventions to the problems encountered with this patient.

4. Design appropriate interventions for common skin problems and types of pain that may be encountered by patients wearing a prosthesis or orthosis.

REFERENCES

1. American Physical Therapy Association. (2001). A guide to physical therapist practice. *Physical Therapy, 81.*
2. Birke, J. A., & Sims, D. S. (1986). Plantar sensory threshold in the ulcerative foot. *Leprosy Review, 57,* 261.
3. Mueller, M. J. (1996). Identifying patients with diabetes mellitus who are at risk for lower-extremity complications: Use of Semmes-Weinstein Monofilaments. *Physical Therapy, 76,* 68–71.

4. Anon. (1998). Foot care in patients with diabetes mellitus (position statement). *Diabetes Care, 21,* S54–55.

5. May, B. (1996). *Amputations and prosthetics.* Philadelphia: F. A. Davis.

6. Anon. (1999). Putting it into practice: A guide with questions and answers. *PT Magazine,* 40–44.

7. Smith, A. G. (1982). Common problems of lower extremity amputees. *Orthopedic Clinics of North America, 13,* 569–578.

8. Bowker, J. H., & Michael, J. W. (1992). *Atlas of limb prosthetics.* St Louis: Mosby Year Book.

9. Sipski, M. L., & Alexander, C. J. (1997). *Sexual function in people with disabilities and chronic illness (p. 294).* Gaithersburg, MD: Aspen.

10. Yang, T. T., Gallen, C. C., Ramachandran, V. S., Cobb, S., Schwartz, B. J., & Bloom, F. E. (1994). Noninvasive detection of the cerebral p in the adult human somatosensory cortex. *Neuro Report, 5,* 701–704.

11. Aglioti, S., Bonazzi, A., Cortese, F. (1994). Phantom lower limb as a perceptual marker of the neural plasticity in the mature human brain. *Proceedings of the Royal Society of London, 255,* 273–278.

12. Wartan, S. W., Hamann, W., Wedley, J. T. R., & McColl I. (1997). Phantom pain and sensation among British veteran amputees. *British Journal of Anaesthesia, 78,* 652–659.

13. Sherman, R., Sherman, C., & Parker, L. (1984). Chronic phantom and stump pain among American veterans: Results of a survey. *Pain, 18,* 83–95.

14. Smith, D. G., Ehde, D. M., Legro, M. W., Reiber, G. E., del Aguila, M., & Boone, D. A. (1999). Phantom limb, residual limb, and back pain after lower extremity amputations. *Clinical Orthopaedics and Related Research, 361,* 29–38.

15. Reiber, G. E., Boyko, E. J., & Smith, D. G. (1995). Lower extremity foot ulcers and amputation in diabetes. In M. I. Harris, C. C. Cowie, M. P. Stern, et al. (Eds), Ed 2. *Diabetes in America* (2nd ed., pp. 409–428) (NIH Publication No 95-1468.). Washington, DC: National Institutes of Health.

16. Broyles, N. (1991). *For the new amputee (p. 7).* Durham, NC: American Academy of Orthotists and Prosthetists.

17. Gailey, R. S. (1994). *One step ahead: An integrated approach to lower extremity prosthetics and amputee rehabilitation.* Miami: Advanced Rehabilitation Therapy.

18. Sherman, R. A., Sherman, C. J., & Bruno, G. M. (1987). Psychological factors influencing chronic phantom limb pain: An analysis of the literature. *Pain, 28,* 285–295.

19. Blankenbaker, W. L. (1977). The care of patients with phantom limb pain in a pain clinic. *Anesthesia and Analgesia, 56,* 842–846.

20. Simanski, C., Lempa, M., Koch, G., Tiling, T., & Neugebauer, E. (1999). Therapy of phantom pain with salmon calcitonin and effect on postoperative patient satisfaction. *Chirurg, 70,* 674–681.

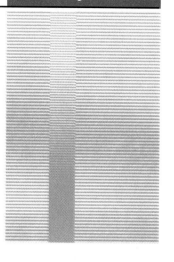

THE TEAM APPROACH
AND FINANCIAL ISSUES

Objectives

1. Delineate the roles of each team member in the care of patients with an amputation and those needing an orthosis
2. Describe the goals and procedures of a prosthetic/orthotic clinic
3. Differentiate the paths to becoming certified as a prosthetist or orthotist
4. Compare the different functional levels used by Medicare for an individual with an amputation
5. Discuss the issues surrounding reimbursement for therapeutic shoes and selected prosthetic and orthotic devices.

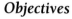

This chapter is divided into the following sections:

Team Approach to Intervention

A team approach is optimal in rehabilitation of a patient requiring a prosthesis or orthosis. A well-coordinated team may assist in maximizing the patient's potential for successful recovery.[1,2] The team should include the physician, prosthetist, orthotist, physical and occupational therapist, vocational rehabilitation counselor, social worker, psychologist, recreation therapist, dietician, nurse, patient, and patient's family or support network. Table 3-1 lists the functions of each of these practitioners.

Integrating each profession into the rehabilitation team can be challenging. However, each team member can provide input regarding case management.[1] The key to any team is communication. Effective communication among team members is vital to optimal patient care. Maximum patient benefits can be achieved by a cohesive team effort that decreases the duration of rehabilitation and significantly improves quality of life.

Ideally, the rehabilitation team, including a physical therapist, should meet with the prospective patient who will need a prosthesis

Table 3-1. Functions of Prosthetic/Orthotic Clinic Team Members

Practitioner	Function
Physician	Often the clinic leader; coordinates decision making; prescribes prostheses or orthoses; may refer patients to physical therapy or other disciplines
Prosthetist	Designs, fabricates, and fits prostheses for persons who have lost a limb due to an injury or disease
Orthotist	Designs, fabricates, and fits orthoses to support limbs or spine affected by muscle or ligament weakness, paralysis, or lack of muscle control
Physical therapist	Examines, evaluates, and provides interventions for patients needing a prosthesis or orthosis; makes recommendations regarding various components
Occupational therapist	Prescribes exercises to increase dexterity, coordination, strength, and endurance; assists clients in performing activities
Vocational rehabilitation counselor	Evaluates employment possibilities; arranges for home modifications, vocational retraining, and job placement
Social worker	Liaison with third-party payers, various agencies, and financial coordinator; may assist with social, housing, and financial adjustments; may provide counseling to patient and family
Psychologist	May assist with coping skills or facilitating emotional adjustment
Recreation therapist	Assists in developing a healthy leisure lifestyle, which may involve activities such as swimming, skiing, or wheelchair sports
Dietician	Assesses nutritional needs; develops and implements nutritional programs to promote good health
Nurse	Assesses and implements medical needs of the patient
Family/support network	Support groups such as the Amputee Coalition of America, United Cerebral Palsy Association, or the Spina Bifida Association of America may be of assistance to the patient and family
Patient	The team leader

or orthosis. Purposes of this preprosthesis or preorthosis meeting may include

- Establishing rapport between the patient and the practitioner
- Educating the patient regarding preprosthesis or preorthosis intervention and the fit of the prosthesis or orthosis
- Reducing patient anxiety
- Assisting the patient in setting realistic functional goals

At this meeting, range of motion and strengthening exercises, functional activities, skin care precautions, and residual limb wrapping (in cases of amputation), may be reviewed. Adaptive equipment and home/work modification determinations may also be made for patients. Early-intervention strengthening and flexibility exercises may prevent weakness and deformity. An introduction to functional activities, proper skin care, and (if necessary) residual limb wrapping may result in achieving independence with a prosthesis or orthosis.

Unfortunately, referral to the rehabilitation team may be delayed because of concern about wound healing. This delay is sometimes seen with patients with diabetes or peripheral vascular disease (PVD). Some believe that movement of the residual limb may contribute to stress on the incision and delay healing. As a result, joint contractures, residual limb edema, weakness, and overall debilitation may occur. Therefore, education by rehabilitation professionals is important to secure early, appropriate referrals. Rehabilitation should not be delayed until the residual limb completely heals. Prolonged immobility may lead to aerobic deconditioning, joint contractures, and skin breakdown.[3]

The importance of the team approach has been documented in a number of studies. Gibson states that the team leader should always be the patient. The patient should have clear expectations of the rehabilitation process.[1] Skillman et al, in a study of patients on a vascular surgery service, including those who underwent amputation, found shorter hospital stays and lower costs over a 4-year period with use of a team approach.[4] Pohjolainen et al. concluded that prosthetic fitting could be improved by better liaison between the surgery and rehabilitation staff and a close team approach.[5] Coletta reported that a coordinated approach to medical, surgical, and rehabilitative care can have a positive effect on functional outcomes after lower extremity amputation.[6] Ham et al., in a study of patients after amputation, showed that team management reduced hospital stays by 20 days and increased the long-term effectiveness of rehabilitation.[7] Schaldach found that use of a multidisciplinary clinical pathway reduced the length of stay and costs in a patient population with lower-extremity amputation. In this study, done over 6 years, length of stay was reduced from 11 to 8 days, with a rehabilitation-focused, goal-oriented plan to return patients home.[8] Likewise, Mikulaninec, in a study of individuals who had lower extremity amputation for arterial occlusive disease, also found a 2-day shorter hospital stay (18.95 vs. 16.95 days) after implementation of a multidisciplinary pathway. This study found that coordination of inpatient care, education of patients and family members, effective discharge planning, and follow-up decreased costs.[9]

The goals of a team approach in a prosthetic/orthotic clinic include

- A coordinated pattern of intervention that ensures a unified approach to a plan of care
- Team and patient education in which team members can learn from each other as well as the patients learning from team members

In clinical situations in which a prosthetic/orthotic clinic is not available, the physical therapist may serve in the role of coordinating care. This coordination may involve a number of activities. Ensuring that impairments such as strength or joint contractures are minimized before prosthetic or orthotic fitting and confirming that the patient is physically and psychologically able to use a prosthesis or orthosis are examples of roles of care coordination. A physical therapist may interact with a hospital discharge planner to determine whether a patient needs home health or subacute center rehabilitation. Effective communication between the physical therapist and prosthetist or orthotist concerning specific components can facilitate earlier patient independence.

Procedures of a Prosthetic/Orthotic Clinic

The procedures of a prosthetic/orthotic clinic are outlined in Figure 3-1. Each of these procedures is described as follows:

1. Preprescription examination—the patient may be examined for impairments and functional abilities by use of an evaluation system described in Chapter 2
2. Prescription—the clinic team may recommend specific prosthetic or orthotic components
3. Prefitting intervention—if appropriate, the patient may be referred for strengthening, range of motion, functional ability training, or residual limb wrapping

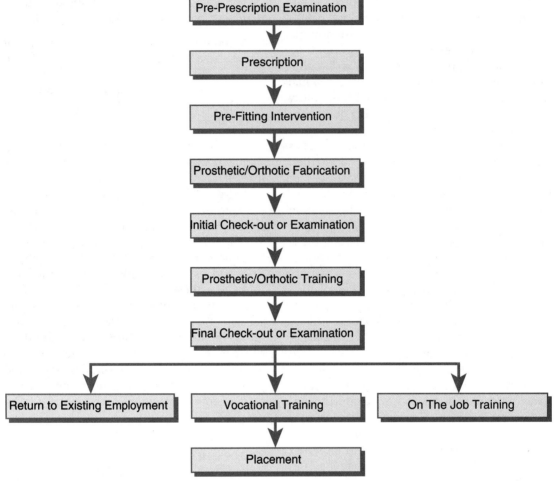

Figure 3-1. Procedures of a prosthetic/orthotic clinic. (Adapted from Berger, N., & Fishman, S. (1990). *Lower limb prosthetics (p. 123–130)*. New York: Prosthetic Orthotic Publications.)

4. Prosthetic/orthotic fabrication—the prosthesis or orthosis is completed according to the clinic prescription
5. Initial checkout or examination—the temporary or initial prosthesis or orthosis is delivered to the patient and compared with the clinic prescription; suggestions for gait training and optimal use of the prosthesis or orthosis can be made at this time
6. Prosthetic/orthotic training—if the prosthesis or orthosis is found to be satisfactory at the initial checkout or examination, the pa-

tient may be referred to physical therapy for gait training
7. Final checkout or examination—the patient is reassessed for successful use of the definitive or final prosthesis or orthosis; at this time, the patient may be either referred for job retraining or given clearance to return to existing employment[10]

An appreciation of the team approach, the functions of a coordinated prosthetic/orthotic clinic, and reimbursement guidelines is necessary to provide optimal care. Likewise, knowledge of the educational requirements and training leading to prosthetic and orthotic certification may result in more-effective interaction with these professionals.

Education and Certification of Prosthetists and Orthotists

Prosthetics and orthotics is a profession that combines specialized clinical and technical skills. Professionals in this field design, fabricate, and fit prostheses and orthoses to help persons lead more independent, active lives. An individual may be certified as either an orthotist, a prosthetist, or both.

Education

The first undergraduate curriculum leading to a bachelor of science in prosthetics and orthotics was started at New York University in 1963. Educational programs are now accredited by the National Commission on Orthotic and Prosthetic Education (NCOPE) and the Commission on Accreditation of Allied Health Programs (CAAHEP)[11] In 1999, there were seven programs accredited by NCOPE/CAAHEP that offered prosthetics/orthotics baccalaureate and postbaccalaureate degrees in the United States. There were three programs at the associate degree level. Persons with an associate degree work under the supervision of a certified orthotist or prosthetist.

Certification

Certification is attained through two organizations, the American Board for Certification (ABC) in Orthotics and Prosthetics or the Board for Orthotist/Prosthetist Certification (BOC). The ABC was established in 1948 and the BOC in 1984. Both organizations promote high professional standards and high quality facilities. Prosthetists and orthotists who have met the rigorous professional credentialing standards of the ABC in orthotics and prosthetics are awarded certification and use the titles CO (certified orthotist), CP (certified prosthetist) and CPO (certified orthotist/prosthetist). More than 3200 orthotic and prosthetic practitioners are currently certified by the ABC.[11] Those who achieve BOC certification use the title BOC certified practitioner.

The ABC describes three ways, or paths, to become eligible for certification as an orthotist and/or prosthetist Table 3-2.[11] Physical therapists have used path 2 to become certified as an orthotist and/or prosthetist. There currently are over 100 NCOPE-accredited residency programs in the United States.[11]

After completion of core studies and clinical training, practitioners must successfully complete a series of three comprehensive examinations to earn certification in orthotics or prosthetics by either the ABC or BOC.[11,12] These comprehensive examinations include:

1. A written test of multiple choice questions
2. A written simulation of clinical practice case scenarios
3. A clinical demonstration assessing design and fitting skills

For either certification, practitioners are required to abide by a code of professional ethics and to complete mandatory continuing education requirements. For the ABC, those in a single discipline (CO or CP) must obtain a minimum of 75 professional continuing-education credits (PCEs) within each 5-year certification cycle. Those with dual disciplines (CPO) must obtain a minimum of 100 PCEs within 5 years.[13] For BOC certification, 15 professional continuing-education credits each year are required.[12] Additional resources for prosthetic and orthotic educational and certification information are shown in Resource Box 3-1. Whether an individual has either certification makes no difference in reimbursement. Many prosthetic and orthotic practitioners have been "grandfathered" into certification. These practitioners do not have a bachelor's degree but have passed the certification examinations and have a number of years of experi-

Table 3-2. Three Paths to Becoming Certified As a Prosthetist/Orthotist According to the American Board of Certification (ABC)

Path	Education	Experience
1	Baccalaureate degree in orthotics or prosthetics from a program accredited by CAAHEP	A 12-month NCOPE-accredited residency program
	Baccalaureate degree in orthotics or prosthetics from a program accredited by NCOPE	1900-hour clinical experience supervised by an ABC-certified practitioner
2	Baccalaureate degree in any major, plus an orthotic and/or prosthetic certificate from a CAAHEP-accredited program	A 12-month NCOPE-accredited residency program
	Baccalaureate degree in any major, plus an orthotic and/or prosthetic certificate from a NCOPE-accredited program	1900-hour clinical experience supervised by an ABC-certified practitioner
3	Foreign degree equivalent to a baccalaureate in orthotics and prosthetics	1900-hour clinical experience supervised by an ABC-certified practitioner
	Foreign degree equivalent to a baccalaureate in any major; plus, an orthotic and/or prosthetic certificate from a CAAHEP accredited program	A 12-month NCOPE-accredited residency program
	Foreign degree equivalent to a baccalaureate in any major; plus an orthotic and/or prosthetic certificate from an NCOPE-accredited program	1900-hour clinical experience supervised by an ABC-certified practitioner

From NCOPE. (1999). Orthotic and Prosthetic Educational Programs. National Commission on Orthotic and Prosthetic Education (NCOPE), 1650 King Street, Suite 500, Alexandria, VA 22314.

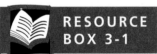

RESOURCE BOX 3-1

The National Commission on Orthotic and Prosthetic Education (NCOPE)
  1650 King Street, Suite 500
  Alexandria, VA 22314
  (703)-836-7114
  email: opncope@aol.com
The American Board for Certification in Orthotics and Prosthetics (ABC)
  1650 King Street, Suite 500
  Alexandria, VA 22314
  (703)-836-7114
  email: opcertmail@aol.com
The Board for Orthotist/Prosthetist Certification
  506 W. Fayette St.
  Century Building
  Suite 200
  Baltimore, MD 21201

National Association for Advancement of Orthotics and Prosthetics
  1275 Pennsylvania Avenue
  Washington, DC 20004-2404
  (202)-624-0064
The American Academy of Orthotists and Prosthetists (AAOP)
  1650 King Street, Suite 500
  Alexandria, VA 22314
  (703)-836-7114
  Web site: http://www.oandp.com/academy
Government resources regarding prosthetics and orthotics are available at
  Web site: http://www.pubmedcentral.nih.gov

ence. In addition to certification, many states have licensure in prosthetics and orthotics. Eventually, certification and/or licensure may be a requirement for reimbursement. Physical therapists should encourage patients to receive services from only certified and/or licensed prosthetic and orthotic professionals.

Employment Settings

Prosthetists and orthotists may own their own business as a sole proprietor or work as an employee in a hospital, rehabilitation center, research facility, or private business. Many large institutions such as children's hospitals or rehabilitation centers provide prosthetic and orthotic services with an internal staff. In addition, government agencies and device manufacturers employ prosthetists and orthotists to conduct research. Depending on geographic location, company size, experience, and other factors, certified prosthetic and orthotic practitioners can earn between $40,000 and $60,000 annually. Practitioners who own their own business can earn substantially more.[11]

Financial Issues

Since physical therapists are often involved in the prescription of a prosthesis or orthosis, a brief discussion of financial issues is warranted. For those with private insurance, reimbursement rates vary widely, depending on the specific policy. Private insurance reimbursement guidelines for prostheses or orthoses are usually covered under durable medical equipment (DME) rules. Clinic members *must* be aware of this coverage, since recommendation of a specific prosthesis or orthosis will depend on potential insurance company reimbursement. Usually an insurance company will pay for a new prosthesis every 3 to 5 years. A new prosthesis or orthosis will most likely be approved sooner in cases of ill-fitting caused, for example, by weight gain or loss. Approval will often be granted when the patient's ability has

changed. For example, with progressive weakness, a patient who has an ankle–foot orthosis may need a knee–ankle–foot orthosis. A study done in the United Kingdom of 104 individuals with transtibial amputation over a 10-year period found that on average, a new prosthesis was needed every 2 years. One major repair to the prosthesis was needed every 5 years and two minor repairs were needed per year.[14] Even though Medicaid receives some federal government funding, it is a state-managed program. Medicaid coverage varies widely from state to state. In the United States, pediatric prostheses and orthoses are usually covered under Medicaid, private insurance, no fault insurance if the injury was due to a motor vehicle accident, or a court settlement from a traumatic event.

Medicare Functional Levels for Amputation

In many clinical settings, most of the patients seen for prostheses, orthoses, or shoe fittings will have Medicare reimbursement. Medicare requires that the prescribing physician and the prosthetist document the patient's potential functional level as a means of determining medical necessity and thus reimbursement. Medicare requires a functional level for reimbursement for foot or knee prosthetic components. The clinic team may interview the patient regarding past activities, current level of function, and goals for the future. Based on this information, a functional level is assigned to the patient. Patients are approved for particular prosthetic components on the basis of this functional level. The approved prosthetic components for each functional level are described in Chapters 8 and 9. The functional levels are described in Table 3-3.[15,16]

Medicare Reimbursement Example

As an example of Medicare reimbursement criteria, Medicare provides reimbursement for a single pair of extra-depth shoes and three pairs

Table 3-3. Medicare Functional Levels

Level	Description
0	Does not have the ability or potential to ambulate or transfer with or without assistance, and a prosthesis does not enhance his or her quality of life or mobility.
1	Has the ability or potential to use a prosthesis for transfers or ambulation on level surfaces at a fixed cadence; typical of the household ambulator
2	Has the ability or potential for ambulation with the ability to transverse low-level environmental barriers such as curbs, stairs, or uneven surfaces; typical of the limited community ambulator
3	Has the ability or potential for ambulation with variable cadence; typical of the community ambulator who has the ability to transverse most environmental barriers and may have vocational, therapeutic, or exercise activity that demands prosthetic use beyond simple locomotion; typical of the unlimited community ambulator
4	Has the ability or potential for prosthetic ambulation that exceeds basic ambulation skills, exhibiting high impact, stress, or energy levels; typical of the prosthetic demands of the child, active adult, or athlete.

Adapted with permission from Marshall Labs LTD. Syracuse, NY (February 1996). *Reference for prosthetic prescription.*

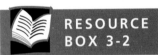

RESOURCE BOX 3-2

Criteria for Medicare Reimbursement for Shoes, Inserts, and/or Shoe Modifications
1. The patient has a diagnosis of diabetes mellitus
2. The patient has one or more of the following conditions:
   a. Previous amputation of the other foot or part of either foot
   b. History of previous foot ulceration of either foot
   c. History of preulcerative calluses of either foot
   d. Peripheral neuropathy with callus formation of either foot
   e. Foot deformity of either foot
   f. Poor circulation in either foot
3. The certifying physician, either an MD or DO, must confirm numbers 1 and 2 above and must demonstrate that the patient is receiving care for diabetes and needs therapeutic shoes.

From Durable Medical Equipment Regional Carrier. (March 1998). *Supplier manual* (Chapter 20). DMERC, Region A.

of inserts or one pair of custom-molded shoes plus two additional pairs of inserts per year. These options are provided to patients with diabetes and high-risk feet who meet the criteria shown in Resource Box 3-2.[17] An extra-depth shoe has a full-length heel-to-toe filler that, when removed, provides a minimum of 3/16 inch of additional depth. This depth is necessary to accommodate custom-molded or customized inserts. A custom-molded shoe is constructed over a positive model of the patient's foot.[17] A prescribing physician, who may be a podiatrist, medical doctor (MD) or doctor of osteopathy (DO), actually orders the therapeutic shoes.

Costs and Reimbursement

The cost of a prosthesis or orthosis varies widely depending on the degree of disability, activity needs of the wearer, and the types of components and materials used. Cost is determined by the sophistication of the components and the types of materials used for construction. Ultralight materials and acrylic resin socket finishes increase the cost of a prosthesis.

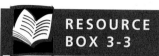

RESOURCE BOX 3-3

Information Contained in a Letter of Justification

Patient demographic information (e.g., name, age, social security number, address)

Patient's diagnosis

Specific components of the prosthesis or orthosis that are needed

Present functional or activity level of the patient

What the patient will be able to do with the requested prosthesis or orthosis

What the patient will not be able to do if the requested prosthesis or orthosis is not approved

Possible cost savings of the prosthesis or orthosis (e.g., patient may not need a wheelchair, may not need home health aide assistance, may be able to live independently)

The cost of a prosthesis includes components, materials, labor, office visits, and adjustments. This cost typically covers adjustments needed for 90 days. If the volume of the residual limb changes greatly because of weight loss or gain, an additional adjustment charge may be made. These costs vary widely, depending on new materials and technology.

A letter of justification is often needed by insurance companies for reimbursement for a prosthesis or orthosis. Information that must be contained in these letters will vary, depending on the individual insurance company. An insurance company may require that a physician complete the letter of justification. Other companies may require documentation by a physical therapist or prosthetist or orthotist. An example of information contained in a letter of justification is in Resource Box 3-3. Some insurance carriers may reimburse the prosthetic/orthotic facility at a higher rate than the federal government or Medicare rate. If a prosthetic/orthotic facility accepts Medicare assignment, they are obligated to provide the patient with a prosthesis or orthosis at the Medicare allowable. The facility may not bill the patient an additional charge above the Medicare allowable rate. The patient or supplemental insurance is responsible for the other 20% of the allowable rate. Medicare allowable rates for selected prostheses and orthoses are shown in Table 3-4.[19] However, these rates vary by region.

These materials and finishes result in a lighter prosthesis or orthosis that is highly durable. The cost of a transtibial prosthesis ranges from $4,000 to $16,000; the cost of a transfemoral prosthesis ranges from $5,500 to $40,000.[18]

Table 3-4. Medicare Allowable Fees for Selected Prostheses and Orthoses in Year 2000		
Base Code	**Descriptor**	**Medicare Allowable Fee**
L1960	Ankle–foot orthosis (AFO), molded plastic, solid ankle	$525.00
L1970	AFO, molded plastic, with ankle joint	$671.00
L2036 + L2182	Knee–ankle–foot orthosis (KAFO), molded plastic with drop lock knee joints	$1889.00
L5300 + many other codes[a]	Transtibial prosthesis	$4000.00+
L5320 + many other codes[a]	Transfemoral prosthesis	$5500.00+

From American Orthotic and Prosthetic Association. (2000). Medicare fee manual. American Orthotic and Prosthetic Association, 1650 King Street, Suite 500, Alexandria, VA 22314.

[a] Other codes may include total contact socket, type of construction, suspension, foot, liner, and socks

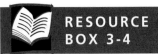

RESOURCE BOX 3-4

The Barr Foundation

The Barr Foundation
c/o Storage USA
3090 NW 2nd Avenue
Suite #693
Boca Raton, FL 33431
Phone: (516)-394-6514
email: http://www.oandp.com/barr

Those who cannot afford the cost of a prosthesis or orthosis have various options for payment. An individual may apply for Medicaid funding. Medicaid approval for the device is based on need and income level. Local or national organizations such as the Muscular Dystrophy Association or the American Cancer Society may be of assistance. The Barr Foundation is a tax-deductible, nonprofit national organization that often pays for prostheses (Resource Box 3-4).

KEY POINTS

- The team approach is optimal in rehabilitation of a patient requiring a prosthesis or orthosis.
- The goals of a team approach in a prosthetic/orthotic clinic include a coordinated pattern of intervention and team and patient education.
- Prosthetic and orthotic educational programs exist at the associate, baccalaureate and postbaccalaureate levels.
- Certification may be achieved through either the American Board for Certification (ABC) or the Board for Orthotist/Prosthetist Certification (BOC).

- Prosthetists and orthotists may own their own business or work as an employee in a hospital, rehabilitation setting, research facility, or private business.
- In the United States, the prosthetic firm is reimbursed by Medicare for particular prosthetic knee or ankle components on the basis of the patient's functional level.
- The cost of a prosthesis or orthosis varies widely depending on the degree of disability, activity needs of the wearer, and the types of materials used.

CRITICAL THINKING QUESTIONS

1. Discuss the advantages of the team approach in the rehabilitation of a patient requiring a prosthesis or orthosis.

2. Assess ways in which a physical therapist could improve communication when a prosthetic/orthotic clinic is not available.

3. Relate the role of a physical therapist in each procedure of a prosthetic/orthotic clinic.

4. Differentiate the educational and certification options for orthotists and prosthetists.

5. Define the five Medicare functional levels.

REFERENCES

1. Gibson, P. M. (2000). The power of teamwork. *Rehab Management, 13*, 36–37.
2. Rosen, C., Miller, A. C., Pitten-Cate, I. M., Bicchieri, S., Gordon, R. M., & Daniele, R. (1998). Team approaches to treating children with disabilities: A comparison. *Archives of Physical Medicine and Rehabilitation, 79*, 430–434.
3. Pinzur, M. S. (1997). Current concepts: Amputation surgery in peripheral vascular disease. *Instructional Course Lectures, 46*, 501–509.
4. Skillman, J. J., Paras, C., Rosen, M., Davis, R. B., Ducksoo, K., Kent, K. C. (2000). Improving cost efficiency on a vascular surgery service. *American Journal of Surgery, 179*, 197–200.

5. Pohjolainen, T., Alaranta, H., Wikstrom, J. (1989). Primary survival and prosthetic fitting of lower limb amputees. *Prosthetics and Orthotics International, 13,* 63–69.

6. Coletta, E. M. (2000). Care of the elderly patient with lower extremity amputation. *Journal of the American Board of Family Practice, 13,* 23–24.

7. Ham, R., Regan, J. M., & Roberts, V. C. (1987). Evaluation of introducing the team approach to the care of the amputee: The Dulwich Study. *Prosthetics and Orthotics International, 11,* 25–30.

8. Schaldach, D. E. (1997). Measuring quality and cost of care: Evaluation of an amputation clinical pathway. *Journal of Vascular Nursing, 15,* 13–20.

9. Mikulaninec, C. E. (1992). An amputee critical path. *Journal of Vascular Nursing, 10,* 6–8.

10. Berger, N., & Fishman, S. (1990). *Lower limb prosthetics (p. 123–130).* New York: Prosthetic Orthotic Publications.

11. NCOPE. (1999). Orthotic and Prosthetic Educational Programs. National Commission on Orthotic and Prosthetic Education (NCOPE), 1650 King Street, Suite 500, Alexandria, VA 22314.

12. Board for Orthotist/Prosthetist Certification. *The advantage is experience.* Available at http://www.bocusa.org. Accessed December 26, 2000.

13. American Board for Certification in Orthotics & Prosthetics. (December 1999). *The practitioner book of rules.*

14. Datta, D., Vaidya, S. P., & Alsindi, Z. (1999). Analyses of prosthetic episodes in trans-tibial amputees. *Prosthetics and Orthotics International, 23,* 9–12.

15. Marshall Labs LTD. (February 1996). *Reference for prosthetic prescription.* : Marshall Labs LTD.

16. Romo, H. D. (1999). Specialized prostheses for activities. *Clinical Orthopaedics and Related Research, 361,* 63–70.

17. Durable Medical Equipment Regional Carrier. (March 1998). *Supplier manual* (Chapter 20). DMERC, Region A.

18. Weed, R. O., Sluis, A. (1997). *Life care planning for the amputee: A step-by-step guide (p. 119).* Boca Raton, FL: CRC Press LLC.

19. American Orthotic and Prosthetic Association. (2000). *Medicare fee manual.* American Orthotic and Prosthetic Association 1650 King Street, Suite 500, Alexandria, VA 22314.

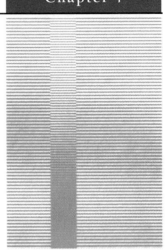

Chapter 4

PSYCHOSOCIAL ISSUES OF PATIENTS
WITH PROSTHESES AND ORTHOSES

Objectives

1. Characterize the psychologic losses a patient needing a prosthesis or orthosis may experience
2. Differentiate among the stages of adjustment
3. Analyze specific factors that may affect psychologic reactions
4. Compare and contrast the reactions of young children, adolescents, and the elderly to the need for a prosthesis or orthosis
5. Discuss common sexuality issues affecting individuals who use a prosthesis or orthosis
6. Determine when a patient should seek professional help
7. Discuss the signs of successful adaptation to disability
8. Describe the common concerns of Americans with a disability
9. Describe the use rates of orthoses and prostheses

This chapter is divided into the following sections:

Physical therapists and physical therapist assistants are involved in the daily examination and intervention of patients requiring a prosthesis or orthosis. Physical therapists and physical therapist assistants understand the psychologic losses and reactions patients and their families may experience. Patient/family concerns and use rates of prostheses and orthoses are also important considerations.

♦♦♦

General Concepts of Psychologic Losses

The psychologic reactions of patients after amputation or an event requiring the use of an orthosis can be both varied and complex.

Potentially, a triple insult may occur, involving loss of function, loss of sensation, and loss of body image.[1] These losses force the patient and family to face life in a new manner with changed or reversed roles. One's perception of wholeness may be changed forever, leading to fragmentation. This feeling of fragmentation is intensified by lowered self-esteem due to body image distortion, changes in employment status, decreased social interaction, and decreased independence.[2] Dependence on others becomes a patient and family focus.

Current societal measures emphasize physical perfection through perceived body images and the perception of others. Negative perceptions may lead to social isolation.[3] If an individual with a prosthesis or orthosis has difficulty accepting his or her body, this nonacceptance may be projected onto others. Alienation from others may result. Positive correlations between body image and increased self-esteem and life satisfaction and decreased anxiety and depression have been found. The more negative one feels about one's body, the less satisfied he or she is with life.[4]

Individuals who have been involved in a traumatic event may experience reactions such as flashbacks, panic, fear of sleep, hostility, and thoughts of suicide.[5] Posttraumatic stress disorder (PTSD) is a well-described psychologic phenomena. A diagnosis of PTSD is made if the traumatic event is persistently reexperienced through flashbacks, thoughts, or dreams.[6]

Stages of Adjustment

Learning the stages of adjustment can help the therapist understand and anticipate the different emotions patients may experience. It also allows use of common terminology among the prosthetic or orthotic clinic team members. These stages of adjustment may vary, depending on whether the amputation or an event requiring the use of an orthosis was traumatic or elective.

Traumatic Injury

Reactions to a loss of normal function may be divided into various stages. Not every individual with a prosthesis or orthosis will experience all these stages or will experience them in the same order.

1. Shock is the initial reaction to an immediate and violent physical injury such as an amputation or spinal cord injury. Shock sometimes results in mental disorientation, psychologic numbness, and depersonalization.
2. Anxiety is a panic-like behavior that occurs after realization of the magnitude of the injury. Anxiety may be manifested by purposeless overactivity, shortness of breath, and increased pulse rate.
3. Denial is a defense mechanism against the painful realization of the extent of the injury. An individual in denial minimizes the implications of the injury and pays selective attention to facts that support a self-imposed distortion of reality.
4. Depression occurs after the initial realization of the magnitude of the injury. Sadness and grief are expected responses after a major injury. However, depression is a serious disabling condition that may affect recovery and independence.[6] Depression may be represented by isolation, despair, and feelings of helplessness and hopelessness.
5. Internalized anger is demonstrated by feelings of guilt and bitterness regarding one's behavior and health practices. Self-injury and suicide may result from this internalized anger.
6. Externalized hostility is shown by anger directed at other persons such as family members or health-care professionals. Externalized hostility is more evident with increasing length of time from the onset of the accident or disease.
7. Acknowledgment is portrayed in increasing acceptance of the disability. The individual regards himself or herself as an individual

with a disability and decides how this new self will adjust in the world.

8. Adjustment is the final phase of the adaptation process, characterized by reestablishing a positive self-image, pursuing vocational or social goals, and attempting to overcome obstacles that result from the disability.[7]

Awareness of these stages will help the prosthetic or orthotic clinic team members interact appropriately with the patient or, if indicated, refer the patient to counseling services. For example, a patient with a spinal cord injury who is in a denial stage may be unwilling to learn proper application of an orthosis. In this instance, counseling may be indicated before intensive physical rehabilitation activities can be taught effectively. A patient with a transfemoral amputation who is depressed may not be ready for intensive gait training. In this instance, contact with a support network may aid psychologic adjustment. A home visit involving a multidisciplinary rehabilitation team may allow preparation to deal with potential barriers to independence and aid in the psychologic adjustment after injury or illness.

Elective Procedure

Stages of adjustment for an elective procedure include the following:

1. The preoperative stage begins with the realization that the loss of limb or the loss of function is a possibility. Grief is the universally identified reaction of those who are about to lose a limb. Concerns about pain, financial difficulties, general health, and future functional abilities at home or at work add to the grief process. However, those undergoing amputation after an unsuccessful, painful, extended treatment of a lower extremity affected by gangrene or infection may see amputation as a relief.[8]

2. The immediate postoperative rehabilitation stage brings the realization that a normal level of function is no longer possible. This stage is characterized by denial gradually replacing grief. Euphoric mood, regression, and withdrawal are sometimes seen. Depression, disorganization, tearfulness, despair, insecurity, concentration difficulties, social withdrawal, insomnia, and self-blame may be experienced. The rehabilitation stage can be made more complex by surgical limb revision or further disability such as another cerebral vascular accident.

3. The return home stage causes mixed reactions. Leaving the hospital signifies recovery; however, the patient is abruptly faced with a decrease in hospital supportive help.[9] The return home stage is marked by reorganization or reconstruction in which one constructs new views of oneself and the world and by attempts to obtain maximum functional potential.[10,11]

Challenges for the young individual may include identity, sexuality, and social acceptance. Challenges for the older individual may include livelihood, functional capacity, and interpersonal relationships. Individuals who have more-difficult psychologic adjustment following disability include younger adults, unmarried persons, and those with a history of alcoholism.[12] In addition, individuals with an amputation in whom phantom limb and pain persist tend to have greater adjustment problems.[13] Conversely, those who regard their health and social support as good and have higher functional abilities and successful stress-reducing mechanisms have better psychologic adjustments.[7,14]

A large part of the psychologic reaction to the return home stage is due to environmental influences. Counseling is available to assist in the emotional adjustments to disability. However, formal psychiatric intervention is needed in only a few cases. Supportive interventions by the family and health-care team members assist in the adjustment process. A home and worksite visit with architectural barrier elimination suggestions may assist in the adjustment process. With proper support and aggressive rehabilitation, this final stage can result in successful social adjustment.

Factors That Affect Psychologic Adjustment

Many factors influence adjustment to amputation or an event requiring the use of an orthosis. These include the following:

Economic and Vocational Factors

Patients with a disability who cannot do their former jobs and who are facing a loss of income will have more adjustment problems.

Psychosocial Support

Individuals with an excellent family and peer support system will have fewer problems with psychologic adjustment.

Reason for the Disability

Individuals suffering a traumatic or accidental limb loss may react with varying forms of denial.[15] Those undergoing an elective amputation for the cure of malignancy may benefit from the amount of time for preparation and exploration of alternatives. These patients often exhibit realistic expectations and cooperation.[10] In contrast, disability caused by the negligent care or behavior of others often produces self-doubt and bitterness.[16] Litigation can also complicate the process of recovery.

Preparation Time

Individuals who have had adequate warning and preparation adjust better in the immediate postoperative stage; those with traumatic events tend to react negatively or with denial.[9] Conversing with members of a support group may be helpful. A support group provides a safe environment in which to discuss grief and loss as well as lifestyle integration.[17] Individuals who have more experience with a prosthesis or orthosis may be able to advise the prospective patient on functional abilities and architectural barrier elimination. Peer visitation may occur preoperatively or pre–hospital admission or postoperatively or post–hospital admission. Patients who have had an amputation feel that speaking to another such patient before and after surgery is helpful for education, alleviating fear, promoting emotional catharsis, and gaining a sense of being understood.[6,17] Discussion topics of support groups may include[17,18]

Coping with grief and loss
Lifestyle alterations
Use and care of the prosthesis or orthosis
Working with prosthetists, orthotists, and rehabilitation personnel
Selecting adaptive equipment
Preventing complications
Managing travel experiences
Sexuality

It may also be helpful for patients to contact organizations dedicated to their particular disability. Some of these organizations are listed in Resource Box 4-1.

Prosthetic or Orthotic Rehabilitation

The earlier a prosthesis or orthosis is used after the disabling event, the less psychologic distress is observed. If prosthetic or orthotic application is absent or delayed, greater apprehension, melancholy, and self-consciousness are often noted.[19]

Age

Reactions of children, adolescents, and the elderly to the need for a prosthesis or orthosis vary.

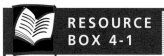

RESOURCE BOX 4-1

Organizations That Provide Information Regarding Disability

Amputee Coalition of America
  900 East Hill Avenue Suite 285
  Knoxville, TN 37915
  (888)-267-5669
  www.amputee-coalition.org
Amputee Resource Foundation of America
  6480 Wayzata Boulevard
  Golden Valley, MN 55426
  www.amputeeresource.org
The War Amputations of Canada
  2827 Riverside Drive
  Ottawa, Ontario K1V OC4 Canada
  (613)-731-3821
National Rehabilitation Information Center
(NARIC)
  1010 Wayne Avenue Suite 800
  Silver Spring, MD 20910-3319
  (800)-346-2742
  www.naric.com
National Spinal Cord Injury Association
  8701 Georgia Avenue Suite 500
  Silver Spring, MD 20851
  (301)-588-6959
  www.spinalcord.org

Association of Children's Prosthetic and
Orthotic Clinics (ACPOC)
  222 South Prospect Avenue
  Park Ridge, IL 60068
  (708)-698-1632
  www.acpoc.org
National Association of Developmental
Disabilities Councils (NADDC)
  1234 Massachusetts Avenue NW, Suite 103
  Washington, DC 20005
  (202)-347-1234
  www.igc.apc.org/naddc
National Clearinghouse of Rehabilitation
Training Materials
  5202 Richmond Hill Drive
  Stillwater, OK 74078-4080
  (800)-223-5219
  www.nchrtm.okstate.edu
Muscular Dystrophy Association
  3300 East Sunrise Drive
  Tucson, AZ 85718
  (520)-529-2000
  www.mdausa.org
United Cerebral Palsy Association
  1660 L Street NW, Suite 700
  Washington, DC 20036
  (800)-872-5827
  www.ucpa.org

Reactions of Children

The reactions of young children to an amputation or event requiring the use of an orthosis may differ from those of adolescents or adults. These reactions are outlined in the Pediatric Perspective Box.

Reactions of Adolescents

Adolescents experience a broad range of emotional reactions to the need for a prosthesis or orthosis. These emotional reactions may in-

clude shock, fear, anger, denial, sadness, grief, depression, shame, guilt, and self-pity. Amputation or an event requiring use of an orthosis is often associated with anxiety, social isolation, and depression, which may affect the adolescent's social life and free-time activities.[22] Parental acceptance of the adolescent's feelings will affirm the validity of emotional reactions, which can accelerate the adjustment process.[23] An adolescent must engage in a process of reconstructing a positive body image and self-concept. However, this reconstruction is more complex since, frequently, no preinjury or preillness positive body image and self-concept has been developed. In contrast, the adult has already established a body image and self-concept. Adolescents may experience fear at the reaction of friends and classmates. Trepidations regarding mobility, architectural barriers, dress, and social life may also be felt. An adolescent's ability to adjust depends on many factors including self-esteem, severity of disability and complications, support systems, and prior life experiences. Empathy, acceptance, and love assist in the adjustment process and minimize emotional scars.[23]

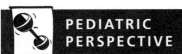

PEDIATRIC PERSPECTIVE

Reactions of Children to an Amputation or Event Requiring the Use of an Orthosis

Children who experienced traumatic events that led to the need for a prosthesis or orthosis often show more feelings of inferiority and depression than children whose need is from congenital causes.[7] However, children who have undergone limb amputation for cancer treatment have a high degree of adjustment as measured by functional independence levels and by social, educational, and occupational achievements.[20] Overall, children and adolescents often show resilience to acquired disability.[21] Some parents react with acceptance to their child's changed status, whereas others exhibit feelings of guilt, rejection, and overprotection.[7] Psychologic interventions may be necessary for both parents and child.

Reactions of Adults

Like adolescents, adults experience a range of emotions to an event requiring the use of a prosthesis or orthosis. Studies have shown no difference in emotional distress between limb-sparing surgery and amputation. Likewise, little disruption of positive body-image feelings have been found after amputation. A study of 65 patients who had been treated for malignant bone tumors and had been in remission for at least 1 year compared limb-sparing surgery with amputation. Results showed no significant differences in educational and occupational status, functional limitations, pain intensity, emotional distress, rehabilitation experience, and overall satisfaction with the surgical procedure.[24] Likewise, a British study of 107 patients attending a limb-fitting clinic found little disruption in body image, anxiety, or depression. Younger patients who sustained traumatic amputations exhibited more anxiety and a more-negative body image. This study found moderate satisfaction with the prosthesis.[25]

Reactions of the Elderly

Anywhere from 20 to 80% of elderly individuals return home after lower extremity amputation rehabilitation. Success rates are based on the level of amputation, co-morbidities, and support systems.[26] Possible social isolation is a particular concern with the elderly.[27] It is important to distinguish depression from cognitive disorders. Cognitive disorders in the elderly such as dementia are commonly mistaken for depression.[6] Reactions of the elderly to an amputation or an event requiring the use of an orthosis are outlined in the Geriatric Perspective Box.

Social Support System

The complications of disability can be lessened by involving family members in patient interventions and providing flexible hours to accommodate family member visitations. In addition, frequent communication regarding the rationale for decisions, shared decision

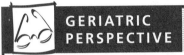

GERIATRIC PERSPECTIVE

Reactions of the Elderly to an Amputation or Event Requiring the Use of an Orthosis

The elderly demonstrate a greater incidence of psychopathology than any other age group.[28] Elderly individuals who are suddenly disabled may have physical, psychologic, and social problems as a result of the disability. These may be compounded by their decreasing physical and mental capabilities and the lack of social support of normal aging.[28] A loss of control over environmental factors may have many negative complications that interfere with independence. These complications include

- Confusion/disorientation
- Agitation
- Forgetfulness
- Becoming fearful
- Feelings of isolation
- Concentration difficulties
- Withdrawal
- Depression

making, and counseling may be helpful.[29] As a result of managed care and cost containment, the average hospital inpatient stay is shortened, requiring many patients to continue their rehabilitation at home with the support of family members. The average length of inpatient stay is discussed in Chapter 3, "The Team Approach and Financial Issues." Home health physical therapy is often needed. Family members need to observe the patient in a hospital or rehabilitation setting to learn tasks, determine activities the patient can safely perform, and assist in setting outcomes and discharge planning.

Sexuality

Sexual counseling is an important component in the rehabilitation of people with disability. Few patients with amputation receive information or advice from the health professionals regarding amputation and its effect on sexuality. Rehabilitation professionals are often uncomfortable talking to patients about sexuality.[6] One study found that fewer than 10% of those with amputations received information on sexuality.[10] The nature of the relationship between a physical therapist or physical therapist assistant and a patient may allow the opportunity to address sexuality issues or provide resource information. A model of sexual counseling has been developed for all health-care professionals, termed PLISSIT. This acronym refers to permission, limited information, specific suggestions, and intensive therapy. Rehabilitation personnel may, once they have the patient's permission, offer limited information regarding sexuality. Moving to the next levels of specific suggestions and intensive therapy involves referral for counseling.[6]

The advanced age of many individuals who have undergone an amputation is often a factor in the lack of sexuality information. Society may view these individuals as having little interest in continuing sexual activity. However, research has not supported this perception of the elderly having little sexual interest.[30]

Sexuality after a disability may be affected for both psychological and physical reasons. Psychological issues affecting sexual function include an altered body image, depression, and anxiety about disease progression.[27] Patients with conditions such as multiple sclerosis or spinal cord injury often require orthoses. Several studies have investigated the effect of these conditions on disability. One study of individuals with multiple sclerosis reported that 91% of men and 72% of women experienced sexual performance changes ranging from a mild loss of sensation to severe impairment.[31] Males with spinal cord injury experience greatly reduced reproductive capacity and sexual function. Conversely, a female with spinal cord injury has relatively unimpaired reproductive capacity, although sexual function is impaired. In a study of individuals between ages 45 and 60 who experienced a cerebral vascular accident, 60% of the men and 70% of the women reported a decrease in sexual behavior.[31] Diabetes or the presence of a tumor treated with chemotherapy or radiation also affect sexuality.

There is debate about the effect of amputation on sexuality. One study of 39 males with a recent amputation and independent levels of prosthesis use found that 77% reported substantial decrease of sexual intercourse frequency. This decrease in frequency of sexual activity was greater in men who were unmarried, those with a transfemoral amputation, and with those experiencing phantom pain.[32] Conversely, in a study of 131 individuals with amputation, 65% reported no change in sexual function.[33] However, this latter study stated that most of the subjects had considerable time to adjust to their amputation, although no mean or range of time from amputation was given. This study also found that those with transfemoral amputations had greater problems adjusting to sexuality issues.[33] One study compared sexual adjustment of 85 individuals who underwent either transtibial or transfemoral amputations and found no significant difference in sexual desire between the two groups.[33]

Resumption of sexual activity assists with self-esteem and self-confidence, which facilitate successful rehabilitation.[33] Individuals who require the use of a prosthesis or orthosis may benefit from sexual counseling and support group interaction.

Seeking Professional Help

When grieving becomes destructive and the patient with a prosthesis or orthosis is not adjusting well, professional counseling may be indicated. Patients may display the following signs that indicate a need for professional help:

- Continual thoughts of self-destruction, including suicide
- Failure to provide for basic needs—failing to take care of health, staying withdrawn, or becoming nonfunctional; for example, a patient with a spinal cord injury may neglect weight shifts to prevent skin pressure sores or a patient who wears a prosthesis may neglect proper skin hygiene
- Engaging in substance abuse, including prescription drugs, alcohol, or illegal drugs
- Mental disorders, including concentration difficulties, persistent anxiety, hallucinations, or inability to function[23]

Psychologic interventions such as counseling or medications for patients with high levels of social discomfort may be implemented to decrease the incidence of depression.[12]

Successful Adaptation to Disability

Successful adaptation to disability is often an evolving process. A physical therapist or physical therapist assistant may observe some of the following behaviors in an individual with a prosthesis or orthosis, which may indicate a successful adaptation to disability.

- Less self-involvement and more interest in others and in the surroundings
- Increased confidence
- Taking charge of life rather than allowing external factors to control one's life
- Return to work or hobbies
- Focus on new activities and skills
- Renewal of friendships and cultivation of new experiences
- Memories of life before the disability no longer trigger associations with grief, sadness, or guilt
- Increased acceptance of impairment and feelings of independence[23]

Successful adaptation to disability may lead to reintegration in to the community as well as improved quality of life.

Community Reintegration

Health-care consumers often become involved with support and advocacy groups. Joining a support group may involve a peer self-help group such as an amputee support network. Joining an advocacy group may involve being active in reducing social prejudice, discrimination, and architectural barriers. Many individuals with a prosthesis or orthosis have become involved in lobbying for optimal health-care legislation to enhance the quality of life for people with disabilities. Successful advocacy may be demonstrated by activities such as developing a homepage to highlight successes and problems with use of a prosthesis or orthosis.[34]

Through the efforts of the individuals with disabilities, the Americans with Disabilities Act (ADA) was enacted in 1990 by the United States Government. The ADA legally prohibits discrimination based on physical or mental disability in the areas of employment, public services, transportation, public accommodations, and telecommunications. The ADA applies to worksites with 15 or more employees and is enforced by state and local civil rights agencies and the Equal Employment Opportunity Commission (EEOC). Reasonable accommodations including architectural barrier elimination must be made for a person with a disability. This legislation allows many individuals with a disability, including those with a prosthesis or orthosis, to fully participate in and contribute to society.[23]

Concerns of Americans with Disabilities

A survey of 13,000 Americans with disabilities in 319 communities in 10 states provided information about their concerns. Eighteen issues were identified as major problems. The five issues that most individuals were concerned about are presented in Table 4-1.[31] Individuals using prostheses or orthoses share these concerns about health-care access, financial means, coordination of benefits, disability rights and advocacy, and accessibility.

Health-care access and expense—Consumers with disability sometimes cannot purchase health insurance because of the disability or expense. In addition, health insurance often does not cover supplies, medications, or therapies needed by the disabled.

Financial concerns—Consumers with a disability who are on a fixed income often cannot afford high utility bills. Because of their medical needs, they cannot survive without utilities to operate equipment.[31]

Coordination of social services benefits—Consumers with a disability were often concerned that social service agencies failed to inform them about all services available through their own agencies or provide assistance through other agencies.[31]

Disability rights and advocacy—The survey found that many with disability were unaware of legal rights and pending legislation. It was felt that training in forming advocacy groups was needed.[31]

Often lack of knowledge of new prosthetic or orthotic components is also a concern. In a Canadian survey of 2176 individuals with amputation, the most important concerns were the

Table 4-1. Concerns of Americans with a Disability

Concerns	Frequency of Response (%)
Health-care access and expense	89
Financial concerns	89
Coordination of social services benefits	88
Disability rights and advocacy	88
Accessibility to commercial services	87

Adapted from Nagler, M. (1993). *Perspectives on disability* (pp. 227–228). Palo Alto, CA: Health Markets Research.

lack of information about new prostheses, modifications to existing prostheses, or new fitting techniques. Lack of a source of information from other individuals with amputation and lack of adaptive equipment for recreation were other areas identified.[35] In a Japanese study of individuals with amputation, patients felt that they had not been adequately informed about the prognosis after amputation. The authors state that possibly information and advice regarding these topics were communicated but not retained by the patients. They advocated using written material and involving family members to increase retention of information.[22] In a study of 92 persons with lower limb amputations in Seattle, Washington, areas of concern were fit of the prosthetic socket, functioning of the prosthesis, and adaptation to life with the prosthesis. This study found that the respondents were well served by their prostheses, and the authors advocated additional patient education to alleviate these areas of concern.[36] In a survey of support groups throughout the United States, individuals with amputation were concerned about the lack of available information on new technologies. Respondents identified the prosthetist, support groups, and pamphlets as important sources of this information.[37] Computer technology and accessing websites of the organizations listed in Resource Box 4-1 may provide valuable information and support from individuals who have experienced similar disabilities.

Accessibility to Commercial Services

Accessibility of businesses, restaurants, and public restrooms was a concern expressed in this survey. Also, accessibility to the worksite is often a concern. One study found that patients with an amputation considered reintegration to work activity unsatisfactory, even though self-worth perception, home mobility, and psychologic adjustments were rated satisfactory.[38] Referral to vocational rehabilitation agencies may facilitate reintegration to work by providing assistance in job modification or retraining.

Use of Orthoses and Prostheses

Prosthesis use has been widely studied. In contrast, little has been written about the use of orthoses. For individuals with neurologic deficits, the wheelchair may be a more effective, less energy-consuming mechanism of locomotion. Studies of the use of the reciprocating-gait orthosis (RGO) among pediatric patients with spina bifida showed that 52% of the patients averaged 25.8 months of use but did not persist with long-term use of the RGO.[39] Likewise, in a study of adults with spinal cord injury, at a follow-up of 5.4 years, 71% were classified as nonusers of their RGO.[40] In another study of adults with spinal cord injury, only 12% used the RGO outside the home.[41] Only one study was found regarding the use of an orthosis for an orthopedic deficit. In a study of 49 knee injuries, 71% of the respondents continued to wear their Townsend Knee Orthosis 2 years after injury.[42]

Even though the use of prostheses has been widely studied, results have varied. Prosthesis use appears to be lower in the United States than in Canada or Australia. In a United States study of 55 vascular disease patients, 50 years of age or older, who underwent either transfemoral or through-knee amputations, only 44% wore their prostheses every day.[43] Neither gait factors, cause of amputation, nor hip range-of-motion at discharge predicted continued prosthetic use. This study found that most patients achieved their maximum function by the time of discharge from the rehabilitation program. Continued gains after discharge were only made by a few patients.[43] In another survey, of 157 patients with lower extremity amputation in the southern United States, 56% became functional ambulators.[44]

Prosthesis use rates appear to be higher in other countries than in the United States. High prosthesis usage rates were seen in a survey of 396 patients with unilateral amputations in Quebec, Canada. In this study, 85% of the respondents were prosthetic wearers; 53% used their prosthesis for most of their indoor activities, while 64% did so for most outdoor activities. This study found that the presence of arthritis in the sound limb was negatively related to prosthetic use. Long delays in prosthetic fitting, prolonged gait training, cardiac and respiratory problems, and constant residual limb pain were significantly related to disuse.[45] In a survey of 52 individuals with lower limb amputations in Australia, prostheses were used by 94% of the respondents, with 72% using their prostheses all day. The number of individuals returning home after amputation was 93%. This high percentage was due in part to government funding for home modifications. A positive result of amputation was reflected in the comments of some of the respondents who reported loss of pain and a feeling of well-being resulting from the amputation.[46] Likewise, a study of 88 children with congenital or acquired amputations of the lower limbs in the Netherlands found high use rates. In this study, 93% were able to walk more than 100 meters, 94% could apply and remove their prostheses, and 90% attended a regular school.[47]

From these studies, it appears that increased use of orthoses and prostheses is a result of various factors. These include early fitting, decrease in pain and associated medical problems, psychologic counseling, support group interactions, and home and work modifications. A physical therapist may be an advocate for many of these factors that increase use rates. For those patients with severe pain or associated medical problems, an orthosis or prosthesis may not be practical.

KEY POINTS

- The psychologic reactions of patients after amputation or an event requiring the use of an orthosis are both varied and complex.

- Positive correlations have been found between body image and increased self-esteem and life satisfaction and decreased anxiety and depression. The more negative one feels about one's body, the less satisfied he or she is with life.

- There are various stages of adjustment one may go through after a traumatic injury or after an elective procedure.

- Reactions of young children, adolescents, and the elderly to traumatic events requiring the need for a prosthesis or orthosis may vary.

- The type of disability one has may have a mild or a devastating impact on sexuality.

- There are specific signs that may be present after a disability that would lead one to seek professional help.

- There are specific behaviors that may show successful adaptation to disability.

- The Americans with Disabilities Act (ADA), enacted in 1990 by the United States Government, prohibits discrimination based on physical or mental disability in the areas of employment, public services, transportation, public accommodations, and telecommunications.

- Those with neurologic deficits appear to have lower use rates for their orthoses than those with orthopedic deficits. Prosthesis use appears to be lower in the United States than in Canada or Australia.

CRITICAL THINKING QUESTIONS

1. A triple insult may occur involving a loss of function, sensation, and body image after an event requiring the use of a prosthesis or orthosis. Consider ways in which your present life might be changed by this triple insult.

2. Compare and contrast psychologic reactions involved with a traumatic injury with those of an elective procedure.

3. Characterize factors that may affect successful psychologic adjustment.

4. Evaluate adjustment difficulties that may indicate that a patient needs professional counseling.

5. Explain signs that may indicate successful adaptation to disability.

6. Analyze typical concerns that those with a disability may have.

REFERENCES

1. Bowker, J. H., & Michael, J. W. (1992). *Atlas of limb prosthetics*. St Louis: Mosby Year Book.
2. Kashani, J., Frank, R., Kashani, S., Wonderlich, S., & Reid, I. (1983). Depression among amputees. *Journal of Clinical Psychiatry, 44,* 256–258.
3. Van der Velde, C. (1985). Body images of one's self and of others: Developmental and clinical significance. *American Journal of Psychiatry, 142,* 527–537.
4. Breakey, J. W. (1997). Body image: The lower-limb amputee. *Journal of Prosthetics and Orthotics, 9,* 58–66.
5. Frierson, R., & Lippmann, S. (1987). Psychiatric consultation for acute amputees. *Psychosomatics, 28,* 183–189.
6. Fitzpatrick, M. C. (1999). The psychologic assessment and psychosocial recovery of the patient with an amputation. *Clinical Orthopaedics and Related Research, 361,* 98–107.
7. Livneh, H., & Antoniak, R. F. (1997). *Psychosocial adaptation to chronic illness and disability (pp. 19–22, 172–180).* Gaithersburg, MD: Aspen.
8. Williamson, V. C. (1992). Amputation of the lower extremity: An overview. *Orthopaedic Nursing, 11,* 55–65.
9. Bradway, J. K., Malone, J. M., Racy, J., Leal, J. M., & Poole, J. (1984). Psychological adaptation to amputation: An overview. *Orthotics and Prosthetics, 38,* 46–50.
10. Williamson GM, & Walters AS. (1996). Perceived impact of limb amputation on sexual activity. A study of adult amputees. *Journal of Sex Research, 33,* 221–230.
11. Reinstein, L., Ashely, J., & Miller, K. H. (1978). Sexual adjustment after lower extremity amputation. *Archives of Physical Medicine and Rehabilitation, 59,* 501–504.
12. Rybarczyk, B. D., Nyenhuis, D. L., Nicholas, J. J., Schulz, R., Alioto, R. J., & Blair, C. (1992). Social discomfort and depression in a sample of adults with leg amputations. *Archives of Physical Medicine and Rehabilitation, 73,* 1169–1173.
13. Parkes, C. M. (1972). Components of the reaction to loss of a limb, spouse, or home. *Journal of Psychosomatic Research, 16,* 343–349.
14. Walters, J. (1981). Coping with a leg amputation. *American Journal of Nursing, 81,* 1349–1352.
15. Noble, D., Price, D., & Gilder, R., Jr. (1954). Psychiatric disturbances following amputation. *American Journal of Psychiatry, 111,* 609.
16. Kolb, L., & Brodie, K. (1984). *Modern clinical psychiatry* (10th ed., pp. 574–576). Philadelphia: W. B. Saunders.
17. Jacobsen, J. M. (1998). Nursing's role with amputee support groups. *Journal of Vascular Nursing, 16,* 31–34.
18. Page, N., & Rowe, J. (1998). Other amputees are the greatest help in dealing with limb losses. *British Medical Journal, 317,* 682.
19. Malone, J. M., Moore, W. S., Goldstone, J., & Malone, S. J. (1979). Therapeutic and economic impact of a modern amputation program. *Annals of Surgery, 189,* 798.
20. Boyle, M., Tebbi, C. K., Mindell, E. R., & Mettlin, C. J. (1982). Adolescent adjustment to amputation. *Medical and Pediatric Oncology,* 301–312.
21. Tyc, V. L. (1992). Psychosocial adaptation of children and adolescents with limb deficiencies: A review. *Clinical Psychology Review, 12,* 275–291.
22. Watanabe, Y., McCluskie, P. J., Hakim, E., Asami, T., & Watanabe, H. (1999). Lower limb amputee patients satisfaction with information and rehabilitation. *International Journal of Rehabilitation Research, 22,* 67–69.
23. Winchell, E. (1995). *Coping with limb loss.* Garden City Park, NY: Avery Publishing Group.
24. Hudson, M. M., Tyc, V. L., Cremer, L. K., Luo, X., Li, H., Rao, B. N., Meyer, W. H., Crom, D. B., & Pratt, C. B. (1998). Patient satisfaction after limb-sparing surgery and amputation for pediatric malignant bone tumors. *Journal of Pediatric Oncology Nursing, 15,* 60–69.
25. Fisher, K., & Hanspal, R. (1998). Body image and patients with amputations: Does the prosthesis maintain the balance. *International Journal of Rehabilitation Research, 21,* 355–363.
26. Cutson, T. M., & Bongiorni DR. (1996). Rehabilitation of the older lower limb amputee: A brief review. *Journal of the American Geriatric Society, 44,* 1388–1393.
27. Coletta, E. M. (2000). Care of the elderly patient with lower extremity amputation. *Journal of the American Board of Family Practice, 123,* 23–34.

28. Solomon, K. (1989). Psychosocial dysfunction in the aged: Assessment and intervention. In O. Jackson, Ed. *Physical therapy of the geriatric patient* (2nd ed.). New York: Churchill Livingstone.

29. Jackson-Wyatt, O. (1992). Age related changes in amputee rehabilitation. *Topics in Geriatric Rehabilitation, 8,* 1–12.

30. Sipski, M. L., & Alexander, C. J. (1997). *Sexual function in people with disability and chronic illness* (pp. 294–299). Gaithersburg, MD: Aspen.

31. Nagler, M. (1993). *Perspectives on disability* (pp. 227–228). Palo Alto, CA: Health Markets Research.

32. Reinstein, L., Ashley, J., & Miller, K. H. (1978). Sexual adjustment after lower extremity amputation. *Archives of Physical Medicine and Rehabilitation, 59,* 501–504.

33. Medhat, A., Huber, P. M., & Medhat, M. A. (1990). Factors that influence the level of activities in persons with lower extremity amputation. *Rehabilitation Nursing,* 13–18.

34. Montan, K. (2000). Internet as a meeting place concerning partial foot amputations. *Prosthetics and Orthotics International, 24,* 85.

35. Chadderton, H. C. (1983). Consumer concerns in prosthetics. *Prosthetics and Orthotics International, 7,* 15–16.

36. Legro, M. W., Reiber, G., del Aguila, M., Ajax, M. J., Boone, D. A., Larsen, J. A., Smith, D. G., & Sangeorzan, B. (1999). Issues of importance reported by persons with lower limb amputations and prostheses. *Journal of Rehabilitation Research and Development, 36,* 155–163.

37. Nielsen, C. C. (1991). A survey of amputees: functional level and life satisfaction, information needs, and the prosthetist's role. *Journal of Prosthetics and Orthotics, 3,* 125–129.

38. Nissen, S. J., & Newman, W. P. (1992). Factors influencing reintegration to normal living after amputation. *Archives of Physical Medicine and Rehabilitation, 73,* 548–551.

39. Guidera, K. J., Smith, S., Raney, E., Frost, J., Pugh, L., Griner, D., & Ogden, J. A. (1993). Use of the reciprocating gait orthosis in myelodysplasia. *Journal of Pediatric Orthopedics, 13,* 341–348.

40. Sykes, L., Edwards, J., Powell, E. S., & Ross, E. R. (1995). The reciprocating gait orthosis: Long-term usage patterns. *Archives of Physical Medicine and Rehabilitation, 76,* 779–783.

41. Franceschini, M., Baratta, S., Zampolini, M., Loria, D., & Lotta, S. (1997). Reciprocating gait orthoses: A multicenter study of their use by spinal cord injured patients. *Archives of Physical Medicine and Rehabilitation, 78,* 582–586.

42. Jennings, J. M., Barringer, W. J., & Trexler, G. S. (1995). Clinical outcomes of the Townsend Knee Orthosis. *Journal of Prosthetics and Orthotics, 7,* 87–90.

43. Beekman, C. E, & Axtell, L. A. (1987). Prosthetic use in elderly patients with dysvascular above knee and through knee amputations. *Physical Therapy, 67,* 1510–1516.

44. Moore, T. J., Baron, J., Hutchinson, F., Golden, C., Ellis, C., & Humphries, D. (1989). Prosthetic usage following major lower extremity amputation. *Clinical Orthopaedics and Related Research, 238,* 219–224.

45. Gauthier-Gagnon, C., Grise, M. C., & Potvin, D. (1999). Enabling factors related to prosthetic use by people with a transtibial and transfemoral amputation. *Archives Physical Medicine and Rehabilitation, 80,* 706–713.

46. Jones, L., Hall, M., & Schuld, W. (1993). Ability or disability? A study of the functional outcome of 65 consecutive lower limb amputees treated at the Royal South Sydney Hospital in 1988–1989. *Disability and Rehabilitation, 15,* 184–188.

47. Boonstra, A. M., Rijnders, L. J., Groothoff, J. W., & Eisma, W. H. (2000). Children with congenital deficiencies or acquired amputations of the lower limbs: Functional aspects. *Prosthetics and Orthotics International, 24,* 19–27.

Chapter 5

BIOMECHANICAL IMPLICATIONS OF PROSTHETICS AND ORTHOTICS

Susan D. Miller, PT, MS

Objectives

1. Correctly use biomechanical terminology related to the design, application, and use of prostheses and orthoses
2. Differentiate between kinematics and kinetics
3. Apply principles of the load/deformation curve and stress/strain principles to the fitting a prosthesis or orthosis
4. Differentiate among various forces that apply to prosthetics and orthotics
5. Describe the effects of posture, gravity, and alignment on prostheses and orthoses
6. Explain the characteristics of normal gait
7. Explain the role of the ground reaction force vector in gait as it relates to the use of prosthetic and orthotic devices
8. Describe common gait deviations seen with the use of a prosthesis or orthosis

This chapter is divided into the following sections:

One primary purpose for prescribing an orthosis or a prosthesis for an individual is to improve the performance of functional activities and mobility, including ambulation. To select, fabricate, fit, or train an individual in the use of an orthosis or prosthesis, a practitioner must possess a basic understanding of biomechanical principles, normal alignment, movement, and forces acting on the body or body segment. In addition, an understanding of normal gait and common gait deviations is important. These important background concepts are discussed in this chapter in preparation for a more in-depth look at various prosthetic and orthotic devices in the chapters to follow.

Kinematics

Kinematics is the biomechanical term used to describe the motion of a body or object. While ignoring the forces that might produce motion, kinematics delineates the type, quantity, location, and direction of motion. Each of these are addressed in this section.

Types of Motion

One can differentiate types of motion as rotary (angular), translatory, or curvilinear (Fig. 5-1).[1] In a pure sense, rotary motion occurs around a fixed axis. The joints in the human body do not really rotate around a fixed axis. Therefore, we often simplify human motion, describing it as pure rotation. By convention, these rotary motions are flexion/extension, abduction/adduction, medial/lateral rotation, pronation/supination, and plantarflexion/dorsiflexion. Translatory motion is movement in a straight line. In the body, this motion is typically compression, distraction, or gliding. **Translation** of a body segment may also occur by rotation of proximal segments moving a distal segment along a straight line. Curvilinear motion occurs as an object rotates about an axis and is moved through space at the same time. Kicking a ball is an example. It involves knee rotation while the hip moves the knee through space, with the foot describing a parabolic path. Coincidentally, the ball also moves in a curvilinear fashion as it rotates about its own axis as it moves through space.

Quantity, Location, and Direction of Motion

Quantity of rotary motion is given in radians or, more typically, degrees. (One radian is equal to 57.3°.) Rotary motion of the joints of the body is measured in degrees, using a goniometer. Linear distance such as the number of centimeters, inches, feet, etc. quantifies translatory

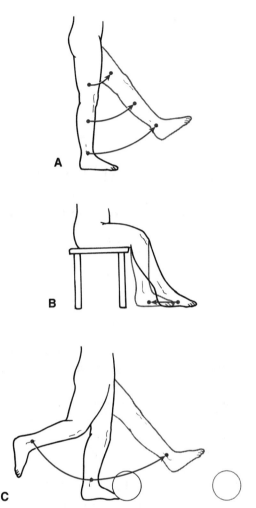

Figure 5-1. Types of motion. **A.** Rotary motion: each point in the extremity moves through the same angle in the same time. **B.** Translatory motion: each point in the segment moves through the same distance, in parallel, at the same time. **C.** Curvilinear motion: distal points move in a parabolic path as the distal segment is translated through space while rotating about its axis.

motion. **Speed,** the displacement per unit time, also quantifies motion. For example, miles per hour or centimeters per second are examples of using speed to quantify linear motion. When used to quantify rotary motion, it is called angular speed, expressed as degrees per second.

Location of motion in the body is described with reference to the horizontal (transverse), frontal (coronal), and sagittal planes (Fig. 5-2) formed by the intersection of the *x, y,* and *z* axes. Rotary motion occurring within these planes occurs about an axis perpendicular to the plane. Note that motion within the plane does not indicate direction. In the case of joint motion, the direction is indicated by the terminology, for example, flexion versus extension or abduction versus adduction.

Axes of Joint Motion

The number of axes of motion indicates the **degrees of freedom** available for a joint. For example, a ball-and-socket joint has three axes of motion and three degrees of freedom, while a hinge joint has one axis and one degree of freedom.

The reality of joint motion is that none of the joint axes fall truly along the cardinal plane axes. A joint may revolve around an axis that

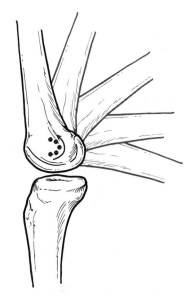

Figure 5-3. Pathway of the instant axis of rotation for the knee joint. (Adapted from Soderberg, G. L. (1997). *Kinesiology application to pathological motion* (2nd ed.). Baltimore: Williams & Wilkins.)

crosses all three planes in the coordinate system, thus giving a combination movement. For instance, the motion we call dorsiflexion not only includes dorsiflexion, but eversion and abduction as well. In addition, joint motion does not occur about a stationary pin–type axis. Instead, the location of the axis of motion may vary from one instant in time to another instant in time. At the knee, for example, the axis moves a considerable extent throughout the range of motion of flexion/extension. If the **instant axis of rotation** (IAR) is plotted throughout the range of motion, it traces a somewhat parabolic pathway on the femoral condyle (Fig. 5-3).[2]

Kinematic Chains

Another important concept to understand is a **kinematic chain.** In considering the lower extremity, the pelvis, hip, knee, ankle, and foot are linked together, and for the upper extremity,

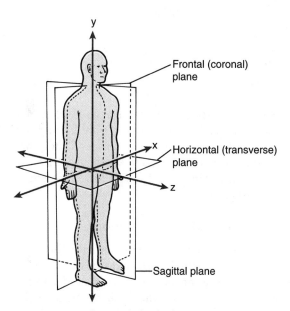

Figure 5-2. Planes of the body. Horizontal (transverse) plane, frontal (coronal) plane, and sagittal plane

the shoulder, elbow, wrist, and hand are linked together. Each of these is analogous to a kinematic chain in engineering. A kinematic chain has the effect of increasing the number of degrees of freedom available for the distal joints through the summation of the number of degrees of freedom of each of the more-proximal joints. This summation of the degrees of freedom makes more combination of movements of the whole extremity possible and allows more-skilled activity and smooth motion. Movement of either the shoulder or elbow alone would not allow for bringing the hand to the mouth or reaching the back pocket. However, as a kinematic chain with four degrees of freedom (three for the shoulder plus one for the elbow), the hand can be positioned appropriately.

A kinematic chain can be either open or closed. In an open kinematic chain, the distal segment (hand or foot) is not fixed; the joints of the extremity can move independently or in an unpredictable combination with another joint. Bringing the hand to the mouth or back pocket as mentioned above would be open kinematic chain movement. In a closed kinematic chain, the distal segment is fixed. Movement at one joint of the kinematic chain imposes motion at another joint in a relatively predictable manner. For example, when standing with the foot planted on the ground, if you bend the knees, the ankle must dorsiflex and the hip will flex. This is in contrast to the open kinematic chain where you can bend the knee without any motion occurring at the hip or ankle (Fig. 5-4). Another example of the predictable motion of a closed kinematic chain is supination of the foot in standing resulting in lateral rotation of the hip or pronation of the foot resulting in medial rotation of the hip. In a closed chain, loss of motion at one joint will almost certainly affect other joints in the chain. If there is limited dorsiflexion at the ankle, to bear weight on the foot, there are two options. Either the individual will bear weight on the toe, resulting in hip and knee flexion, or to get the foot flat on the ground, the knee will hy-

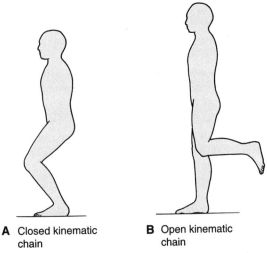

A Closed kinematic chain   **B** Open kinematic chain

Figure 5-4. Kinematic chain. **A.** Closed kinematic chain. Hip flexion and ankle dorsiflexion accompany knee flexion in a closed kinematic chain. **B.** Open kinematic chain. Hip and ankle motion are independent of knee flexion in an open kinematic chain.

perextend. In either case, the position of the proximal joints in the closed kinematic chain are predictable (Fig. 5-5).

Implications of Principles of Kinematics for Lower Extremity Prosthetics and Orthotics

The kinematic concepts discussed thus far have implications for the selection, fit, and use of prosthetic and orthotic devices. There are several questions related to kinematics that one should ask when looking at a lower extremity orthosis or prosthesis.

Orientation of Axes of Motion

Does the orthosis or prosthesis have the same orientation as the human joint in the x, y, and z planes? Are the axes of motion similar to the anatomic axes? For the limb to move in its normal path of motion, the axes must be aligned similarly. This is not always easy to accomplish. As seen above in Figure 5-3, even a joint with one axis does not move exactly like a device with a pin-type axis. When an orthosis with a single axis is used at the knee, that axis will align with the knee for only a small part of the knee range of motion. Orthoses with polycentric joints have been designed to try to better match the instantaneous centers of rotation of the knee. These mechanical polycentric joints are described in Chapter 15. A transfemoral prosthesis may also have a polycentric axis of motion at the knee. Prosthetic polycentric knees are described in Chapter 9. Since an individual with a transfemoral amputation has lost his or her knee, the concern is not matching the axis of the device to the knee, but rather understanding the fact that the type and location of axes will affect the movement and stability of the prosthetic limb.

Range of Motion

Does the orthotic or prosthetic device allow normal range of motion in any one plane? If not, what are the effects on the adjacent joints? Because of the closed kinematic chain, whether you are looking at a distal or proximal joint, adjacent joints are likely to be affected. Looking distally, the prior example of limited dorsiflexion is again pertinent, since an orthosis or a prosthetic foot may be locked in plantarflexion, with results at the knee similar to those seen in Figure 5-5. Looking proximally for example, a device preventing the hip from extending to neutral would most likely result in knee flexion too.

Degrees of Freedom

Does the orthotic or prosthetic device provide the same number of degrees of freedom as the normal joint? If not, the function of the joint will be affected. For example, some prosthetic feet, such as SACH feet, allow plantarflexion/dorsiflexion, but do not allow pronation/supination. This will affect the interface of the foot with the ground. Adaptation to uneven terrain is diminished, and forces may be transferred to the residual limb in the case of a prosthesis or to a weakened limb in the case of an orthosis.

Is the purpose of the device to control or limit the motion of a joint? If so, how many degrees of freedom are normally available at the joint, and how many require control or limitation of movement? If a joint with three degrees of freedom requires control in all three directions and the device only controls one or two, joint instability or deformity may still occur in the uncontrolled planes. For example, if an individual needs control for plantarflexion/dorsiflexion, inversion/eversion, and abduction/adduction of the foot, but an orthosis only controls plantarflexion/dorsiflexion, joint instability might still occur in the other two planes.

What effect will limiting the degrees of freedom of one joint have on other joints in the kinematic chain? For both orthotic and prosthetic devices, one must remember that if the degrees of freedom of a proximal joint are limited, it ultimately affects the degrees of freedom of the distal limb, because of the concept of the kinematic chain. Imagine the diminished options for foot placement in three dimensional space if an orthosis blocked all hip movement.

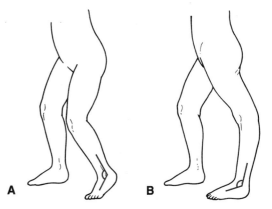

Figure 5-5. Limited dorsiflexion at the ankle. If the ankle can not dorsiflex normally, either **A.** the individual will weight bear on the toe or **B.** the knee must hyperextend to get the foot flat on the ground.

Kinetics

Unlike kinematics, kinetics takes forces into account. Simply stated, a force is the push or pull of one object or material on another. All forces are **vector** quantities with a point of application, direction or action line, and magnitude (Fig. 5-6). In applying kinetics to the human body, we must consider both external forces acting on the body and internal forces created within the body. The typical external forces are **inertia**, gravity, **ground reaction forces**, and **friction**. Additionally, a push or pull by another person or an object, including wind and water, is also considered an external force. The suspension of a prosthesis would be an example of an external object exerting a force on the body. Typical internal forces include those created by muscles, ligament pull, the push of one bone on another, or again, friction. Some of these forces are dealt with in more detail below in this chapter.

Stress

The amount of **stress** placed on the body or object is determined by the magnitude of the force and the size of the area to which the force is ap-

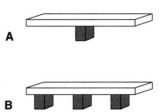

Figure 5-7. Stress on a cube. A. The stress on the cube is equal to the weight of the bar divided by the area of the top of the cube. B. The three cubes are of the same material, equal distance apart. The supporting area is three times the supporting area in A. Therefore, in B, the stress on the middle cube is one-third the original stress.

plied. Thus stress is equal to the force per area $(S = F/A)$. Note the similarity to the formula for pressure $(P = F/A)$. A small force over a given area will create less stress (or pressure) than a large force over the same size area. Similarly, a force applied over a small area will create more stress (or pressure) than a force applied over a large area. In Figure 5-7A, a steel bar is resting on a cube. The stress on the cube is equal to the weight of the bar divided by the area of the top of the cube. If two more identical cubes are added at equal distance from the first, as in Figure 5-7B, the supporting area is three times that of the single cube. The stress on the first cube is therefore only one-third of the original stress on the cube.[3] Using a rocker-bottom sole to increase the surface area and thereby decrease the stress on the metatarsal heads is an application of this principle. A rocker-bottom sole is described in Chapter 16. Another application of this principle is the use of a total surface-bearing (TSB) socket for an individual with a transtibial amputation to distribute the stress/pressure of the prosthesis over a larger area of the residual limb.[4] Further information on this type of socket is located in Chapter 8.

Deformation

Stress may deform the object. If **deformation** occurs, it could be a change in length, width, or general shape. Tissues, as well as materials

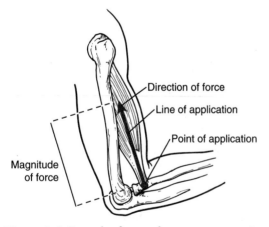

Figure 5-6. Example of a muscle as a vector quantity. Note the point of application, the direction, and action line. The magnitude of the force is represented by the length of the arrow.

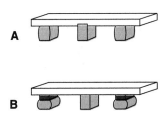

Figure 5-8. Stress on a cube when the cubes are not of the same material. **A.** The two end cubes are made of rubber, the middle of steel. A relief has been cut in the middle of the bar to accommodate the firmer steel cube. Without the relief, the less firm rubber cubes would deform, leaving the steel cube to bear more of the stress. **B.** The rubber cubes are even softer, compressing more easily. Further accommodation is made by building up the bar on the ends over the rubber cubes. The combination of the relief and the buildup on the ends of the bar helps to distribute the pressure evenly despite the difference in firmness of the materials used for the cubes.

used in orthotics and prosthetics, vary in their ability to resist deformation. For example, bone and cartilage respond differently, as do aluminum and steel. The resistance offered by a tissue or material as it deforms from an external force is called **stiffness**. If we return to the example of the cubes above and substitute soft-rubber cubes on the ends and a steel cube in the middle, the pressure would not be distributed evenly. Most of the load would be sup-

ported by the steel cube. This is a good analogy for the force applied to the residual limb by a prosthesis. The bone, being stiffer than the surrounding soft tissue, bears the brunt of the load. Again using the cube analogy, the load could be more equally distributed by cutting a relief in the steel bar (Fig. 5-8A). If this did not suffice to equalize the load, building up the steel bar at the ends would help (Fig. 5-8B).

Implications for Prosthetics and Orthotics

Living tissue is complicated in that tissue health requires circulation as well as neural input. One must consider the ability of the neurovascular system to withstand pressure. If you occlude the vessels, creating ischemia, tissue damage may result. Similarly, nerve damage may result from pressure on the nerves. The nerves and blood vessels are pressure sensitive. Therefore, load distribution is very important. The same principles described above can be used to help equalize pressure on a residual limb with tissues of varying firmness or to relieve pressure on pressure-sensitive tissues. Figure 5-9 presents a circular socket that matches the shape of the residual limb. If the tissue is of uniform stiffness, the stress (pressure) will be uniform. In Figure 5-9B, the residual limb is not of uniform stiffness or

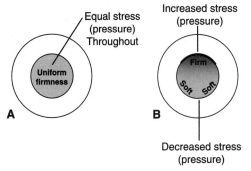
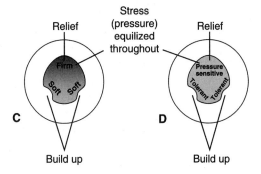

Figure 5-9. Stress on the residual limb from the prosthesis. **A.** The hypothetical situation in which the residual limb is of uniform firmness and the socket matches the circular shape of the limb. **B.** A residual limb of nonuniform firmness and a socket that matches the circular shape of the limb. This would result in increased stress on the firm areas of the residual limb. **C.** The same residual limb with a socket designed to equalize the pressures over the firm and soft areas. **D.** The same socket design used to accommodate pressure-sensitive areas and pressure-tolerant areas.

firmness, therefore the stress would not be uniform. To equalize the stress, the inner part of the socket could have reliefs cut over the firm tissues and built up over those less firm, as in Figure 5-9C. The same principle could be applied to pressure-sensitive and pressure-tolerant areas (Fig. 5-9D). The patellar tendon bearing (PTB) socket described in Chapter 8 is an example of a design that uses pressure-sensitive and pressure-tolerant areas. Not only is this pressure-sensitive and pressure-tolerant concept important for the socket, but in both orthotics and prosthetics, the relationship of force, area, and the ability of tissue to tolerate stress must be taken into account when determining the location and size of suspensions. Locating a narrow strap over a superficial nerve or a major blood vessel might result in damage to the nerve or tissues supplied by the blood vessel. The consequences would be even greater if there is preexisting compromise of the neural or vascular system from conditions such as diabetes or peripheral vascular disease. A good working knowledge of human anatomy and the principles of stress and deformation are very important for the selection and fit of orthotic and prosthetic devices.

Load/Deformation Curve

In addition to variance in stiffness, tissues and materials vary in the ability to return to their original shape after removal of a load. This ability to return to original shape after the removal of the load is **elasticity**. Permanent deformity occurs when the load exceeds the material's ability to return to its original shape. The point where this occurs is the **yield point**. Some materials tolerate deformation after the yield point more than other materials. This is the **plasticity** of the material. The relationship between load and deformation for a particular material can be plotted on a curve (Fig. 5-10). In the graph, the slope of the curve in the elastic region indicates the stiffness of the material; the stiffer the material, the steeper the slope. The size of the area

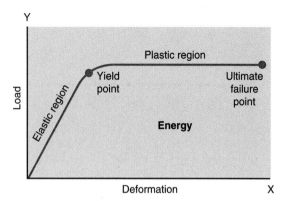

Figure 5-10. Load/deformation curve. Note the yield point that demarcates the elastic region from the plastic region. Note also the ultimate failure point. (Adapted from: Nordin, M., & Frankel, V. H. (2001). *Basic biomechanics of the musculoskeletal system* (3rd ed.). Philadelphia: Lippincott Williams & Wilkins.)

under the entire curve indicates the strength of the material in terms of energy storage, or energy buildup in the material as the load is applied; the greater the area, the more energy results.[5] A material that tolerates considerable deformity before failure is **ductile**, while one that tolerates little deformity before failure is **brittle**. For example, a soft metal is ductile, whereas glass is brittle. Plastic laminate is more brittle, and silicone is more ductile. These characteristics may affect the choice of materials used in the fabrication of orthoses or prostheses. In actuality, there is really a continuum between brittle and ductile. Comparing ligaments, cartilage, and bone, ligaments tolerate deformation more than cartilage, and cartilage can deform more than bone.[1] Different woods, metals, and plastics vary in ductility. This characteristic affects the choice of materials used in the fabrication of an orthosis or prosthesis.

Stress/Strain Curve

According to Sears, the relative change in dimensions or shape of a body subjected to stress is **strain**.[6] The relationship between stress and

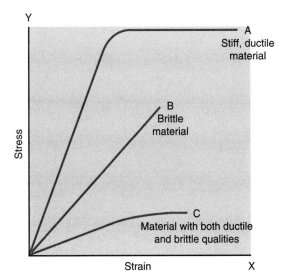

Figure 5-11. Stress/strain curve. Note the difference in the shape of the curve for the three materials. Material A is stiffest, with the steepest curve. It also is ductile, with a long plastic region before failure. Material B is brittle, with no plastic region before failure. Both A and B materials are linear in the elastic region; material C is nonlinear in the elastic region. Material C continues to deform in the plastic region before failing.

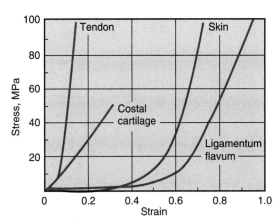

Figure 5-12. Stress/strain plots for various human connective tissues tested in uniaxial tensions. (Reprinted with permission from Barbenel, J. C., Evans, J. H., & Jordan, M. M. (1978). Tissue mechanics. *English Medicine, 7,* 5.)

strain can also be plotted on a graph (Fig. 5-11). The stress/strain graph varies for different tissues of the body (Fig. 5-12). The shape of the curve upon unloading is also important. If the return curve is congruent, all of the energy from loading is returned upon unloading. Some materials exhibit a lack of congruence for the curves for increasing stress and decreasing stress. (Fig. 5-13). This is called **hysteresis**. Vulcanized rubber, for example, displays this phenomenon. The work required to deform the material is greater than the work done by the material in returning to its original shape. The area between the curves represents the energy dissipated, usually in the form of heat, within the elastic material. Materials with a larger area between the curves are good for absorbing vibration and shock.[6] Materials may be selected for parts of an orthosis or prosthesis, especially prosthetic feet, based upon the ability to either

return energy or absorb energy. Also, remember that one material would not work for all individuals, because the load or stress placed on the material would be different from, for example, a light individual and a heavy individual. A case in point would be the firmer heel of a SACH prosthetic foot for a heavier individual versus a less-firm material for a lighter individual.

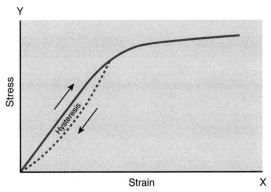

Figure 5-13. Hysteresis is demonstrated by noncongruent curves for loading a material and unloading the material when plotting the stress/strain curve.

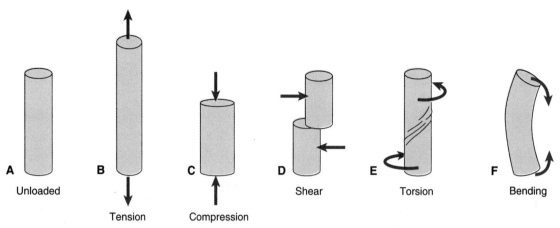

Figure 5-14. Unloaded in comparison to five types of forces. A. Unloaded. B. Tension. C. Compression. D. Shear. E. Torsion. F. Bending.

Types of Forces

In general, forces applied to an object fall into one of five types or a combination of these types (Fig. 5-14). These are

1. Tension
2. Compression
3. Shear
4. Torsion
5. Bending

Tension and Compression Forces

Both tension and compression are forces applied in a direction perpendicular to the surface or a plane within an object.[7] Tensile forces pull apart or stretch; compression forces push or press together. Tensile forces result in elongation and narrowing deformation; compression results in a shortening and widening of the dimensions. Avulsion fractures and sprains are examples of injuries due to primarily tensile forces. On the other hand, vertebral body fractures and joint pain from osteoarthritis commonly result from compression forces. Orthotic devices are frequently used to protect tissues from tensile and compressive forces and provide a counteracting force. A specific exam-

ple might be the use of unloader orthosis or a lateral-wedged insole to counter the compressive load (force) on the medial compartment of the knee of an individual with osteoarthritis.[12] Additional examples of compressive and tensile forces are given below in this chapter.

Shear Forces

A shear force is applied in a direction parallel to the surface or a plane within an object.[7] When a shear force is applied to an object, shear stress and strain are created. The object deforms internally in an angular manner (Fig. 5-15). Shear forces are also present when a ma-

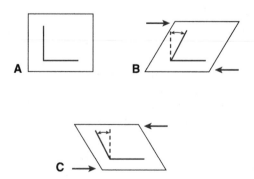

Figure 5-15. Shear loading results in an internal deformation as demonstrated by the change in angle.

terial is under tensile or compressive loading (Fig. 5-16). Clinically, the application of a shear or tangential force can cause shear stress and strain on weight-bearing surfaces, for example, under the sole of the foot or between skin and the surface in sitting. One complication of a poorly fitted orthotic or prosthetic device is the creation of shear between the device and the skin. Internally, shear can occur between muscle and fascia or bone. Shear forces may also distort blood vessels, restricting blood and lymph flow.[8]

Another internal shear force occurs when muscles contract and pull on bone, as illustrated by the quadriceps pull on the tibia. Not only does the quadriceps create a rotary force, it also creates an anterior shear of the tibia on the femur (Fig. 5-17). Like the quadriceps, the hamstrings create both a rotary force and a shear force, but in this case rotary and shear forces are opposite to those of the quadriceps. In the normal knee, the cruciate ligaments counter these shear forces. When a cruciate is

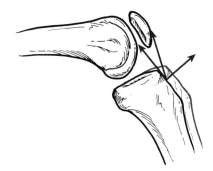

Figure 5-17. Shear force occurring between the tibia and femur. Because the knee does not have a fixed pin axis, the force perpendicular to the tibia is not just rotary. The quadriceps also shears the tibia forward on the femur.

lax or torn, the shear increases. One purpose of an orthosis is to provide a force to counter the shear created at a joint, especially in the absence of normal anatomic restraints. This is especially true at the knee.

Torsion Forces

A torsion force tends to twist a body, and a bending force occurs when there is not direct support for the force applied to the object. Again, Figure 5-14 depicts a torsion force. A spiral fracture is an example of an injury from a torsion force. Some knee orthoses are designed to control torsion-type forces. These derotational orthoses are discussed in Chapter 15.

Bending Forces

Bending forces occur about an axis. With these forces, tensile stresses and strains occur on the convex side of the bend, and compressive stresses and strains occur on the concave side. An example of this can be seen in the femur in weight bearing (Fig. 5-18). Either three or four forces may produce bending (Fig. 5-19). With a three-point system, the axis for bending is the point in the middle. The application of this three-point bending principle to spinal orthoses is clearly demon-

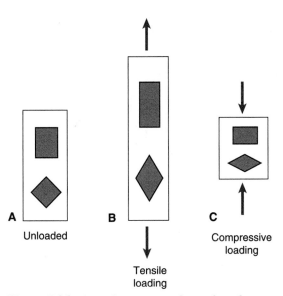

Figure 5-16. Shear also occurs with tensile and compression loading as demonstrated by the internal angular deformation.

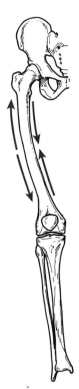

Figure 5-18. Bending force on the femur. When loaded, the femur has tensile stresses and strains on the convex side and compressive stresses and strains on the concave side.

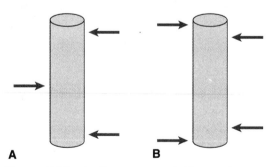

A   **B**

Figure 5-19. Bending systems. A. Three-point system. B. Four-point system.

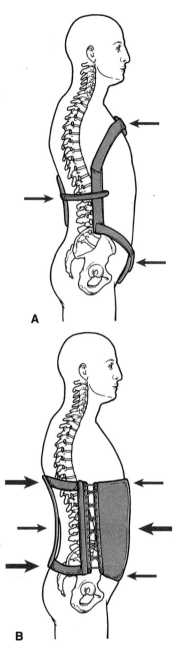

A

B

Figure 5-20. Application of three-point spinal orthoses. A. Jewett brace with one three-point system. B. Knight brace with two three-point systems.

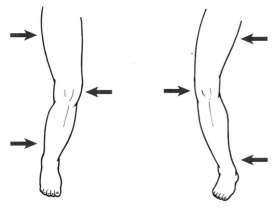

Figure 5-21. Application of three-point system for varus or valgus control of the knee.

strated in Figure 5-20. Lower extremity applications can be seen in Figures 5-21 and 5-22. For a system to be in equilibrium, the sum of the magnitude of the two forces must be equal to the one countering force. The magnitude of the countering forces is inversely proportional to the perpendicular distance from the axis force. If the two forces are equidistant from the single force, each of the two will be one-half that of the single force. Another way of looking at the bending moment is the longer the orthosis, the greater the leverage. **Torque,** or the ability of a force to rotate a lever, is equal to the force times the perpendicular distance from the axis. Therefore, with a given force applied to the lever, the farther from the axis the force is applied, the greater the torque created. In the case of the three-point system, however, this would mean that the single force would also have to be greater to counter the other two. This can create uncomfortable strain unless the size of the straps or pads is significantly increased, since, as discussed above, the stress on the skin is determined by the area over which the force is applied.

A four-point bending system, makes use of two force couples. A force couple consists of two forces in opposite directions that cause rotation about an axis.[1] For the system to be in equilibrium, one force couple must be countered by another force couple of equal magnitude. An example of an orthosis

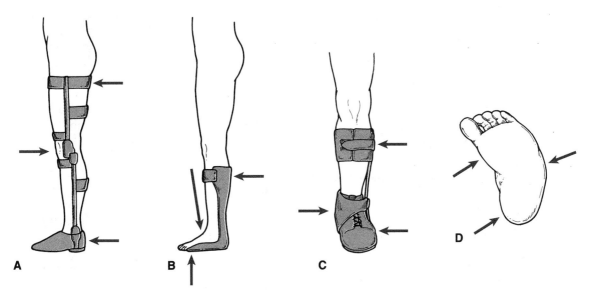

Figure 5-22. Additional three-point system examples of lower extremity orthoses.

using a four-point bending force is shown in Figure 5-23.

Viscoelasticity

Viscoelasticity is another biomechanical concept that is important in the application of prostheses and orthoses. Viscoelastic materials, such as the connective tissues of the body, exhibit some of the characteristics of both elasticity, as discussed above, and viscosity. Viscous substances have the ability to resist loads that produce shear. Viscoelastic materials may be used in prosthetics or orthotics for this reason, that is, to reduce shear and pressure.[8] Liners for a transtibial prosthesis use viscoelastic materials. Two commercially available viscoelastic materials used in foot orthotics are Sorbothane (Sorbothane, Inc., Kent, OH) and Viscolas (Chattanooga Corp., Chattanooga, TN).[9]

Forces applied to viscous or viscoelastic materials exhibit time- and rate-dependent properties. For example, the viscosity of synovial fluid varies inversely with joint velocity or rate

of shear.[1] As the joint velocity increases, the viscosity decreases, producing less resistance to movement. Another example of the rate dependency of viscoelastic materials is the loading of bone at a high rate versus a low rate. The slope of the stress/strain curve is steeper, representing an increase in stiffness, at the higher rate of loading. The area under the stress/strain curve for a high rate of loading is therefore greater than that for a low rate of loading, that is, the energy buildup is greater. If the failure point is reached under high-rate loading, that energy is dissipated, with the potential for comminution or significant damage to the surrounding soft tissue.[5]

Creep

Viscoelastic materials demonstrate the characteristic of **creep**, the increase in strain with time under a constant load.[7] The deformation is time dependent. Even though the load is constant, the material continues to deform until a state of equilibrium is reached. Constant loading, whether compressive or tensile, subjects joints and surrounding structures to the effects of load and creep. An example of the application of this principle is the use of a spring-loaded static orthosis such as a Dynasplint to reduce a contracture or alter tissue length. Constant loading of tissues of the body as well as materials for orthoses and prostheses may, at times, create excessive deformation. Even repetitive loading may subject a joint, orthosis, or prosthesis to damage if there is not time to recover the original dimensions before being subjected to another loading cycle.[1] In living material, damage occurs if the fatigue process outpaces the process of repair.[5] A case in point is a stress fracture of the second metatarsal. This is sometimes referred to as a "march fracture," as it often occurs as a result of a long march or another repetitive activity such as increased running mileage or long ballet exercise.[10] In this case, the repetitive loading causes bone deformation and fatigue exceeding the rate of repair.

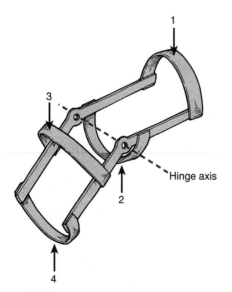

Figure 5-23. Example of a four-point system in a knee orthosis.

Posture, Gravity, and Alignment

Posture, gravity, and alignment affect the proper functioning of a prosthesis or orthosis.

Posture

Posture is the alignment of the body segments in space. We can look at posture statically (i.e., maintaining a position) or dynamically. *Dynamic posture* refers to postures in which the body or its segments are moving. In either case, to maintain upright posture, the body must counteract the effect of gravity or other forces acting upon it. The effect of gravity on the body is typically countered by internal forces, that is, the pull of muscles, ligaments, capsules, other soft tissue, and bone pushing on bone. The nervous system also plays a critical role. The nervous system must be capable of receiving, processing, and interpreting information to provide an appropriate output. An intact nervous system provides a sense of proprioception and muscles contracting with the appropriate pattern and timing.

Line and Center of Gravity

Gravity is a predictable force. The line of gravity (LOG), or action line, is always vertical, pointing toward the center of the earth. The point of application for gravity is a hypothetical point in the center of the mass of the object. The point where gravity appears to act is called the *center of gravity* (COG). The geometric center of a symmetric object is the COG. With an asymmetric object, the COG is the point around which the mass is evenly distributed. Think of the COG as the balance point of the object. In the human body, the COG lies approximately anterior to S2 (Fig. 5-24). The human body is made up of many movable segments. Each segment

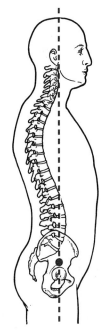

Figure 5-24. Location of the COG. In the average adult, the COG lies anterior to S2.

may be considered to have its own COG. If these segments were fixed in relation to each other, the COG would not change as those segments were moved in space. They are, however, free to move in relation to each other. As a result, the combined COG is not in a fixed location. The mass of the segments remains the same; therefore, the force of gravity remains the same. Nonetheless, the combined COG will be in a different location due to the rearrangement of the segments. In actuality, this point does not have to lie within the body (Fig. 5-25).

Altering the proportional mass of the limb, as might occur with quadriceps atrophy or with a disproportionate gain of weight in the thighs, will also alter the combined COG of the limb. In the first example, the COG would shift distally; with the second example, the COG would shift proximally. In the case of a lower-limb orthosis, for example, we must consider the weight applied to a limb in com-

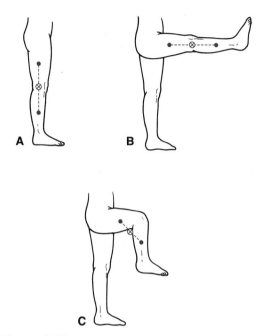

Figure 5-25. COG of segments and combined COG. A. Location of COG of thigh segment and lower leg segment and the combined COG of the two. B. Unchanging relationship as they are translated through space by hip flexion. C. Changing relationship as the knee is flexed. Note that the combined COG does not lie within the body.

per body mass to shift the COG back toward the midline.

For the best stability, the LOG should pass through the base of support. The larger the base of support, the more stable the person. The larger base of support gives the LOG more freedom to move without exceeding the limits of the base. The base of support can be increased by changing the position of the feet or by adding a cane or crutches (Figs. 5-26 and 5-27). In ambulation, a wide base of support is more stable, but there are other consequences in terms of efficiency of movement and energy costs. Energy costs of a prosthesis are described in Chapter 7.

Effect of Gravity

To determine the effect of gravity on the body, we must look at the relationship of the LOG to the axis of the joint. When the LOG passes through the axis of the joint, gravity has a linear effect, either a compression or tensile force (Fig. 5-28). If it does not pass through the axis of the joint, a moment, or torque, is created. The magnitude of the moment is proportional to the perpendicular distance from the axis of

bination with the weight of the limb itself. The more distally the weight of the orthosis is applied, the more distal the combined COG will be. The heavier the orthosis, the closer the COG will be to the orthosis. The effect on the COG of a limb is also obvious with an amputation. The limb loses distal mass, and the COG again moves proximally. When wearing a prosthesis that weighs less than the original limb, the new resulting combined COG of the limb will lie more proximally than that of the original limb. In addition, the overall COG of the body will shift up and away from the side of the prosthesis (toward the uninvolved limb, which has more mass). An individual with an amputation may lean the trunk toward the uninvolved side, rearranging the up-

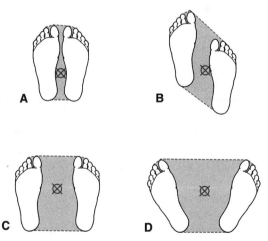

Figure 5-26. Base of support. The size of the base of support varies with a change in foot position.

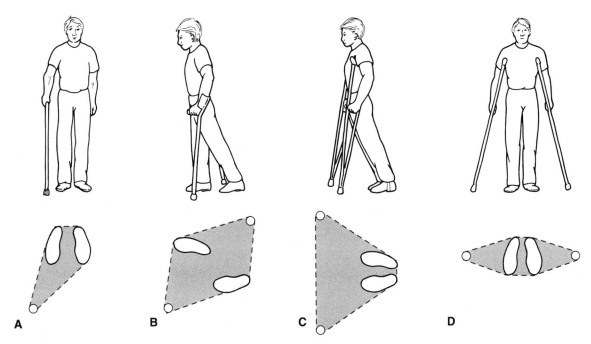

Figure 5-27. Base of support. The size of the base of support varies with the use of a cane or crutches and with placement of the assistive device.

the joint to the LOG. This distance is the **moment arm** (Fig. 5-29). The greater the moment arm, the greater the torque or rotary force. The most torque is generated when the line of force is perpendicular to the lever arm. In that case, the moment arm is equal to the distance along the lever arm from the axis to the force line (Fig. 5-30). The smaller the moment arm, the less the torque and greater the linear force created. Comparing erect standing to the bent-knee posture, there is a smaller moment arm in erect standing and a much longer moment arm at the hip, knee, and ankle with the bent-knee posture (Fig. 5-31). With the longer moment arms, there is more tendency for the hip and knee to flex and the ankle to dorsiflex. To counter the effects of gravity, more torque must be created by the muscles. When the muscles are unable to create this torque because of weakness or loss of neural control, orthoses might be used to provide forces to counter the gravitational torque.

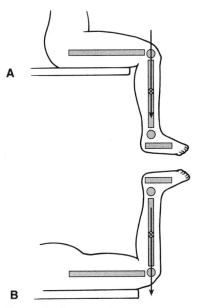

Figure 5-28. Linear force of gravity created when the LOG passes through the axis of the joint. A. Tensile force. B. Compressive force.

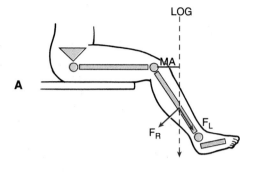

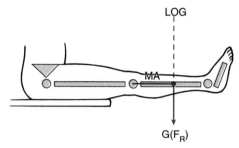

Figure 5-30. Maximum torque. The maximum torque or moment is created when the force is applied perpendicular to the lever arm. That is, the force of gravity is all rotary with no linear component.

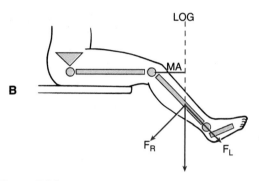

Figure 5-29. Gravitational moment created when the LOG does not pass through the axis of the joint. The magnitude of the moment (torque) is proportional to the perpendicular distance from the axis of the joint to the LOG. The magnitude of the moment is smaller in A than in B. F_R, rotary component; F_L, linear or translatory component of the LOG.

The torque of a muscle is equal to the force of contraction times the perpendicular distance from the axis to the line of application or line representing the line of pull of the muscle; that is, $T_M = F \times D$. Torque is increased by either increasing the magnitude of the force of contraction or increasing the moment arm. Again, the moment arm would be longest when the line of application of the force is perpendicular to the lever arm. Rarely, if ever, does the force line of the muscle pass through the joint axis or run perpendicular to the lever arm. This means that the force generated by the muscle will have both a rotary and a linear effect. In the bent-

knee posture described above, the linear effect results in compression at the joints (Fig. 5-32).

When two objects are in contact, they exert a force on each other. When gravity acts down through the body with the body in contact with the ground, there is an equal and opposite force of the ground on the body. This vector is

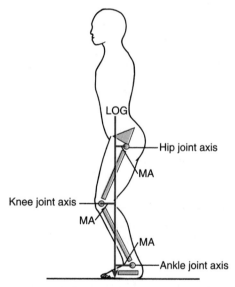

Figure 5-31. LOG and gravitational moments created by the bent-knee posture. With this posture, the perpendicular distance from the axes of the joints to the LOG is greater than in erect standing. Therefore, the gravitational moments are greater in the bent-knee posture.

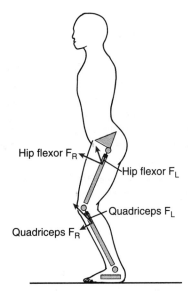

Figure 5-32. Components of hip flexor and knee extensor muscular forces in bent-knee posture.

the **ground reaction force vector** (GRFV) (Fig. 5-33). The GRFV will be a factor when we look at normal gait. It is also a factor when aligning a prosthesis. *Alignment* in this case refers to the placement of the prosthetic units in relation to each other.

Transtibial Prosthesis Alignment

Prosthetic alignment is performed in two phases, a bench or **static alignment** according to established guidelines and a dynamic alignment to fine-tune the device to achieve an optimal gait pattern.[11]

Static Alignment

Static alignment of the transtibial prosthesis is based on the alignment of the socket and foot. In this case, static alignment uses a plumb line from the center of the posterior wall of the socket to a location about ½ inch lateral to the center of the heel. This alignment maintains a fairly normal base of support and loads the

more–pressure-tolerant areas on the medial residual limb rather than the fibular head region. In the sagittal plane, a plumb line should fall from the center of the lateral wall of the socket to just anterior to the front edge of the heel (Fig. 5-34).[11]

Static alignment of the transtibial socket usually includes flexion of the socket 5 to 10°. A socket with vertical walls would increase the likelihood of the prosthesis sliding off because of gravity when the foot is off the ground or the residual limb sliding down when the foot is on the ground. Sliding of the prosthesis could increase shear between the prosthesis and the skin of the residual limb. In addition to decreasing slippage, flexion of the socket allows greater exposure of the patellar tendon for weight bearing. The inward bulge of the PTB prosthesis is less steeply inclined than the walls of the socket and provides additional weight-bearing surface (Fig. 5-35). As you know, for an object to remain in equilibrium, a force must have an equal and opposite force. Therefore, since the anterior bulge provides a larger

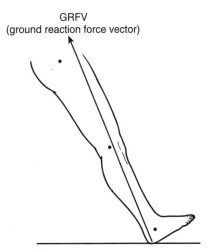

Figure 5-33. GRFV during gait. (Adapted from Levangie, P. K., & Norkin, C. C. (2001). *Joint structure and function, A comprehensive analysis* (3rd ed.). Philadelphia: F. A. Davis.)

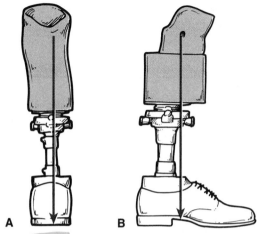

Figure 5-34. Static alignment for a transtibial prosthesis. **A.** In the frontal plane, the plumb line should fall from the center of the posterior wall of the socket to about $\frac{1}{2}$ inch lateral to the center of the heel. **B.** In the sagittal plane, the plumb line should fall from the center of the lateral wall of the socket to the breast of the heel.

horizontal vector component, the posterior wall of the prosthesis must supply a counterforce to prevent the residual limb from sliding down and backward.

Because of the factors mentioned above in the chapter, the residual limb will not tolerate full weight bearing on the distal end of the tibia. When the alignment and fit of the socket, whether PTB or TSB, do not provide enough relief of forces on the distal tibia, other methods of reducing the load may be tried. For example, liners made of materials demonstrating hysteresis, such as urethane, might help to transfer the load or absorb shock.[4] Bars, such as the patellar tendon bar used in a Syme prosthesis, may also be used to transfer some of the load and relieve pressure on the distal end of the residual limb.

Dynamic Alignment

If the forces from the residual limb downward on the prosthesis and the GRFV from below act along the same straight line, the prosthesis will

not rotate or change its angular relationship to the residual limb. However, if those forces are not along the same line, there is a tendency for the prosthesis to rotate. The fit of the socket is crucial to resist the rotation during gait. If the foot is placed too far medially, the prosthesis will tend to rotate and exert more pressure on the proximal medial residual limb and the distal lateral residual limb (Fig. 5-36). If the foot is placed too far laterally, the prosthesis will exert more pressure on the fibular head and the distal medial residual limb (Fig. 5-37).

Rotation can also occur in the anterior/posterior direction, with the socket exerting force on the distal anterior residual limb and proximal posterior residual limb when the foot hits the ground and again before the toe leaves the ground. If the prosthetist aligns the foot too far posteriorly, in relation to the socket, these pressures will be exaggerated (Fig. 5-38). At times during walking, the forces tend to rotate the socket so that pressure is exerted on the distal posterior residual limb and the proximal

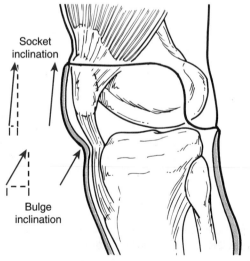

Figure 5-35. Inclination of the bulge of the PTB socket. The bulge provides more surface for weight bearing than the wall of the socket. Note the relatively longer horizontal component of the vector. (Adapted from Berger, N., & Fishman, S. (1998). *Lower limb prosthetics*. New York: Prosthetic Orthotic Publications.)

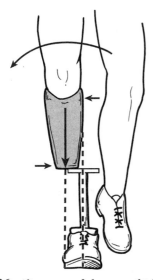

Figure 5-36. Alignment of the transtibial prosthesis in the sagittal plane, placing the foot medial to the socket. This placement tends to cause a rotation of the socket (lateral thrust) that then places pressure on the proximal medial residual limb and distal lateral residual limb.

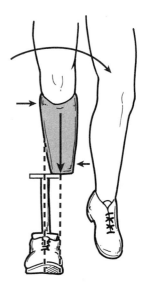

Figure 5-37. Alignment of the transtibial prosthesis in the sagittal plane placing the foot lateral to the socket. This placement tends to cause a rotation of the socket (medial thrust) that then places pressure on the fibular head of the residual limb and distal medial residual limb.

anterior residual limb. If the prosthetist aligns the foot too far anteriorly in relation to the socket, these pressures will be exaggerated (Fig. 5-39). One purpose of a supracondylar strap is to counter the rotational forces in this direction and decrease these pressures on the residual limb.[3] As you can see from this discussion, the alignment of the prosthesis and fit of the socket are critical to countering the forces acting on the limb.

Transfemoral Prosthesis Alignment

As with the transtibial prosthesis, the prosthetist uses both static and dynamic alignment phases. The application of the biomechanical principles is somewhat similar to that with the transtibial prosthesis, albeit complicated by the intervening mechanical knee joint and loss of muscle control for the knee of a transfemoral prosthesis

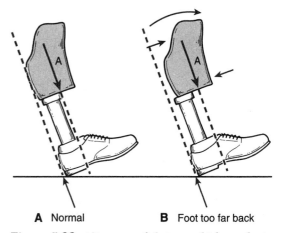

A Normal   **B** Foot too far back

Figure 5-38. Alignment of the transtibial prosthesis in the frontal plane. **A.** Normal alignment. **B.** Foot placed too far backward in relation to the socket. This placement tends to cause a rotation of the socket that then places pressure on the distal anterior part of the residual limb and proximal posterior part of the residual limb.

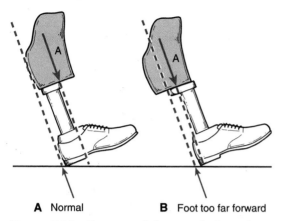

A Normal   **B** Foot too far forward

Figure 5-39. Alignment of the transtibial prosthesis in the frontal plane. **A.** Normal alignment. **B.** Foot placed too far forward in relation to the socket. If the force through the socket fell posterior to the GRFV, the prosthesis would tend to rotate and place pressure on the distal posterior part of the residual limb and proximal anterior part of the residual limb.

Static Alignment

With an average-length residual limb, as seen from a posterior view, static alignment of the prosthesis provides for the center of the heel to fall just under the point of contact of the ischial tuberosity with the socket. (Fig. 5-40).[11] In the sagittal plane, a **TKA line**, that is, trochanter–knee–ankle line, is used for static alignment (Fig. 5-41A). The T mark is a point transferred to the lateral wall of the socket from a mark 1 inch anterior to the posterior medial corner of the inside of the socket (Fig. 5-41B), the K is the knee axis, and the A is where the bolt attaching the prosthetic foot to the ankle is located.[13] By using the TKA line, the GRFV is aligned to stay anterior to the knee joint, producing an extension moment. This extension moment helps to ensure prosthetic knee stability during weight bearing in gait. In the horizontal plane, the prosthetist typically aligns the knee bolt so that it is 5° externally rotated from the line of progression. This allows the foot to swing straight forward in gait.

The distal femur, like the distal tibia, does not tolerate full weight bearing. A horizontal surface would provide the best weight-bearing support to decrease the load on the distal femur. An ischial seat as in a quadrilateral socket or the posterior wall in an ischial containment socket helps to provide this horizontal surface for weight bearing. The line of gravity for the body falls anterior to the ischium. Because of this, the pelvis would tend to rotate anteriorly without a counterforce provided by the anterior wall of the socket. For this reason, the prosthetist will create an anterior wall in a quadrilateral socket that is approximately $2\frac{1}{2}$ inches higher than the posterior wall to help keep the ischium on the shelf. The inner surface of the anterior wall also bulges inward, which helps to keep the ischium on the posterior shelf.

Static alignment also angles the socket in both the sagittal and frontal planes. Normally, the socket is flexed about 5°. In the quadrilateral socket, this alignment helps to keep the ischial tuberosity on the shelf and, more importantly, helps the gluteus maximus and

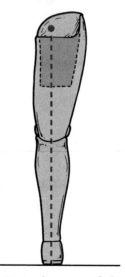

Figure 5-40. Static alignment of the transfemoral prosthesis in the frontal plane. The center of the heel lies directly under the ischial seat contact.

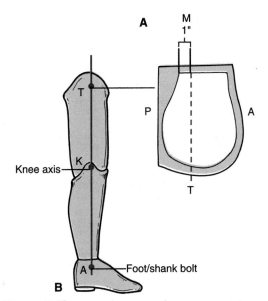

Figure 5-41. A. Static alignment of the transfemoral prosthesis using the TKA line. *T* is a mark transferred from a point one inch anterior to the posteromedial corner of the inside of the socket. **B.** *K* is the center of the knee, and *A* is the ankle bolt attaching the foot to the shank.

femur tends to become more vertical because of the imbalance of forces between the abductors and adductors. Statically aligning the socket in adduction helps to position the femur in a more anatomic plane and also helps to maintain the length/tension ratio for the gluteus medius. Therefore the adduction also helps the gluteus medius to develop a better force of contraction.[3]

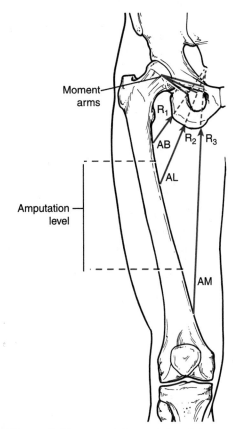

Figure 5-42. Line of force of the adductor magnus (AM), adductor longus (AL), and adductor brevis (AB). Note the relative length of the moment arms for each of these muscles. A short residual limb leaves only the adductor brevis attaching normally to the femur. A longer residual limb leaves both the adductor brevis and the adductor longus. The adductor magnus has the longest moment arm, and its normal attachment to the femur is lost in both cases.

hamstrings generate better hip extension forces, which are needed to control the prosthetic knee. If the socket was set in extension, the line of force would tend to pass behind the knee when standing. This would tend to make the knee buckle or flex. The individual with a transfemoral amputation lacks quadriceps control, so stability must be built into the alignment of the prosthesis.

In the frontal plane, the socket is also typically adducted 7°. While it is easy to comprehend how a transfemoral amputation affects the hamstrings and rectus femoris as two joint muscles, the effect on the adductors may be less obvious. The adductor magnus has the longest moment arm, followed by the longus, and then the brevis (Fig. 5-42). Remember that the muscles with the longest moment arm generate the most torque. The shorter the residual limb, the more loss of adductor torque.[14] The

Dynamic Alignment

As with the transtibial prosthesis, the force applied to the socket by the residual limb is not typically along the same line as the GRFV. Therefore, angular rotation tends to occur between the socket and residual limb. An inset (medially placed) foot applies pressures to the same part of the residual limb as described with the transtibial prosthesis, that is, on the proximal medial residual limb and the distal lateral residual limb. If the foot is outset (laterally placed), the prosthesis will exert more pressure on the proximal lateral residual limb and the distal medial residual limb. The greater the inset or outset, the greater the tendency to change the angular relationship to the residual limb.[3] Dynamic alignment, using an adjustment shank or adjustable prosthesis, may be necessary for an individual to decrease rotation of the prosthesis, improve comfort, or correct other gait deviations.

Normal Gait

Before a practitioner can select an appropriate orthosis or prosthesis to facilitate ambulation for an individual or correct accompanying gait deviations, the practitioner must first have a good understanding of normal gait. Secondly, an understanding of common gait deviations and their causes is very important.

Gait can be defined as the translation of the body from one point to another by way of bipedal motion.[15] In both walking and running there is a rhythmic displacement of body parts that maintains the person in constant forward progression.[16] Gait can be described from both a kinematic and a kinetic standpoint.

Kinematics of Gait

Kinematically speaking, we can use distance variables, time variables, the sequence of events, the functional significance of the events, and joint angles or range of motion to describe gait.

Distance Variables

First, we will look at the definitions of the distance variables. A pictorial representation of these variables is found in Figure 5-43. Stride length is the linear distance between the point of initial contact by one foot to the next point of initial contact of the same foot.[1,17] In normal gait, typically the distance from heel contact to ipsilateral heel contact is measured. Therefore, there is a right stride length and a left stride length in normal gait. These should be approximately equal. According to Perry, normal stride length averages 1.41 meters, with men having a higher average (1.46 meters) than women (1.28 meters). Children reach nearly an adult stride length at about 11 years of age.[17] Step length is the distance between the sequential points of initial contact by opposite feet.[1,17] Again, there is a right and a left step length. The normal width of the base of sup-

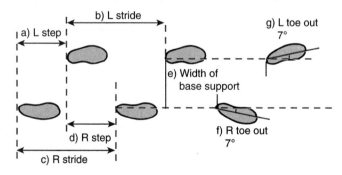

Figure 5-43. Distance variables of gait. *a*, Left step length. *b*, Left stride length. *c*, Right stride length. *d*, Right step length. *e*, Width of base of support. *f*, Right toe-out. *g*, Left toe-out.

Table 5-1. Sequence of Events in Gait Cycle

Stance Period

Phase	Description	Percentage of Gait Cycle
Initial contact	When the foot hits the ground	0–2
Loading response	Until the opposite foot leaves the ground	0–10
Midstance	Until the body is over and just ahead of the support	10–30
Terminal stance	To toe-off	30–50
Preswing	Just after heel-off to toe-off	50–60

Swing Period

Phase	Description	Percentage of Gait Cycle
Initial swing	Until maximum knee flexion occurs	60–73
Midswing	Until the tibia is vertical	73–87
Terminal swing	Until initial contact	87–100

port ranges between 1 and 5 inches, averaging 3 inches.[1,17] The width of the base of support is the linear distance from the center of the heel of one foot to the center of the other heel. Another parameter to measure is the degree of **toe out**. This is the angle formed by the line of progression of the foot and the intersection of a line drawn from the second toe to the center of the heel. The normal toe out is about 7° at normal walking speed. The angle decreases as the speed of walking increases.[1]

Time Variables

The time variables include the time it takes to complete a stride, the stride duration, and the time it takes to complete a step, the step duration. **Cadence** is another time variable. Cadence is defined as the number of steps per unit of time (either a second or minute).[1] If the steps are shorter, the cadence increases at a given velocity. The average cadence for men is about 100 steps per minute and for women about 116 steps per minute.[1] When the cadence reaches about 180 steps per minute, it represents running rather than walking. The mechanics of running are described in Chapter 14.

The **velocity** of walking can be defined as the speed of walking in a designated direction.[17] Practically speaking, the velocity and the speed of gait are the same, since typically we walk in a forward direction. This rate of linear forward motion is equal to the cadence times the step length, or the distance walked per unit time. The speed of gait is measured in centimeters per minute and is increased by either increasing the cadence or increasing the step length.[1] The normal, comfortable walking speed is referred to as *free speed*. *Slow speed* and *fast speed* are just that, slower than the free speed and faster than free speed, respectively.[1]

Sequence of Events

Gait can be described by looking at the sequence of events that occur during a stride or one **gait cycle.** There are two primary periods of gait: stance and swing. Each of these can be subdivided into several phases. *Stance* is the period of gait in which some part of the foot is on the ground, and *swing* occurs when the foot is in the air. Stance makes up 60% of the gait cycle, and swing represents the other 40%. The sequence of events of the gait cycle are summarized in Table 5-1 and Figure 5-44.

Normal Gait Cycle
Right Limb is Reference

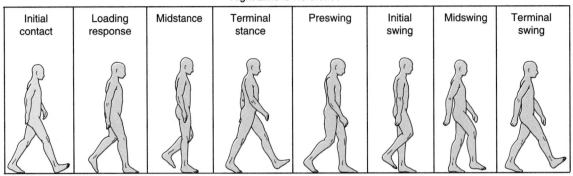

| Initial contact | Loading response | Midstance | Terminal stance | Preswing | Initial swing | Midswing | Terminal swing |

Figure 5-44. Phases of the gait cycle.

As the right limb is going through the gait cycle, the left is going through its own gait cycle. There is a period of time when both lower extremities are in contact with the ground. This represents double stance, or double support. **Double stance** occurs during loading response on one side and preswing on the other. Each of these phases equals 10% of the gait cycle, so the total time in double stance equals 20% of the gait cycle. **Single stance**, or support, is the time when only one extremity is on the ground. In single stance the opposite limb is in swing, so single stance must also equal 40% of the gait cycle. Table 5-2 demonstrates what is happening on the left side as the reference limb on the right is going through the gait cycle.

Functional Significance of Events

Perry refers to three basic tasks of gait:[17]

- Weight acceptance
- Single-limb support
- Limb advancement

The relationship of these tasks to the periods and phases of gait are summarized in Table 5-3. The primary accomplishments during weight acceptance are stability, forward progression, and shock absorption. Weight acceptance includes the phases of initial contact and loading response. During these phases, the body pivots over the heel, the **heel rocker** (Fig.5-45A). Single-limb support includes midstance and terminal stance. During these

Table 5-2. Summary of Gait Phases

R	0–10% (10%)	10–30% (20%)	30–50% (20%)			50–60% (10%)	60–73% (13%)	73–87% (14%)	87–100% (13%)
R	Initial & loading	Midstance	Terminal stance			Preswing	Initial swing	Midswing	Terminal swing
L	Preswing	Initial swing	Midswing		Terminal swing	Initial & loading	Midstance	Terminal stance	
L	0–10% (10%)	10–23% (13%)	23–37% (14%)	37–50% (13%)		50–60% (10%)	60–80% (20%)	80–100% (20%)	

Key: Swing ▓   Stance ☐

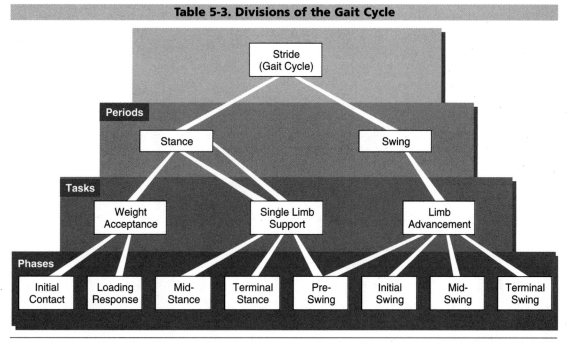

Table 5-3. Divisions of the Gait Cycle

Reprinted with permission from Perry, J. (1992). Gait analysis normal and pathological function (Table 2.1). Thorofare, NJ: Slack.

phases, the body pivots over the ankle, the **ankle rocker** (Fig. 5-45b), continuing the forward progression. Preswing and all of the swing phases constitute limb advancement. In preswing, the body pivots over the forefoot, the **forefoot rocker** (Fig. 5-45c). The rockers assist the progression of the body over the supporting foot.[17] During swing-limb advancement, in addition to moving the limb forward, the major accomplishment is foot clearance.

Range of Motion

The range of motion of the hip, knee, ankle, and subtalar joints accompanying the phases of gait can be found in Table 5-4. For normal gait to occur, the hip must be able to move from 10° of extension to 30° of flexion. Maximum hip extension occurs in preswing, and maximum hip flexion occurs in terminal swing. The knee moves through a range of approximately 0° to 60° of flexion. Maximum extension is typically

at initial contact but may occur again in terminal stance; maximum flexion occurs during initial swing. The ankle traverses 20° of plantarflexion to 10° of dorsiflexion. Maximum

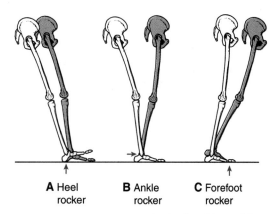

Figure 5-45. Pivoting over the heel, ankle, and forefoot. **A.** Heel rocker. **B.** Ankle rocker. **C.** Forefoot rockers. (Adapted from Perry, J. (1992). *Gait analysis normal and pathological function.* Thorofare, NJ: Slack.)

Table 5-4. Phases of Gait: Joint Position and Moments

	Initial Contact	Loading Response	Midstance	Terminal Stance	Preswing	Initial Swing	Midswing	Terminal Swing
% of gait cycle	0–2%	0–10%	10–30%	30–50%	50–60%	60–73%	73–87%	87–100%
Rocker phase		Heel rocker	Ankle rocker	Ankle rocker	Forefoot rocker			
Hip moment	Flexion	Flexion	Flexion to extension; adduction	Extension; adduction	Extension			
Hip angle	30° flexion	30–25° flexion	25° flexion to 0°	0° to 10–20° extension	10–20° extension	to 20° flexion	to 30° flexion	30° flexion
Pelvis position	Left backward rotation; neutral lateral tilt	Left backward rotation; neutral lateral tilt	Neutral rotation; neutral coronal; left pelvic drop	Moving into left forward rotation; left pelvic drop	Left forward rotation; neutral lateral tilt	Left forward rotation; right pelvic drop	Neutral coronal; right pelvic drop	Left backward rotation; right pelvic drop
Knee moment	Extension; valgus	Flexion; valgus	Flexion to extension	Extension	Extension to flexion	Gravity extending; acceleration	Gravity linear distracting	Gravity flexing; deceleration
Knee angle	0°	0–15° flexion	15° flexion to 5° flexion	5° flexion to 0°	0° to 30° flexion	to 60° flexion	to 30° flexion	0°
Ankle moment	Plantarflexion; valgus	Plantarflexion; valgus	Plantarflexion to dorsiflexion	Dorsiflexion	Dorsiflexion	Gravity plantarflexing	Gravity plantarflexing	Gravity plantarflexing
Ankle angle	Neutral	0 to 15° plantarflexion	15° plantarflexion to 5–10° dorsiflexion	5° dorsiflexion to 0°	0 to 20° plantarflexion	10° plantarflexion	Neutral	Neutral
Subtalar position	Supination	Rapid pronation	In pronation but supinating	Neutral to supination	Supination	Supination to neutral	Neutral	Neutral to supination

plantarflexion occurs during preswing at toe-off, and maximum dorsiflexion occurs during midstance as the tibia moves over the foot. Some 4 to 6° of pronation and 4 to 6° of supination are required for normal gait. Peak pronation occurs in midstance, and peak supination in early preswing. About 55° of extension is required at the metatarsophalangeal (MTP) joints in preswing. If these ranges are not available at each of the joints of the lower extremity, gait deviations will result.[1]

Other Factors Affecting Gait

Many factors besides joint mobility can affect normal gait. Among these are age, anthropometrics, strength, cardiovascular status, habit, psychological status, type of clothing, and footwear. The effect of age is poignantly clear when comparing the unsteady gait of a baby first learning to walk with the mature gait of a young adult. Young children have a higher cadence than adults, and many geriatric adults have a slower free speed. Psychological state, including depression and the fear of falling, is known to affect gait. Both of these states tend to cause a decrease in speed. The effect of clothing on gait is most obvious in the limited step length when a woman wears a tight skirt. Slippery soles on shoes alter the step length, and heavy boots increase the energy expenditure. Anthropometric characteristics such as height and size may affect the stride length and other variables of gait. Height, size, and distribution of mass also affect the location of the COG.

Movement of the Center of Gravity

As the body moves through space, the COG describes a sinusoidal path in both the sagittal and horizontal planes. In the vertical plane, the COG is at a low during the two double-stance phases and at a high at right midstance and again at left midstance. Horizontally, COG is farthest right at right midstance, in the middle during the two double-stance phases, and farthest left at left midstance. The COG in a typi-cal adult male displaces about 2.3 cm in each direction, for a total 4.6 cm displacement.[17]

Kinetics of Gait

The primary external forces acting on the body in normal gait are gravity and the ground reaction force. Muscles function to counteract these forces and to accomplish the forward progression of the body.

Gravity

The greater the excursion of the COG, the greater the muscular effort needed, and the greater the energy required. Historically, several factors have been described that diminish the excursion of the COG, thereby increasing the efficiency of gait.[1,16] Limitation of the side-to-side excursion of the COG relies on keeping the feet closer together. The angulation between the shaft of the femur and the head and neck, as well as the angle between the femur and tibia, helps to keep the supporting feet closer to the midline. If the femur and tibia were not angled in this manner, the feet would be farther apart, and an individual would have to shift his or her body laterally for the limb to accept the weight.[17,18] There is a tradeoff between energy cost and stability. A wider base of support would increase stability but result in an increase in the side-to-side excursion of the COG and thus increase energy cost.

When the right limb is in single support, the left is in swing. During swing of the left limb, the pelvis drops about 4° on the left side. This has the effect of keeping the COG from going as high during midstance. Knee flexion of the stance limb also helps to keep the COG from rising higher. Rotation of the pelvis in the horizontal plane throughout the gait cycle helps to keep the COG from dropping lower. As the swing limb moves forward, the pelvis rotates forward on that side, extending the reach of the limb. (*Note:* forward rotation of the pelvis on the left is accomplished by medial hip rotation on the right, and vice versa.) Without the pelvic rotation, the femur would have to flex more to get the same reach of the limb. The consequence would be a lower COG.

Motion of the ankle/foot complex also plays a very important role in limiting the vertical excursion of the COG. If you observe the axis of the ankle joint from the side, it is high at initial contact, lowers as the foot is flat, and then rises again in preswing. Remember that the COG is lowest during double support (loading response and preswing). When the knee flexes at initial contact, the ankle joint axis is higher. After initial loading, the knee begins to extend, raising the COG, but the foot is on the ground, and the ankle joint axis is lower. In preswing, the knee is again flexing, which would lower the COG. However, the heel comes off the ground and the ankle axis rises. The net result is a smoothing of the motion of the COG.

While some studies[17-19] have questioned the validity of some of these factors, the fact remains that the greater the excursion of the COG, the more muscular effort needed and the more energy required for gait. Lack of motion at one of the lower extremity joints, whether from deformity, application of an orthosis, or the design of a prosthesis, and lack of muscular control will affect the ability to modulate the motion of the COG.

Ground Reaction Force

The ground reaction force plays a large role in gait. The magnitude and direction of the torques created by the GRFV change as the segments of the body move through the gait cycle. The lower-extremity joint angles and the moments created by the GRFV throughout the gait cycle are summarized in Table 5-4. See Figure 5-46 for a diagrammatic representation of the effects of the GRFV in the sagittal plane. Muscles function to counteract the ground reaction forces (as well as gravity) and to accomplish the forward progression of the body. When muscles cannot function to counter the GRFV or gravity, the application of an orthosis

may be appropriate to control the limb position in relation to the force vector.

Role of Muscles

A brief discussion of the role of the muscles is needed to understand normal gait and its implication for orthoses and prostheses.

Period of Stance

At initial contact, the critical event for normal gait is heel contact first. The ankle should be in neutral dorsi/plantarflexion, with some supination upon hitting the ground. A plantarflexion moment then occurs that is controlled eccentrically by the anterior tibialis. At the hip, a flexor moment exists at initial contact. To restrain this moment, both the hamstrings and gluteus maximus are active. At the knee, there is an extensor moment at initial contact. Both the quadriceps and hamstrings are active to ensure a stable knee for accepting the weight of the body. In the frontal plane, there is a valgus thrust at the knee upon initial contact. The gracilis, vastus medialis, and semitendinosus act medially to help control this thrust.[1] A pronation moment exists in the foot because the GRFV falls on the lateral aspect of the heel. The posterior tibialis comes in to control this pronation moment. Pronation is the loose-packed position of the subtalar joint. When the subtalar joint is pronated, the midtarsal joint is free to pronate or supinate to adjust to the ground surface in the loading phase.

Once the foot hits the ground, loading response occurs. In this phase, the critical events are hip stability and controlled knee flexion and plantarflexion for shock absorption. The moment at the knee changes to a flexion moment. The hamstring action decreases, and the gluteus maximus action increases to continue hip control and to extend the hip. The quadriceps is needed to control the knee flexion eccentrically. At the ankle, the dorsiflexors continue to control the plantarflexion moment, and they also start to advance the tibia over the

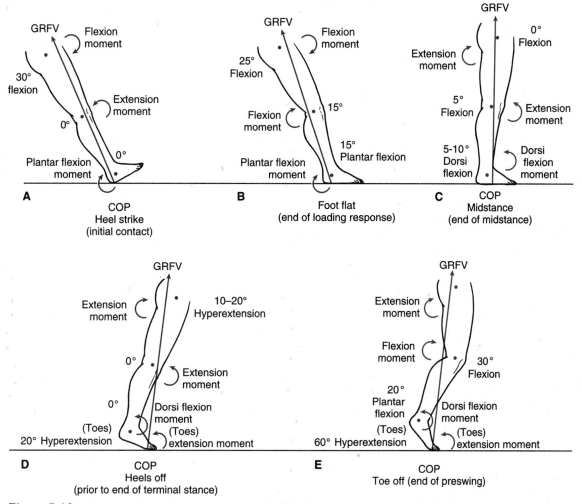

Figure 5-46. GRFVs. **A.** At initial contact. **B.** At end of loading response. **C.** At end of midstance. **D.** At end of terminal stance. **E.** At end of preswing. Note the relationship of the GRFV to the axis of the hip, knee, and ankle in each phase. Since the GRFV is not passing through the axes of the joints, a torque or moment is created. (Adapted from Levangie, P. K., & Norkin, C. C. (2001). *Joint structure and function, A comprehensive analysis* (3rd ed.). Philadelphia: F. A. Davis.)

foot. In the frontal plane, the gluteus medius and minimus are both active to provide pelvic stability. The foot is rapidly pronating. Since the limb is in closed chain, the pronation imposes medial rotation on the tibia. The posterior tibialis continues to control the pronation eccentrically. In addition, the biceps femoris works at the knee to control the medial rotation of the tibia, imposed by the pronation.

From the end of loading response to the end of midstance, the GRFV changes in orientation at the hip, knee, and ankle. In other words, it goes from anterior of the hip to posterior, from posterior to the knee to anterior, and from posterior to the ankle to anterior. (Additional information on the GRFV is included in Chapters 8 and 9 on transtibial and transfemoral components.) The hip extensors become less active as the vector moves posteriorly to the hip axis. In early midstance, the quadriceps is active as it extends the knee, but it becomes less active as the vector passes anterior to the knee. At the ankle, passive dorsiflexion would occur. The critical event in this phase is controlled tibial advancement. The gastrocsoleus serves as this control. This has the added benefit of maintaining the knee extension by keeping the tibia from going forward. If the knee is flexed, the vector would likely shift behind the knee. In the frontal plane, the gluteus medius and minimus are functioning on the stance side to prevent the pelvis from dropping too far on the swing-limb side. These muscles, along with the tensor fascia lata, initiate the forward rotation of the pelvis to assist in the swing-limb advancement. The foot, although pronated, begins to supinate. The peroneus longus comes into play to stabilize the first ray on the ground, keeping it from lifting with the supinating foot.

In terminal stance, the hip extension moment increases, and the tensor fascia lata helps to restrain the extension at the hip. The GRFV is moving farther over the front of the foot. The gastrocsoleus contracts strongly to stabilize the advancing tibia and to raise the heel. The heel rise is a critical event in this phase. In the frontal plane, the body begins to "fall" toward the opposite limb, and the adductor magnus fires to control the fall. The foot continues into supination. With the subtalar joint in the closed packed position of supination, the midtarsal joint follows, helping to create a more rigid foot lever.

In preswing, the GRFV passes posterior to the axis of the hip. The adductor longus and rectus femoris work to counter this vector and to initiate the hip flexion needed for swing. At the ankle, the gastrocsoleus decreases activity, allowing the tibia to advance. As a result of the advancement of the tibia over the foot, the vec-

tor at the knee moves posterior to the knee, and the knee flexes. This passive knee flexion is a critical event. The rectus femoris prevents the knee from flexing too much. In the frontal plane, the body continues to fall toward the other limb, with continuing adductor restraint.

Period of Swing

During swing, there is no longer a GRFV, because the foot is not in contact with the ground. Gravity is the primary external force consideration. Throughout swing, there is a tendency for the pelvis to drop on the swing side. You will remember from the discussion on the stance phases that the abductors of the stance limb are responsible for countering this frontal plane moment. During initial swing, the critical event is hip flexion to 15° and knee flexion to 60°. The iliopsoas works to flex the hip and accelerate the thigh. The sartorius, gracilis, and short head of the biceps, particularly, function to flex the knee. The sartorius also assists the hip flexors. At the ankle, gravity would tend to plantarflex the foot. This is countered by the muscles of the anterior compartment of the leg. This phenomena continues throughout all the swing phases. Muscle action countering gravity is particularly critical in midswing. Without the muscles of the anterior compartment, the toe would tend to drag on the ground. The other critical event in midswing is hip flexion to 25°. To accomplish this, the hip flexors continue to contract. In midswing, the knee passively extends with the relaxation of the knee flexors. The lower leg acts much like a pendulum.

In terminal swing, the critical event is knee extension to prepare for a stable landing. The knee extensors function at the end of this phase to ensure that the knee is extended. Deceleration of the limb is also needed to prepare for accepting the body weight. To accomplish this, the hip extensors contract. The posterior part of the gluteus medius may contract to rotate the femur laterally, keeping the toe pointed more straight ahead. At this point, the cycle would start again as the foot contacts the ground.

Common Gait Deviations

Each of the most common causes of gait deviations are to be considered. These are

- Muscle weakness
- Deformity (bony or soft tissue)
- Impaired control including sensory loss
- Fear or anxiety
- Pain
- Ill-fitting or poorly aligned orthosis or prosthesis

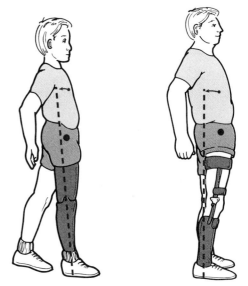

Figure 5-48. Posterior trunk lean altering the position of the GRFV in relation to the hip joint axis. This creates more extension moment at the hip and increases hip joint stability.

Weakness

Gait deviations due to muscle weakness are numerous. Frequently, with muscle weakness individuals may try to rearrange the segments of the kinematic chain or the position of the trunk to manipulate the position of the LOG or the GRFV in relation to the joint axes. It is common to see individuals lean the trunk to make up for lower-extremity weakness. The direction of the lean depends on the weakness present. Weakness of the gluteus medius may result in a lateral trunk lean toward the side of weakness. Leaning the trunk toward the weakness brings the LOG closer to the joint axis (Fig. 5-47). This decreases the moment-arm associated with the forces. A shorter moment arm means less torque, and in turn, the muscle does not have to generate as much force to counter the torque. Using the same premise, a person with hip extensor weakness may lean the trunk posteriorly (Fig. 5-48). In this case, leaning posteriorly may actually change the GRFV from a flexor moment to an extensor moment, obviating the

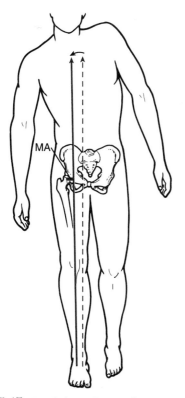

Figure 5-47. Trunk lean altering the position of the GRFV in relation to the hip joint axis and decreasing the moment arm at the hip.

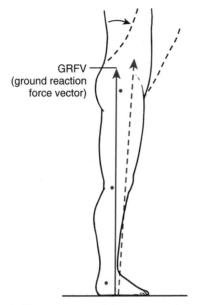

GRFV
(ground reaction
force vector)

Figure 5-49. Anterior trunk lean moving the position of the support line and GRFV more anterior in relation to the knee joint axis. This creates more extension moment at the knee and increases knee stability.

Weakness around the ankle joint may also cause common gait deviations. Weak dorsiflexors might result in foot-slap on loading if they are unable to control the plantarflexion moment eccentrically. In swing, weak or absent dorsiflexors would result in toe-drop. Weakness of the plantarflexors shows up in two places. One, there is a lack of control of the advancing tibia in stance, and excessive knee flexion is seen. Second, there would be loss of heel-off for terminal stance. Excessive pronation on loading and throughout midstance may result from weakness of the posterior tibialis. Weakness of the peroneals results in excessive varus at the subtalar joint. There is a loss of some stabilization of the forefoot during stance, allowing the medial foot to lift off the ground as the foot is supinating.

need for the gluteus maximus to work. An anterior trunk lean is more often due to weakness in the quadriceps than the hip flexors. Leaning the trunk forward can move the GRFV anterior to the knee to give an extension moment, adding stability to the knee (Fig. 5-49). Generally, with weak quadriceps or an unstable prosthetic knee, the individual will try to limit the amount of knee flexion during stance.

Weak muscles can cause other common postural and gait deviations. For example, weak abductors on the stance limb can result in increased pelvic drop on the swing side. This is relative adduction of the stance limb and relative abduction of the swing limb. Another example related to the pelvis is an exaggerated lordosis or an anterior pelvic tilt that may result from weakness of the abdominals. The abdominals and hip extensors normally work as a force couple to tilt the pelvis posteriorly. If either are weak, it essentially allows the pelvis to "fall" into an anterior pelvic tilt.

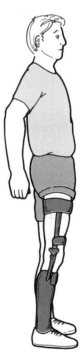

Figure 5-50. Long limb created by a manual lock on an orthosis.

Orthoses are often used to help compensate for weak muscles. One example is an orthosis with a posterior stop used to prevent the excessive plantarflexion that results from weakness of the dorsiflexors. The use of an orthosis with a locking knee joint to compensate for weak quadriceps is another illustration (Fig. 5-50).

Individuals with amputations are also subject to gait deviations due to muscle weakness. Weakness of the residual limb with poor muscle tone can result in rotation of the soft tissue and prosthesis over the underlying bone. The consequence might be a **whip** at toe-off, or excessive foot rotation. Additional gait deviations of individuals with amputations are explored in Chapters 8 and 9 on transtibial and transfemoral components.

Deformity

Deformity is another source of gait deviations. Many deformities create a leg length difference. Whether the difference is a true anatomic leg length discrepancy or something that effectively creates a leg length difference, walking may be affected. A short limb can be created by a hip flexion contracture, a knee flexion contracture, fracture healing, congenital or growth factors, etc. Remember that if one lower extremity is short, the other is essentially long, and vice versa. A limb can be effectively lengthened in several ways. At the ankle, insufficient dorsiflexion, as occurs with weakness of the dorsiflexors or contracture of the plantarflexors, effectively lengthens the limb. At the hip and knee, insufficient flexion can prevent shortening the limb in swing, thereby creating a "long" limb.

Whatever the cause of the long limb, it is more difficult to clear the ground during swing. An individual has several options to accommodate the long limb (Fig. 5-51). One is to raise the pelvis on the swing side, by either hip hiking or by a lateral trunk lean opposite the long limb. The long limb can be circumducted in swing to get clearance, or alternatively, the limb can be cleared by excessively flexing the hip and knee. An individual may also choose to vault on the shorter limb side to clear the long limb. Going up on the toe on the stance side es-

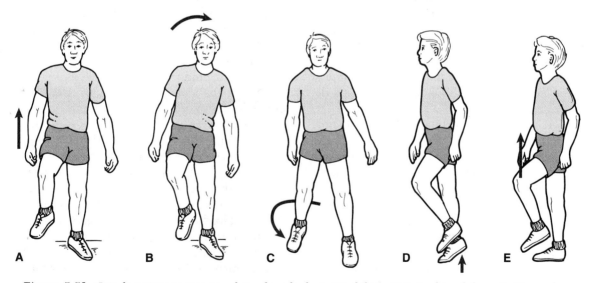

Figure 5-51. Gait deviations to accommodate a long limb. **A.** Hip hiking. **B.** Lateral trunk lean. **C.** Circumduction. **D.** Vaulting. **E.** Excessive hip and knee flexion.

sentially increases the length of the shorter limb. In double stance, a wide walking base may help accommodate a longer limb. For smaller differences in length, an individual may accommodate by pronating the foot on the long side and supinating the foot on the short side.

In the sagittal plane, hip flexion, knee flexion, and plantarflexion contractures are more common than hip extension, knee extension, and dorsiflexion contractures. A hip flexion contracture of 15° or less may be accommodated by an increased anterior pelvic tilt or increased lumbar lordosis.[17] An individual with more contracture might lean the trunk forward. An anterior lean shifts the COG forward and necessitates greater extensor muscle activity during stance. If the trunk maintains more-normal vertical alignment, then, due to the closed kinematic chain, the knee typically flexes to compensate for the flexed hip. This requires increased quadriceps activity during stance. Progressing down the chain, when increased knee flexion exists, to obtain foot-flat, there will be excessive dorsiflexion as might be seen with a crouched gait. An individual may also accommodate for the excessive hip and knee flexion by plantarflexing. With this option the heel will not touch the ground. A knee flexion contracture would result in similar compensations at the foot during stance and would also result in hip flexion. A knee flexion contracture may limit the reach of the limb at the end of terminal swing, resulting in decreased step length.

At the ankle, a plantarflexion contracture may cause several gait deviations. The effective lengthening of the limb from a plantarflexion contracture is discussed above. In the presence of a significant plantarflexion contracture, an individual may be forced to land on the toe or flat foot rather than the heel at initial contact. If the foot is flat, the knee will hyperextend because of the posteriorly directed tibia, as was seen in Figure 5-5. Limited dorsiflexion at the talocrural joint may also lead to excessive pronation or calcaneal valgus during stance.

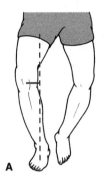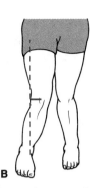

Figure 5-52. GRFV in the presence of varus and valgus at the knee resulting in **A.** increased varus moment and **B.** increased valgus moment.

When more dorsiflexion is needed than the talocrural joint can provide, the subtalar and midtarsal joints often attempt to compensate through pronation. Pronation is considered a triplanar motion, which includes eversion, abduction, and dorsiflexion components. Therefore the degrees of dorsiflexion gained by pronating add to the dorsiflexion available at the talocrural joint.

In the frontal plane, gait can be affected by deformities of varus or valgus at the knee, such as those seen with osteoarthritis. Varus and valgus deformities can alter the width of the base of support. In some cases, varus and valgus deformities at the knee can result in varus and valgus deformities of the calcaneus and forefoot as the individual adjusts the foot position to get the foot flat on the floor. The moment created by the GRFV passing through a joint with a varus or valgus deformity is greater than that in a normally aligned joint (Fig. 5-52). This increased moment tends to worsen the deformity and stress the collateral ligaments of the knee or the ankle. Lax ligaments might also lead to a valgus or varus deformity. Disturbed loading of the joint surfaces may result from varus and valgus deformities. A lateral trunk lean may help to unload the medial compartment with a varus knee deformity. Conversely, a lateral trunk lean (as seen with hip abductor weakness) may create a valgus deformity at the knee.[17] An orthosis may be used to counter the moments of gravity or the GRFV, thereby preventing the deformity from worsening. For example, an unloader orthosis as discussed in Chapter 15 is designed to alleviate the varus moment.[12] Frontal-plane deformities at the hip tend to be contractures of the abductors or adductors. Contractures in this plane can result in alteration of the base of support, circumduction, or lateral trunk lean. Deformities of scoliosis may result in pelvic obliquity in the coronal plane. The hip on the low side is in more abduction, and the hip on the high side is adducted more. This may result in abnormalities in walking.

In the horizontal plane, contractures can occur in the medial or lateral rotators of the hip. These contractures can affect the degree of toe-in or toe-out. Rotation contractures will affect the degree of forward and backward pelvic rotation. A right medial rotation contracture would limit the left backward rotation of the pelvis, while a right lateral rotation contracture would limit the left forward rotation of the pelvis (Fig. 5-53). As discussed above in this chapter, these motions help to give adequate step length without excessive movement of the COG. Rotary deformities at the hips can also result in pronation or supination gait deviations because of the obligatory motion in the closed kinematic chain. The opposite is also true. Deviations of pronation or supination can result in gait deviations affecting rotations at the hips. These deviations may be even more exaggerated with running. See Chapter 14 for a discussion on the use of these orthotics to correct some of the deviations in this plane.

Impaired Control and Sensory Loss

Pathologic states involving either upper or lower motor units can cause gait deviations. Central nervous system lesions as in cerebral palsy, cerebral vascular accident, or spinal cord injury also affect gait. In fact, in some instances, there is such significant paralysis or lack of control that gait is impossible. In other instances, orthoses can compensate for the loss of voluntary control of the muscles. The level of a spinal cord lesion is critical for determining functional ambulation. Lesions in the lower thoracic spine may allow household ambulation with the use of orthoses and assistive devices.[22] Adults are unlikely to have func-

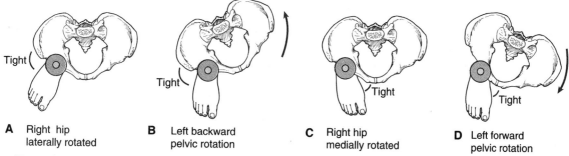

A Right hip laterally rotated **B** Left backward pelvic rotation **C** Right hip medially rotated **D** Left forward pelvic rotation

Figure 5-53. Relationship of hip rotational contractures to pelvic forward and backward rotation. A. Hip lateral rotation, pelvis in frontal plane. B. Hip lateral rotation with foot pointing straight ahead results in left backward rotation of the pelvis. If the medial rotators are tight, lateral rotation is limited, and in this case, the left backward rotation of the pelvis would be limited (unable to assume the position of B). C. Hip medial rotation, pelvis in frontal plane. D. Hip medial rotation with foot pointing straight ahead results in left forward rotation of the pelvis. If the lateral rotators are tight, medial rotation is limited, and in this case, the left forward rotation of the pelvis would be limited (unable to assume the position of D).

tional ambulation without the hip flexors that are innervated by lumbar segments L1 through L4. A spinal cord lesion at L1-2 results in loss of position sense to the lower extremity, including the hip. To maintain an upright position, an exaggerated lordosis and passive hip extension are typically used. This is not possible if there is a hip flexion contracture or if overrecruitment of the flexor muscles prevents hip extension.

An individual with a spinal cord lesion at L3-4 will typically have hip flexor function.[22,23] However, this lesion classically results in loss of everything with an L4 innervation and below. There is loss of hip extension musculature and loss of all foot control, including the anterior tibialis. Orthosis control of the foot and ankle is needed not only because of the motor loss, but also because foot and ankle sensation and proprioception are severely impaired. Development of contractures of the hip flexors, knee flexors, and plantarflexors would make it difficult to use the passive hip extension for stabilization of the hips.

A spinal cord lesion at L5-S1 spares the anterior tibialis and quadriceps. However, there is still involvement of the gluteus maximus and medius and the gastrocsoleus. As a result, hip extensor and ankle plantarflexion stability during stance is decreased. A calcaneal deformity is likely to develop because of the muscle imbalance. Stabilization of the ankle with an orthosis to restrict dorsiflexion will allow the patient to use trunk lordosis to lock the hips.

After a cerebral vascular accident, many individuals will exhibit abnormal movement patterns. The gait deviations observed will depend on the nature of the movement patterns. With what has been traditionally called a flexor synergy, there is likely to be an increased anterior tilt, along with excessive hip and knee flexion and excessive dorsiflexion and valgus in the swing phase. With an extensor synergy, a posterior pelvic tilt occurs along with excessive hip and knee extension and excessive plantarflexion and varus. In general, central nervous sys-

tem involvement, whether from cerebral palsy, multiple sclerosis, cerebral vascular accident, or another disorder, may result in overrecruitment of muscles. For example, quadriceps overactivity results in excessive knee extension, peroneal overactivity leads to excessive calcaneal valgus, and adductor overactivity causes excessive adduction. This increased recruitment of muscles contributes to deviations in the phases of gait in which the muscle normally provides eccentric control or when the overactivity impedes the function of opposing muscles.

In the case of peripheral nerve damage, motor and/or sensory damage may result. Weakness or paralysis of the muscles supplied by the nerve occurs. The gait deviations that occur depend on the particular nerve injured. For example, a tibial nerve lesion would cause weakness or paralysis of the whole posterior compartment of the leg and the intrinsic muscles of the sole of the foot. The gastrocsoleus and posterior tibialis, two important muscles for normal gait would be lost.

With sensory loss and the loss of joint proprioception, the ability to know when the feet are in contact with the floor and to know where joints are in space is lost. To compensate, a person may try to look at his or her feet. However, this forward trunk lean, as we have seen, changes the GRFV and makes it more difficult for weak muscles to control the moments about the joints. Instead, the person without sensory input may walk with a wide base of support and excessive hip and knee extension to try to ensure stability of those joints. Lack of joint input may lead to either excessive varus or valgus of the foot. Speed of walking is typically slower. A person with an amputation must rely on the sensory input from the residual limb, a factor that may affect the individual's confidence in gait. Again, the cadence for individuals with amputations is lower than normal. For a person with a transtibial amputation, the average cadence is 96 steps per minute and for one with a transfemoral amputation, 70 steps per minute.

Fear and Anxiety

Typically, fear and anxiety are related to a fear of falling. As mentioned above, an increase in the base of support provides more stability. Thus, fear of falling may lead to a wide base of support. This larger base of support gives the LOG more freedom to move without exceeding the limits of the base. Another common reaction when an individual feels insecure is a decreased step length. Think of your reaction when you walk on an icy sidewalk or wet tile. Most individuals decrease the cadence and step length of their gait. With different step lengths, the components of forces acting on the heel are different (Fig. 5-54).

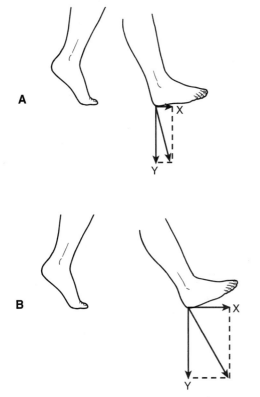

Figure 5-54. Reduced horizontal component of forces acting at the heel with a small step length, **A.** compared with the horizontal component of forces acting with a longer step length, **B.**

Fear and anxiety are particularly pertinent contributors to gait deviations among those with amputations. Vaulting may occur if there is a fear of stubbing the toe of the prosthesis during swing. If there is a lack of confidence in the prosthesis, the individual may try to get off the limb quickly, resulting in an uneven step length. Again, fear of buckling of the prosthetic knee in a transfemoral prosthesis may result in **terminal impact.** With this gait deviation, the prosthetic shank comes to a sudden stop with a visible and possibly audible impact as the knee reaches full extension.[24] Another deviation related to the fear of not having the prosthetic knee extended for heel strike is foot-slap. Foot-slap results when the individual tries to drive the prosthesis into the walking surface forcibly to ensure extension of the knee. Fear and anxiety can also cause an uneven arm swing. While this is not an exhaustive list of the gait deviations that can occur, it does demonstrate the effects that fear, anxiety, and insecurity can have on gait.

Pain

A painful limb can cause gait deviations ranging from subtle to major. The natural response to pain is to try to move away from it, to take the weight or pressure off the painful area. For example, an individual with pain of the distal residual limb may bend the trunk laterally to get more weight off the area, and an individual with pain from a high medial brim in a quadrilateral socket may abduct the limb to take the pressure off the painful area. Pain can lead to deformity, as occurs when a contracture develops because motion is painful or when a joint is swollen causing pain and limitation of motion. Additionally, pain can lead to weakness from disuse or inhibition.

With the application of orthoses or prostheses, pain can develop from the stress and strain of the device on the tissues of the body. The forces applied to the body may exceed the tolerance of the tissue, leading to pain and gait eviations. To avoid this, the principles discussed above in the chapter must be considered in fitting the orthoses and prostheses. Careful planning is required to determine the best location to apply forces and the size of the area over which the forces should be applied.

Design, Materials, Alignment, and Fit of Prostheses

The design and materials used for a prosthesis may cause gait deviations. Materials used in the prosthesis will affect deformation and the energy absorbed or returned, with a resulting impact on gait. Table 5-5 summarizes some of the deviations due to materials used in prosthetic feet.

Design, alignment, and fit of the prosthesis may also contribute to leg length differences. These leg length discrepancies may occur in a number of ways. A poorly constructed prosthesis may be too long or too short. A residual limb that fits too far into the socket or one that does not fit into the socket far enough, as occurs with too much edema or weight gain, can create a leg length discrepancy. Other discrepancies can be caused by an extension aid that is too tight, excessive friction in a prosthetic knee, or a foot set in too much plantarflexion. Each of these effectively lengthens the leg. The gait deviations that result are similar for individuals with or without amputations.

In the coronal plane, an individual with an amputation may have a valgus malalignment of the prosthesis if the shank is placed in a valgus position in relation to the thigh. As with genu valgus of the individual without an amputation, a wide base of support may result. Additionally, the individual with an amputation may experience a **lateral whip** at toe-off.

Deformities an individual with an amputation may possess are likely to have more-dire effects on gait, because the prosthesis cannot compensate for deformities in the same way as an anatomic part. For example, in the presence of a hip flexion contracture, a prosthetic foot cannot dorsiflex in the same way as an anatomic foot. This may result in instability of the prosthetic knee.

The gait deviations observed with transtibial amputations generally are

- Between heel-strike and midstance: excessive knee flexion or absent or insufficient knee flexion
- At midstance: lateral trunk bend to the prosthetic side
- Between midstance and toe-off: early knee flexion (drop-off) or delayed knee flexion
- Swing phase: foot whips and pistoning of the residual limb in the socket

Table 5-6 depicts deviations due to alignment of the transtibial prosthesis, while Table 5-7 identifies gait deviations due to alignment

Table 5-5. Deviations Due to Materials and Alignment Prosthetic Feet	
Heel cushion too hard may cause	Heel cushion too soft may cause
Foot rotation	Foot-slap
Excessive knee flexion	Absent or insufficient knee flexion
Plantar flexion bumper too hard may cause	Plantarflexion bumper too soft may cause
Foot rotation	Foot-slap
Excessive knee flexion	Absent or insufficient knee flexion
Dorsiflexion bumper too hard may cause	Dorsiflexion bumper too soft may cause
Delayed knee flexion	Early knee flexion (drop-off)

Table 5-6. Deviations Due to Alignment of the Transtibial Prosthesis

Posterior displacement of the keel may cause
  Early knee flexion (drop-off)

Anterior displacement of the keel may cause
  Delayed knee flexion

Excessive dorsiflexion of prosthetic foot may cause
  Excessive knee flexion
  Early knee flexion (drop-off)

Excessive plantarflexion of prosthetic foot may cause
  Absent or insufficient knee flexion
  Delayed knee flexion
  Circumduction

Excessive medial placement of foot may cause
  Excessive lateral thrust of prosthesis

Foot too far anterior in relation to the socket may cause
  Absent or insufficient knee flexion
  Delayed knee flexion

Foot too far posterior in relation to the socket may cause
  Excessive knee flexion
  Early knee flexion (drop-off)

Excessive posterior tilt of socket may cause
  Delayed knee flexion

Excessive anterior tilt of socket may cause
  Early knee flexion (drop-off)
  Excessive knee flexion

Table 5-7. Deviations Due to Materials and Alignment of Transfemoral Prosthesis

Insufficient friction in knee may cause
  Excessive heel rise in swing
  Vaulting
  Terminal impact
  Uneven step length

Excessive friction in knee may cause
  Insufficient heel rise in swing
  Circumduction

Extension aid too loose may cause
  Excessive heel rise
  Uneven step length

Extension aid too tight may cause
  Insufficient heel rise
  Terminal impact
  Circumduction
  Vaulting

Socket fits too loosely may cause
  Foot rotation

  Pistoning

Socket too small, causing the ischial tuberosity to rest above brim, may cause
  Circumduction

Table 5-8. Deviations Due to Components and Alignment of Orthoses

Components or Alignment	Deviation
Locks	
Knee locked	Circumduction
	Hip hiking
	Vaulting
	Posterior trunk lean
	Wide base of support
Inadequate knee lock	Excessive knee flexion
	Hyperextended knee
	Anterior trunk lean
Inadequate hip lock	Posterior trunk lean
Dorsiflexion/plantarflexion stops and assists	
Inadequate dorsiflexion stop	Delayed/absent shift of weight over forefoot
	Flat-foot contact
	Excessive knee flexion
Inadequate dorsiflexion assist	Toe drag
	Circumduction
	Hip hiking
	Vaulting
	Foot-slap
	Toe contacts first rather than heel
Inadequate plantarflexion stop	Toe-drag
	Circumduction
	Hip hiking
	Vaulting
	Foot-slap
	Toe contacts first rather than heel
	Hyperextended knee
Plantarflexion stop	Excessive knee flexion
Shoes	
Inadequate traction from sole	Flat-foot contact
Inadequate heel lift	Trunk lean
	Toe contacts first rather than heel— ipsilateral side
	Hyperextended knee—contralateral side
	Excessive knee flexion—contralateral side
	Wide base of support—contralateral side

Table 5-8. Deviations Due to Components and Alignment of Orthoses (continued)	
Components or Alignment	*Deviation*
Uprights	
Excessive height of medial upright of knee–ankle–foot orthosis (KAFO)	Lateral trunk lean Wide base of support
Uprights aligned incorrectly in horizontal plane	Excessive internal (external) rotation of limb
Bands	
Excessively concave calf band	Hyperextended knee
Lack of pelvic band or rotation control straps	Excessive internal (external) rotation of limb
Joint Position	
Excessive abduction of hip joint of hip–knee–ankle–foot orthosis (HKAFO)	Lateral trunk lean Wide base of support

or materials for the individual with a transfemoral amputation. The most common gait deviations for this individual are[24]

- Lateral trunk bending
- Wide walking base
- Circumduction
- Vaulting
- Swing-phase whips
- Foot rotation at heel-strike
- Foot-slap
- Uneven heel-rise
- Terminal impact
- Uneven step length
- Exaggerated lordosis

Most of these are discussed above. These gait deviations can also be revisited in the chapters on transtibial and transfemoral components.

Design, Materials, Alignment, and Fit of Orthoses

The design, materials, alignment, and fit of orthoses may also contribute to gait deviations. Some of these are summarized in Table 5-8.[25]

Additional information is presented in the chapter on lower extremity orthotics for the neurologic patient.

KEY POINTS

- In summary, it is important to have an understanding of biomechanical terminology and the effects of posture, gravity, and alignment related to prosthetics and orthotics.

- Many factors determine whether an individual will have normal gait.

- These factors include a combination of internal and external forces acting on the body, neural control, and mental state.

- When orthoses or prostheses are used, the principles of biomechanics must be followed to make appropriate selection of materials, fabrication, and application of the devices.

- If gait deviations occur, good problem-solving and critical-thinking skills are needed to determine if the deviation is due to habit, anatomic or physiologic factors, or the orthosis or prosthesis.

CRITICAL THINKING QUESTIONS

1. Compare and contrast open and closed kinematic chains.

2. Give examples of tension, compression, internal and external shear forces, torsion, and bending types of forces that may occur with the wearing of a prosthesis or orthosis.

3. Discuss the effects of moment arms on torque or rotary force.

4. Define

Ground reaction force vector
Stride length
Step length
Toe-out
Cadence
Gait cycle
Double and single stance
Heel, ankle, and forefoot rocker

5. Describe the six determinants of gait.

6. Give examples of how a specific muscle weakness, deformity, impaired control and sensory loss, fear and anxiety, or pain may cause a specific gait deviation.

7. Analyze how each of the common gait deviations presented in Tables 5-6, 5-7, and 5-8 may occur.

REFERENCES

1. Levangie, P. K., & Norkin, C. C. (2001). *Joint structure and function, A comprehensive analysis* (3rd ed.). Philadelphia: F. A. Davis.
2. Frankel, V. H., Burstein, A. H., & Brooks, D. B.. (1971). Biomechanics of internal derangement of the knee. Pathomechanics as determined by analysis of the instant centers of motion. *Journal of Bone and Joint Surgery, 53A,* 945.
3. Berger, N., & Fishman, S. (1998). *Lower limb prosthetics.* New York: Prosthetic Orthotic Publications.
4. Fergason, J., & Smith, D. G. (1999). Socket considerations for the patient with a transtibial amputation. *Clinical Orthopaedics and Related Research, 361,* 76–84.

5. Nordin, M., & Frankel, V. H. (2001). *Basic biomechanics of the musculoskeletal system* (3rd ed.). Philadelphia: Lippincott Williams & Wilkins.
6. Young, H. D., Freed, R. A., Sandin, T. R., & Ford, A. L. (2000). *Sears and Zemansky's university physics* (10th ed.). San Francisco: Addison-Wesley.
7. Soderberg, G. L. (1997). *Kinesiology application to pathological motion* (2nd ed.). Baltimore: Williams & Wilkins.
8. Redford, J. B., Basmajian, J. V., & Trautman, P. (1995). *Orthotics: Clinical practice and rehabilitation technology.* New York: Churchill Livingstone.
9. Nawoczenski, D. A., & Epler, M. E. (1997). *Orthotics in functional rehabilitation of the lower limb.* Philadelphia: W. B. Saunders.
10. McCormack, A. P., & Hoppenfeld, S. (2000). Forefoot fractures. In S. Hoppenfeld & V. L. Murthy (Eds.), *Treatment & rehabilitation of fractures (p. 486).* Philadelphia: Lippincott Williams & Wilkins.
11. Shurr, D. G., & Cook, T. M. (1990). *Prosthetics & orthotics.* Norwalk, CT: Appleton & Lange.
12. Crenshaw, S. J., Pollo, F. E., & Calton, E. F. (2000). Effects of lateral wedged insoles on kinetics at the knee. *Clinical Orthopaedics and Related Research, 375,* 185–192.
13. Picken, R. R. (1986). The above knee prosthesis. In L. A. Karacoloff (Ed.), *Lower extremity amputation.* Rockville, MD: Aspen.
14. Gottschalk, F. (1999). Transfemoral amputation, biomechanics and surgery. *Clinical Orthopaedics and Related Research, 361,* 15–22.
15. Gillis, M. K. (1989). Observational gait analysis. In R. M. Scully & M. R. Barnes (Eds.), *Physical therapy.* Philadelphia : J. B. Lippincott.
16. Inman, V. T., Ralston, H. J., & Todd, F. (1994). Human locomotion. In J. Rose & J. G. Gamble (Eds.), *Human walking* (2nd ed.). Baltimore: Williams & Wilkins, 1994.
17. Perry, J. (1992). *Gait analysis normal and pathological function.* Thorofare, NJ: Slack.
18. Bowker, J. H., & Michael, J. W. (1992). *Atlas of limb prosthetics. Surgical, prosthetic, and rehabilitation principles. American Academy of Orthopaedic Surgeons* (2nd ed.). Philadelphia: Mosby Year Book.
19. Gard, S. A., & Childress, D. S. (1999). The influence of stance phase knee flexion on the vertical displacement of the trunk during normal walking. *Archives of Physical Medicine and Rehabilitation, 80,* 26–32.
20. Gard, S. A., & Childress, D. S. (1997). The effect of pelvic list on the displacement of the trunk during normal walking. *Gait & Posture, 5,* 233.

21. Pandy, M. G., & Berme, N. (1989). Quantitative assessment of gait determinants during single Stance via a three dimensional model. Part I: Normal gait. *Journal of Biomechanics, 22,* 717.

22. Schmitz, T. J. (2001). Traumatic spinal cord injury. In S. B. O'Sullivan & T. J. Schmitz (Eds.), *Physical rehabilitation assessment and treatment* (4th ed., p. 899). Philadelphia: F. A. Davis.

23. Atrice, M. B., Morrison, S. A., McDowell, S. L., & Shandalov, B. (2001). Traumatic spinal cord injury. In D. A. Umpred (Ed.), *Neurological rehabilitation* (4th ed.). Philadelphia: Mosby.

24. Berger, N. (1992). Analysis of amputee gait. In J. H. Bowker & J. W. Michael (Eds.), *Atlas of limb prosthetics surgical, prosthetic, and rehabilitation principles, American Academy of Orthopaedic Surgeons* (2nd ed.). Philadelphia: Mosby Year Book.

25. Edelstein, J. E. (2001). Orthotic assessment and management. In S. B. O'Sullivan & T. J. Schmitz (Eds.), *Physical rehabilitation assessment and treatment* (4th ed., p. 1048). Philadelphia: F. A. Davis.

Prostheses

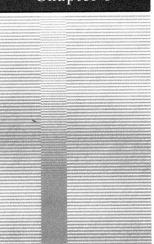

Chapter 6

CLINICAL USE OF DRESSINGS AND BANDAGES

Objectives

1. Compare and contrast the indications for, and advantages and disadvantages of, various types of residual limb dressings
2. Apply the principles of proper wrapping of transtibial and transfemoral residual limbs
3. Compare and contrast the advantages and disadvantages of elastic bandages and shrinkers
4. Describe the components of, and indications for, the immediate postoperative prosthesis (IPOP)
5. Explain methods of skin care for both the residual and sound limb to a patient with an amputation
6. Describe ways to care for the prosthetic socket, insert, shrinkers, and socks

This chapter is divided into the following sections:

An integral part of the care of a patient with an amputation is bandaging of the residual limb. Some physical therapists are also involved in the application of dressings used soon after amputation. *The Guide to Physical Therapist Practice* in "Practice Pattern, Impaired Motor Function, Muscle Performance, Range of Motion, Gait, Locomotion, and Balance Associated with Amputation" (4J) discusses supportive devices that have an impact on various goals and outcomes. These impacts include those on pathology (e.g., edema), on impairments (e.g., improving integumentary integrity), on functional limitations (e.g., independence in activities of daily living). and on disabilities (e.g., independent self-care).[1] This chapter discusses types of dressings, ways to achieve residual limb compression, skin care, and care of the prosthetic socket, insert, shrinkers, and socks.

♦♦♦

Dressings

Dressings can contain postoperative drainage. They also control postoperative edema and facilitate prosthetic fitting. Any delay in prosthetic fitting because of excessive edema is both frustrating and costly for the patient with an amputation and the rehabilitation team. Prospective payment and managed care emphasize the need to prevent edema and manage it in an effective and timely manner.

When the patient with an amputation is in the recumbent position, capillary pressure is 15-20 mm Hg. If the bandage results in pressures below the capillary pressure, little resistance to edema formation is provided. Conversely, if the bandage is applied too tightly, blood flow may be impeded.[2]

Goals for dressings after amputation are listed in Resource Box 6-1.

Dressings after amputation have been used for hundreds of years. Early dressings applied to the residual limb consisted of small buckets of tar used in the Peloponnesian wars, lint, sea sponges and pig's bladders.[2] Today, dressings used after amputation include soft, semirigid, rigid, air splint, and silicone liners.

Soft Dressing

The **soft dressing** consists of gauze, cotton padding, and an elastic bandage. Advantages of the soft dressing include low cost, ease of application, and easy inspection of the wound. Disadvantages of this type of dressing include

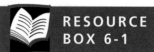

RESOURCE BOX 6-1

Goals for Dressings after Amputation

- Protect from infection
- Contain or reduce edema
- Protect the residual limb from trauma
- Provide attachment of prosthetic devices to permit early walking in some cases.

poor control of edema, slippage, inadequate trauma protection, and, if not applied evenly, creation of a tourniquet effect. Slippage over the wound and soft tissue can create pain and cause blisters. In one study, soft dressings did not contain residual limb edema after transtibial amputation, which resulted in increases in both volume and circumference.[4] Despite these disadvantages, the soft dressing is the most commonly used dressing postoperatively. A soft dressing is depicted in Figure 6-1.

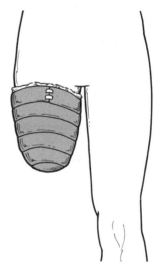

Figure 6-1. Soft dressing consisting of gauze, cotton padding, and an elastic bandage.

Semirigid Dressing

The **semirigid dressing** uses an **Unna paste bandage,** which is a combination of zinc oxide, gelatin, glycerin, and gauze. This dressing is often placed over a thin layer of gauze that covers the incision. Pads may be used to cushion bony prominences. Once applied over the residual limb, the dressing acts as a soft liner that maintains the shape of the residual limb. The semirigid dressing is changed every 2–3 days. The Unna paste bandage lacks flexibility, and folds must be avoided to prevent areas of high pressure. Consequently, the bandage must be cut periodically during application.[5] Strips of the bandage are applied from posterior to anterior, to protect the distal end of the residual limb. Figure-8 bandages and diagonal strips can be applied with more tension distally to help shape the residual limb. Finally, the bandage is covered with gauze or stockinette to protect the patient's clothing. One roll of bandage is usually sufficient for a patient with a transtibial amputation. Two rolls may be needed for a large transfemoral residual limb.[6,7] The adhesive qualities of Unna paste make the semirigid dressing self-suspending.[8] With good residual limb healing, the semirigid dressing is often used for only 2 to 3 weeks. Because of the effective containment qualities of the semirigid dressing, ambulation with full weight bearing with a prosthesis is often accomplished in 5–6 weeks.[9] Although semirigid dressings are typically made of Unna paste, they may consist of polyethylene. Swanson described a polyethylene semirigid dressing that weighs 6–7 ounces and is used with a shrinker.[10] The semirigid dressing is shown in Figure 6-2.

Advantages of the semirigid dressing include being comparatively inexpensive, having better edema control than soft dressings, and minimal **pistoning,** or up-and-down move-

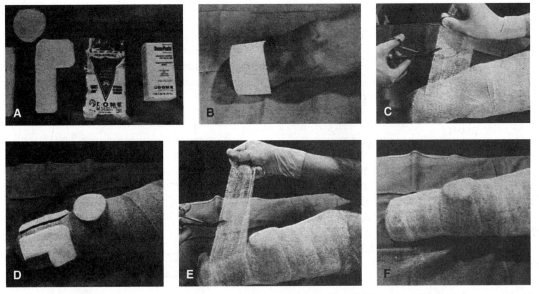

Figure 6-2. Semirigid dressing (Photo courtesy of Ghiulamila, R. I. (1972).) Semirigid dressing for postoperative fitting of below knee prosthesis. *Archives of Physical Medicine and Rehabilitation 53,* 186-189.) A. Unna paste bandages and felt pads. B. Gauze placed over the incision. C. One Unna paste bandage is applied. D. Pads are used to cushion bony prominences. E. Second Unna paste bandage is applied to hold the pads in place. F. Completed semirigid dressing.

ment of the bandage on the residual limb. Unna paste never completely hardens but has enough support to shape the residual limb. It remains secure during functional mobility and range-of-motion exercises. Disadvantages include the need for trained personnel to apply the dressing, and improper application fails to promote adequate circulation. Other disadvantages are the lack of easy inspection of the amputation site to monitor healing and its unsuitability for incontinence.

Rigid Dressing

The **rigid dressing** consists of plaster or fiberglass used in combination with felt, cotton, or polyurethane pads. Rigid dressings may be applied either in the recovery room after amputation or after the incision has healed and the sutures have been removed.

Components

Components of a rigid dressing are as follows:

- Lycra spandex sock placed directly over the residual limb
- Sterile lamb's wool
- Relief pads for the tibia, patella, and fibular head, to avoid areas of high pressure
- Elastic plaster
- Regular plaster
- Waist belt and suspension strap

The Lycra spandex sock is pulled over the distal end of the residual limb, and sterile lamb's wool is placed over the distal end to allow wound drainage. Relief pads are placed on the patella, on both medial and lateral sides of the tibial crest, and on the fibular head, to avoid abnormal pressure on these bony prominences. Elastic plaster is then applied, followed by regular plaster. A suspension strap is encased in the plaster and attached to a waist belt. Plaster is removed from the patella to avoid a pressure sore. Plaster drying time is 12–24 hours.[11]

The rigid dressing is typically changed every 3–10 days.[4] Prevention of postoperative edema

and excellent shaping of the residual limb are advantages of this dressing. Use of the rigid dressing resulted in less pain and better wound healing and edema control in patients with amputation due to arteriosclerosis.[12] The rigid dressing is shown in Figure 6-3. Disadvantages of this dressing include difficult access for inspection of the incision site, not being suited for incontinence, and the need for highly skilled personnel to apply and remove the dressing. In addition, a cast cutter is required for rigid dressing removal. Patients with precarious circulation are not candidates for rigid dressings, since the wound and surrounding area are not easily visualized. One study investigating the effects of a rigid dressing found that 9 of 12 patients with transtibial amputation due to arteriosclerosis had either pain, fever, or elevated white blood cell counts requiring removal of the rigid dressing. Five of these patients had to have revision to the transfemoral level, while the remaining four had a protracted hospital course.[13]

Immediate Postoperative Prosthesis (IPOP)

The rigid dressing may be attached to a pylon and foot to allow ambulation soon after surgery. This combination of rigid dressing, **pylon**, and

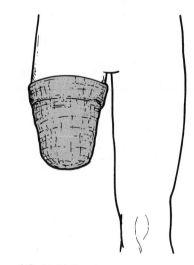

Figure 6-3. Rigid dressing.

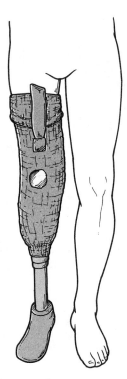

Figure 6-4. Immediate postoperative prosthesis (IPOP).

foot was developed in the late 1960s and is called an **immediate postoperative prosthesis (IPOP)**.[10] A fiberglass cast for the rigid dressing, rather than the plaster cast, reduces the weight of the IPOP. The pylon is usually made of aluminum, steel, or plastic. An IPOP can provide the psychologic and physiologic benefits attributed to walking. It can also result in a shorter hospital stay, reduce the severity of phantom pain, and assist in attaining a positive psychologic effect after amputation. With the use of an IPOP, the patient sees a pylon and artificial foot rather than an absent leg. Patients with transtibial and knee disarticulation IPOPs may weight bear, using an assistive device, 5–21 days following surgery.[14,15] The IPOP is shown in Figure 6-4. Typically, 20 lb of weight is optimal to begin weight bearing on the IPOP[16] (Fig. 6-5).

Advantages of the IPOP are listed in Resource Box 6-2. Disadvantages of the IPOP may include impaired healing and lack of easy in-

spection of the incision site to monitor healing. Falls or injury due to early ambulation are also a possibility. An IPOP is most often used, following trauma, for younger patients who have good balance and skin condition.

Contraindications

Contraindications to the use of an IPOP include

- History of slow healing
- Extreme obesity

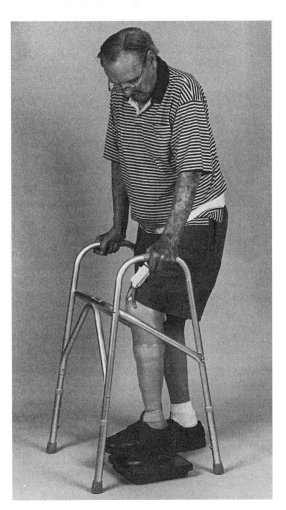

Figure 6-5. Patient with an amputation determining the optimal pressure for weight bearing.

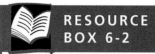

RESOURCE BOX 6-2

Advantages of the Immediate Postoperative Prosthesis

- Control and shaping of the residual limb
- Protection of the surgical site
- Improved healing time
- Maintenance of residual and sound limb and upper body strength
- Reduction of contracture development
- Maintenance of cardiovascular status
- Early return to balance and ambulation
- Social and emotional
- Shorter hospital stay
- Shorter overall recovery time
- Quicker identification of patient functional levels

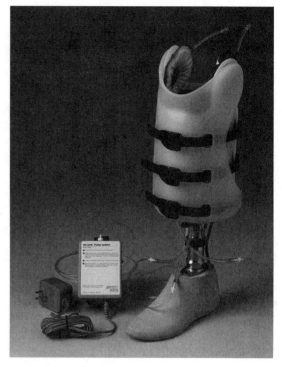

Figure 6-6. The Aircast AirLimb, a noncustom IPOP. (Photo courtesy of Aircast Inc.)

- Excessive preoperative edema
- Lack of 45 days of preoperative ambulation[16]

A noncustom IPOP is also available. This device, which is lighter than fiberglass or plaster, contains air bladders that may be inflated to accommodate the size of the residual limb. This version of the IPOP is preferable for patients with diabetes, since its ease of removal allows skin integrity visualization.[16] This noncustom IPOP is shown in Figure 6-6.

Removable Rigid Dressing (RRD)

When sutures are removed from the amputated limb, a removable rigid dressing (RRD) may be used. The RRD consists of a plaster shell, socks, a stockinet sleeve, and a thermoplastic supracondylar cuff. The RRD can be made in approximately 45 minutes with materials commonly found in a hospital physical therapy department.[17] The components of the RRD are depicted in Figure 6-7. The patient applies the sock, the plaster shell, the stockinet sleeve, and finally the thermoplastic supracondylar cuff

with Velcro closure. The stockinet is folded down over the supracondylar cuff and held in place by the cuff Velcro strap.[18] The RRD is primarily used for a patient with a transtibial amputation. It allows easy assessment of the surgical site, good shrinkage, and protection of the residual limb against accidental trauma. Weight bearing with the RRD against a surface such as a chair seat or raised platform will prepare the patient for eventual weight bearing in a prosthesis.[19] However, ambulation using the RRD is not recommended.[3,20] The RRD is worn full time except for bathing and inspection of the residual limb. The RRD does not extend proximal to the knee so that knee flexion contractures are minimized. As the residual limb shrinks, socks are added to ensure a better fit between the residual limb and the RRD. The use of the RRD has significantly reduced the incidence of skin breakdown and distal edema, produced fast residual

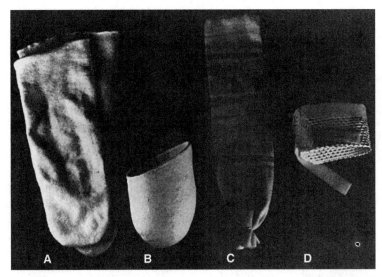

Figure 6-7. Components of the removable rigid dressing (RRD). **A.** Prosthetic sock. **B.** Plaster cast. **C.** Stockinette with one end tied. **D.** Thermoplastic supracondylar suspension cuff with Velcro closure. (Photo courtesy of Wu, Y., Keagy, R. D., Krick, H. J., Stratigos, J. S., Betts, H. B. (1979). An innovative removable rigid dressing technique for below-the-knee amputation. *Journal of Bone and Joint Surgery, 61A*, 724-729.)

limb shrinkage, and shortened time to ambulatory discharge by 90 days.[18,21]

Disadvantages of the RRD are not being suited for incontinence and the need for the patient or caregiver to apply and remove the RRD. A patient who is not motivated or who is confused may easily remove the RRD, which may result in residual limb edema. As a result, prosthetic fitting could be delayed.

Air Splint

The **air splint** was originally designed as an emergency splint to stabilize fractures. Advantages of the air splint include visualization of, and easy access to, the incision; provision of uniform pressure over the residual limb; and ease of use. The air splint is usually applied 2–10 days after the amputation.[22] Application of the air splint is as follows: the patient wears a sock on the residual limb to absorb moisture and prevent skin maceration; the air splint is placed over the residual limb; the air splint is zipped to secure it around the residual limb; the

hose is attached to a pump; a distal-to-proximal measured pressurization occurs as the bladder is inflated to a pressure of 25 mm Hg. with a pump; and finally, the hose is disconnected. More air can be added if residual limb edema is reduced. The air splint is shown in Figure 6-8.

Studies have found that the use of the air splint facilitates early ambulation and balance training and allows partial weight bearing on the recently amputated limb. An assistive device such as crutches or a walker is necessary for partial weight bearing ambulation.[23,24] The use of the air splint allows continuous limb support and protection, minimizes edema, and reduces the occurrence of hematomas in the residual limb.[25] Disadvantages of the air splint include difficulty with weight bearing and a buildup of heat, especially in warmer climates.

Silicone Liners

Recently, prosthetists have used the **silicone liner** to control edema. The silicone liner is inverted and rolled on the residual limb.[3] The

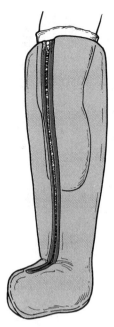

Figure 6-8. Air splint (bony prominences such as the patella and shaft of the tibia are padded to avoid skin breakdown).

liner's roll-on design is often less traumatic to the suture line than the fabric pull of the shrinker sock (described later in this chapter). The silicone liner is described further in Chapter 8 on transtibial components. Disadvantages of the silicone liner are similar to those of the air splint, i.e., difficulty with weight bearing and a build-up of heat, especially in warmer climates. The silicone liner is shown in Figure 6-9.

Research Studies

The literature comparing one dressing with another is sparse, with conflicting results. MacLean and Fick, in a study comparing patients who had a semirigid dressing with those with a soft dressing, found that the semirigid-dressing group required less than half as much time to prosthetic fitting as those with a soft dressing. This study concluded that patients may be ready for prosthetic fitting sooner if

treated with semirigid dressings instead of soft dressings.[6] In another study, Mueller showed statistically significantly more residual limb shrinkage with the RRD than with a soft dressing. In addition, pain was minimized in the RRD group, possibly because of the rigid protection against bumping of the residual limb. Patients with bilateral transtibial amputations found that transfers were easier with use of the RRD because they were able to push down on the ends of the residual limbs to extend the hips with no pain.[14] Vigier et al., in a study of 56 subjects, found a shorter average healing time and shorter average length of hospital stay with the RRD group than with a group using an elastic compression bandage.[26] Cutson et al., in a study of elderly patients with transtibial amputation secondary to vascular disease, found the use of the RRD to be a safe method of residual limb shrinkage. They stated that the time from surgery to prosthetic gait training was reduced (although the amount of time was not stated), without risk of wound compromise.[27]

A study of 182 mostly elderly patients with a transtibial amputation secondary to diabetes, compared soft dressings, rigid dressings, and an IPOP. Mooney et al. showed that the rigid dressing and use of an IPOP improved the patient's physical and mental attitude, did not deter

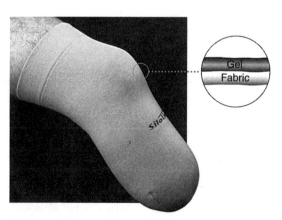

Figure 6-9. Silicone liner used to control edema. (Photo courtesy of Silipos Inc.)

wound healing, and decreased time to receipt of the definitive prosthesis. However, they found that immediate ambulation may deter wound healing and should be delayed for several weeks.[28] Harrington and Esses studied patients with transtibial amputations in Canada and found that the use of an immediate postoperative pylon contributed to control of edema and promoted earlier fitting of the definitive prosthesis.[29]

Conversely, in a study of 51 patients with a transtibial amputation secondary to vascular disease, Baker et al. found little difference in wound healing between a rigid dressing and a soft dressing. Complete wound healing was 85% using rigid dressing and 83% using soft dressings.[30] In an animal study, Frogameni et al. found no significant difference in residual limb wound approximation, interstitial edema, or the presence of granulation tissue, between rigid and soft dressings.[31] Kane and Pollock, in a study of 52 patients with transtibial amputations, showed no statistically significant differences between use of the IPOP or soft dressing in regard to postoperative hospitalization time, functional recovery, postoperative pain, morbidity, or mortality.[32]

In summary, the differing results of these studies comparing dressing effectiveness may be due to a variety of causes including patient selection, number of subjects studied, prior patient factors such as reason for amputation and risk factors such as smoking, the effect of different antibiotics, and the presence of a coordinated team approach. Excellent resources concerning dressings and general information on prosthetics and orthotics are contained in Resource Box 6-3.

Compression of the Residual Limb

After the incision is healed and the sutures removed (usually 10–21 days post-operatively), a patient will discard the dressing and use a compression device. **Elastic wraps** or **shrinkers** are commonly used compression devices to con-

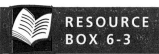

RESOURCE BOX 6-3

Resources Regarding Dressings and Prosthetics and Orthotics in Journal of Prosthetics and Orthotics

Editorial Office
635 Executive Drive
Troy, MI, 48083 USA
(248)-588-7480
http://www.oandp.org/educ/pub/jpo
    A global resource for orthotics and prosthetics information containing industry and educational addresses and websites is available at http://www.oandp.com

tain residual limb edema. When the residual limb edema has decreased a preparatory or adjustable prosthesis is prescribed.

Indications for the use of compression devices include

1. Controlling edema; in some patients edema is difficult to manage because of changes associated with diabetes, hypertension, and peripheral vascular disease
2. Reducing an **adductor roll** in transfemoral cases
3. Shaping the residual limb
4. Acclimating the residual limb to pressure as a preparation for prosthetic fitting
5. Assisting in prevention of residual limb contractures
6. Desensitizing the residual limb

Patients should be instructed in application of the elastic wraps or shrinker early in the postoperative period and advised to avoid skin friction, which may lead to shear pressure sores.[33] Generally, elastic bandages are 3, 4, and 6 inches wide. They are available in double rolls with Velcro closure, which makes application easier than attempting to use two separate bandages (Fig. 6-10). The use of elastic bandages creates a pressure gradient, with higher pressure distally and lower pressure proximally. The patient may need to bandage the residual limb indefinitely because of edema fluctuations. In the preprosthetic phase, the bandage should be worn 24 hours a day, except for bathing. The patient's ability to wrap the residual limb independently depends on many factors, including cognition, vision, upper extremity and residual limb range of motion, strength, sensation, proprioception, coordination, psychosocial factors, family support, and proper education. Visser, in a study of 22 individuals with lower extremity amputation, found that only 49% had received instruction in bandaging the residual limb.[34]

Principles of Compression

The following principles should be used when wrapping a residual limb:

- Distal pressure should exceed proximal pressure, otherwise a bulbous or hourglass

appearance may result in the residual limb. This may delay healing and result in prosthetic fitting difficulties.
- Pressure should be applied on the oblique turns, as in a figure-8 wrap. Circular turns with pressure may result in an undesired tourniquet effect.
- The medial and lateral aspects of the end portion of the residual limb should not be included in the same turn. Otherwise, slippage of the bandage on the residual limb results.
- The bandage should be reapplied about every 4 hours. A bandage should never be left on for more than 24 hours without rewrapping.
- Wrinkles in the bandage should be avoided as much as possible to prevent skin injury.
- Metal clips should never be used to secure a bandage on an insensitive limb. Tape should be used instead.
- If the bandage causes aching, burning, or numbness, it should be removed, the site inspected, and the residual limb rewrapped.

Transtibial Wrapping

Individuals with a transtibial amputation use two or three 4-inch bandages that extend above the knee. Extending the bandage above the knee is imperative, to secure the bandage and minimize slipping of the residual limb. If the patella is covered with the bandage, edema around the patella is minimized. However, knee movement may loosen the bandage. Often, a patient with a recent transtibial amputation will cover the patella with the bandage. Other patients who are moving the knee in rehabilitation and transfer activities will keep the patella uncovered. Techniques of wrapping include the figure-8, recurrent, and circular start methods.

Figure-8 Wrap

With a figure-8 procedure, the first bandage is started at either the proximal medial or proximal lateral aspect of the residual limb

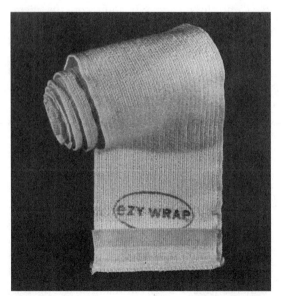

Figure 6-10. Double roll bandage with Velcro closure.

and brought diagonally over the limb to the distal area. The second bandage is brought down over the opposite aspect of the residual limb. Subsequent layers overlap these first two bandages; i.e., the third bandage over the first, the second over the fourth etc. Distal pressure should exceed proximal pressure. The bandage should extend approximately 3 inches proximal to the patella. Bandages that do not extend proximal to the patella will easily slip off the residual limb. A figure-8 wrap for the transtibial amputation is shown in Figure 6-11.

Recurrent Wrap

A recurrent bandage may also be used for a transtibial amputation and may be applied from anterior to posterior or side to side. The recurrent bandage may be easier for the patient to apply than a figure-8 bandage. An anterior incision is common with most transtibial amputations. Therefore, to avoid distracting pressure on the incision, the bandages should be brought from posterior to anterior over the distal end.[35] After the initial recurrent wrap, subsequent wraps may use a figure-8 pattern. A recurrent wrap is

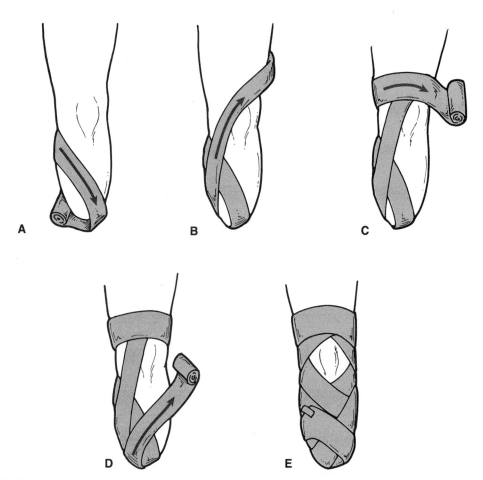

Figure 6-11. Figure-8 wrap for the transtibial amputation. **A.** First wrap may extend from proximal medial to distal lateral. **B.** Second wrap may extend from proximal lateral to distal medial. **C.** Third wrap may overlie first wrap. **D.** Bandage is loosely wrapped approximately 3 inches proximal to the knee. **E.** Completed wrap.

also extended proximal to the knee. The recurrent wrap is shown in Figure 6-12.

Circular Start

A third wrapping method for the transtibial residual limb is called the circular start. This method involves starting the bandage above the knee with a loose circular wrap that anchors the bandage. A figure-8 pattern may then be used to cover the residual limb. Anchoring above the knee first minimizes the tendency for the bandage to slip. Figure 6-13 depicts a wrap with the patella left uncovered.

Transfemoral Wrapping

A patient with a transfemoral amputation may use two to three 4- or 6-inch bandages, depending on the size of the residual limb. The part of the bandage around the waist and hip is called a **spica**. It is often preferable to start the transfemoral wrap with a hip spica before wrapping the residual limb. The hip spica helps to prevent the bandage slipping off the residual limb. The hip spica should be wrapped securely around the waist and hip but not tight enough to result in a tourniquet effect. Since patients with transfemoral amputations are prone to hip external rotation contractures from lying in bed, the hip spica should pull the residual limb into internal rotation. The hip spica may be started at the residual limb greater trochanter and brought over the abdomen and around the waist. It is then extended to the proximal medial part of the residual limb to pull the residual limb into internal rotation. The transfemoral wrap is shown in Figure 6-14.

The transfemoral bandage should be brought high up in the groin to avoid an ad-

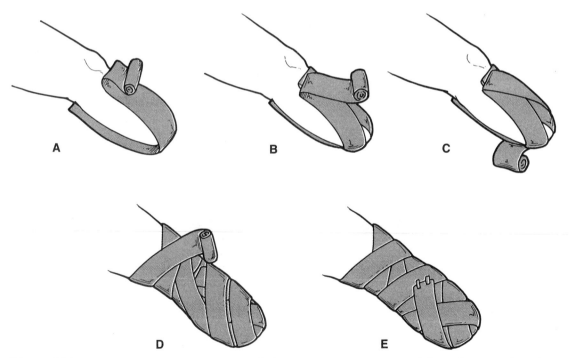

Figure 6-12. Recurrent wrap. **A.** First wrap extends from posterior to anterior. **B.** A figure-8 wrap is then done. **C.** Figure-8 wrap is continued. **D.** Bandage is loosely wrapped approximately 3 inches proximal to the knee. **E.** Completed wrap.

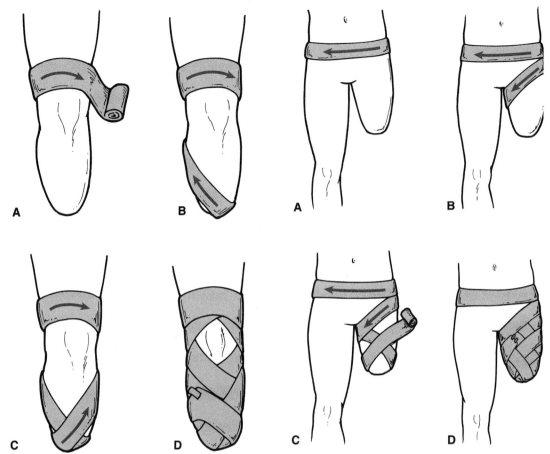

Figure 6-13. Circular start wrap. A. A loose circular wrap is placed over the knee to anchor the bandage. B. A figure-8 wrap extending over the lateral distal end of the residual limb. C. A figure-8 wrap extending over the medial distal end of the residual limb. D. Completed wrap with patella left unwrapped.

Figure 6-14. Transfemoral wrap. A. Start over the bandage over the left greater trochanter and extend the bandage over the patient's abdomen. B. Hip spica goes around waist and is extended high in the groin to help prevent an adductor roll. The bandage pulls the hip into internal rotation. C. Residual limb is wrapped with a figure-8 pattern. D. Completed wrap.

ductor roll. The presence of an adductor roll is painful for a transfemoral prosthesis wearer when the adductor roll is caught between the pubic ramus and the medial wall of the quadrilateral socket (Fig. 6-15). To decrease this adductor roll, patients may use a template, which may be a piece of orthoplast or plastic. This template is placed over the skin in the groin area, and the bandage is wrapped over it (Fig. 6-16).

Transmetatarsal and Syme Wrapping

In most cases, since marked edema is not present, a transmetatarsal amputation does not need to be wrapped with an elastic wrap or bandage. Wrapping a Syme residual limb should use the principles of compression reviewed above in this chapter. The wrapping of a Syme residual limb should extend to the superior calf region, below the knee.

136

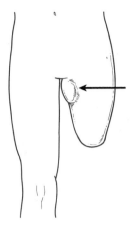

Figure 6-15. Presence of an adductor roll due to incorrect bandaging.

Shrinkers

Because of the difficulty of applying elastic bandages, the use of a shrinker is often more practical. Most patients with transfemoral amputations use a shrinker rather than elastic wraps (Fig. 6-17). Shrinkers are used after sutures are removed. Commercially made shrinkers for hemipelvectomy/hip disarticulation patients are also available (Fig. 6-18).

There are few studies comparing elastic bandages with shrinkers. Manella showed that the shrinker decreased residual limb volume more than the elastic bandages did. In fact, residual limb volume increased over the 4-week test period for the elastic bandage group. However, this study had a small sample of 12.[36]

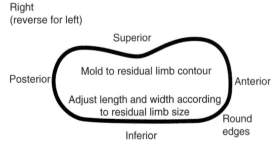

Figure 6-16. A template placed over the adductor roll and under the transfemoral wrap.

Right
(reverse for left)

Superior

Posterior

Mold to residual limb contour

Adjust length and width according to residual limb size

Anterior

Round edges

Inferior

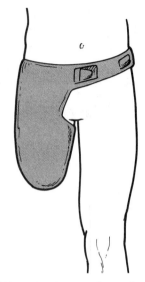

Figure 6-17. A shrinker may be used instead of elastic wraps.

Spandex

Spandex may also be considered a shrinker. Fitting difficulties with elastic bandages and conventional shrinkers have led some investigators to use modified Spandex shorts as an alternative in cases of high transfemoral or hip disarticulation amputations. The Spandex shorts can be sewn with cotton thread to serve as a shrinker around the end of the residual limb. They may be worn under the prosthesis.[24]

Summary

The advantages and disadvantages of elastic bandages compared with shrinkers are outlined in Pros and Cons Box 6-1 and Pros and Cons Box 6-2.

Removable Protective Socket

Another way to provide compression and to protect the residual limb from trauma is by the use of a removable protective socket. This socket may be used with elastic wraps or

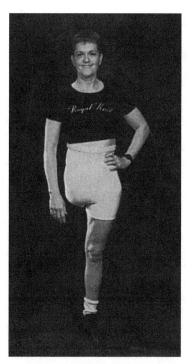

Figure 6-18. A shrinker may be used for a patient with a hemipelvectomy or hip disarticulation. (Photo courtesy of Royal Knit Inc.)

shrinkers. The removable protective socket is a custom-fitted device made of thermoplastics. This socket

- Protects the wound from traumatic impact such as falls
- Allows easy access for wound inspection and dressing changes
- Decreases the incidence of knee flexion contractures
- Shapes the residual limb and establishes early prosthetic socket tolerance
- Adjusts to volume changes in the residual limb
- Is lightweight and easy to apply and remove

An example of the removable protective socket is the FloTech Tor. A Universal Frame Outer Socket (UFOS) can be put over the FloTech Tor to enable weight bearing (Fig. 6-19).

PROS & CONS
BOX 6-1

Elastic Bandages

Advantages
- Readily available
- Inexpensive
- Can provide a gradient pressure
- Promotes tapered shape to the residual limb

Disadvantages

- Loses its elasticity over time
- Difficulty in application especially for a patient with a transfemoral amputation
- Must be changed frequently to maintain adequate pressure
- Possibility of a tourniquet effect
- Wrinkles and slipping may cause irregular pressure

PROS & CONS
BOX 6-2

Shrinkers

Advantages
- Easier to use, especially with a transfemoral amputation
- Slipping minimized because the hip spica aids suspension
- Better compliance than with elastic bandages

Disadvantages

- Increased expense
- Multiple shrinkers may be needed as the residual limb loses edema
- Do not prevent an adductor roll
- May be uncomfortable over sensitive or open areas

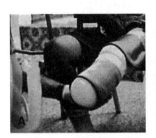
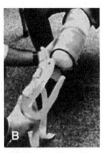

Figure 6.19. A. Example of a removable protective socket. B. Example of a weight-bearing socket. (Photos courtesy of Flo-Tech.)

Skin Care

Proper skin care is critical to prevent further complications that may affect the sound and residual limbs. For those who wear a prosthesis, confining a residual limb in an airless chamber with accumulated heat and perspiration can promote bacterial growth. After amputation, the residual limb is often irritated and prone to injury and infection. In addition, irritation from the rubbing of the prosthetic socket may cause skin infections. Care of the skin is a vital part of rehabilitation. A daily inspection and cleansing routine should become as regular as brushing one's teeth.

Skin Care for the Residual Limb

The guidelines in Resource Box 6-4 regarding residual limb care may be shared with the patient.

Skin Warning Signs

Patients with amputation should be instructed to look for the following skin warning signs:

- Color changes of the skin, including erythema lasting longer than 15 minutes
- Elevation of skin temperature

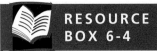

RESOURCE BOX 6-4

Skin Care for the Residual Limb

- The residual limb should be washed with a fragrance-free soap and patted dry, preferably at night to allow the skin to dry thoroughly before wearing the prosthesis. Fully rinse the skin with warm (not hot) water to eliminate a soapy film, which may cause skin irritation. Towel dry gently after cleaning. Apply a small amount of fragrance-free skin lotion to the entire residual limb. Keeping the skin supple helps lessen the formation of calluses and abrasions. Excessive lotion may clog hair follicles.
- Cologne or perfumed lotion should not be used, since they may irritate the skin.
- If the patient cannot visualize all areas of the residual limb, a mirror may be used for inspection.
- The healed incision scar should be mobilized to keep tissue from adhering.
- If a small open wound occurs, a hydrocolloid dressing (DuoDERM) held in place by the prosthetic sock may be used. Adhesive bandages may also be used. Adhesive bandages tend to roll, however, and are more effective if placed longitudinally over the wound. Patients with skin insensitivity may need to refrain from wearing the prosthesis until the wound heals.

- Blisters or open skin areas
- Pain in the leg, either at rest or while walking
- Edema
- Corns or calluses
- Dry cracks in the skin

Advise the patient to consult the physician if any of these warning signs are present. Because of the increased risk for another amputation, patients should also be instructed in proper skin care for the sound limb. Proper skin care is especially important for an insensitive limb.

Sound-Limb Care Guidelines

The following guidelines regarding sound limb care may be shared with the patient:

- Wash feet daily using lukewarm water. Rinse thoroughly and dry gently. Don't rub; pat the skin dry.
- Inspect feet and shoes daily. Feet should be inspected for signs of skin breakdown such as cuts, scratches, bruises, blisters, or cracks between the toes. If your eyesight is poor, have someone else check.
- Inspect shoes before putting them on. Shoes should be inspected to determine if linings are smooth and to make sure that construction material is not bunched and foot powder has not accumulated. Turn each shoe over in the morning to determine if an object has fallen into it during the night.
- Do not use strong chemicals on feet such as iodine or foot deodorants. Check with the physician before using chemical agents for removal of corns or calluses.
- Never walk barefoot, even when going to the bathroom at night.
- Avoid extreme temperatures. Use a portion of the body other than the feet such as the inner forearm, to test bath water temperature or have someone else check. Avoid external heat sources when the feet are cold. Heating pads, heat lamps, hot water bottles, heat registers, and car heaters can be dangerous. Woolen socks or down slippers may help maintain body heat.
- Avoid elastic or dyed socks, use white cotton instead. Avoid stockings that bind at the toes or at the top. Watch for pressure from seams.
- Break in new shoes gradually. Do not wear a new shoe more than 1–2 hours without checking for pressure areas on the feet. Do this for 7–10 days until the shoe is broken in. Have shoes fitted properly. Avoid pointed shoes. A high toe-box should be used with claw or hammer toes.
- Trim toenails straight across, do not round the corners. Look for ingrown toenails and fungal infections. Seek medical attention if a nail or foot injury occurs. Often a podiatrist may need to trim the toenails.
- Do not bear weight on a blistered foot.
- If appropriate, advise anyone caring for your feet that you have a vascular problem or diabetes.[37]

Care of Prosthetic Shrinkers, Socks, Inserts, and Sockets

Prosthetic socks are often worn over the residual limb and inside the socket of the prosthesis. Prosthetic socks add cushioning, reduce friction between the residual limb and the socket, and replace lost volume in the socket due to shrinking of the residual limb (Fig. 6-20). As the residual limb changes size, socks can be added or removed.[38] Prosthetic socks are available in various thicknesses often called *ply*. If a sock is made with one

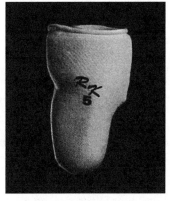

Figure 6.20. A prosthetic sock. (Photo courtesy of Royal Knit Inc.)

strand of yarn, it is designated a 1-ply sock, if knitted with two strands, the sock is 2-ply, and so on. Today 3- and 5-ply socks are most commonly used.[39] The top of the sock may have a color-coded thread indicating ply size. Prosthetic socks can be made of wool, cotton, or acrylic synthetics. Wool socks are often used because of their excellent cushioning and absorbent qualities. After washing, wool becomes full, resulting in excellent cushioning between the residual limb and liner or socket. However, some patients may be allergic to wool and complain of itching. Acrylic socks have the advantage of wicking away moisture from the skin and helping to prevent blisters. Lycra spandex can be blended with acrylic materials to thicken the sock fabric and still provide stretchability and enhance skin protection.

Shrinkers, socks, inserts, and sockets may absorb body oils and perspiration and so may harbor fungi and bacteria. The following instructions regarding care of the prosthetic socket, insert, shrinkers, and socks may be given to a patient:

Care of Shrinkers and Socks

The care of shrinkers and socks is shown in Resource Box 6-5.

Care of Inserts

- Wipe out daily, using warm water and mild soap. Rinse thoroughly.
- Allow the insert to dry thoroughly. Damp skin put in an insert is likely to swell and become irritated.
- Inspect the insert daily for cracks or rough areas.

Care of the Socket

- The inside of the socket should be cleansed weekly. Wash the socket with warm water

---

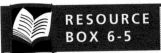

RESOURCE BOX 6-5

Care of Shrinkers and Socks

- In hot, humid weather, socks need to be changed more frequently during the day.
- Wash daily in warm water, using mild soap. The best time to wash the shrinker and socks is at night.
- Cotton and nylon socks can be machine washed and dried.
- Rinse wool socks thoroughly; do not twist or wring. Air dry by laying flat. Do not hang to dry or machine dry.
- Allow shrinkers and socks to dry completely inside and out.
- If the sock dries with a "dog ear," or a distal lateral or medial pocketing, a rubber ball or 2-liter bottle may be inserted to restore shape.

- If the sock cannot be identified by the color of the thread at the top of the sock, it is helpful to mark the number of plies on the top of the sock with a laundry marker.
- When socks are applied, make sure there are no wrinkles in the socks that might cause pressure areas.
- If a seam is present in the sock, rotate it away from bony prominences.
- Wearing the fewest number of socks to achieve the desired ply will help reduce bunching and wrinkling of the socks. For example if four plies are needed, do not wear four separate 1-ply socks but rather one 3-ply sock and one 1-ply sock.

and mild soap. The best time to cleanse the socket is at night.

- Allow the socket to dry thoroughly.[40]

KEY POINTS

- Dressings are used to control postoperative edema and facilitate prosthetic fitting. Dressings may consist of soft, semirigid, rigid, removable rigid, air splint, or silicone liners.

- An immediate postoperative prosthesis (IPOP) consists of a rigid dressing, pylon, and foot. The IPOP allows early ambulation.

- Compression of the residual limb helps control edema, shape, acclimatize to pressure, prevent contractures, desensitize, and reduce an adductor roll in transfemoral cases. Compression may be accomplished by the use of elastic bandages, shrinkers, or spandex.

- Proper skin care is critical to prevent further complications that may affect the residual and sound limbs.

CRITICAL THINKING QUESTIONS

1. Differentiate among the advantages and disadvantages of soft dressings, semirigid dressings, rigid dressings, an IPOP, the RRD, the air splint, and the silicone liner.

2. Explain the rationale for the principles of proper wrapping of transtibial and transfemoral residual limbs.

3. Given a patient with an amputation, evaluate whether the patient would be better served with an elastic wrap bandage or a shrinker.

4. Instruct a patient in proper wrapping of a transtibial or transfemoral residual limb.

5. Describe proper methods of skin care and ways to care for the prosthetic socket, insert, shrinkers, and socks.

REFERENCES

1. American Physical Therapy Association. (2001). A guide to physical therapist practice. *Physical Therapy, 81.*
2. Murdoch, G. (1983). The postoperative environment of the amputation stump. *Prosthetics and Orthotics International, 7,* 75–78.
3. Barner, K. (1999, June/July). Faster functioning. *Rehab Management,* 42–47.
4. Golbranson, F. L., Wirta, R. W., Kuncir, E. J., Lieber, R. L., & Oishi C. (1988). Volume changes occurring in postoperative below knee residual limbs. *Journal of Rehabilitation Research and Development, 25,* 11–18.
5. Fish, S. L. (1976). Semirigid dressing for stump shrinking. *Physical Therapy, 56,* 1376.
6. MacLean, N, & Fick, G. H. (1994). The effect of semirigid dressings on below-knee amputations. *Physical Therapy, 74,* 668–673.
7. Ghiulamila, R. I. (1972). Semirigid dressing for postoperative fitting of below knee prosthesis. *Archives of Physical Medicine and Rehabilitation, 53,* 186–189.
8. Laforest, N. T., & Regon, L. W. (1973). The physical therapy program after an immediate rigid dressing and temporary below knee prosthesis. *Physical Therapy, 53,* 497–501.
9. Sterescu, L. E. (1974). Semirigid (Unna) dressing of amputations. *Archives of Physical Medicine and Rehabilitation, 55,* 433–434.
10. Swanson, V. M. (1993). Below knee polyethylene semirigid dressing. *Journal of Prosthetics and Orthotics, 5,* 10–15.
11. Burgess, E. M., & Zettl, J. H. (1969). Amputations below the knee. *Artificial Limbs, 13,* 1–12.
12. Nicholas, G. G., & DeMuth, W. E. (1976). Evaluation of use of the rigid dressing in amputation of the lower extremity. *Surgery, Gynecology and Obstetrics, 143,* 398–400.
13. Kerstein, M. D., Zimmer, H., & Dugdale, F. (1975). Rigid dressings: Poor results. *Connecticut Medicine, 39,* 690–691.
14. Mueller, M. J. (1982). Comparison of removable rigid dressings and elastic bandages in preprosthetic management of patients with below-knee amputations. *Physical Therapy, 62,* 1438–1441.
15. Burgess, R., Romano R., & Zettl, J. (1998). *The management of lower extremity amputations* (book on CD-ROM). Seattle: Prosthetics Research Study.

16. Wu, Y., Keagy, R. D., Krick, H. J., Stratigos, J. S., & Betts, H. B. (1979). An innovative removable rigid dressing technique for below-the-knee amputation. *Journal of Bone and Joint Surgery, 61A,* 724–729.

17. Richter, K. J., Hurvitz, E. A., & Girardot, K. (1988). Rigid removable dressing in a case of poor wound healing. *Archives of Physical Medicine and Rehabilitation, 69,* 128–129.

18. Ullendahl, J. E. (1988). Patient care booklet for below-knee amputees. *American Academy of Orthotists and Prosthetists,* 6–7.

19. Gandhavadi B. (1987). Porous removable rigid dressing for complicated below-knee amputation stumps. *Archives of Physical Medicine and Rehabilitation, 68,* 51–53.

20. Pinzur, M. S. (1997). Current concepts: Amputation surgery in peripheral vascular disease. *Instructional Course Lectures, 46,* 501–509.

21. Continuing Education Course (1999, November 13). *Concepts in orthotics & prosthetics.* San Francisco: California Chapter of the American Physical Therapy Association.

22. Rausch, R. W. & Khalili, A. A. (1985). Air splint in preprosthetic rehabilitation of lower extremity amputated limbs. *Physical Therapy, 65,* 912–914.

23. Bonner, F. J., & Green, R. F. (1982). Pneumatic air-leg prosthesis: Report of 200 cases. *Archives of Physical Medicine and Rehabilitation, 63,* 383–385.

24. Little, J. M. (1971). A pneumatic weight bearing temporary prosthesis for below-knee amputees. *Lancet, 1,* 271–273.

25. Barraclough, B. H., Coupland, G. A. E., & Reeve, T. S. (1972). Air splints used as immediate postoperative prostheses after long posterior flap below knee amputation. *Medical Journal of Australia, 2,* 764–767.

26. Vigier, S., Casillas, J. M., Dulieu, V., Rouhier-Marcer, I., D'Athis, P., & Didier, J. P. (1999). Healing of open stump wounds after vascular below-knee amputation: Plaster cast socket with silicone sleeve versus elastic compression. *Archives of Physical Medicine and Rehabilitation, 80,* 1327–1330.

27. Cutson, T. M., Bongiorni, D., Michael, J. W., & Kochersberger, G. (1994). Early management of elderly dysvascular transtibial amputees. *Journal of Prosthetics and Orthotics, 6,* 62–66.

28. Mooney, V., Harvey, J. P., McBride, E., & Snelson, R. (1971). Comparison of postoperative stump management: plaster vs. soft dressings. *Journal of Bone and Joint Surgery, 53A,* 241–249.

29. Harrington, I. J., & Esses, S. I. (1984). Use of a pylon for early ambulation after below knee amputation: A preliminary report. *Canadian Journal of Surgery, 27,* 500–502.

30. Baker, W. H., Barnes, R., & Shurr, D. G. (1977). The healing of below-knee amputations: A comparison of soft and plaster dressings. *American Journal of Surgery, 133,* 716–718.

31. Frogameni, A. D., Booth, R., Mumaw, L., & Cummings, V. (1989). Comparison of soft dressing and rigid dressing in the healing of amputated limbs of rabbits. *American Journal of Physical Medicine and Rehabilitation, 68,* 234–239.

32. Kane 3d, T. J., & Pollak, E. W. (1980). The rigid versus soft postoperative dressing controversy: A controlled study in vascular below-knee amputees. *American Surgeon, 46,* 244–247.

33. Pandian, G., & Kowalske, K. (1999). Daily functioning of patients with an amputated lower extremity. *Clinical Orthopaedics and Related Research, 361,* 91–97.

34. Visser C. (1998). Knowledge and skill of patients with regard to amputation stump bandaging, prior to a prosthesis. *South African Journal of Physiotherapy, 54,* 8–10.

35. May B. (1996). *Amputations and prosthetics: A case study approach.* Philadelphia: F. A. Davis.

36. Manella, K. (1981). Comparing the effectiveness of elastic bandages and shrinker socks for lower extremity amputees. *Physical Therapy, 61,* 334–337.

37. Wagner, F. W., Jr. (1981). The dysvascular foot: A system for diagnosis and treatment. *Foot and Ankle, 2,* 64–122.

38. Shurr, D. G. *Patient care booklet for above-knee amputees.* American Academy of Orthotists and Prosthetists. 27, Alexandria VA.

39. Field, M. (1996, August/September). All socks aren't White House cats. http://www.amputee-coalition.org.InMotion 6. Accessed October 2, 2001.

40. Anon. (1998). *Care guide for lower limb prosthesis.* Marshall Labs, Syracuse NY.

Chapter 7

DEVELOPMENT OF AN

EXERCISE/FUNCTIONAL PROGRAM

Objectives

1. Describe the purposes of exercise for a patient with an amputation or a patient needing an orthosis
2. Demonstrate various positions a patient should adopt to avoid joint contractures
3. Design a specific flexibility and strengthening program for a patient with an amputation or for a patient needing an orthosis
4. Fabricate a desensitization program for a patient with a hypersensitive limb
5. Plan a progression of cardiovascular and ambulation activities for a patient with an amputation or for a patient needing an orthosis to achieve optimal independence
6. Differentiate the energy expenditure of individuals with various levels of amputation compared with able-bodied individuals
7. Given a patient with an amputation or a patient needing an orthosis, design appropriate functional activities

This chapter is divided into the following sections:

E xercises are an integral part of rehabilitation and facilitate the ability to transfer independently, perform functional activities, and use a prosthesis most efficiently. The *Guide to Physical Therapist Practice* defines therapeutic exercise as a systematic performance of planned movements, postures, or activities to accomplish a variety of general purposes. Physical therapists select, prescribe, and implement exercise activities for a variety of purposes. These general purposes include

1. Remediating or preventing impairments
2. Enhancing function
3. Reducing risk of injury
4. Optimizing overall health
5. Enhancing fitness and well-being[1]

Since the conditions that require an orthosis vary widely, they are not a point of emphasis in this chapter. These conditions may range from increased muscle tone, which may be seen with neurologic conditions such as cerebral palsy or a cerebrovascular accident, to decreased muscle tone, which may be seen with a peripheral nerve injury. Instead, this chapter emphasizes exercises and functional activities for the patient with an amputation. Many of these exercises and functional activities may also apply to the patient needing an orthosis. This chapter reviews the purposes of exercise, positioning, the types of exercise, preparatory ambulation, energy expenditure, and functional activities.

Ideally, a patient who will be undergoing an elective amputation can meet with members of the prosthetic clinic team before surgery. The team may discuss residual-limb pain, phantom pain and limb, and the rehabilitation process, including exercises and time frames for prosthetic fitting. The team approach is discussed in detail in Chapter 3. This meeting may help to alleviate many fears regarding the surgical procedure and the rehabilitation process. In many areas of the United States, a support network is active, allowing a patient to speak directly with an individual who has previously undergone an amputation. This individual should be selected on the basis of similarities of amputation level, outside interests, age, and gender. This patient-to-patient perspective will do much to lessen fears and aid communication with the clinic team.

Purposes of Exercise

The purposes of exercise for the patient with an amputation or the patient needing an orthosis are outlined in Resource Box 7-1.

Types of Exercises

Types of exercises a patient with an amputation or, if appropriate, a patient who needs an orthosis may perform are described as follows.

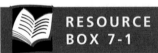

RESOURCE BOX 7-1

Purposes of Exercise for the Patient with an Amputation or Needing an Orthosis

- Increase circulation
- Increase upper- and lower-extremity strength
- Increase ROM
- Prevent contractures or correct existing contractures
- Decrease sensitivity of the residual limb
- Develop coordination
- Reduce edema and promote healing
- Promote mobility and self-care
- Increase cardiorespiratory fitness

These exercises may be done before the prosthesis is received (preprosthetic phase) or, if appropriate, before the orthosis is received (preorthosis phase).

Positioning

Positioning, an important part of a patient's exercise program, is done to prevent shortening of soft tissue and joint contractures. Joint contractures may result from muscle imbalance. In a transfemoral amputation, the hip flexors and abductors tend to be stronger than the hip extensors and adductors. In the transtibial amputation, the knee flexors tend to be stronger than the knee extensors.[2] Use of a wheelchair and sitting up in bed contribute to flexion deformities of the hip and knee. Therefore, the supine and prone positions are recommended to attempt to avoid hip and knee joint contractures. In addition, in cases of a transtibial amputation, sitting with the knee extended is encouraged. If possible, patients with an amputation should lie prone intermittently to foster hip extension and knee extension. However, care must be taken with the prone position with elderly patients or those with a cardiac history, because of respiratory or circulatory problems.

The following positions may be used to prevent joint contractures:

When lying supine, make sure the hips and knees are straight. The patient should lie on a firm surface and avoid pillows under the residual limb. The legs should be held close together (Fig. 7-1).

When prone, pillows should be avoided under the hips, and the hips should be kept flat on a firm surface. The knees should be kept straight, and the legs close together. The patient should lie prone or on either side for up to 15 minutes, four times a day. This position will extend the hip and the knee (Fig. 7-2).

When side-lying, the hip should be kept in a neutral position (Fig. 7-3). The patient

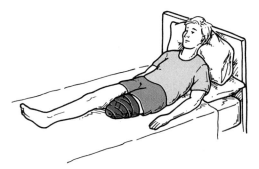

Figure 7-1. Supine position with hips and knees straight.

should not sleep with large pillows between the legs or under the back. Pillows in these positions foster hip flexion and abduction contractures.

A patient with a transtibial amputation, when sitting, should use a sliding board or another firm surface under the residual limb to promote knee extension. A board may be

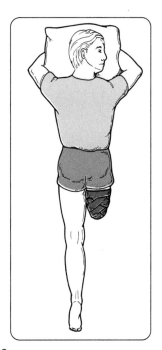

Figure 7-2. Prone position with knees straight and legs held close together.

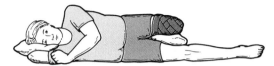

Figure 7-3. Side-lying position with residual-limb hip and knee straight. A small pillow between the legs keeps the affected hip in a neutral position.

constructed similar to the one depicted in Figure 7-4. This board measures 8 inches wide and 20 inches long, with the distal half padded with 2 inches of foam. To decrease the chance of knee flexion contractures, prolonged sitting or side-lying with the knees bent should be avoided. The affected knee should be kept straight, and crossing the legs should be avoided. A knee immobilizer may be used to facilitate residual-limb knee extension. A swing-away leg support as part of the wheelchair may also be used to prevent knee flexion contractures (Fig. 7-5).

Flexibility

Flexibility or stretching exercises to help prevent muscle shortening and subsequent joint contractures should be done in a slow,

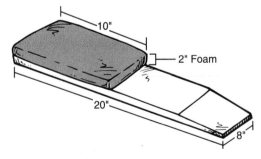

Figure 7-4. Wheelchair insert to foster residual-limb knee extension. The proximal beveled part of the insert is put under the patient's wheelchair cushion and buttock. The foam part of the insert is put under the distal residual limb.

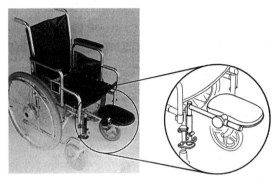

Figure 7-5. A wheelchair swing-away support for residual-limb knee extension. (Photo courtesy of Gerber Chair Mates.)

controlled manner. Manual stretches may be done using hold-relax or contract-relax proprioceptive neuromuscular facilitation (PNF) techniques. (PNF techniques are explained later in this chapter.) The stretching positions should be held for at least 20 seconds.[2] Various flexibility exercises that a patient may do alone or with a therapist or family member providing the stretch are illustrated as follows:

Hip flexor stretches may be done in the prone or supine positions. In the prone position, the sound foot may be put on the floor and the elbows straightened to extend the affected hip farther (Fig. 7-6A). Flexion of the knee with extension of the hip will cause a stretch of the rectus femoris muscle over two joints. The supine hip flexor stretch is done in a position in which the affected hip is extended off the side of the bed or table. The knee on the sound side is flexed toward the trunk. This position is also called the Thomas Test position (Fig. 7-6B). A therapist or family member may assist in this stretch, as illustrated in Figure 7-6C.

Hamstring stretches may be performed in the supine or long-sitting position (Fig. 7-7). In the long-sitting position, the hamstrings

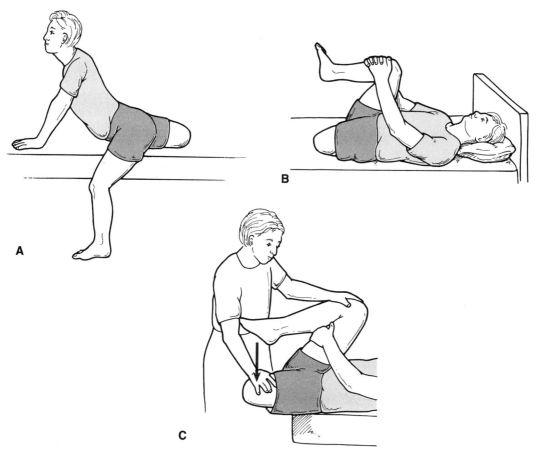

Figure 7-6. Hip flexor stretch. A. Prone position. B. Supine position (Thomas test position). C. Therapist or family member providing the stretch.

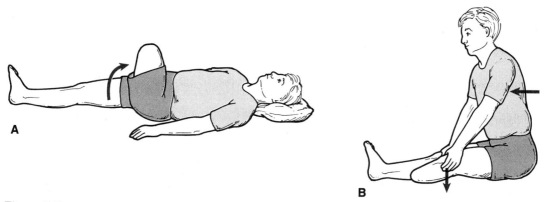

Figure 7-7. Hamstring stretch. A. Supine position. B. Long-sitting position.

be stretched over the hip and the knee
h additional trunk flexion.

Quadriceps stretches may be done in either the supine or prone positions (Fig. 7-8). In the prone position, hip extension and knee flexion will stretch the rectus femoris muscle at both the hip and knee joints.

Desensitization Activities

Desensitization activities are important to accustom the residual limb to weight bearing and for prosthetic wear. For a patient who requires an orthosis, desensitization exercises may decrease skin hypersensitivity. This desensitization may be necessary before the patient can tolerate the pressure of an orthosis. Desensitization activities should only be performed over a well-healed incision with a patient who has undergone an amputation. Desensitization activities may include[3,4]

- Massage. Using fragrance-free lotion over the area of tenderness can help decrease skin irritation. Care should be taken not to stress the healing incision. Lotion should only be applied at night to ensure that the residual limb is dry during the day when wearing a prosthesis or dressing.
- Rubbing and tapping. This is a way to toughen or decrease skin sensitivity. The residual limb may be gently tapped or rubbed with a dry wash cloth. The patient may progress to more-rigid objects such as a rolled-up newspaper or a vibrator. These techniques may also decrease phantom limb sensation or pain.
- Friction massage. This may prevent adherence of scar tissue and may be performed when the incision is healed. Adherent tissue is common along the incision line and over the distal aspects of the residual limb. Friction massage may minimize skin breakdown, especially during ambulation activities.[5]
- Mild weight bearing. When the residual limb is ready for weight bearing, a towel used as a sling may be put around the distal aspect of the residual limb and pressure applied. This towel pressure will prepare the residual limb for the pressures of weight bearing. Supported standing in the parallel bars or with a walker also results in graded weight bearing through the residual limb (Fig. 7-9).
- Coordination exercises. These may assist in desensitizing the residual limb. Coordination exercises may also facilitate controlled movement of the residual limb and, ultimately, the prosthesis. Activities such as moving the residual limb up and down and progressing to drawing figure-8s, pictures, numbers, and letters with the residual limb may be done.

Strengthening Exercises

Strengthening exercises are a vital component of an exercise program to enable the patient with an amputation or the patient needing an orthosis to gain sufficient strength to perform functional activities and to ambulate efficiently.

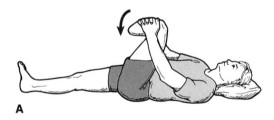

A

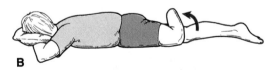

B

Figure 7-8. Quadriceps stretch. **A.** Supine position (the rectus femoris muscle is not stretched in this position). **B.** Prone position (the rectus femoris muscle is stretched in this position).

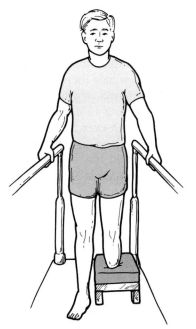

Figure 7-9. Supported standing applying graded weight-bearing through the residual limb.

The following general guidelines may be helpful for the patient with an amputation or the patient needing an orthosis who is beginning a muscle-strengthening exercise program:

- The patient should have physician clearance before exercising, especially before beginning weightlifting activities.
- The patient must start slowly and increase gradually. Exercises should be done slowly and with control. Jerking movements should be avoided. Concentration should focus on the specific muscle group being exercised. The quality of the exercise should be emphasized over the quantity.
- The patient should stop or cut back any exercise that causes sharp or burning pain except for mild muscular pain.
- The weight or number of repetitions should be increased when the exercise feels easy. The isotonic regimens that are explained later in this chapter may be used as a guide.

- If soreness or discomfort persists more than a few days, the patient may be exercising too hard or progressing too fast. Many variables may be built into a mechanical-resistance exercise program. These variables include the intensity of the exercise, frequency, mode or type, speed, and the position of the patient during exercise.[6]

Types of Strengthening Exercises

Types of strengthening exercises include isometric, isotonic, PNF, and isokinetic. Each of these is described in detail as follows.

Isometric

Isometrics is a static form of exercise that occurs when a muscle contracts without an appreciable change in its length or without visible joint motion.[7] Although there is no physical work (force times distance) performed during an isometric exercise, a great amount of tension and force output are produced by the muscle. Ideally, isometric contractions should be held against resistance for at least 6 seconds. This time allows peak tension to develop.[6] Gluteal sets are an example of an isometric contraction of the hip extensor gluteus maximus muscles. A patient may perform gluteal sets on postoperative day 1 or 2 (Fig. 7-10).

A brief, repetitive isometric exercise (**BRIME**) regimen is an extension of the original research on isometrics. A patient with an amputation may use this regimen, which consists of up to 20 maximum contractions, each held for 6 seconds. A 20-second rest after each contraction as well as rhythmic breathing during the contractions is recommended, to prevent increases in blood pressure.[8]

In the early postoperative phase, isometrics may be the only exercise that is tolerated by the patient. To improve strength throughout the

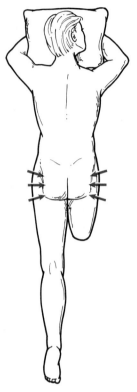

Figure 7-10. Isometric gluteus maximus contraction in a prone position. (These contractions may be done in any position.)

range of motion (ROM), multiple-angle isometrics may be performed. Multiple-angle isometrics are indicated in the presence of chronic inflammation or painful movement of the body part, especially just after amputation or injury. Gains in strength will occur only at, or closely adjacent to, the training angle.[9] Some investigators have found a physiologic overflow that only occurs a total of 20° from the training angle (10° in either direction). Therefore, to strengthen a muscle at 90° of knee flexion, training should occur between 80 and 100° of knee flexion.[10]

In summary, isometric exercises are beneficial in the early rehabilitation process when other types of exercise may be too painful. The

BRIME and the multiple-angle isometric exercises, because of their multiple components, are best given to the motivated patient who is able to follow complex instructions. However, isometric exercises may increase systolic blood pressure.[7] Because many patients with an amputation or requiring an orthosis have cardiac problems, isometric exercises should be used with caution, and the patient should be instructed not to hold his or her breath during the isometric contraction.

Isotonic

Isotonics is a type of exercise that is carried out against a constant or variable load as a muscle lengthens or shortens through the available ROM. Concentric exercise is muscle shortening; eccentric exercise is muscle lengthening. Isotonic exercises the patient may perform are illustrated in the next several figures.

Hip extension. The patient is supine with a towel placed under the residual limb. The residual limb is depressed firmly into the towel, raising the buttocks off the resting surface. Additional resistance may be provided by placing a weight on the pelvis. The

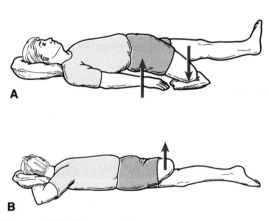

Figure 7-11. Hip extension exercise. **A.** Supine position. **B.** Prone position.

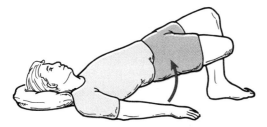

Figure 7-12. Bridging exercise for sound-limb hip extension.

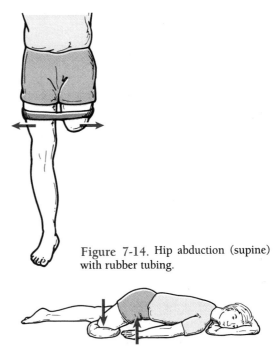

Figure 7-14. Hip abduction (supine) with rubber tubing.

patient may also strengthen the hip extensors in a prone position (Fig. 7-11).

Bridging. The patient is supine, with the sound knee at 90° of flexion. The foot is pushed into the resting surface, raising the hips upward. This exercise results in sound-limb hip extensor contraction. The residual limb should be raised upward until both hips are of equal height (Fig. 7-12).

Hip abduction in a side-lying position is described in Figure 7-13.

Hip abduction strengthening may be done using rubber tubing in which the patient pulls the residual limb away from the sound limb Figure 7-14.

Hip flexion with the patient prone is described in Figure 7-15.

Hip adduction with the patient lying on the sound side is described in Figure 7-16.

Knee extension with the patient prone is described in Figure 7-17.

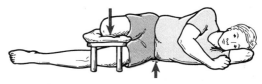

Figure 7-15. Hip flexion exercise. The patient is prone with a towel under the residual limb. The residual limb is depressed firmly into the towel, raising the pelvis off the resting surface.

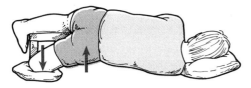

Figure 7-13. Hip abduction exercise. The patient lies on the amputated side with a towel under the residual limb. The sound limb rests on a stool that is placed in front of the hips. The residual limb is depressed firmly into the towel, raising the hip of the residual limb.

Figure 7-16. Hip adduction exercise. The patient lies on the sound side with a pillow-covered stool placed over the sound limb and under the residual limb. The residual limb is depressed firmly into a stool, raising the hip of the sound side off the resting surface.

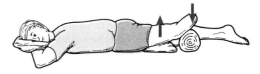

Figure 7-17. Knee extension exercise. The patient is prone, with a towel under the distal residual limb. The distal residual limb is pushed into the towel, extending the knee.

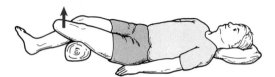

Figure 7-18. Short-arc quad exercise for knee extension.

The patient may also perform short-arc quad (Fig. 7-18) and straight leg-raise (Fig.7-19) knee-extension exercises.

Knee flexion. The patient is supine with a towel under the distal residual limb. The patient pulls back into the towel, slightly bending the knee (Fig. 7-20A). The patient may also lie prone and flex the knee against gravity (Fig. 7-20B).

In a study of 30 subjects with diabetes mellitus and transmetatarsal amputation, Salsich and Mueller found a relationship between hip and knee strength and increased function. They advocated emphasis on strengthening hip and knee strength to improve function.[11]

Isotonic Regimens

Various isotonic regimens have been developed.

DeLorme Technique

Also termed *progressive resistive exercise* (PRE), this technique uses a term known as *repetition maximum* (RM). An RM is the greatest amount of weight a muscle can move through the ROM

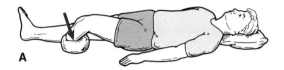

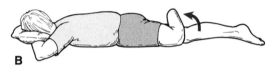

Figure 7-20. Knee flexion exercise. A. Supine. B. Prone.

a specific number of times. The procedure for the DeLorme technique is as follows:

1. Determine the 10 RM.
2. Perform the following:
   10 repetitions at one-half of the 10 RM
   10 repetitions at three-fourths of the 10 RM
   10 repetitions at the full 10 RM
3. The patient performs all three bouts at each exercise session, with a brief rest between bouts.[6]

Oxford Technique

The Oxford technique is the reverse of the DeLorme system. This technique decreases the possible detrimental effects of fatigue. The procedure for the Oxford technique is as follows:

1. Determine the 10 RM.
2. Perform the following:
   10 repetitions at the full 10 RM
   10 repetitions at three-fourths of the 10 RM
   10 repetitions at one-half of the 10 RM
3. The patient performs all three bouts at each exercise session, with a brief rest between bouts.[6]

Either the DeLorme or the Oxford technique is a suitable strengthening regimen for the motivated patient. Investigators have recommended a baseline of 6 to 15 RM to improve strength.[5] Thus, it may be helpful for patients

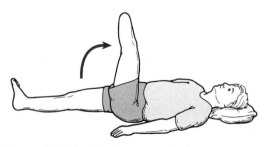

Figure 7-19. Straight-leg exercise for knee extension.

with an amputation or who need an orthosis to perform at least 6 RM of an exercise to strengthen a muscle.

If the patient is unable to grasp the multiple concepts of these regimens, many clinicians advocate three sets of 10 repetitions. Incremental weights are added when 30 repetitions are performed easily.[6]

Upper-Extremity Strengthening

Upper extremity strengthening is often necessary to enable the patient with an amputation or one who needs an orthosis to perform activities such as bed positioning; bed, commode, and tub transfers; and eventual ambulation. Upper-extremity strengthening often uses an isotonic form of exercise. Various equipment may be used for upper-extremity strengthening including dumbbells, cuff weights, and rubber tubing. Soup cans or socks filled with stones or coins may be used as weights in a home setting. These upper-extremity strengthening exercises may progress in difficulty from short sitting to long sitting to, finally, a standing position. The different positions will challenge a patient in a variety of postures.

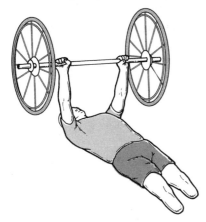

Figure 7-21. Wheelchair barbell exercise to strengthen the triceps and pectoralis major muscle groups. Adapted from Gailey, R. S. & Gailey, A. M. (1994). *Stretching and Strenghtening for Lower Extremity Amputees.* Miami, FL: Advanced Rehabilitation Therapy.

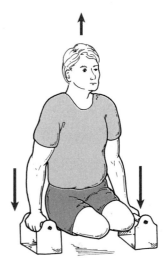

Figure 7-22. Dip exercises to strengthen the latissimus dorsi and triceps muscles.

Upper-extremity exercises are depicted in the following figures:

A wheelchair barbell raise may be used to strengthen the triceps and the pectoralis major muscle groups. In this exercise, the patient is supine, with the wheelchair barbell placed at chest level. The hands are placed a shoulder-width apart, and the barbell is raised upward (Fig. 7-21).

Dip exercises or seated pushups will strengthen the latissimus dorsi and triceps muscles. The patient pushes downward into blocks or small footstools, slowly raising the buttocks off the resting surface (Fig. 7-22).

Sitting trunk-rotation exercises with a wand and progressing to placing objects such as cones on various surfaces may be used to increase trunk stability. Sitting trunk-rotation exercises involve the patient grasping a wand with both palms facing down. The wand is raised to shoulder height and the patient rotates the trunk while keeping the pelvis stationary (Fig. 7-23). Raising the wand overhead or placing the wand behind the head displaces the center of gravity and

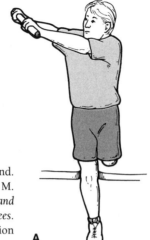
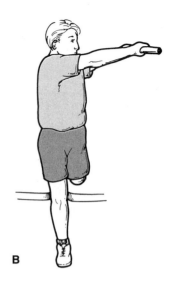

Figure 7-23. Trunk rotation with wand. Adapted from Gailey, R. S. & Gailey, A. M. (1994). *Balance, Agility, Coordination, and Endurance for Lower Extremity Amputees.* Miami, FL: Advanced Rehabilitation Therapy.

A   B

makes this activity more difficult. Objects placed on a variety of surfaces permit reaching across the body and picking up a cone from, for example, a surface on the right side and placing it on a surface on the left side (Fig. 7-24). Placing the cones farther away increases the difficulty.

Ball-throwing exercises may be done either in short sitting, long sitting, or a standing position to increase trunk stability and coordination. Throwing may be done either underhand or overhand. Overhand throwing is more difficult because of the greater displacement of the center of gravity. The ball may be thrown progressively farther away from the patient to challenge balance further (Fig. 7-25). Patients with excellent balance may perform throwing activities while standing on a balance or wobble board, wearing the prosthesis (Fig. 7-26).

These activities to increase trunk strength and coordination are first done from the sitting position, which is the easiest. The patient can

Figure 7-24. Trunk rotation with object placement. Adapted from Gailey, R. S. & Gailey, A. M. (1994). *Balance, Agility, Coordination, and Endurance for Lower Extremity Amputees.* Miami, FL: Advanced Rehabilitation Therapy.

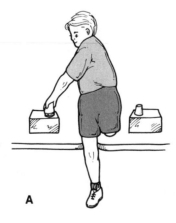
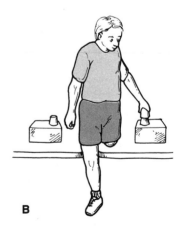

A   B

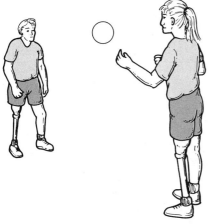

Figure 7-25. Ball throwing in a standing position. Adapted from Gailey, R. S. & Gailey, A. M. (1994). *Balance, Agility, Coordination, and Endurance for Lower Extremity Amputees*. Miami, FL: Advanced Rehabilitation Therapy.

then progress to the more-difficult positions of quadruped, kneeling, and ultimately standing. Adaptation of exercises for pediatric and geriatric patients is found in the Pediatric and Geriatric Perspective Boxes, respectively.

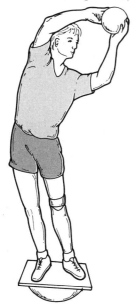

Figure 7-26. Ball throwing standing on an unstable surface.

Proprioceptive Neuromuscular Facilitation (PNF)

PNF is an exercise made popular by the works of Kabat, Knott, and Voss in the 1950s.[12] PNF techniques can improve strength and motor control of the trunk and limbs to enhance functional abilities such as ambulation, transfers, and bed mobility.

PNF techniques are an excellent form of exercise for the patient with an amputation and, if muscle tone is not increased, for the patient needing an orthosis. One example of a PNF technique is **rhythmic stabilization**. This technique involves alternating isometric contrac-

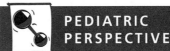

PEDIATRIC PERSPECTIVE

Adaptation of Exercises for the Pediatric Patient

To increase compliance with an exercise program, the following activities may be helpful for the pediatric patient.

- Incorporation of exercises into play activities
- Allowing choices regarding number of repetitions, sequencing of exercises, ways to perform the exercise
- Opportunity to get siblings or friends involved in doing or assisting with the exercises
- Use of positive reinforcements such as stickers
- Support group involvement such as amputee networks or organizations that pertain to a certain condition such as the Muscular Dystrophy Association
- Daily journals to track exercise compliance
- Age-appropriate written exercise programs with graphics

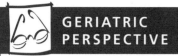

GERIATRIC PERSPECTIVE

Adaptation of Exercises for the Geriatric Patient

The geriatric patient, besides having physical problems that necessitated an amputation or an orthosis, may also have cognitive difficulties such as decreased memory, attention, concentration, or organizational skills. In addition, depression is common with aging and may affect compliance with a home exercise program. One *must* reinforce exercises with the patient's family and/or caregivers. Short durations of exercise for 5 minutes, four to six times a day may be needed with concentration difficulties. Both verbal and written communication of the purposes of the exercises or functional activities

as well as frequency may improve compliance. Other physical problems such as decreased vision and tactile sensation may make exercise more difficult.

Many geriatric patients will be seen in a home health setting. This setting may necessitate creative uses of equipment on the part of the physical therapist or physical therapist assistant. Adaptations in the home such as the use of countertops, weights made of reclosable bags filled with stones or dried beans, and cookie sheets to provide a reduced friction board for lower-extremity exercises may be needed.

tions against resistance, with no motion intended.[13] Careful grading of the therapist resistance to the patient's "hold" contractions may strengthen trunk musculature. For example, the patient assumes a quadruped position. First the therapist pushes the patient away

while the patient resists the movement; then the therapist pulls the patient toward him or her while the patient resists the movement. Patients must not be overpowered by so much resistance that the position cannot be maintained (Fig. 7-27). When patients can easily maintain

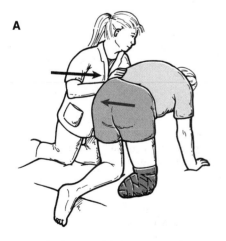
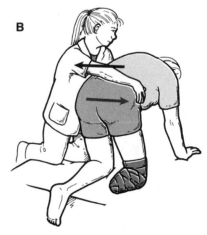

Figure 7-27. Rhythmic stabilization—quadruped position. A. The therapist pushes the patient away while the patient resists the movement. B. The therapist then pulls the patient toward while the patient resists the movement.

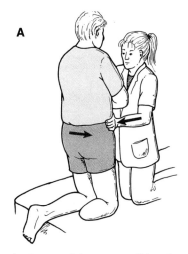
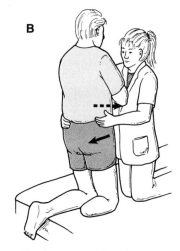

Figure 7-28. Rhythmic stabilization—tall kneeling position. A. The therapist pushes the patient away while the patient resists the movement. B. The therapist then pulls the patient toward while the patient resists the movement.

a quadruped position with resistance, they may progress to tall kneeling (Fig. 7-28). Both of these techniques may assist in functional activities such as getting up from the floor.

Slow reversal is another PNF technique that involves an isotonic contraction in one diagonal pattern, with changes in direction performed alternately at a point in the range where strength and control are limited. An isometric contraction may be performed at the end of each active command by the therapist resisting strongly but not overpowering the patient. Examples of slow reversal are pelvic anterior elevation which assists the patient in a motion of hip flexion. In this case the anterior, superior, and elevation motions of the pelvis are resisted by the therapist (Fig. 7-29). Pelvic posterior depression assists the patient with a motion of hip extension. In this case the posterior, inferior, and depression motions of the pelvis are resisted by the therapist (Fig. 7-30).

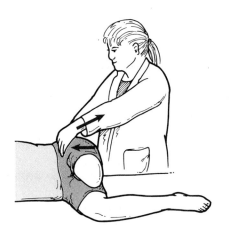

Figure 7-29. Pelvic anterior elevation resistance.

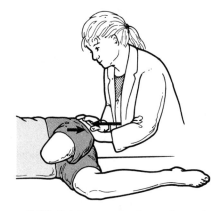

Figure 7-30. Pelvic posterior depression resistance.

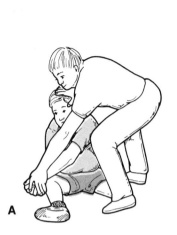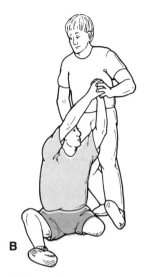

Figure 7-31. Resisted upper-extremity diagonal exercises. **A.** Upward diagonal resistance. **B.** Downward diagonal resistance. Adapted from Gailey, R. S. & Gailey, A. M. (1994). *Balance, Agility, Coordination, and Endurance for Lower Extremity Amputees.* Miami, FL: Advanced Rehabilitation Therapy.

Pelvic control will also assist in bed mobility and balance.

PNF techniques may also involve the upper trunk and upper extremity. Resistance to upper-extremity, trunk, and neck movements may be applied in an upward or downward diagonal chopping pattern (Fig. 7-31). These activities may assist in better trunk rotation control, which is important in functional activities and ambulation.

Resisted diagonal rotation using rubber tubing or sport cords may be done in a PNF pattern to increase upper- extremity and trunk strength. In this exercise, the rubber tubing or sport cord is secured to an immovable object such as a heavy table leg. The patient grasps the rubber tubing and pulls up and across the body, rotating at the waist. The elbows and wrists should stay in a slightly extended position. The patient slowly returns the rubber tubing to the starting position (Fig. 7-32).[14] Rubber tubing may also be attached to either leg to facilitate strengthening or better balance. If the tubing is attached to the residual limb, strengthening in PNF patterns may be done. If the tubing is attached to the sound limb, the patient must stand on the prosthesis facilitating balance.

PNF exercises are most appropriate as a means of strengthening and increasing coordination and flexibility for the motivated patient who is able to follow directions closely. The reader is encouraged to consult PNF textbooks for additional ways in which these techniques may be used with a patient with an amputation.

Isokinetics

Isokinetics is a type of exercise in which movement occurs at a constant speed but a variable resistance. Isokinetics is an accommodating resistance exercise. Many isokinetic machines are capable of concentric and eccentric training. Because of the patient's limited mobility and difficulty in transferring to a narrow bench, isokinetics may initially be a difficult mode of exercise. However, adjustments in the machine such as shortening the resistance arm are readily made (Fig. 7-33).

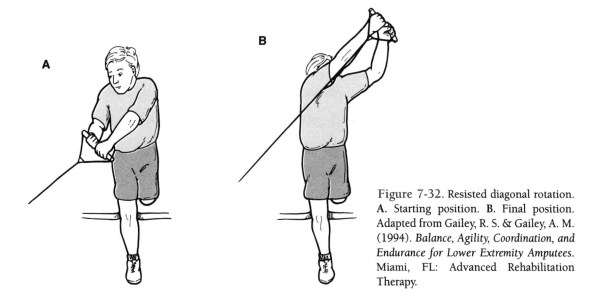

Figure 7-32. Resisted diagonal rotation. A. Starting position. B. Final position. Adapted from Gailey, R. S. & Gailey, A. M. (1994). *Balance, Agility, Coordination, and Endurance for Lower Extremity Amputees.* Miami, FL: Advanced Rehabilitation Therapy.

Cardiovascular Activities

Cardiovascular activities may be tailored to improve endurance and allow more-efficient functional activities of daily living. These activities may be done in either a pre-prosthesis/preorthosis phase or postprosthesis/postorthosis phase. Cardiovascular status must be optimal to allow a symmetric, energy-efficient gait. Factors including **duration,** fre-

quency, **intensity,** and **mode** or type may be changed according to the needs and abilities of the patient. The American College of Sports Medicine addresses duration and frequency issues by recommending a duration of 20–30 minutes, 3–4 days per week to produce cardiovascular improvements.[15] Deconditioned patients may need to break this 20–30 minutes of time into smaller periods, such as two 10-minute or four 5-minute sessions. Many pa-

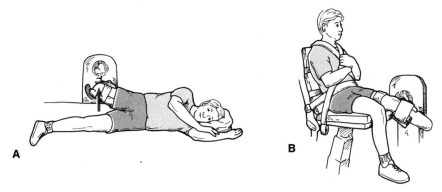

Figure 7-33. Use of an isokinetic device. A. Hip abduction. B. Knee extension. Adapted from Gailey, R. S. & Gailey, A. M. (1994). *Strengthening and Stretching for Lower Extremity Amputees.* Miami, FL: Advanced Rehabilitation Therapy.

tients with amputation or needing an orthosis are not healthy; therefore, exercise progression that stresses the cardiovascular system should be done slowly.

Healthy individuals should exercise at 55–90% of maximal heart rate. Maximal heart rate is determined by the number 220 minus the person's age. For example, a 60-year-old patient's maximal heart rate is 160 (220–60). Cardiovascular improvements may be produced by maintaining a heart rate between 88 (55% times 160) and 145 (90% times 160) beats per minute for 20–30 minutes, 3–4 days a week. Exercise intensity can be increased by adding resistance, increasing speed, or changing terrain, as in inclines or hills. The more intense the exercise, the shorter the duration.

The mode is the type of exercise that is most suited for the patient with an amputation. The use of an upper- extremity ergometer will, in most cases, rapidly increase heart rate. Swimming is an excellent exercise for those patients with an amputation or an orthosis who have sensitive residual limbs and may need to minimize weight-bearing impact. The warm-up period associated with cardiovascular endurance should last 5-10 minutes. The warm-up period increases muscle blood flow, muscle temperature, and neural conduction and may decrease the chances of muscle injury during exercise. A cool-down period of the same duration (5–10 minutes) often consists of stretching exercises.[12]

Early Postamputation Activities

The following exercises and functional activities may be done 1-3 days after amputation:

- Isometrics—gluteal and quadriceps sets and abdominal strengthening.
- Active range of motion (AROM) of unaffected limbs. Affected-limb hip AROM can be done on postoperative days 1–3 by patients with transtibial amputation. Positioning, as described earlier, is emphasized

in this early rehabilitation, to prevent contractures.
- Upper-extremity strengthening, such as dips or seated push-ups are important for latissimus dorsi and triceps strengthening to facilitate transfers. Upper-extremity ergometry is a useful strengthening and endurance activity.
- Bed mobility, sitting tolerance, and transfer training are often begun on postoperative day 2.

Transfer training may be done in a number of ways. These include bed-to-wheelchair transfers leading with the sound extremity. The therapist, using proper body mechanics, blocks the patient's sound knee and, by grasping the patient's pelvis, assists the patient with a stand-pivot transfer (Fig. 7-34).[16]A patient may use a transfer board to transfer from wheelchair to bed or to a car (Fig. 7-35). A patient with bilateral amputations may use a forward/backward transfer (Fig. 7-36). Patients with bilateral amputations often use a specialized wheelchair, sometimes called an amputee wheelchair. This wheelchair has the wheel axis posterior to the center support to allow better balance (Fig. 7-37).

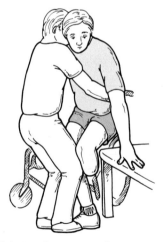

Figure 7-34. Stand-pivot transfer.

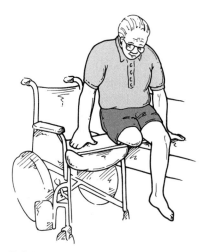

Figure 7-35. Use of a transfer board.

Classes

Whenever available, class and pool programs are appropriate adjuncts to a patient's program because they allow variety as well as interaction with others with an amputation or an orthosis. Classes may be done as part of an inpatient rehabilitation program or later in the

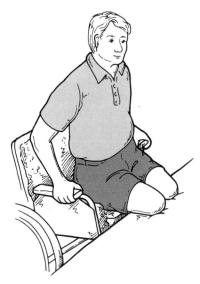

Figure 7-36. Forward/backward transfer for a patient with bilateral amputations.

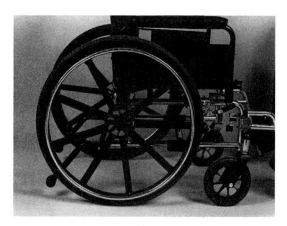

Figure 7-37. Specialized wheelchair with a posterior wheel axis used for a patient with bilateral amputations.

rehabilitation process, on an outpatient basis. Classes in advanced upper-extremity strengthening use resistance, balance, mobility, and endurance. Wheelchair mobility skill classes build endurance and develop skills needed to negotiate a wheelchair both indoors and outdoors. Use of the pool may be contraindicated for those with open lesions, incontinence, or allergic reactions to chlorine. In addition, problems with edema may be exacerbated with a warm-water pool.

Immediate Postoperative Prosthesis (IPOP) Protocols

Rigid dressings and IPOP are reviewed in Chapter 6. The following protocols serve as a guide in the management of a patient with an IPOP due to vascular disease, diabetes, or trauma.

Amputation Due to Vascular Disease or Diabetes

The patient with a rigid dressing performs straight leg raising; gluteal, quadriceps, and hamstring isometrics; and transfer skills until the first cast change at 5–7 days. If wound healing is satisfactory, a new rigid dressing with an IPOP is applied and weight bearing is started at 20–30 lb. Most patients are discharged to home after the first week. The rigid dressing is changed weekly by the prosthetist, and weight bearing is advanced by approximately 30 lb each week. When the residual-limb circumference is the same for 1–2 weeks and wrinkles have returned to the skin, the rigid dressing is no longer needed. Shrinkers or elastic bandages are then applied, and the prosthetist begins fabrication of the first prosthesis. This process may take up to 4–6 months.[16]

Amputation Due to Trauma

The patient with trauma performs the same activities initially as the patient with vascular disease or diabetes. However, an IPOP is applied initially rather than just a rigid dressing. Weight bearing at 20–30 lb is often started the day after amputation. As with the patient with vascular disease or diabetes, the rigid dressing is changed weekly by the prosthetist, and weight bearing is advanced by approximately 30 lb each week. When the residual limb circumference is the same for 1–2 weeks and wrinkles have returned to the skin, the rigid dressing is no longer needed. Shrinkers or elastic bandages are applied, and the prosthetist begins fabrication of the first prosthesis. This process usually takes between 3 and 6 weeks.[17]

Duration of Rehabilitation

The duration of rehabilitation varies, depending on a number of factors including patient specifics and the clinical setting. However, it is common for hospital discharge to occur 5 days after amputation. The time that a patient with an amputation performs certain activities will vary, based on the type of dressing used postoperatively and the cognition, strength, motivation, and other comorbidities that patient possesses. Resource Box 7-2 lists a timeline of activities that a typical patient with an amputation may perform.

Ideally, a patient should not be discharged until independence is achieved in transfers, activities of daily living, and home exercises. Patients who can transfer independently and have transportation are typically seen in an outpatient setting.[10] Those who have poor balance and are elderly may benefit from intensive short-term rehabilitation at a rehabilitation or extended-care facility. Family education in assistive care is an important component of early prosthetic rehabilitation. Home program exercises may be given to both the patient and the family. A patient with an amputation will often take the prosthesis home when application or removal of the prosthesis can be done independently. Taking the prosthesis home allows the patient to become accustomed to it. Even though the patient may not be able to stand safely with the prosthesis, it can be used in transfers. Before facility discharge, a home visit should be made to determine if architectural modifications or equipment may be necessary for the patient.

Ambulation Activities

For patients using a soft dressing after amputation, a cast for a temporary socket is often fabricated during weeks 6–8 postamputation. Ambulation activities with a prosthesis often begin during weeks 10–11 after amputation. Ambulation activities with an orthosis usually begin immediately after the orthosis is received.

Skin problems should be anticipated in patients with peripheral vascular disease or diabetes. Therefore, initially, the patient should wear the prosthesis or orthosis for only a 15-minute period. If the skin appears abraded or fragile, the 15-minute period should be shortened. The patient with a prosthesis should then rest for 15 minutes with a shrinker or elastic wrap in place to avoid residual-limb

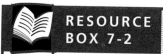

RESOURCE
BOX 7-2

Timeline of Activities the Patient with an Amputation May Perform

Acute postoperative (1–2 days): Elevation of the limb for the first 24-48 hours, isometric muscle strengthening, gentle ROM, a patient wearing an IPOP may begin weight bearing. Positioning to avoid contractures is done. Positioning principles are explained to patient and family. Bed mobility and transfer activities are begun. Home evaluation and equipment needs are assessed.

Preprosthetic (3–6 weeks with IPOP, 6-8 weeks or longer with soft or other types of dressings): When dressings are not needed, the patient and family are instructed in bandaging or use of a shrinker. Skin care precautions are explained. Desensitization and coordination exercises of the residual limb are done. More aggressive upper and lower-extremity strengthening and ROM exercises are started. Cardiovascular activities are also begun. Ongoing functional activities including gait training and stairs are initiated. Patient education and preparation for the use of the prosthesis and its care may occur.

Prosthetic (time varies with type of dressing and comorbidities associated with a specific patient, may extend from 6 weeks to 6 months): Use of a temporary or preparatory prosthesis and finally a definitive prosthesis is begun. Balancing, ambulation, and functional training activities are done with the prosthesis. Floor-to-chair transfers and other functional activities should be done with and without the prosthesis.

---

edema. Ideally, a schedule of 15 minutes wearing the prosthesis or orthosis and 15 minutes of rest should continue during the first several days of initial prosthesis or orthosis wear. Weight bearing on the prosthesis, with an assistive device, can be limited to 25 to 40 lb initially. This amount of weight bearing may be determined by using a scale under the prosthetic foot. Weight bearing on the orthosis depends on the patient's condition and reason for needing the orthosis.

Specific ambulation activities consist of the following:

Finding the center of gravity within the base of support—The patient, holding onto the parallel bars, may shift the body weight from side to side, working toward maintaining balance. The use of a mirror may assist in proper weight shift (Fig. 7-38).

Forward-and-backward weight shift—Forward-and-backward shifts with small movements may progress to larger movements. Patients may begin by using the parallel bars with palms flat and progress to support with one hand and then to using no hands. The patient must not grasp the parallel bars, since this reduces the weight on the prosthesis. Supporting the weight with a flat palm allows some support, yet enables the patient to place most of the weight onto the prosthesis (Fig. 7-39).

Compliant surface—Patients may progress to weight-shifting exercises on a compliant surface such as a piece of foam, wheelchair cushion, or minitrampoline. The use of a compliant surface will challenge balance

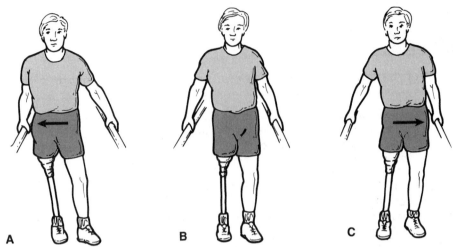

Figure 7-38. Side-to-side weight shift. Adapted from Gailey, R. S. & Gailey, A. M. (1994). *Balance, Agility, Coordination, and Endurance for Lower Extremity Amputees.* Miami, FL: Advanced Rehabilitation Therapy.

further and lead to better stability in weight bearing (Fig. 7-40).[14]

Early ambulation—Patients must practice taking steps with the prosthetic leg, avoiding circumduction and abduction of the prosthesis. Stride length may be varied with each step. Progression to ambulating with a narrow base of support (2-4 inches) will further challenge balance. In early prosthetic training, individuals with good cardiovascular status and balance may ambulate using crutches and a swing-through gait. Those with poor balance may ambulate using a walker. The walker, however, reinforces an abnormal gait pattern characterized by short steps, forward lean, and poor arm swing. A walker is also difficult to maneuver in tight spaces and on stairs.

Sidestepping—Sidestepping may be done for gluteus medius strengthening, which helps

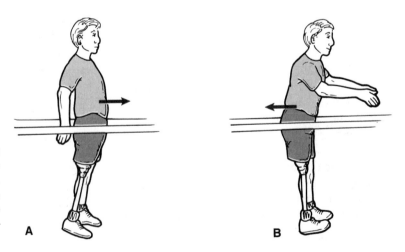

Figure 7-39. Front-and-back weight shift. Adapted from Gailey, R. S. & Gailey, A. M. (1994). *Balance, Agility, Coordination, and Endurance for Lower Extremity Amputees.* Miami, FL: Advanced Rehabilitation Therapy.

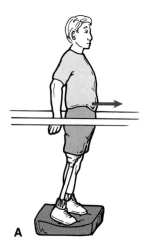

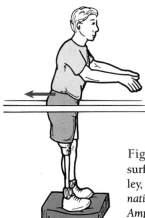

A   B

Figure 7-40. Weight shift on a compliant surface. Adapted from Gailey, R. S. & Gailey, A. M. (1994). *Balance, Agility, Coordination, and Endurance for Lower Extremity Amputees*. Miami, FL: Advanced Rehabilitation Therapy.

in navigation in tight quarters such as church pews or narrow stall doors.

Stool stepping—Stool stepping involves the patient stepping onto a 8-inch stool with the unaffected leg as slowly as possible. This may be a difficult activity to perform initially because of weakness and loss of balance and coordination. Patients may start by holding onto the parallel bars with palms flat and progress from single-hand support to no hand support (Fig. 7-41).

Balance challenging—Balance challenging promotes trunk stability. The patient is asked to maintain proper standing stability while the therapist's hands are placed on either side of the shoulders and the patient is gently pushed. The patient may be challenged at the pelvis in a rhythmic stabilization PNF technique to promote hip stability or at the prosthetic socket to promote knee stability (Fig. 7-42). Progression to resisted gait training may be done to ensure pelvic rota-

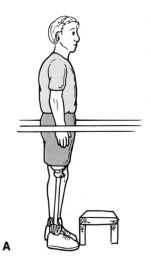

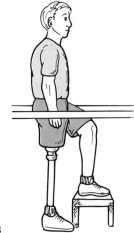

A   B

Figure 7-41. Stool stepping leading with the unaffected leg. Adapted from Gailey, R. S. & Gailey, A. M. (1994). *Balance, Agility, Coordination, and Endurance for Lower Extremity Amputees*. Miami, FL: Advanced Rehabilitation Therapy.

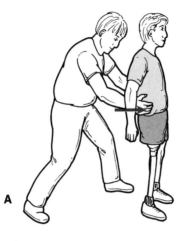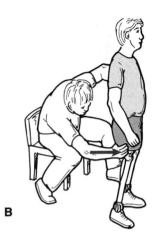

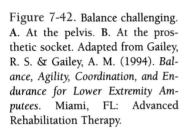
Figure 7-42. Balance challenging. A. At the pelvis. B. At the prosthetic socket. Adapted from Gailey, R. S. & Gailey, A. M. (1994). *Balance, Agility, Coordination, and Endurance for Lower Extremity Amputees.* Miami, FL: Advanced Rehabilitation Therapy.

tion and improve pelvic and trunk disassociation. Resisted gait training may ensure a more natural cosmetic gait.

Resisted ambulation—Resisted ambulation using a cable column machine may also strengthen pelvic and hip motions (Fig. 7-43).

Equipment

When discharged from the hospital or a rehabilitation facility, a patient with an amputation or needing an orthosis may need the equipment listed in Practical Application Box 7-1.

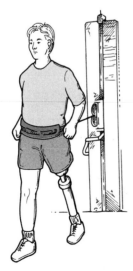
Figure 7-43. Resisted walking using a cable column.

Energy Expenditure

Individuals with an amputation expend more energy than the able-bodied at any ambulation speed. Energy-cost studies have indicated that for able-bodied individuals, a symmetric gait of 1.3 meters per second or 80 meters per minute is an optimal method and speed. Energy costs of ambulation in individuals with lower-extremity amputation are given in Table 7-1[8,19] As Table 7-1 shows, the knee joint is a major determinant in the energy cost of ambulation.[20] In one study of 24 male subjects with transtibial amputation, individuals with a vascular cause for amputation had lower stance duration and lower ground reaction forces than those with a traumatic cause for amputation.[21]

Individuals with amputation use adaptations to compensate for the missing limb. The reduction in push-off in terminal stance by the prosthetic foot is partially compensated by an increase in hip extensor activity.[22] Cocontraction of the hamstrings and quadriceps has been found in midstance, possibly for increased knee stability.[21,23] Newer prosthetic components and sockets have been developed to decrease the energy costs of ambulation. However, despite biomechanical designs of energy absorption in newer prosthetic feet, energy costs of ambulation have not been significantly reduced.[22]

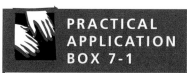

PRACTICAL APPLICATION BOX 7-1

Equipment That May Be Needed at Home by a Patient with an Amputation or Needing an Orthosis

Bathroom items

- Raised toilet seat
- Grab bars around toilet and tub
- Hand shower
- Long-handled sponge
- Bedside commode
- Tub seat

Other items

- Wheelchair, cushion, antitip bars
- Sliding board
- Ramp or outside railings
- Stair lift
- Driving adaptation of gas and brake for a right lower-extremity amputation
- Hand controls for bilateral amputations

Individuals with a well-fitted prosthesis and a satisfactory gait have significantly lower physiologic energy demand than those with an amputation who use crutches and no prosthesis. In a study of nine subjects with transtibial amputations who used a three-point-crutch gait pattern, those using a prosthesis had significantly lower rate of energy expenditure, heart rate, and oxygen cost than those without a prosthesis. Since the use of a prosthesis results in less exertion than not using a prosthesis, patients who cannot ambulate with crutches should not necessarily be denied a prosthesis.[24] Based on the results of this study, nonambulatory patients, if given a prosthesis, may become successful ambulators.

Few energy-expenditure studies have been performed on individuals with bilateral ampu-

tations. The individual with a bilateral amputation expends more effort than the individual with a unilateral amputation. Individuals with more-distal amputations expended less energy than those with more-proximal amputations. In addition, those with traumatic, bilateral transtibial amputations had a faster walking speed than those with a vascular cause (67 vs. 40 m/min).[25] The energy demands of ambulation for an individual with bilateral transfemoral amputations is 280% higher than that of unimpaired subjects.[26]

Harness-supported treadmill ambulation has been used with individuals with amputation. In a study of seven individuals with transtibial amputation, 40% body-harness-supported ambulation at a speed of 1.34 m/sec resulted in significantly lower energy expenditure and lower heart rates.[27] The investigators in this study recommended harness-supported treadmill ambulation in early prosthetic training when energy expenditure savings would be advantageous.

Functional Activities

The functional activities listed in Table 7-2 must be mastered by the patient with an amputation to reach an independent functional level.[3] Many

Table 7-1. Energy Expenditure of Ambulation in Individuals with Lower-Extremity Amputations	
Amputation Level	**Amount by Which Energy Expenditure Exceeds That of Able-Bodied Persons (%)**
Transtibial	9–20
Transfemoral	45–70
Bilateral transtibial	41
Bilateral transfemoral	Up to 300

Adapted from Kumar, V. N. Normal locomotion and prosthetic gait deviation. In S. N. Banerjee (Ed.). (1982). Rehabilitation management of amputees (pp. 237–254). Baltimore: Williams & Wilkins, and Murray, D., & Fisher, F. R. (1982). *Normal gait. Handbook of amputations and prostheses (pp. 28–31).* Ottawa: University of Ottawa.

Table 7-2. Description of Activities for Independent Functioning

Activity	Plan of Accomplishment
Ascending stairs	Patient leads with the sound foot, ascending one or two stairs at a time (Fig. 7-44)
Descending stairs	Patient leads with the prosthesis, one step at a time; more-agile patients may be able to descend step over step (Fig. 7-45).
Ascending inclines	Ascending inclines is illustrated in Figure 7-46

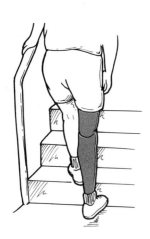

Figure 7-44. Stair ascent leading with the sound leg.

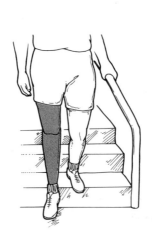

Figure 7-45. Stair descent leading with the prosthesis.

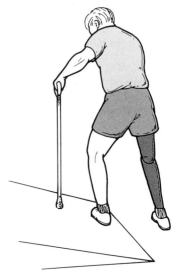

Figure 7-46. Incline ascent leading with the sound leg. The patient leads with sound foot. Sufficient hip flexion of the residual limb is necessary to prevent the prosthetic toe from catching. In cases of weakness, ascent may be on a diagonal, leading with, and taking a longer step with, the sound leg.

Descending inclines	Descending inclines is illustrated in Figure 7-47
Picking up an object	Picking up an object is depicted in Figure 7-48
Clearing an obstacle: direct approach	Patient leads with the sound leg and forcibly flexes the residual limb hip to clear the obstacle (Figure 7-49)

Table 7-2. Description of Activities for Independent Functioning (Continued)

Activity	Plan of Accomplishment

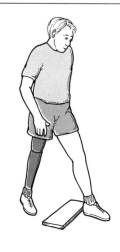

A

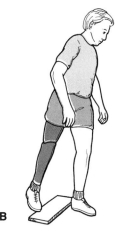

B

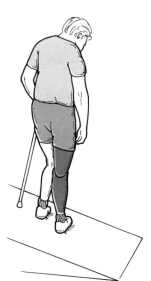

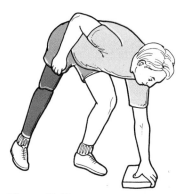

Figure 7-47. Incline descent leading with the prosthesis. The patient leads with the prosthesis, taking a shorter step than usual. The prosthesis is kept behind the sound leg to increase the base of support. The hip of the residual limb must be forcibly extended on initial contact to maintain knee stability.

Figure 7-48. Picking up an object. The prosthetic foot is placed behind the sound foot while maintaining body weight on the sound leg. The hips are flexed to allow grasping of an object. This position avoids flexing the prosthetic knee, which may lead to instability.

Figure 7-49. Clearing an obstacle—direct approach. The patient leads with the sound leg and forcibly flexes the residual-limb hip to clear the obstacle.

Clearing an obstacle: side approach	The side approach to clearing an obstacle is shown in Figure 7-50

Table 7-2. Description of Activities for Independent Functioning (Continued)

Activity	Plan of Accomplishment

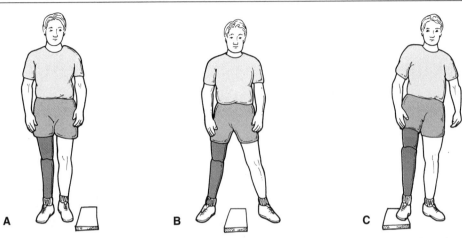

Figure 7-50. Clearing an obstacle—side approach. The sound limb is placed nearer the obstacle and swung over the obstacle first, followed by the prosthesis. The side approach to clearing an obstacle requires controlled weight-shifting from the sound to the residual-limb side.

Falling	The steps involved in breaking a fall are depicted in Figure 7-51

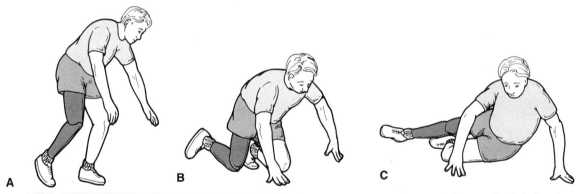

Figure 7-51. Falling. An attempt should be made during a fall to throw the weight toward the sound side by bending at the waist, breaking the fall if possible with the hands, and rolling onto the sound side.

Sitting on the floor	Sitting on the floor is similar to a controlled falling maneuver as shown in Figure 7-51; the prosthesis is placed a half-step behind the sound foot, with the body weight on the residual limb; while bending at the waist, the arms are outstretched, both hips and knees are flexed, and a pivot to the sound side is done
Rising from the floor	There are several methods a patient wearing a prosthesis may use to rise from the floor; one method is described in Figure 7-52

Table 7-2. Description of Activities for Independent Functioning (Continued)

Activity	Plan of Accomplishment

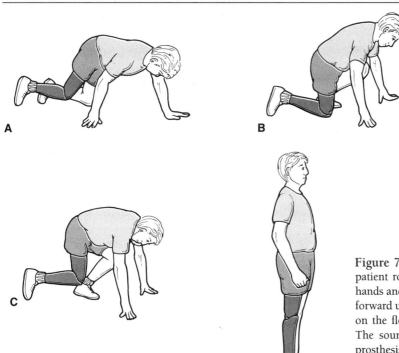

Figure 7-52. Rising from the floor. The patient rolls to the sound side, onto the hands and knees. The sound leg is placed forward under the trunk with the foot flat on the floor in a half-kneeling position. The sound knee is extended while the prosthesis is brought forward. An object such as a chair or a counter may provide support and make this activity easier.

| Driving | A patient with a right lower-extremity amputation may need to have the brake and gas pedals switched to move the gas pedal closer to the left sound leg; hand controls are necessary for patients with bilateral lower-extremity amputations (Fig. 7-53); two-door cars offer more front seat leg room than four-door cars; resources for driving controls and mobility products are listed in Practical Application Box 7-2 |

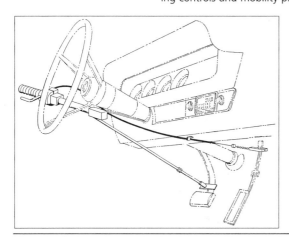

Figure 7-53. Driving hand controls. (Reprinted with permission from Wells Engberg Co.)

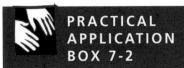

PRACTICAL APPLICATION BOX 7-2

Resources on Driving Controls

Braun Corporation
  P.O. Box 310
  Winamar, IN 46996
  (219)-946-6153
  Mobility products and driving controls
EMC Inc.
  2001 Wooddale Blvd
  Baton Rouge, LA 70806
  (504)-926-2403
  Manufacturer of driving controls
I.D.S.
  580 T.C. Jester
  Houston, TX 77007
  (713)-846-1460
  Manufacturer of driving controls
Manufacturing and Production Services Corporation
  7948 Ronson Road
  San Diego, CA 92111
  (800)-243-4051
  Manufacturer of driving controls
Wells Engberg Inc.
  P.O. Box 6388
  Rockford, IL 61125
  (800)-642-3628
  Manufacturer of driving controls
Wrightway
  P.O. 460907
  Garland, TX 75046
  (800)-241-8839
  Manufacturer of driving controls

of these activities also apply to a patient wearing an orthosis. It is beyond the scope of this book to include functional activities for each condition that may necessitate an orthosis.

KEY POINTS

- Positioning is done to prevent shortening of soft tissue and subsequent joint contractures.

- Flexibility exercises should be done in a slow, controlled manner, and a stretch should be held for 20 seconds.

- Desensitization activities accustom the residual limb to weight bearing and to eventual wearing of the prosthesis.

- Types of strengthening exercises include isometric, isotonic, upper-extremity, PNF, isokinetic, and cardiovascular.

- Individuals with an amputation expend much more energy than the able-bodied during ambulation activities.

- Ambulation activities may progress from maintaining balance to independent performance of functional activities such as inclines, stairs, and getting up from the floor.

LABORATORY ACTIVITIES

1. Given the fact that in most patients with transfemoral amputation, the hip flexors and abductors tend to be stronger than the hip extensors and adductors, what type of positioning and what type of strengthening exercises would you recommend for such a patient. Simulate this positioning and types of strengthening exercises on a classmate.

2. A patient with a transtibial amputation tends to have stronger knee flexors than knee extensors. What type of positioning and what type of strengthening exercises would you recommend for this patient. Simulate this positioning and types of strengthening exercises on a classmate.

3. Design an activity program for a patient with a hypersensitive extremity that would be appropriate for a particular patient with an amputation or one needing an orthosis. Be able to explain the rationale for this desensitization program. Simulate these desensitization activities on a classmate.

4. Differentiate among the types of strengthening exercises that would be appropriate for a particular patient with an amputation or one needing an orthosis.

5. Design an exercise program for a patient 1–3 days after amputation

6. Simulate ambulation activities that would be appropriate for a patient with a new prosthesis. Progress these activities from easiest to hardest. Simulate these ambulation activities on a classmate.

7. Design a functional activity training program that would be appropriate for a patient with a new prosthesis or orthosis. Progress these activities from easiest to hardest. Simulate these functional activities on a classmate.

REFERENCES

1. American Physical Therapy Association. (2001) A guide to physical therapist practice. *Physical Therapy, 81.*

2. Shurr, D. G. (1999). *Patient care booklet for above-knee amputees (p. 6).* Alexandria, VA: American Academy of Orthotists and Prosthetists.

3. Rehabilitation Institute of Chicago. (1985). *Lower extremity amputation.* Rockville, MD: Aspen.

4. Mensch, G., & Ellis, P. M. (1986). *Physical therapy management of lower extremity amputations.* Rockville, MD: Aspen.

5. Hertling, D. & Kessler, R. M. (1996). Management of common musculoskeletal disorders (3rd ed., p. 276). Philadelphia: J. B. Lippincott.

6. Kisner, C., & Colby, L. A. (1996). *Therapeutic exercise* (3rd ed., pp. 70–90). Philadelphia: F. A. Davis.

7. Prentice, W. E. (1990). *Rehabilitation techniques in sports medicine* (3rd ed., p. 77). St Louis: Times Mirror/Mosby.

8. Gerber, L., & Hicks, J. (1990). Exercise in the rheumatic diseases. In Basmajian (Ed.). *Therapeutic exercise (p. 333).* Baltimore: Williams & Wilkins.

9. Lindh, M. (1979). Increase of muscle strength from isometric quadriceps exercise at different knee angles. *Scandinavian Journal of Medicine, 11,* 33.

10. Knapik, J. J., Mawadsely, R. H., & Ramos, M. U. (1983). Angular specificity and test mode specificity of isometric and isokinetic strength training. *Journal of Orthopaedic and Sports Physical Therapy, 5,* 58.

11. Salsich, G. B., & Mueller, M. J. (1997). Relationships between measures of function, strength, and walking speed in patients with diabetes and transmetatarsal amputation. *Clinical Rehabilitation, 11,* 60–67.

12. Hall, C. M., & Brody, L. T. (1999). *Therapeutic exercise moving toward function.* Philadelphia: Lippincott Williams & Wilkins.

13. Adler, S. S., Beckers, D., & Buck, M. (1999). PNF in practice: *An illustrated guide* (2nd ed.). Berlin: Springer.

14. Gailey, R. S., & Gailey, A. M. (1994). *Stretching and strengthening for lower extremity amputees.* Miami, FL: Advanced Rehabilitation Therapy.

15. American College of Sports Medicine. (1990). Position stand: The recommended quantity and quality of exercise for developing and maintaining cardiorespiratory and muscular fitness in healthy adults. *Medicine and Science in Sports and Exercise, 22,* 265-274.

16. Engstrom, B., & Van Deven, C. (1985). *Physiotherapy for amputees: The Roehampton approach.* New York: Churchill Livingstone.

17. Smith, D. G., & Fergason, J. R. (1999). Transtibial amputations. *Clinical Orthopedics and Related Research, 361,* 108-115.

18. Kumar, V. N. (1982). Normal locomotion and prosthetic gait deviation. In S. N. Banerjee (Ed.). *Rehabilitation management of amputees (pp. 237–254).* Baltimore: Williams & Wilkins.

19. Murray, D., & Fisher, F. R. (1982). *Normal gait. Handbook of amputations and prostheses (pp. 28-31).* Ottawa: University of Ottawa.

20. Waters, R. L., Perry, J., Antonelli, D., & Hislop, H. (1976). Energy cost of walking of amputees: The influence of level of amputation. *Journal of Bone and Joint Surgery, 58A,* 42–46

21. Hermodsson, Y., Ekdahl, C., Persson, B. M., & Roxendal, G. (1994). Gait in male trans-tibial amputees: A comparative study with healthy subjects in relation to walking speed. *Prosthetics and Orthotics International, 18,* 68–77.

22. Czerniecki, J. M. (1996). Rehabilitation in limb deficiency. Gait and motion analysis. *Archives of Physical Medicine and Rehabilitation, 77,* S3–8.

23. Winter, D. A., & Sienko, S. E. (1988). Biomechanics of below knee amputee gait. *Journal of Biomechanics, 21,* 361–367.

24. Gonzalez, E. G., Corcoran, P. J., & Reyes, R. L. (1974). Energy expenditure in below knee amputees: Correlation with stump length. *Archives of Physical Medicine and Rehabilitation, 55,* 111–119.

25. Waters, R. L. (1992). Energy *Expenditure of Amputee Gait (pp.* 381-387). In J. H. Bowker, & J. W. Michael (Eds.). *Atlas of limb prosthetics.* St Louis: Mosby Year Book.

26. Huang, C. T., Jackson, J. R., Moore, N. B., Fine, P. R., Kuhlemeier, K. V., Truahg, G. H., & Saunders, P. T. (1979). Amputation: Energy cost of ambulation. *Archives of Physical Medicine and Rehabilitation, 60,* 18–24.

27. Hunter, D., Cole, E. S., Murray, J. M., & Murray, T. D. (1995). Energy expenditure of below-knee amputees during harness-supported treadmill ambulation. *Journal of Orthopaedic and Sports Physical Therapy, 21,* 268–276.

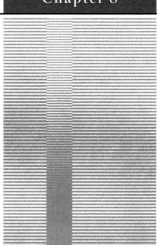

Chapter 8

TRANSTIBIAL COMPONENTS—
CLINICAL DECISION MAKING

Objectives

1. Differentiate postoperative, temporary, and definitive prostheses and describe when they are used in the rehabilitative process
2. Describe conventional and computer-aided fabrication of a prosthesis
3. Differentiate various types of prosthetic feet and suspensions and give a rationale for their use with a particular patient
4. Contrast the areas of weight bearing and areas of relief of a patellar tendon bearing (PTB) socket
5. Describe the indications for different liners
6. Describe the examination or checkout procedures for a transtibial prosthesis
7. Given a patient with a transtibial amputation, develop a prescription recommendation for prosthetic components
8. Recommend prosthetic and musculoskeletal corrections that may be made for a particular gait deviation

This chapter is divided into the following sections:

P hysical therapists, as part of the prosthetic clinical team, or in consultation with a prosthetist need to possess an understanding of prosthetic componentry to recommend the optimal prosthetic components for an individual with an amputation. There are numerous prosthetic components available, with ongoing research to design more-efficient components. The information in this chapter on transtibial components and in the next chapter on transfemoral components covers many of the most common prosthetic components used. One must know the advantages and disadvantages of a prosthetic component. The *Guide to Physical Therapist Practice* in the practice pattern "Motor Function, Muscle Performance, Range of Motion, Gait, Locomotion, and Balance Associated with Amputation" (4J) refers to interventions with prosthetic devices.[1] Regional differences and philosophies may alter the prosthetic components that are recommended. These chapters are not intended to be inclusive but representative of commonly used components.

◆◆◆

Types of Prostheses

There are three types of prostheses appropriate for different stages after amputation. These include postoperative prostheses, temporary prostheses, and definitive prostheses.

Postoperative Prostheses

A **postoperative prosthesis** may be an immediate postoperative prosthesis (IPOP). These are often used for younger patients, usually after a traumatic injury. A detailed description of an IPOP is given in Chapter 6 (see Fig. 6-4).

Temporary Prostheses

A **temporary prosthesis** consists of the socket, pylon, and foot. The temporary prosthesis allows early ambulation and promotes residual limb shrinkage. A temporary prosthesis is usually used for 3–6 months following the date of amputation. A type of temporary prosthesis, an adjustable prosthesis, is used for early gait training and dynamic alignment (Fig. 8-1). The adjustable prosthesis can be modified so that the foot is moved in a medial, lateral, anterior, posterior, inversion, or eversion direction. Transtibial prosthesis alignment is described in Chapter 5 on biomechanics. Modifications to the adjustable prosthesis may correct gait deviations, increase energy efficiency, and make ambulation more cosmetic and comfortable. Use of a temporary prosthesis enables the wearer to weight bear and significantly reduces edema. A temporary prosthesis may be converted to a definitive or final pros-

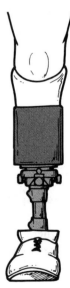

Figure 8-1. Adjustable prosthesis used in early gait training under the supervision of a physical therapist. (Adapted from a drawing by Campbell Childs Inc.)

thesis with cosmetic modifications made by the prosthetist.

A temporary prosthesis may also consist of a removable protective prosthetic socket. This socket may be integrated into a modular pre-fabricated preparatory prosthesis for controlled weight bearing and gait training.

Definitive Prostheses

A **definitive prosthesis** is recommended when the patient's residual limb no longer has marked volume changes. The patient may be ready for the definitive prosthesis 3–9 months after amputation. The average life span of a de-finitive prosthesis is 3–5 years. Replacement may be needed due to residual limb atrophy, weight gain or loss, or excessive wear of the prosthesis.

Types of Design

Definitive prostheses may have either an en-doskeletal (modular) or exoskeletal design. The endoskeletal design is more common. Temporary and postoperative prostheses are al-ways endoskeletal. Each of these design types is described as follows.

Endoskeletal or Modular Design

The **endoskeletal or modular design** in-cludes an anatomically shaped soft-foam cover designed to look and feel like skin. The plastic laminate socket is connected to the foot by a stainless-steel, titanium, aluminum, or carbon **pylon.** The material used in the py-lon varies, depending on the needs of the in-dividual with an amputation. Stainless steel is the heaviest of these materials and is typically used for a patient who weighs more than 225 pounds. Titanium is lightweight and approx-imates the strength of stainless steel. Alu-minum is the least expensive and is not as

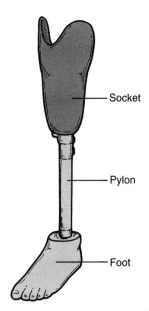

Figure 8-2. Endoskeletal or modular design prosthe-sis depicting socket, pylon, and foot.

strong as titanium. Carbon is used when a foot such as the Flex foot (described below in this chapter) is used.

The endoskeletal or modular design is de-picted in Figure 8-2. The advantages of the endoskeletal or modular design include being adjustable and lightweight. A temporary pros-thesis is always an endoskeletal design. The en-doskeletal design permits new sockets to be made as the volume in the residual limb de-creases, without altering the entire prosthesis. It is more cost effective to reuse components such as the pylon, suspension, and foot while replacing only the socket.[2] The more debili-tated individual generally requires a very light-weight endoskeletal and stable prosthesis. Shock-absorbing components (consisting of high-density bumpers, springs, or fluid fill) may be placed in the endoskeletal pylon at ei-ther the proximal end (attached to the socket) or the distal end (attached to the foot). A shock-absorbing component, the Total Shock, is shown in Figure 8-3. Nylon hose is the traditional finishing material for covering the prosthesis. Custom prosthetic skins that are matched to color and hair of the wearer are becoming more popular. These custom prosthetic skins increase cosmetic appearance, but they may interfere with prosthetic joint functioning and are expensive (Fig. 8-4). Some patients have elected to leave the endoskeletal prosthesis uncovered, which allows the joints to function optimally.[3] An endoskeletal transfemoral prosthesis with foam covering often is difficult to flex when sitting or in swing phase. This prosthesis should be stored initially with the prosthetic knee joint in the bent-knee position. Any endoskeletal prosthesis with a prosthetic skin should be covered with plastic to minimize tearing when storing.

Exoskeletal Design

An **exoskeletal design** has a hard outer cover made of plastic laminate. This design may be needed for occupations that require great durability, such as farming or construction work. Occupations involving high heat such as steel mills also may require an exoskeletal design. When not in use, the prosthesis should be laid

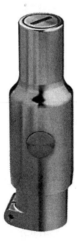

Figure 8-3. Total Shock shock-absorbing unit. (Reprinted with permission from Ossur.)

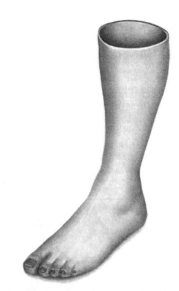

Figure 8-4. New Skin. (Reprinted with permission from Kingsley Manufacturing Co.)

flat to avoid breakage or cracking. This design is depicted in Figure 8-5.

Fabrication

Conventional and computer-aided (CAD/CAM) are two methods of fabricating a prosthesis.

Conventional Fabrication

A conventional method of fitting a residual limb for a prosthesis involves fabricating a negative impression and subsequent positive mold. A prosthetist will take length and circumferential measurements of both the residual and sound limbs. The cast of the residual limb creates the negative impression (Fig. 8-6). This negative impression is then filled with plaster to create a positive mold that represents the patient's residual limb. Addition of material to the positive mold relieves prosthetic socket pressure over bony prominences and tender areas. Conversely, subtraction of material results in increased pressure over ar-

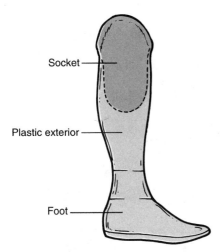

Figure 8-5. Exoskeletal design prosthesis depicting socket, plastic exterior, and foot.

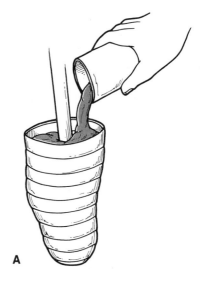

A

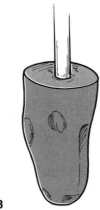

B

eas that can accept more weight bearing (Fig. 8-7). For example, pressure is increased in the PTB transtibial prosthesis by removing material from the positive mold at the following areas: patellar tendon, pretibial muscles, tibial flare, popliteal area, and calf musculature. Conversely, pressure is relieved by adding material to the positive mold in the following areas: tibial crest, distal portion of the tibia, fibular head, hamstring tendons, and patella. A

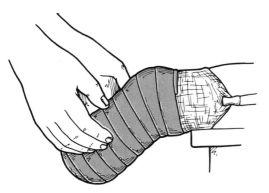

Figure 8-6. Negative mold. (Adapted from a drawing For the New Amputee by American Academy of Orthotists and Prosthetists, Alexandria, VA.)

Figure 8-7. Positive mold. A. Plaster poured into negative mold to create a positive mold. B. Positive mold after shaping. (Adapted from a drawing in For the New Amputee by American Academy of Orthotists and Prosthetists, Alexandria, VA.)

socket and liner are then built over the positive mold. A transparent diagnostic test socket may be used to determine if total contact of the residual limb is occurring. The socket is attached to an adjustable preparatory prosthesis. Static and dynamic alignments are done for a definitive prosthesis. Finally, shaping and finishing are completed.

Computer-Aided Fabrication

An alternative method of prosthesis fabrication uses a **computer-aided design/computer-aided manufacturing system (CAD/CAM)**. This system has been used on a clinical basis in the United States since the early 1990s. This system has three parts:

1. A probe or digitizer that converts information from the negative impression of the residual limb into computer data; the digitizer converts the location of each landmark into numerical data and records the dimension of the entire negative impression (Fig. 8-8).
2. A software system that enables the prosthetist to look at an exact replica of the patient's residual limb on the computer screen
3. A carver that reads the computer image of the residual limb and carves a positive plaster mold (Fig. 8-9)

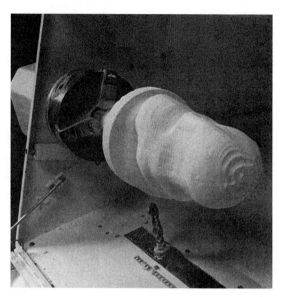

Figure 8-9. Positive mold in CAD/CAM.

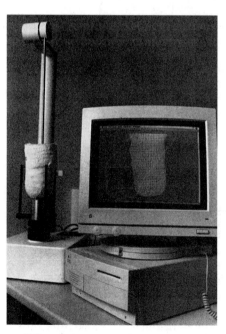

Figure 8-8. Digitizer in the CAD/CAM fabrication method.

Advantages of computer-aided fabrication over conventional fabrication are as follows:

- It decreases the need for cast modifications and thus is a time saver
- If an individual has torn a liner, a new liner may be made without a new positive mold being constructed
- A printout showing volume changes in the residual limb that necessitate modifying the socket or liner can be used to justify insurance reimbursement
- Patient education regarding normal area discoloration over weight-bearing areas and concerns about discoloration that occur over areas of relief in the PTB socket

Disadvantages of the computer-aided system are increased initial cost and the training that is needed to operate the system. As in conventional fabrication, the socket is attached to the adjustable temporary prosthesis, and static alignment, dynamic alignment, shaping, and finishing are done.

Prosthetic Feet

Prosthetic feet should provide the following functions:

1. Joint simulation
2. Shock absorption
3. Stable weight-bearing base of support
4. Muscle simulation
5. Cosmetically pleasing appearance[4,5]

Prosthetic feet may be divided into a number of categories. One categorical system is as follows:

1. Conventional
2. Dynamic response
   a. Nonarticulated
      i. Long keel
      ii. Short keel
   b. Articulated[6]

Conventional Feet

Five types of conventional foot–ankle assemblies are discussed below.

Single-Axis Foot

The articulated single-axis foot includes an internal keel, a molded foam-rubber shell, a metal single-axis joint, and plantarflexion and dorsiflexion bumpers. An articulated foot ankle assembly refers to the presence of a prosthetic ankle joint. A keel is the hard inner part of the prosthetic foot, similar to the bones and ligaments of the anatomic foot. The single-axis foot allows 5–7° of dorsiflexion and 15° of plantarflexion. This limited motion suffices for level-floor ambulation but does not allow for walking on a steep incline.[7] Minimal inversion and eversion occur through the flexibility of the rubber sole. Components of this single-axis foot include a dorsiflexion bumper that substitutes for an eccentric contraction of the gastrocnemius–soleus and a plantarflexion bumper that substitutes for an

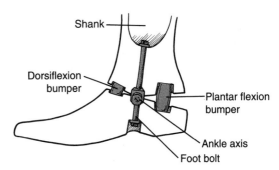

Figure 8-10. Single-axis foot. (Adapted from *Lower limb prosthetics* (1998). New York: Prosthetic Orthotic Publications.)

eccentric contraction of the anterior tibialis (Fig. 8-10).

Advantages and disadvantages are listed in Table 8-1.[7]

Multiple-Axis Foot

The articulated multiple- or functional-axis foot consists of an internal keel, a molded rubber foot, a central rubber rocker block that allows dorsiflexion and plantarflexion, and a transverse ankle joint that provides inversion, eversion, and rotation. Advantages of the multiple-axis foot include adaptation to walking on uneven ground as well as the ability to walk up a steep incline.[7] The transverse ankle joint provides good shock absorption, thereby lessening shear forces between the prosthesis and skin of the residual limb. The multiple-axis foot is appropriate for golfers, hikers, and those with brittle skin. Advantages and disadvantages are listed in Table 8-1 (Fig. 8-11).[2]

The Solid-Ankle Cushion-Heel (SACH) Foot

The nonarticulated solid-ankle cushion-heel (SACH) foot, introduced in 1956, is one of the most common foot assemblies used.[8] It is frequently used with temporary prostheses. The

Table 8-1. Comparison of Prosthetic Feet

Prosthetic Foot	Cost	Weight	Indication	Advantages	Disadvantages
Single axis	Low	Heavy	Enhances knee stability	Adjustable bumpers; adds to knee stability; allows rapid plantarflexion	Increased maintenance and weight; not cosmetic; moving parts may loosen and become noisy; debris can enter the joint and interfere with function
Multiple axis	Low	Heavy	Accommodates uneven surfaces	Allows multidirection motion; good shock absorption	Less stability on smooth surfaces; increased weight and maintenance
SACH	Low	Medium	General use	Large variety of heel heights available; reliable; less maintenance	Limited dorsiflexion due to the rigid keel; no propulsion at terminal stance
SAFE	Low	Medium	Accommodates to uneven surfaces	Little maintenance required; moisture and grit resistant; adjustable heel heights; pediatric sizes available	Less medial lateral stability; poor push-off at the end of stance phase
STEN	Low	Medium	Smooth stance roll over	Allows much motion; accommodates numerous shoe styles	Heavier and more expensive than SACH
Flex	Very high	Very light	Vigorous sports	Lightweight; vertical jumping allowed; medial lateral stability	High cost, complex fabrication and alignment, difficult heel height changes
Springlite	Very high	Very light	Vigorous sports	Same as Flex, except less expensive	Same as Flex
Seattle	Moderate	Heavy	General sports; active wearer	Dynamic response; improved cosmetic appearance	Increased weight and cost
Carbon Copy II	Moderate	Light	Active wearer; smooth stance roll over	Good medial lateral stability; light weight	Increased cost
College Park True-Step	High	Medium	Accommodates to uneven surfaces; high activity level	Increased stability; adjustable bumpers	Increased maintenance and expense; available only for adult sizes and low-heeled shoes

SACH foot consists of a keel that extends to the toe break and is surrounded by a molded external foam foot. The keel affects stability and push-off. A longer keel adds to foot stability. A shorter keel may lead to reduced stability, resulting in early heel-rise and a shortened stance phase. The wider the keel, the more stable the base of support.[7] The correct size keel is recommended on the basis of the patient's needs (Fig. 8-12).[4]

Plantarflexion is simulated by the SACH compressible heel. At the loading response phase of stance, the heel wedge compresses to simulate plantarflexion. The cushion heel may be ordered in different levels of firmness. Firmness of the heel in the SACH foot depends on

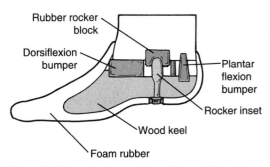

Figure 8-11. Multiple-axis foot. (Adapted from *Lower limb prosthetics* (1998). New York: Prosthetic Orthotic Publications.)

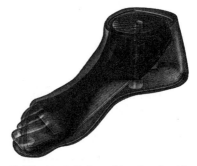

Figure 8-13. SAFE II foot. (Reprinted with permission from Campbell Childs Inc.)

the individual's weight and gait characteristics. Heavier patients need a firmer heel cushion to avoid quick plantarflexion. An extra-firm SACH heel results in a slow initial contact to loading-response phase, while a less firm SACH heel results in a quicker phase. As a result of this less firm SACH heel, the ground reaction force quickly moves forward to provide increased stability. The rubber forefoot provides resistance to toe extension during the late part of stance phase.

Advantages and disadvantages of the SACH foot are listed in Table 8-1.[6,7]

Stationary-Attachment Flexible Endoskeletal (SAFE) Foot

The nonarticulated stationary-attachment flexible endoskeletal (SAFE) foot was introduced in the late 1970s. The SAFE foot keel, a solid-

ankle version of the multiaxis concept, is composed of a rigid polyurethane elastomer section positioned at a 45° angle in the sagittal plane to simulate the human subtalar joint. This foot features two Dacron polyester–fiber plantar bands that force the keel to compress and dorsiflex from mid- to terminal stance. This dorsiflexion ensures a smooth progression over the foot. At preswing, the keel releases, which aids somewhat in push-off.[6,9] Styles include a waterproof foot, heavy-duty construction, and a Syme foot.[9] Advantages and disadvantages are listed in Table 8-1. The SAFE II model foot is a lighter version with molded toes (Fig. 8-13).

STored-ENergy (STEN) Foot

The stored-energy (STEN) foot has a keel that compresses in the loading response to midstance phase of gait, thereby storing energy. The energy is released in the terminal stance to the preswing phase of gait. Advantages and disadvantages of the STEN are listed in Table 8-1 (Fig. 8-14).[10]

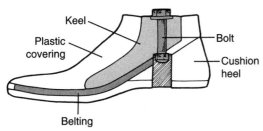

Figure 8-12. SACH foot. (Adapted from *Lower limb prosthetics* (1998). New York: Prosthetic Orthotic Publications.)

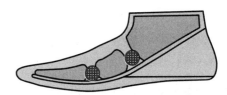

Figure 8-14. STEN foot. (Reprinted with permission from Kingsley Manufacturing Co.)

Dynamic-Response Feet

Dynamic-response, or energy-storing, feet store and release energy with ambulation. They function as sophisticated springs that cushion at initial contact and provide propulsion at terminal stance, enhancing the ability to walk long distances, run, and jump. These feet permit a more normal range of motion and a more symmetric gait. Individuals with more-active lifestyles require dynamic-response feet. Many dynamic-response feet have a split-toe design that mimics inversion and eversion, thereby increasing stability.[11] Dynamic-response feet may include cushioned bumpers at the heel and forefoot and bushings at the ankle to assist in alignment control. These features may dampen shock to the residual limb, resulting in a more natural gait. However, multiple moving parts often require increased maintenance and difficulty with a cosmetic cover design.[11] Conversely, these newer types of feet may provide too much spring for the slow and hesitant walker.

There are many types of dynamic-response feet. They may be divided into nonarticulated and articulated categories. The nonarticulated feet may be further divided into those with long and short keels.[6]

Nonarticulated Long-Keel Feet

A nonarticulated, long-keel design dynamic-response foot may attach to the socket, providing a very responsive prosthetic foot that allows excellent dorsiflexion.[6] Two examples of nonarticulated, long-keel design feet are the Flex Sprint and the Springlite.

Flex Foot

The Flex Foot is a radical departure from the typical foot design. The endoskeletal shank and keel of the Flex Foot consist of carbon fiber composite. The Flex Foot provides maximum energy storing in comparison with other prosthetic feet. The bulk of the weight

is in the socket and socket attachment. As a result, wearers typically perceive the Flex Foot as weighing half as much.[9] The cosmetic cover is fabricated from closed-cell foam that will not absorb water and resists compression damage.

Advantages and disadvantages are listed in Table 8-1. The Flex Foot is the best design for vertical jumping and has performed well for long-distance running as well as other vigorous sports. There are several models of the Flex Foot including the Low Profile available for individuals with a Syme amputation, a split-toe option that enables the foot to function uniformly on uneven terrain, and the Re-flex VSP (Vertical Shock Pylon), which absorbs shock through telescoping tubes and a carbon fiber side spring. The Flex Modular III foot is shown in Figure 8-15.

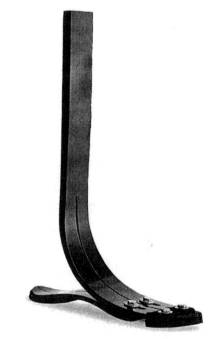

Figure 8-15. Flex Modular III foot. (Reprinted with permission from Flex-Foot Inc.)

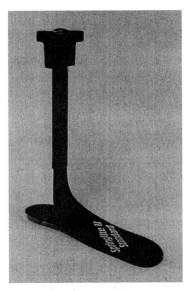

Figure 8-16. Springlite foot. (Reprinted with permission from Springlite)

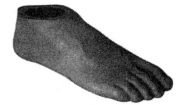

Figure 8-17. Seattle LightFoot. (Reprinted with permission from Seattle Limb Systems)

Springlite Foot

The Springlite Foot is similar in design to the Flex Foot and consists of two layers of carbon and fiberglass filaments surrounded by a soft cover. Advantages and disadvantages are similar to those of the Flex Foot; however, the Springlite Foot is approximately 30% less expensive. Syme and pediatric models are also available (Fig. 8-16).

Nonarticulated Short-Keel Feet

A nonarticulated, short-keel design, dynamic-response foot does not attach to the socket but is attached to a pylon at the ankle. Since they have a shortened keel, they are less responsive and provide less dorsiflexion than the long-keel design. Two examples of this design, the Seattle and Carbon Copy II, are described below.

Seattle Foot

The Seattle foot was developed in the early 1980s at the University of Washington. This was the first foot to provide increased push-off capability in late stance. The Seattle foot was initially developed for runners. The Seattle foot has a lifelike appearance, including vein simulations and a cleft between the great and second toe that allows wearing beach thongs. During mid- to terminal stance, the keel section gradually stores energy that is released at the end of the stance phase. Advantages and disadvantages are listed in Table 8-1. The Seattle Lightfoot is depicted in Figure 8-17.

Carbon Copy II

The Carbon Copy II foot consists of two carbon fiber deflection plates that return energy during walking or running.[10] The Carbon Copy II is designed to support the activities of the physically active ambulator. This foot is sculpted from lightweight materials and contains a strong Kevlar/nylon keel covered by polyurethane foam.[7] The Carbon Copy II is available in a Syme version. Advantages and disadvantages are listed in Table 8-1 (Fig. 8-18).

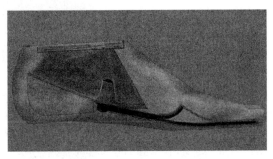

Figure 8-18. Carbon Copy II foot. (Reprinted with permission from Ohio Willow Wood Co.)

Articulated Dynamic-Response Feet

The articulated dynamic-response foot allows significant terrain accommodation as well as plantarflexion, dorsiflexion, inversion, eversion, and torsion absorption. One example of this design is the College Park True Step foot.

College Park True Step Foot

The College Park True Step Foot was designed to mimic the anatomic foot and ankle. The College Park True Step foot contains cushioning bumpers and ankle alignment bushings. Advantages and disadvantages are listed in Table 8-1. The bumpers are easily changed to accommodate different weights, thereby providing the correct resistance for a smooth gait. The College Park True Step foot is shown in Figure 8-19.

Research Studies

The large number of different types of prosthetic feet make it confusing to decide on the best foot for a particular individual.[12] A number of studies have been done to compare the effectiveness of prosthetic feet. However, many of these studies included small samples with a limited number of prosthetic feet. The best foot for a particular patient depends on many fac-

tors, including the activity level of the patient, foot size, weight, features of the particular foot, cost, and insurance reimbursement.[12]

The beneficial effects of dynamic-response feet compared with conventional feet was questioned in a double-blind, randomized study of 10 patients with transtibial amputations. Subjects in this study had no preference for either of the dynamic feet over the conventional feet.[13] A study comparing five feet (Carbon Copy II, STEN, Seattle, SACH, and Flex Foot) involved 17 individuals with transtibial amputations (10 with a traumatic cause and 7 with peripheral vascular disease (PVD)). Results showed that the Flex Foot resulted in significantly greater ankle dorsiflexion and joint torque in terminal stance than the other four feet. However, electromyographic and oxygen consumption results showed no advantages of the dynamic-response feet.[14] In a study of three individuals with transtibial amputations, comparing the Flex Foot to the SACH foot, the only major difference that was found was greater ankle dorsiflexion in late stance by the Flex Foot.[15]

However, dynamic-response feet, including the widely studied Flex Foot, have been preferred in a number of other studies. In a study of seven subjects with transtibial amputation, five different prosthetic feet (Flex Foot, SACH, Car-

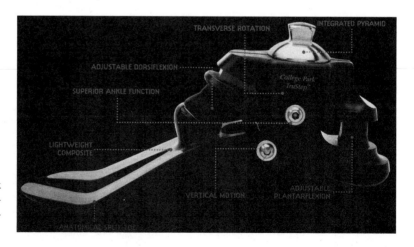

Figure 8-19. College Park True Step. (Reprinted with permission from College Park Industries Inc.)

bon Copy II, Seattle, and Quantum) were compared. The Flex Foot had the lowest sound-limb vertical forces because of its large arc of dorsiflexion motion.[16] This study also found that the sound limb is susceptible to increased vertical forces during loading. On average, the sound limb carries 11% more body weight than the prosthetic limb. If the wearer has an insensitive foot due to PVD or diabetes, this increased load may result in skin breakdown. Increased sound-limb loading was seen for all feet in this study except the Flex Foot, which absorbed a normal load. Therefore, another rationale for the use of a Flex Foot is in cases of preservation of the sound foot.[16] A study of five physically active subjects with unilateral transtibial amputations compared the Flex Foot, SACH foot, and the Re-Flex VSP. Results showed the Flex Foot and Re-Flex VSP to be more efficient in stair climbing than the SACH.[17]

In another comparison of five prosthetic feet, the Flex Foot was found to best simulate the sound limb ascending a four-step staircase. The limited dorsiflexion of the SACH foot resulted in limited tibial advancement and progression of body weight.[18] In a study comparing the effects of four dynamic-response feet, higher prosthetic dorsiflexion moments and increased power at later stance, which could assist in push-off, were found for the Carbon Copy III and the Springlite II feet.[19]

Overall, it appears that dynamic-response feet have definite advantages over conventional feet. The question of how light to make a prosthetic foot was investigated in one study of 15 individuals with transtibial amputations. When the center of mass was changed from distal to proximal, a more-efficient gait resulted. Therefore, low-weight feet and a higher mass were advocated. Designs such as the Flex and Springlite feet have greater proximal and less distal mass. This study concluded that gait parameters such as propulsion due to deceleration of the swing leg require some weight to be effective.[20] Therefore, ultralight prostheses would not provide further advantages in level walking.

In many cases, these research studies have presented conflicting results for the reasons stated above. The answer to what represents the best foot remains elusive. Additional research may determine the best prosthetic foot for a particular activity level.

Shoe Wear

Comments about shoes are contained in Practical Application Box 8-1.

Sockets

The socket is the connection between the residual limb and the foot. There are primarily two sockets used for transtibial amputations, the patellar tendon bearing (PTB) and the total surface bearing (TSB).

Patellar Tendon Bearing (PTB) Socket

The PTB socket is the most commonly used socket for transtibial amputations. The PTB socket offers areas of pressure and areas of re-

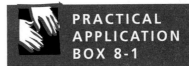

PRACTICAL APPLICATION BOX 8-1

Shoes

Most prosthetic feet are designed with a ¾-inch heel height. Prosthetic wearers may have residual limb complications such as increased pressure or experience instability if the shoe heel height varies much from this ¾-inch height. Shoes should be comfortable, fit the prosthetic foot snugly, and have non-slippery soles.[21]

lief.[2,22] Areas of weight bearing include fleshy or weight-tolerant areas that have a good blood supply to dissipate pressures. The PTB socket uses total contact to avoid pockets of edema. However, primary areas of weight bearing and areas of relief are provided in the PTB socket.

Areas of Weight Bearing

Areas of weight bearing of the PTB socket include

- Patellar tendon
- Flare of the medial tibial condyle and the anteriomedial aspect of the tibial shaft
- Anterolateral aspect (pretibial group) of the residual limb
- Midshaft of the fibula
- Gentle end-bearing if tolerated

Areas of Relief

Areas of relief include bony prominences, areas of poor blood supply, or areas that are near prominent nerves such as the common peroneal. Areas of relief of the PTB socket include

- Anterior and lateral edges of the lateral tibial condyle
- Head and distal end of the fibula
- Crest and tubercle of the tibia
- Anterior distal end of the tibia

An anterior view of areas of weight bearing and areas of relief of the PTB socket is shown in Figure 8-20. Areas of weight bearing are depicted as darkened areas, areas of relief as light areas.

Functions of Patellar Tendon Bearing Socket Walls

The medial wall of the PTB socket extends $1/2$ to 1 inch above the anterior wall. This wall provides a major pressure-tolerant area for the pes anserinus (tendons of the gracilis, semitendinous, and sartorius). The shelf of the tibial condyle is an excellent weight-bearing area, so

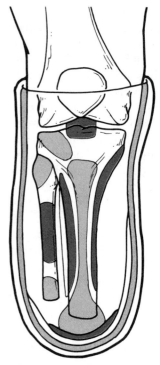

Figure 8-20. PTB socket. Anterior view showing areas of weight bearing and areas of relief.

the socket is shaped to make maximal weight bearing of this area. The proximal aspect of the medial wall supports the femoral condyle and is normally $2\frac{1}{2}$ inches above the medial tibial plateau in height. Together the medial and lateral walls control rotation and provide medial lateral stability.[10]

The lateral wall provides relief for the head of the fibula and the common peroneal nerve. The lateral wall supports the fibular shaft. The lateral wall also exerts comfortable pressure over the shaft of the fibula. Relief is provided for the sensitive fibular head and the distal end of the fibula.[10]

The posterior wall applies an anteriorly directed force to maintain the patient's patellar tendon on the prosthetic patellar bar. The superior border of the posterior wall is $1/2$ inch above the center of the patellar tendon bar, and the lateral and medial sides dip slightly for the hamstring tendons.[10] The top of the anterior wall bisects the patella.

Two variations of the PTB socket design, the supracondylar and the supracondylar/suprapatellar, are discussed below in this chapter, under suspensions. The PTB socket has been in use for more than 40 years, which is a tribute to its efficacy in the management of those with transtibial amputations.[2]

Total Surface Bearing (TSB) Socket

The TSB socket, rather than using areas of weight bearing and areas of relief, distributes pressures more equally throughout the transtibial residual limb.[2] Body weight is borne by the entire surface of the residual limb.[23] The liner of the socket assists in distributing these pressures. The TSB socket is primarily used with the pin/shuttle suspension, discussed later in this chapter.

The choice of socket, the PTB or the TSB, depends on the patient's anticipated activity level, comorbidities, residual-limb condition, and the skill of the prosthetist.[2]

Liners

Some individuals with transtibial amputations may prefer not to wear a liner and instead have the residual limb and sock against the hard PTB socket. This socket without liner is primarily indicated for a residual limb with intact sensation, good soft tissue coverage, and no sharp bony prominences. Advantages and disadvantages of a hard socket without a liner are outlined in Pros and Cons Box 8-1.[4]

Soft liners are recommended for individuals with PVD; those with thin, sensitive, or scarred skin; and patients with sharp bony prominences. The added protection of a soft liner may also benefit the highly active individual.

PROS & CONS BOX 8-1

Hard Socket

Advantages of a hard socket include
• Less bulk
• Easier cleaning
• Fewer perspiration problems

Disadvantages of a hard socket include
• More difficult for the prosthetist to fit and modify
• Less comfortable

Liners are fabricated over the positive mold to fit inside the PTB socket. They act as an interface between the residual limb and socket to provide added comfort and protection.

The advantages and disadvantages of liners are listed in Pros and Cons Box 8-2.

PROS & CONS BOX 8-2

Liner

Advantages of a liner include
• Total contact, which decreases edema
• Modifications may be made more easily in the liner than in the socket

Disadvantages of liners include
• Deterioration over time
• Sanitation due to perspiration absorption
• Difficulties in applying the liner in cases of decreased hand function
• Increased bulk and weight

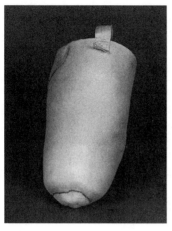

Figure 8-21. Pelite liner.

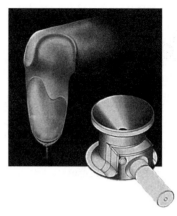

Figure 8-23. Silicone liner with double-walled construction. (Reprinted with permission from Otto Bock Orthopedic Industry Inc.)

Types of Liners

There are several different liners that may be used. Two of the most common types are described below.

Pelite

Pelite is the most commonly used liner for an individual with a transtibial amputation. It is made of a lightweight closed-cell 5-mm polyethylene foam (Fig. 8-21).

Viscoelastic

Viscoelastic liners are suitable for scarred, tender, or bony transtibial residual limbs. These liners feature even pressure distribution, minimal shear forces, and high shock absorption (Fig. 8-22). Some liners are doubled-walled with an adjustable air chamber. This air chamber reduces friction and provides optimal total contact between the socket and the residual limb (Fig. 8-23). Disadvantages of the viscoelastic liner include increased cost and weight.

Application of a liner is described in Practical Application Box 8-2. Care of liners and sockets is discussed in Chapter 6.

Suspensions

Suspensions are used to secure a prosthesis on the residual limb. Selection of the optimal suspension is paramount to achieving efficient and safe prosthetic ambulation. An improperly fitting suspension may result in discomfort, pistoning of the prosthesis around the residual limb, skin breakdown, increased energy consumption, gait deviations, and falls. Seven of

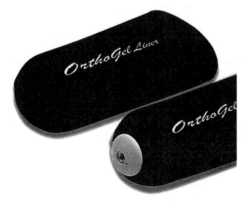

Figure 8-22. Ortho Gel liner. (Reprinted with permission from Otto Bock Orthopedic Industry Inc.)

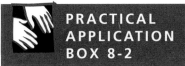

PRACTICAL APPLICATION BOX 8-2

To apply the prosthesis, the patient may apply a nylon sheath, followed by a prosthetic sock, and then the liner. The prosthetic sock is turned inside out, placed over the end of the residual limb, and then gently rolled up the residual limb. There should be no wrinkles in the nylon sheath or prosthetic sock(s), and seams of the sock should not be over bony areas or directly across the scar. Wrinkles or seams over bony areas or the scar may result in tissue breakdown. The liner and then the prosthesis are applied. In addition to tissue discoloration, sock marks on the skin indicate prosthetic socket pressure. If indentations in the skin are too deep, excessive pressure of the socket may exist. Conversely, if there are no sock marks in areas where pressure should be normally occurring, pressure may be maldistributed.

To check for distal total contact, a ball of clay the size of a pea can be put in the bottom of the insert or at the bottom of the hard socket. After the patient stands and shifts body weight over the prosthesis, the clay ball may be removed to see if it has flattened. If it is slightly flattened, there is sufficient distal total contact. If the ball is totally flattened, the distal end of the residual limb may be experiencing too much weight bearing. Reevaluation of the number of prosthetic socks or fit of the prosthetic socket may be indicated. To achieve less weight on the distal end of the residual limb, the number of ply of socks may be increased. If the clay ball remains round after bearing weight, there is no total contact and the number of ply of socks may need to be reduced. Another option to determine total contact, is to place a lipstick mark in the bottom of the socket. If the lipstick appears on the end of the liner, total contact is present. Lack of total contact may lead to distal edema, increased pain, or skin blistering. The skin of the residual limb should be inspected for areas that appear discolored or bruised. If the patient cannot see the distal end of the residual limb, a mirror should be used.

the more common suspensions are described below.

Supracondylar Cuff

The supracondylar cuff is one of the most commonly used suspensions for individuals with transtibial amputations. The supracondylar cuff is suspended above the femoral condyles and the proximal patella. The medial and lateral attachment points of the supracondylar cuff are slightly posterior to the knee, to resist hyperextension or recurvatum forces. The cuff tightens with knee extension and loosens with knee flexion. Placement of these cuff attachment points on the prosthetic socket is critical for suspension throughout the full range of knee flexion.[14] The advantages and disadvantages of this suspension are listed in Table 8-2. The supracondylar cuff is not recommended for short residual limbs, since these limbs need increased surface-contact area and higher walls to control rotation. The supracondylar cuff is also not recommended for individuals with vascular problems. High forces result in the popliteal space, especially when the knee is flexed 90° as in sitting. In addition, the supracondylar cuff may restrict knee flexion, which may result in difficulty with kneeling and sitting in an airplane or taxicab. Since the cuff provides little

Table 8-2. Comparison of Suspensions for the Individual with a Transtibial Amputation

Suspension	Indications	Advantages	Disadvantages
Supracondylar cuff	Simple, durable	Adjustable; ease of application; easy replacement	Not recommended with vascular problemsor short residual limbs; high forces may result with knee flexion in sitting
Supracondylar system (PTB SC)	Short residual limb; medial–lateral instabilities	Minimizes vascular problems	Requires good hand dexterity
Supracondylar suprapatellar system (PTB SC/SP)	Short residual limb; medial–lateral and anterior–posterior ligamentous instabilities	Minimizes vascular problems; supports knee	Kneeling difficulties; poor cosmetic appearance since the anterior wall juts upward when sitting; difficult to fit over heavy thighs
Thigh corset	Excellent stability; short residual limbs; poor knee stability	Decreases weight on the residual limb through side bars; good for occupations where stability is paramount	Poor cosmetic appearance; excessive weight; possible quadriceps atrophy
Waist belt	Auxiliary suspension	Decreases pistoning	Cumbersome; hygiene problems; poor cosmetic appearance
Sleeve	Light weight; may be used as an auxiliary suspension	Improved cosmetic appearance; simple, minimal pistoning	Not durable; increased perspiration; hygiene problems; does not control knee instability; good hand function needed
Pin/shuttle	Scarred or sensitive residual limbs; simple mechanism	Improved cosmetic appearance; eliminates straps around knee; decreased shear forces; minimal pistoning	Same as sleeve; increased expense

support, it is not recommended for patients with knee instability (Fig. 8-24).

Supracondylar System

The supracondylar system, sometimes called a PTB SC, may be either a wedge suspension or a removable medial wall or brim. This suspension is used with a PTB socket that has high medial and lateral walls. The higher medial and lateral walls provide increased surface area for better distribution of pressures in a short transtibial amputation. Therefore, this suspension is often used for residual limbs less than 5 cm in length.[22] The more commonly used wedge suspension, which was introduced in

the United States in the mid-1960s, is incorporated into a removable soft liner by creating a thicker superior medial wall.[22] This buildup over the medial femoral condyle extends proximal to the adductor tubercle. The combination of the high medial and lateral walls and the wedge over the medial femoral condyle provides suspension (Fig. 8-25). A removable wedge, used in cases of a hard socket, is less commonly seen.[24] The supracondylar system may also consist of a proximal medial wall or brim that is removed to allow the residual limb to be inserted into the socket. Laminated into the proximal brim is a steel bar that fits into a channel on the medial aspect of the socket. This allows the medial brim to be removed and

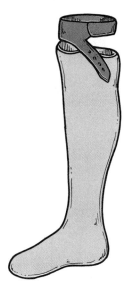

Figure 8-24. Supracondylar cuff suspension. (Adapted from Shurr, D. G., & Cook, T. M. *Prosthetics and orthotics*. Norwalk, CT: Appleton & Lange.)

then replaced.[4] The medial brim may be indicated for heavier individuals and is typically used when no insert is used (Fig. 8-26).

The advantages and disadvantages of this suspension are listed in Table 8-2. Since good hand dexterity is required to apply the supra-

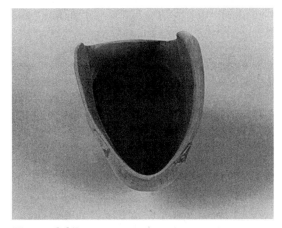

Figure 8-25. Supracondylar system wedge suspension built into the liner (PTB SC). (Adapted from *Lower limb prosthetics* (1998). New York: Prosthetic Orthotic Publications.)

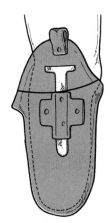

Figure 8-26. Supracondylar system removable brim suspension (PTB SC). (Adapted from *Lower limb prosthetics* (1998). New York: Prosthetic Orthotic Publications.)

condylar system, it may not be appropriate for individuals with diabetes and sensory neuropathy or intrinsic hand weakness.

Supracondylar/Suprapatellar system (PTB SC/SP)

The supracondylar/suprapatellar system (PTB SC/SP) suspension provides increased mediolateral and anteroposterior stability, since the high walls fully encompass the femoral condyles and the patella. This suspension is often indicated for individuals with short residual limbs, since it encompasses more surface area to distribute weight bearing and can resist torsional forces. Individuals with knee ligamentous instability or recurvatum may be ideal candidates for this suspension (Fig. 8-27). The advantages and disadvantages are listed in Table 8-2.

Thigh Corset

Prior to 1958, the thigh corset combined with a waist belt was the most common form of transtibial prosthetic suspension.[4] Today, less than 1% of individuals with a transtibial ampu-

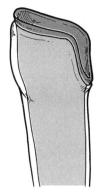

Figure 8-27. Supracondylar suprapatellar system suspension (PTB SC/SP). (Adapted from *Lower limb prosthetics* (1998). New York: Prosthetic Orthotic Publications.)

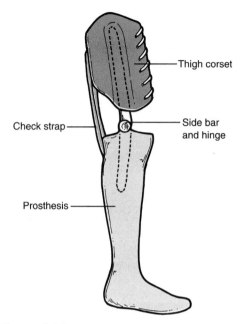

Figure 8-28. Thigh corset suspension. (Adapted from *Lower limb prosthetics* (1998). New York: Prosthetic Orthotic Publications.)

tation use a thigh corset suspension.[24] This suspension may be indicated when maximum stability of the knee is required, which may occur after a traumatic event that results in a transtibial amputation as well as knee ligament damage. The thigh corset provides some shared weight bearing and is indicated when partial unloading of the residual limb is necessary. This is particularly important for patients with recurrent skin breakdowns. Advantages and disadvantages of this suspension are listed in Table 8-2.

The thigh corset may have a check strap added to the posterior part of the prosthesis between the thigh corset and the socket to prevent **terminal impact** (a banging sound as the knee extends) and hyperextension of the knee (Fig. 8-28).[2]

Waist Belt

A waist belt suspension is often used temporarily in the early training of a new patient who is adjusting to the functioning of a prosthesis. It is often used on postoperative or temporary prostheses because it maintains some suspension regardless of residual-limb volume changes.[4] The waist belt consists of 2-inch cotton webbing that is fitted above the iliac crests with an elastic strap extending distally to the supra-

condylar cuff or supracondylar system suspension of the prosthesis. The waist belt resembles an inverted Y strap. As the elastic strap stretches during swing phase, knee extension assistance is provided. However, the elastic strap does not provide uniform suspension throughout the swing phase of gait.[24] Other disadvantages are listed in Table 8-2 (Fig. 8-29).

Sleeve

The sleeve suspension was introduced at the University of Michigan in 1968.[4] Sleeves were formerly made of latex but now are more commonly constructed of neoprene. Silicone and urethane are often used as well. Sleeves fit snugly over the proximal aspect of the prosthesis and are rolled up over the thigh approximately 3 inches above the prosthetic socks. By making contact with the skin, the sleeve makes the socket a sealed chamber.[4] This suspension is widely used because of its simplicity and ease of replacement. The advantages and disadvantages of this suspension are listed in Table 8-2 (Fig. 8-30).[24]

Pin/Shuttle

The pin/shuttle suspension is achieved by rolling a closed end liner of silicone, urethane, or thermoplastic elastomer directly onto the limb. This suspension is often used with a TSB socket. To apply, the sleeve is turned inside out and rolled over the residual limb.[4] The prosthesis then is suspended with a pin or plunger threaded into the distal end of the liner. Unrestricted knee flexion and minimal pistoning make this suspension ideal for many patients.[21] To remove the prosthesis, a button on the locking mechanism is depressed. Prosthetic socks, worn over the liner, may be used with limb volume changes. In a survey of 13 individuals with transtibial amputations who wore a pin/shuttle suspension, this suspension was rated higher than other suspensions in areas

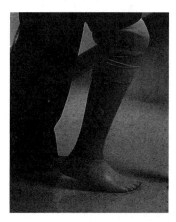

Figure 8-30. Suspension sleeve. (Adapted from *Lower limb prosthetics* (1998). New York: Prosthetic Orthotic Publications.)

including stability, comfort, maintenance, ease of application, and overall preference.[25] The advantages and disadvantages of this suspension are listed in Table 8-2.[26] Fitting this suspension may be difficult with residual-limb bony deformities (Fig. 8-31).

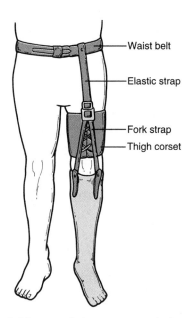

Figure 8-29. Waist belt suspension. (Adapted from *Lower limb prosthetics* (1998). New York: Prosthetic Orthotic Publications.)

Waist belt
Elastic strap
Fork strap
Thigh corset

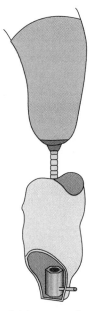

Figure 8-31. Shuttle/pin suspension. (Reprinted with permission from Ossur.)

Summary

The type of suspension to recommend requires clinical decision making based upon the activity level of the patient, ease of application, cost, and insurance reimbursement.

Other Prostheses

The transmetatarsal and Syme amputations are discussed in Chapter 1. The following are descriptions of prostheses that may be used with these amputations.

Transmetatarsal Prostheses

Transmetatarsal amputations may result in an equinus attitude and a distal sensitive end, often leading to skin breakdown. As reviewed in Chapter 1, the shortened foot lacks adequate push-off at terminal stance, causing loss of balance and proprioception.[27] The older transmetatarsal prostheses consisted most commonly of a shoe insert molded under the remaining area of the longitudinal arch. A prosthesis for a transmetatarsal amputation may consist of a rocker sole, a short shoe, a regular shoe, an ankle–foot orthosis (AFO), a shoe insert, or any of these combinations. Figure 1-21 depicts a regular shoe and ankle-foot orthosis (AFO). In a study of 30 subjects with diabetes mellitus and a transmetatarsal amputation, subjects who wore a short shoe and AFO were dissatisfied with ankle motion restriction and cosmetic appearance. In contrast, subjects who wore either a total contact insert and rocker sole or a short shoe with rocker sole had faster walking speeds and higher physical-performance test scores than those wearing regular shoes with a toe filler.[28]

Syme Prosthesis

As reviewed in Chapter 1, a Syme prosthesis lacks a pleasing cosmetic appearance because of the distal end bulge that accommodates the malleoli. The limited space available between the distal portion of the residual limb and the floor severely constrains the type of prosthetic foot that may be used with the Syme prosthesis. As a result, many of the feet associated with the Syme prostheses use a nonarticulated foot such as a SACH. Syme prostheses use a lateral or posterior opening secured by Velcro and a PTB socket for better weight distribution (Fig. 8-32).[4] Some Syme prostheses use a closed double-wall prosthesis with a flexible inner wall that allows expansion so that the bulbous end may be inserted past the expandable portion. The absence of windows allows a more cosmetic and stronger prosthesis. This type of Syme prosthesis with a flexible inner wall cannot be used with extremely bulbous or sensitive residual limbs.[29] Individuals with a Syme amputation may walk on the heel pad without the prosthesis (e.g., for nightly trips to the bathroom).

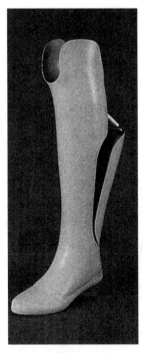

Figure 8-32. Syme prosthesis. (Reprinted with permission from Otto Bock Orthopedic Industry Inc.)

The long-term use of the Syme prosthesis has been shown to be satisfactory. A study of 10 young adults who had a Syme amputation for fibular deficiency when they were children showed that all subjects had an appropriate functional Syme prosthesis and no difficulty with walking or running. In addition, assessment of quality of life and self-esteem was similar to that of adults without amputation.[30]

Prosthesis Wearing Schedule

To minimize skin breakdown and discomfort, it may be helpful for the patient to adopt the following prosthesis-wearing schedule:

Days 1–2: Wear prosthesis for $\frac{1}{2}$ hour in the AM and monitor fit. Allow some ambulation. Repeat in PM.

Days 3–4: Increase AM and PM wearing time to 1 hour.

Days 5–10: Increase AM and PM wearing time to 2 hours.

Days 11–14: Put the prosthesis on in the morning and check skin before lunch. Continue to wear the prosthesis, checking again at dinner and once more before bed.

Day 14: If no problems have been experienced, the prosthesis can be worn on a full-time basis. Nonetheless, the fit of the prosthesis should be checked at least once a day by the wearer or a family member.[31]

Examination (Checkout) Procedure

An **examination (checkout) procedure** serves as a systematic method of examining the patient with an amputation and the prosthesis. The examination or checkout procedure determines whether accepted standards of prosthesis fabrication and fit have been met and, if not, if possible corrective action is needed. During this procedure, the therapist should consider the following:

1. Comfort or fit
2. Stability or function
3. Alignment
4. Appearance
5. Ability to apply and take off the prosthesis[10]

Examination or Checkout of a Transtibial Prosthesis

Standing Position

1. The patient should be comfortable while standing with the midlines of the heels (heel seams) not more than 6 inches apart. If the patient is uncomfortable, the therapist should address the areas that are a problem as discussed below.

2. The anteroposterior alignment of the prosthesis should be satisfactory. The anterior portion of the heel and the ball of the sole should be flat on the floor, and the patient should, with minimal muscular effort, be able to maintain knee stability. One should be able to put a piece of paper no more than $\frac{1}{2}$ inch under the heel and the ball of a new shoe.

3. The mediolateral alignment of the prosthesis should be satisfactory. The shoe should be flat on the floor, and there should be no uncomfortable pressure at the lateral or medial brim of the socket. One should be able to put a piece of paper no more than $\frac{1}{2}$ inch under each side of a new shoe.

4. The prosthesis should be the correct length. To check the length of the prosthesis, palpate one or more of the following landmarks: (a) iliac crests, (b) anterior superior iliac spines, or (c) greater trochanters. Causes of the apparent discrepancy in length may be (a) an excessively plantarflexed or dorsiflexed foot, (b) a residual limb that is either too far or not far enough into the socket because of poor socket fit

or improper donning, (c) a prosthesis of the wrong length. Small plywood boards, $1/4$-inch high, may be placed under the shoe to ensure similar leg lengths.

5. The anterior, medial, and lateral walls should be of adequate height. The anterior brim of the basic PTB prosthesis should extend to the level of the middle of the patella. With a supracondylar cuff suspension, the medial and lateral walls should extend to the epicondyles. With a supracondylar system and supracondylar/suprapatellar suspensions, the side walls should extend above the epicondyles.[10]

Sitting Position

6. The patient should, in most cases, be able to sit comfortably with minimal bunching of soft tissues in the popliteal region when the knees are flexed to 90°. If the patient finds the prosthesis uncomfortable while sitting, it may indicate
   a. Inadequate hamstring channels
   b. Unduly high posterior wall of the socket
   c. Excessive anterior or distal placement of the tabs of the supracondylar cuff[10]
   d. Bunching of the elastic sleeve or shuttle/pin suspension

Walking

7. Performance in level walking should be satisfactory. The patient should be observed from the back, side, and front and any gait deviations noted.
8. The piston action between the residual limb and the socket should be minimal. If the piston action between the residual limb and the prosthesis exceeds $1/4$ inch, additional ply socks, tighter suspension, or a different suspension may be indicated. A mark may be put on the prosthetic sock to note the amount of pistoning between the top of the prosthetic posterior brim and the mark on the sock.

9. Stairs, curbs, and inclines should be ascended and descended satisfactorily. Note knee stability and toe clearance.
10. The ability to kneel should be satisfactory. The patient wearing a prosthesis with supracondylar/suprapatellar suspension probably will be unable to kneel for long, if at all, before experiencing discomfort from the hard anterior brim. If the patient had discomfort sitting with knees flexed to 90°, kneeling will not be tolerated. The same reasons that caused uncomfortable sitting should be investigated.
11. The prosthesis should function quietly. Occasionally, hissing may be heard as air enters and escapes from the socket as the patient walks. This may be associated with piston action caused by inadequate suspension and poor socket fit or with incongruence between the socket and liner.
12. The residual limb should be free from abrasion, discolorations, and excessive perspiration immediately after the prosthesis is removed. Discoloration is to be expected in areas of weight bearing of the PTB socket as discussed previously in this chapter. Discoloration that fades within 10 minutes usually is not cause for concern, provided there is no pain, discomfort, or sensory deficit in the area. To determine the concentration and location of distal pressure, it may be desirable to insert a piece of modeling clay in the bottom of the socket. Flattening of the clay will indicate distal contact.[19]

Prosthetic Prescription

In the United States, Medicare has required the prescribing physician and the prosthetist to document the patient's potential functional level as a means of determining the medical necessity for components. If the patient's ability changes, the functional level can be changed accordingly. Various prosthetic components and, subsequently, reimbursement are allowed according to the patient's functional level. Functional levels do not influence the type of prosthetic suspension recommended. However, functional levels do influence the type of prosthetic feet reimbursed by Medicare.[31,32] The functional levels defined by Medicare are presented in Table 3-3 and are reviewed in Table 8-3 in relation to prosthetic feet reimbursed by Medicare.

Recommendations and Prosthetic Component Guidelines

In recommending components of a prosthesis such as feet, suspensions, or liners for a particular patient with a transtibial amputation, a number of factors must be considered. Awareness of these factors enables an informed decision regarding the optimal prosthetic component for a particular patient. These factors include

- Age—an elderly patient with comorbidities that compromise vascular flow may need the light weight of the endoskeletal or modular prosthesis, while a younger, more active patient may need the durability of an exoskeletal unit.
- Cosmesis—appearance may be more important to some individuals. Prosthetic components may need to reflect this satisfactory cosmetic appearance.
- Climate/geographic location—liners may not be used as much in warmer, more humid climates; suspensions such as a sleeve or pin/shuttle may result in increased perspiration problems in these climates.

Table 8-3. Approved Prosthetic Feet According to Medicare

Medicare Levels	Approved Prosthetic Feet
Level 0 Does not have the ability or potential to ambulate or transfer, with or without assistance, and a prosthesis does not enhance the quality of life or mobility	Noncandidate
Level 1 Has the ability or potential to use a prosthesis for transfers or ambulation on level surfaces at a fixed cadence; patients who are household ambulators or those in an extended care facility are typically included in this category	Conventional feet such as a SACH or single axis
Level 2 Has the ability or potential for ambulation, with the ability to transverse low-level environmental barriers such as curbs, stairs, or uneven surfaces; the limited community ambulator is an example of this level	Conventional feet such as a multiaxis, SAFE, or STEN
Level 3 Has the ability or potential for ambulation with variable cadence; typical of the community ambulator who has the ability to transverse most environmental barriers and may have vocational, therapeutic, or exercise activity that demands prosthetic use beyond simple locomotion.	Dynamic-response feet such as Seattle, Carbon Copy, College Park, Flex Foot, or Springlite
Level 4 Has an ability or potential for prosthetic ambulation that exceeds basic ambulation skills, exhibiting high impact, stress, or energy levels; typical of the prosthetic demands of the child, active adult, or athlete	Dynamic-response feet such as Seattle, Carbon Copy, College Park, Flex Foot, or Springlite

- Level of health—those with skin insensitivity or vascular problems may need additional cushioning or areas of relief. Those with allergies to socket finish may not be able to use a hard socket. Those with knee flexion contractures of more than 25° will have a difficult prosthetic fit.
- Functional status, work, and avocation—a very athletic individual requires a durable prosthesis with specialized components.
- Occupation—a patient who works around high heat such as welding or heavy metal work would be better suited with an exoskeletal prosthesis. The foam covering of a modular prosthesis is not durable in high heat.
- Previous prosthesis—an awareness of problems with the old prosthesis may help avoid difficulties with the new prosthesis[4]
- Insurance reimbursement—certain prosthetic components may not be reimbursed, such as those that correspond to a Medicare functional level.

PEDIATRIC PERSPECTIVE

Prosthetic Component Recommendations

A child with a transtibial amputation will often use a supracondylar cuff suspension. This suspension must be adjusted regularly so that knee ligament stress does not occur as the child grows. Sleeve or pin/shuttle suspensions may be appropriate for the less active child. The active child needs dynamic-response feet to ensure an energetic lifestyle. Endoskeletal prostheses may be adjusted easily as the child grows. The soft covering may be left off to avoid soiling or becoming wet during play activities.

Geriatric and pediatric perspectives regarding prosthetic component recommendations are included in the geriatric and pediatric perspective boxes.

Prosthetic Prescription Cases

It is helpful to consider typical cases in which prosthetic components may be ordered for a particular patient. Additional cases in a *Guide to Physical Therapist Practice* format are presented in Appendix A.[1] Answers to each of these cases are included at the end of the case. The reader should attempt to answer the case, considering which prosthetic component would be best for that particular patient. Use of the prescription guidelines discussed previously may be helpful. For each question, several other components may be correct, not necessarily the component that was recommended. It is important for the reader to be able to give a plausible rationale for the suggested prosthetic component.

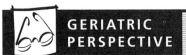

GERIATRIC PERSPECTIVE

Prosthetic Component Recommendations

The elderly patient would benefit from a lightweight suspension such as a sleeve or pin/shuttle suspension. Depending on the residual limb characteristics and comorbidities, either a TSB or PTB socket may be used. The TSB distributes pressures more equally throughout the residual limb, which may be important in cases of skin insensitivity. This may be seen in diabetes or PVD. An endoskeletal prosthesis is almost always used for the elderly patient because of its light weight.

CASE 1

PATIENT/CLIENT HISTORY

General Demographics

Jim Snyder is a 48-year-old welder who had a left transtibial amputation 3 months ago because of a hunting accident.

Employment/Work

Jim plans to continue welding work, which consists of about 4 hours of standing and 4 hours of sitting per day and some kneeling.

General Health

Jim describes himself as being otherwise healthy with no chronic illnesses.

TESTS AND MEASURES

Anthropometric Characteristics

The residual limb is 6 inches (13.2 cm) long, measured from the tibial tubercle. Shrinkage is adequate so that a cylindrical residual limb has been formed. Jim weighs 275 lb.

Integumentary Integrity

The scar over the medial distal end of the residual limb is well healed.

Muscle Performance/Range of Motion

Strength in upper extremities and right lower extremity is graded on manual muscle testing as 5/5, strength in the left hip and knee is 4/5. Range of motion is within normal limits.

Gait, Locomotion, and Balance

Jim is independent in ambulation with axillary crutches more than 500 feet on level surfaces as well as uneven terrain, stairs, and inclines. Even though Jim does not have Medicare insurance reimbursement, he would be classified level 4 (has the ability or potential for prosthetic ambulation that exceeds basic ambulation skills, exhibiting high impact, stress, or energy levels. Typical of the prosthetic demands of the child, active adult, or athlete).

1a. Which socket would you recommend? Why?

1b. Which suspension would you recommend? Why?

1c. Which foot–ankle assembly would you recommend? Why?

1a. The PTB socket is commonly used with transtibial amputations since it has areas of relief and areas of weight bearing. A PTB socket would be suitable in this case. An exoskeletal prosthesis is appropriate around welding and high heat. An endoskeletal prosthesis may also be used without the soft covering. Stainless steel should be used because Jim weighs more than 225 pounds. A Pelite liner will absorb shock and result in a comfortable fit. A shock-absorbing pylon is a recommended feature for an active wearer.

1b. The recommended suspension is a supracondylar cuff. This suspension is adequate for this patient's occupation. A supracondylar system (wedge or brim) or supracondylar/suprapatellar suspension would be uncomfortable when kneeling. A sleeve or a pin/shuttle suspension may not be practical around welding. An auxiliary waist belt may be needed if he is on ladders. Jim does not need the ultimate stability of a thigh corset suspension unless he is doing much climbing in his occupation.

1c. A dynamic-response foot is recommended since Jim is active and fairly young. A dynamic-response foot such as a Flex foot or Springlite foot will result in a more efficient gait than a conventional foot such as a SACH.

CASE 2

PATIENT/CLIENT HISTORY

General Demographics

Nancy Holliday is a 73-year-old homemaker who had a right transtibial elective amputation secondary to PVD.

Employment/Work

Nancy is a retired teacher. She lives in a first floor apartment, her husband assists with household chores.

General Health

She reports hypertension, which is now well controlled with medication. Otherwise she is healthy.

TESTS AND MEASURES

Anthropometric Characteristics

Her residual limb is 5 inches (11 cm) long measured from the tibial tubercle. Shrinkage is adequate, so that a conical residual limb has been formed. Nancy weighs 110 lb.

Integumentary Integrity

Well-healed scar on the right residual limb. No evidence of PVD on the left remaining extremity.

Muscle Performance/Range of Motion

Strength in upper extremities and left lower extremity is graded on manual muscle testing as 4/5, strength in the right hip and knee is 3+/5. Range of motion is within normal limits

Gait, Locomotion, and Balance

Nancy uses a standard walker to ambulate independently 50 feet on level surfaces. She must stop to rest secondary to fatigue. She is unable to climb stairs or inclines or ambulate on uneven terrain without moderate assistance from one person. According to Medicare, Nancy is classified level 2 (has the ability or potential for ambulation with the ability to transverse low-level environmental barriers such as curbs, stairs, or uneven surfaces. The limited community ambulator is an example of this level.).

2a. Which socket would you recommend? Why?

2b. Which suspension would you recommend? Why?

2c. Which foot–ankle assembly would you recommend? Why?

2a. The TSB socket offers the advantage of distributing pressures equally throughout the residual limb. With her history of PVD, this socket would be indicated for Nancy. An endoskeletal prosthesis made with titanium is indicated for energy conservation.

2b. A pin/shuttle suspension is recommended since it offers a soft surface for weight bearing. This suspension is indicated because of the history of PVD. Nancy is retired and not around high-temperature working conditions. She does not have diabetes and has adequate hand function to apply the suspension.

2c. According to Medicare, Nancy is classified level 2; therefore, conventional feet such as a SACH, SAFE, or STEN foot would be appropriate. A multiple-axis foot would not be appropriate because of the weight of the foot and the inability to walk on uneven ground.

C A S E   3

GENERAL DEMOGRAPHICS

Hank Jacquis is an 85-year-old male who had a right transtibial amputation 5 months ago.

Social History

Hank lives with his son, daughter-in-law and their two children. Hank reports that someone is always at home with him.

General Health

Before his right transtibial amputation, Hank was a functional ambulator with a straight cane. He has type I diabetes that is well controlled with insulin injections. Healing of the incision took 4 months.

TESTS AND MEASURES

Anthropometric Characteristics

The residual limb is 3 inches (7.6 cm) long, measured from the tibial tubercle, and has a bulbous appearance. Hank weighs 160 lb.

Integumentary Integrity

Residual limb is well healed. The left foot is insensitive to a Semmes Weinstein monofilament 5.07. (See Fig. 2.3)

Muscle Performance/Range of Motion

Strength in the upper extremities and left lower extremity is 3+/5. Strength in the right hip and knee is 3/5. Bilateral hip flexion is 10–95°, right knee flexion is 20–100°. Bilateral hand function is not impaired.

Gait, Locomotion, and Balance

Hank uses a standard walker to ambulate independently 30 feet on level surfaces. He must stop to rest secondary to fatigue. He is unable to climb stairs or inclines or ambulate on uneven terrain. According to Medicare, Hank is classified level 1 (has the ability or potential to use a prosthesis for transfers or ambulation on level surfaces at a fixed cadence. Patients who are household ambulators or those in an extended care facility are typically included in this category).

3a. Which socket would you recommend? Why?

3b. Which suspension would you recommend? Why?

3c. Which foot–ankle assembly would you recommend? Why?

3a. The PTB socket is commonly used with transtibial amputations since it has areas of relief and areas of weight bearing. This socket will need to be extended on the medial and lateral borders to accommodate the short residual limb. An endoskeletal prosthesis of titanium is indicated because its light weight may result in possible energy conservation.

3b. A PTB SC is indicated because of the short residual limb. A buildup on the medial wall of the Pelite liner would be easier to use than a removable brim or wedge. This suspension is superior to a supracondylar cuff because it minimizes vascular problems that may be associated with diabetes.

3c. According to Medicare, Hank is classified level 1; therefore, a conventional foot such as a SACH would be appropriate. The SACH weighs less than other approved feet for this level such as the single axis.

Gait Analysis of a Patient with a Transtibial Amputation

When analyzing gait, it is helpful to divide the gait cycle into phases and analyze from above to below or below to above. In each phase, the position of the foot, shank, knee, hip, pelvis, and trunk are determined. Phases of the gait cycle and the underlying biomechanical concepts of these gait deviations are discussed in Chapter 5. The following list outlines phases of the gait cycle, gait deviations that are commonly seen during these phases, possible causes of the deviation, and possible corrections.[2]

I. Phase of Gait: Between Initial Contact and Loading Response

Problem: Knee Remains Extended (Ground reaction force vector ((GRFV)) too anterior to the knee)

Possible Causes	Corrections
1. Foot too anterior	1. Move foot posteriorly on an adjustable leg
2. Foot too plantarflexed	2. Move foot into dorsi flexion on an adjustable leg
3. Heel cushion too soft	3. Heel cushion should compress about 3/8 inch; may need firmer heel cushion
4. Heel on shoe too low	4. Add appropriate heel wedge
5. Excessive use of knee extensors or weak quadriceps	5. More intensive strengthening and gait training to decrease the fear of falling

The prosthetist will most likely apply the first four corrections; the physical therapist's responsibility is correction 5.

Problem: Excessive Knee Flexion (GRFV too posterior to the knee)

Possible Causes	Corrections
1. Foot too posterior	1. Move foot anteriorly on an adjustable leg
2. Foot too dorsiflexed	2. Move foot into plantarflexion
3. Heel on shoe too high	3. Decrease the heel wedge or shoe heel height
4. Heel cushion too firm	4. Heel cushion should compress about 3/8 inch
5. Increased pressure against anterodistal tibia	5. Move foot anteriorly or into plantarflexion
6. Weak knee extensors resulting in flexion that is not smooth	6. Quadriceps strengthening

The prosthetist will most likely apply the first five corrections; the physical therapist's responsibility is correction 6.

II. Phase of Gait: Midstance (Ankle Rocker)

Problem: Lateral Trunk Bending to the Prosthetic Side	
Possible Causes	Corrections
1. Prosthesis seems too short	1. Measure leg length or evaluate the need for additional suspension or socks to functionally lengthen the prosthesis
2. Residual limb pain (patient leans away to reduce torque)	2. Evaluate fit and need for additional socks
3. Weak residual limb abductors	3. Design hip abductor–strengthening exercises.

The prosthetist must modify the suspension. The physical therapist can tighten the suspension, add more socks, and design strengthening exercises.

III. Phase of Gait: Between Midstance and Preswing

Problem: Early Knee Flexion (Drop-Off) (GRFV too far posterior)	
Possible Causes	Corrections
1. Excessive posterior displacement of the foot in relation to the socket	1. Move foot more anteriorly
2. Excessive dorsiflexion	2. Move foot more into plantarflexion
3. Prosthetic foot keel is too short	3. Prosthetic foot needs to be reevaluated
4. Excessive socket flexion (may occur with a resolving knee flexion contracture)	4. Decrease socket flexion

The prosthetist will apply all these corrections.

Problem: Delayed Knee Flexion (GRFV too far anterior to the knee)	
Possible Causes	Corrections
1. Foot too anterior	1. Move foot posteriorly
2. Foot too plantarflexed	2. Move foot into dorsiflexion

The prosthetist will apply both these corrections.

IV. Phase of Gait: Swing Phase

Problem: Foot Whips

Foot whips occur during swing phase. A medial whip is present when the heel travels medially at the beginning of swing phase to almost hit the opposite malleolus. A lateral whip occurs when the heel moves laterally.

Footwhips	
Possible Causes	Corrections
1. Suspension cuff not aligned evenly	1. Reevaluate suspension attachment to prosthesis
2. Prosthesis is rotated	2. More socks or more-accurate donning of the prosthesis may be needed

The prosthetist will apply correction 1; the physical therapist correction 2.

Problem: Pistoning of the Residual Limb in the Socket

Pistoning of the residual limb in the socket occurs when there is more than $\frac{1}{4}$ inch difference in the superior aspects of the residual limb and prosthetic socket in swing phase, but in stance phase the differences are less than $\frac{1}{4}$ inch.

Problem: Pistoning of the Residual Limb in the Socket	
Possible Causes	Corrections
1. Suspension inadequate	1. Tighten or modify suspension to provide better support
2. Not enough prosthetic socks	2. Add socks; especially important when the residual limb shrinks because of more-frequent ambulation
3. Prosthesis has been put on incorrectly	3. Reevaluate application of the prosthesis
4. Patient has lost weight	4. Reevaluate need for further prosthetic socks

The prosthetist must modify the suspension. The physical therapist can tighten the suspension or add more socks.

Other Gait Deviations

Other gait deviations may include

1. Vaulting (patient rises up on the toes of the sound foot in midstance) and circumducted gait (patient swings the prosthesis laterally in a wide area during swing phase) are often due to a prosthesis that is too long. These deviations commonly occur when poor suspension causes relative lengthening of the prosthesis.
2. A gluteus maximus gait is present when the patient throws the trunk backward over the hip, typically from initial contact to midstance. This gait deviation serves to extend the hip and is due to either weak hip extensors or a hip flexion contracture.
3. Unequal stride length may be caused by faulty suspension in which the patient is fearful of putting weight on the prosthesis or has painful weight bearing or it can be a habit. Unequal stride length in which a long sound-leg stride and a shorter prosthetic stride occur is a common gait deviation, since an individual with an amputation is fearful of putting weight on the prosthesis.
4. Leading with the prosthetic foot is a function usually of habit and fear. It is more comfortable and secure for the patient when getting up from a chair to lead with the prosthetic foot. In this case, most of the weight is initially put on the unaffected limb and kept off the prosthesis, which the patient may perceive as less stable.

GAIT ANALYSIS PROBLEMS

When analyzing gait deviations, the therapist should attempt to solve these deviations with as few solutions as possible. Many gait deviations may have the same solution. If multiple corrections are done when only one was needed, gait deviations may worsen. As a result, it is advisable to perform only one possible correction at a time. The effect of the correction should then be determined. If the gait deviation is still present, subsequent corrections, one at a time, may then be made. A prosthetist will make prosthetic alignment corrections. The physical therapist and prosthetist collaborate regarding the need for prosthetic or physical therapy corrections to solve a gait deviation.

CASE 1

The following deficiencies were found on evaluation of the right definitive prosthesis with a TSB socket, shuttle/pin suspension, and Flex Foot:

a. Abducted gait (9 inches or 23 cm between heel seams) during stance
b. Lateral bending of the trunk toward the prosthesis during stance
c. Leading with the right foot when starting to walk
d. Gluteus maximus gait seen between initial contact and midstance
e. Increased lumbar lordosis seen between initial contact and midstance
f. Difficulty maintaining stability on right leg during weight bearing

As a physical therapist, which of these deficiencies can you correct?

a and c. An abducted gait and leading with the right foot when starting to walk are typically due to habit or fear. It is more stable for the patient to ambulate with a wide base of support (9 inches or 23 cm) than with the normal 6 inches between heel centers. Likewise it is more comfortable and secure for the patient getting up from a chair to lead with the prosthetic foot. In this case, the patient can put most of the weight on the sound leg first by taking a step with the prosthetic leg. Additional gait training under the supervision of the physical therapist is indicated.

b. Lateral bending of the trunk toward the prosthesis on weight bearing may be due to a weak right gluteus medius causing a compensated Trendelenburg gait. If the patient did not compensate by leaning the trunk over the prosthetic side hip, a falling of the contralateral pelvis or a Trendelenburg gait would result during swing phase. The residual-limb hip abductors must exert a force almost twice as great as gravitational force to prevent lateral drop of the pelvis on the sound side. Another reason for lateral trunk bending is that the prosthetic side may be shorter, causing the patient to trunk bend laterally toward the prosthesis. Prosthetic length should be checked. It is common for the patient to have a shorter prosthetic side due to residual-limb shrinkage. In this case, the patient may need additional socks. Lateral trunk bending may also be caused by pain at the distal lateral end of the residual limb. If this is the cause, referral to a prosthetist may be necessary.

d and e. A gluteus maximus gait and an increased lumbar lordosis may be due to a weak gluteus maximus or a hip flexion contracture. At the beginning of stance, when the gluteus maximus is weak, the patient must extend the trunk over the hip joint. This movement counteracts the flexion moment of the hip. A lordosis frequently results. The patient may be put into a Thomas test position to determine if the hip flexors are tight. The Thomas test position is depicted in Figure 7-6B. The lordosis may also be caused by weak abdominals, tight hip flexors, or lengthened hamstring muscles. Strengthening of the gluteus maximus and abdominals or stretching of the hip flexors may be indicated.

f. Difficulty maintaining stability on the right leg during weight bearing may be due to fear or weakness. The patient is unable to keep the affected-side knee stable because of a fear of falling or weakness in the hip and/or knee extensors. Additional gait training or strengthening of the hip and knee extensors under the supervision of the physical therapist may be indicated.

In summary, a physical therapist would likely be able to correct all these deficiencies.

CASE 2

The following deficiencies were found on initial evaluation of a left transtibial prosthesis on an adjustable leg with a PTB socket, supracondylar cuff suspension, and a SACH foot:

a. Excessive pressure over the fibular head on weight bearing

b. Excessive pressure over the tendon of the semimembranosus on sitting and kneeling
c. Lateral bending of the trunk away from the prosthesis on weight bearing
d. Darkened area over the head of fibula
e. Darkened area over tendon of semimembranosus

As a physical therapist, which of these deficiencies can you correct?

a and d. Excessive pressure over the fibular head on weight bearing may be caused by a foot that is too far laterally. A lateral foot will give excessive pressure over the proximal lateral aspect of the residual limb or, in this case, over the fibular head. The foot can be moved into a more medial position on an adjustable leg. The prosthetist typically makes these corrections. The effects of an outset or lateral foot are discussed in Chapter 5.

b and e. Excessive pressure over the tendon of the semimembranosus and a darkened area over the tendon of semimembranosus on sitting and kneeling may be caused by a tight supracondylar cuff causing excessive medial pressure over the semimembranosus tendon. The patient or therapist may need to loosen the suspension. Otherwise, the prosthetist may need to adjust the placement of the cuff suspension on the prosthetic socket.

c. Lateral trunk bending away from the prosthesis can have several causes such as a prosthetic foot that is too far outset or a weak unaffected-side gluteus medius. This weakness would result in a lateral trunk-bend away from the prosthesis as a compensated Trendelenburg gait pattern. Also lateral trunk bending may be caused by a prosthesis that is apparently too long. This increased length may be due to the fact that the patient is not settled into the prosthesis all the way and may need fewer socks. Either strengthening the unaffected-side gluteus medius or evaluation of prosthesis length is indicated. The physical therapist can apply these corrections. If these are not successful, the prosthetist may need to be consulted.

In summary, a physical therapist could correct deficiency c, and possibly b and e. The prosthetist would correct deficiencies a and d.

KEY POINTS

- Prostheses that may be used in the rehabilitation process include postoperative, temporary, and definitive.

- There are two ways to fabricate a prosthesis, conventional and computer-aided (CAD/CAM).

- Prosthetic feet are divided into conventional and dynamic-response, articulated and nonarticulated categories. Indications, advantages, and disadvantages of many of the most common feet are listed.

- Prosthetic sockets consist of the more common PTB and the TSB.

- The indications, advantages. and disadvantages of different liners and suspensions are outlined.

- An examination (checkout) procedure is a systematic method of examining individuals with an amputation and their prostheses.

- Prescription guidelines such as age, cosmetic appearance, climate, level of health, functional level, type of employment, previous prosthesis, and insurance reimbursement should be used in deciding on a particular prosthesis.

- It is helpful when analyzing gait to divide the gait cycle into various phases and analyze from above to below or below to above.

CRITICAL THINKING QUESTIONS

1. Characterize which feet, according to Medicare reimbursement guidelines, would be approved for a household ambulator, for a limited community ambulator, for a community ambulator, and for a child, active adult, or athlete.

2. Compare which suspensions may be used with each of the two sockets used for transtibial amputations.

3. Review the prosthetic prescription cases. Which other prosthetic components may be used in these cases.

4. Review the gait analysis cases. What other causes could exist for these gait deviations?

5. Refer to case 1 in the Appendix for a comprehensive case in the *Guide to Physical Therapist Practice* format.

REFERENCES

1. American Physical Therapy Association. (2001). A guide to physical therapist practice. *Physical Therapy*, 81.
2. Fergason, J., & Smith, D. G. (1999). Socket considerations for the patient with a transtibial amputation. *Clinical Orthopaedics and Related Research, 361*, 76–84.
3. Uellendahl, J. E. Prosthetic primer: Materials used in prosthetics. http://www.amputee-coalition.org. In Motion 8:1998.
4. Bowker, J. H., & Michael, J. W. (1992). *Atlas of limb prosthetics*. St Louis: Mosby Year Book.
5. May, B. (1996). *Amputations and prosthetics A case study approach*. Philadelphia: F. A. Davis.
6. Romo, H. D. (1999). Specialized prostheses for activities. *Clinical Orthopaedics and Related Research, 361*, 63–70.
7. Edelstein, J. E. (1988). Prosthetic feet state of the art. *Physical Therapy 68*, 1874–1881.
8. Wilson, A. B. (1972). The modern history of amputation surgery and artificial limbs. *Orthopedic Clinics of North America, 3*, 267–285.
9. Michael, J. (1987). Energy storing feet: A clinical comparison. *Clinical Prosthetics and Orthotics, 11*, 154–168.
10. Berger, N., & Fishman, S. (1998). *Lower limb prosthetics*. New York: New York University.
11. Sabolich, S. (2000). Putting your best foot forward. *InMotion 10*, 18–24.
12. Boughton, B. (2000). Prosthetic foot research. Advances in leaps and bounds. *Biomechanics, 7*, 73–80.
13. Postema, K., Hermens, H. J., deVries, J., Koopman, H. F., & Eisma, W. H. (1997). Energy storage and release of prosthetic feet. Part 2: Subjective ratings of 2 energy storing and 2 conventional feet, user choice of foot and deciding factor. *Prosthetics and Orthotics International, 21*, 28–34.

14. Perry, J., & Shanfield, S. (1993). Efficiency of dynamic elastic response prosthetic feet. *Journal of Rehabilitation Research and Development, 30,* 137–143.

15. Wagner, J., Sienko, S., Supan, T., & Barth, D. (1987). Motion analysis of SACH vs Flex-Foot in moderately active below-knee amputes. *Clinics in Prosthetics and Orthotics 11,* 55–62.

16. Snyder, R. D., Powers, C. M., Fontaine, C., & Perry, J. (1995). The effect of five prosthetic feet on the gait and loading of the sound limb in dysvascular below knee amputes. *Journal of Rehabilitation Research and Development, 32,* 309–315.

17. Yack, H. J., Nielsen, D. H., & Shurr, D. G. (1999). Kinetic patterns during stair ascent in patients with transtibial amputations using three different prostheses. *Journal of Prosthetics and Orthotics, 11,* 57–62.

18. Toburn, L., Schweiger, G. P., Perry, J., & Powers, C. M. (1994). Below knee amputee gait in stair ambulation. A comparison of stride characteristics using five different prosthetic feet. *Clinical Orthopaedics and Related Research, 303,* 185–192.

19. Van der Linden, M. L., Solomonidis, S. E., Spence, W. D., Li, N., & Paul, J. P. (1999). A methodology for studying the effects of various types of prosthetic feet on the biomechanics of trans-femoral amputee gait. *Journal of Biomechanics, 32,* 877–889.

20. Lehmann, J. F., Price, R., Okumura, R., Questad, K., deLateur, B. J., & Negretot, A. (1998). Mass and mass distribution of below-knee prostheses: Effect on gait efficacy and self-selected walking speed. *Archives Physical Medicine and Rehabilitation, 79,* 162–168.

21. Broyles, N. (1991). *For the new amputee (p. 20).* Durham, NC: American Academy of Orthotists and Prosthetists.

22. Kapp, S. (1999). Suspension systems for prostheses. *Clinical Orthopaedics and Related Research, 361,* 55–62.

23. Hachisuka, K., Takahashi, M., Ogata, H., Ohmine, S., Shitama, H., & Shinkoda, K. (1998). Properties of the flexible pressure sensor under laboratory conditions simulating the internal environment of the total surface bearing socket. *Prosthetics and Orthotics International, 22,* 186–192.

24. Shem, K. L., Beakey, J. W., & Werner, P. C. (1998). Pressures at the residual limb socket interface in transtibial amputes with thigh lacer slide joints. *Journal of Prosthetics and Orthotics, 10,* 51–55.

25. Periago, R. Z. (1998). Subjective evaluation of the prosthesis of 13 transtibial amputes with the ICEROSS suspension. *Rehabilitacion, 32,* 297–300.

26. Lake, C., & Supan, T. J. (1997). The incidence of dermatological problems in the silicone suspension sleeve user. *Journal of Prosthetics and Orthotics, 9,* 97–104.

27. Koziell, T. (1993). Transmetatarsal amputation management. *PT Magazine,* 50–53.

28. Mueller, M. J., & Strube, J. M. (1997). Therapeutic footwear: Enhanced function in people with diabetes and transmetatarsal amputations. *Archives of Physical Medicine and Rehabilitation, 78,* 952–956.

29. Mazet, R. Jr. (1968). Syme's amputation. *Journal of Bone and Joint Surgery, 50,* 1549.

30. Birch, J. G., Walsh, S. J., Small, J. M., Morton, A., Koch, K. D., Smith, C., Cummings, D., & Buchanan, R. (1996). Syme amputation for the treatment of fibular deficiency. *Journal of Bone and Joint Surgery, 81A,* 1511–1518.

31. Marshall Labs LTD. (1996). Reference for prosthetic prescription.

32. Continuing course (1999, November 13). *Current concepts in orthotics & prosthetics.* San Francisco: California Chapter of the American Physical Therapy Association.

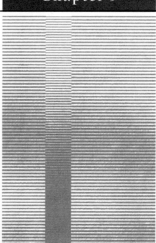

Chapter 9

TRANSFEMORAL COMPONENTS—
CLINICAL DECISION MAKING

Objectives

1. Differentiate the types of prosthetic knees, sockets, and suspensions and give a rationale for their use with a particular patient

2. Describe how you would instruct an individual with an amputation to apply the traditional and roll-on silicone liner suction suspensions and the pelvic band suspensions

3. Describe the examination or checkout procedures for a transfemoral prosthesis

4. Given a patient with a transfemoral amputation, develop a prescription recommendation for prosthetic components

5. Based on patient examination, recommend prosthetic and musculoskeletal corrections that may be made for a particular gait deviation

This chapter is divided into the following sections:

P hysical therapists, as part of the prosthetic clinical team, need to possess an understanding of prosthetic components to recommend or prescribe these components for a particular individual with an amputation. Numerous prosthetic components are available, and there is ongoing research to design more-efficient components. The information in this chapter depicts many of the most common transfemoral prosthetic components used. The *Guide to Physical Therapist Practice* in the practice pattern "Impaired Motor Function, Muscle Performance, Range of Motion,

Gait, Locomotion, and Balance Associated with Amputation" (4J) refers to interventions with prosthetic devices.[1] Regional differences and philosophies may alter the prosthetic components that are recommended. This chapter is not intended to be an inclusive list but representative of commonly used transfemoral components. Prosthetic feet are addressed in the previous chapter. This chapter on transfemoral components begins with a discussion of prosthetic knees.

◆◆◆

Knees

Knee stability is the ability of the prosthetic knee to remain extended and fully supportive during the stance phase of walking. A particular prosthetic knee is often recommended on the basis of the inherent knee stability required. An individual with a long residual limb and good hip extensor muscle strength may use a knee unit with less knee stability than an individual with a short residual limb or weak hip extensors. The extension or stability of a prosthetic knee is related to the individual's ability to generate a hip extension moment at the initiation of initial contact. Knee classifications are divided into axes, friction, braking or locking mechanisms, and microprocessor control.

Types of Knee Axes

Two types of knee axes, the single and the polycentric, are commonly used. They are described as follows.

Single Axis

Single-axis knees consist of a simple hinge mechanism that allows free knee flexion but no swing-phase control. Single-axis knees lack ca-

dence response; therefore, they are indicated for individuals who walk at the same speed. The single-axis knee is illustrated in Figure 9-1.

Polycentric Axis

Most polycentric axes consist of a mechanically complex four-bar linkage that provides more than one point of rotation. A changing instantaneous center of knee rotation occurs, which adds to stability during initial contact and shortening of the shank for toe clearance during swing. One group of polycentric knees swings the shank under the thigh when sitting, allowing equal thigh and shank lengths.[2] An ideal candidate for the polycentric knee is a patient with a knee disarticulation amputation. Other individuals who may benefit from the stability of this knee include those with short transfemoral amputations and those with weak hip extensors. Newer materials such as carbon fiber, titanium, and aluminum have resulted in lighter units. Polycentric knees also lack cadence response; therefore, they are indicated for individuals who walk at the same speed. They are superior to single-axis knees in that they have greater toe clearance at midswing. The Total Knee polycentric axis that creates a locking moment for in-

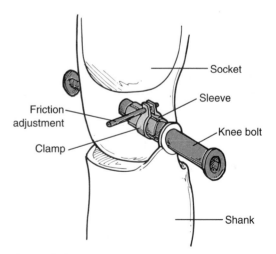

Figure 9-1. Single-axis knee.

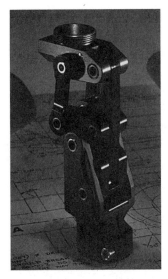

Figure 9-2. Total knee polycentric axis. (Reprinted with permission from Ossur.)

creased knee stability and has a shock absorber is depicted in Figure 9-2.

Types of Friction

Three types of friction are commonly used. These are mechanical, pneumatic, and hydraulic.

Mechanical Friction

A mechanical, constant friction is often used with the single axis knee. Constant friction provides uniform resistance throughout the gait cycle. This friction is adjusted to the individual's normal cadence so the pendulum action of the shank (part of the prosthesis between the knee and ankle) will correspond to that of the opposite limb. The single-axis constant-friction knee is durable and inexpensive. However, this mechanism has many drawbacks. It offers no stance stability and is not cadence responsive because of the constant, nonvarying friction. If the wearer walks more rapidly, vaulting or excessive heel rise may occur. Because of the risk of serious gait devia-

tions, the single-axis constant-friction knee is rarely used.[3] The principal indication for the single-axis constant-friction knee is living in a remote area without access to a prosthetist.[3] If the single-axis constant-friction knee has terminal swing impact or if the prosthetic heel rises more than the normal heel, friction must be increased. If prosthetic heel rises less than the normal heel, friction must be decreased.

Problems with mechanical friction are as follows:

1. Mechanical friction units do not adjust to walking speed. When the cadence increases, resistance decreases, and terminal impact (a banging sound as the knee extends) and excessive heel rise result.
2. Mechanical friction may loosen, requiring adjustment.
3. Debris may enter the system, interfering with function.

As a result of problems with mechanical friction, pneumatic and hydraulic units were developed.

Pneumatic

Pneumatic and hydraulic units solve the problems of mechanical-friction knees by offering minimal resistance at the initiation of movement but increasing resistance as the speed and the force of movement increase. These units are therefore cadence responsive. This responsiveness provides less resistance to movement at lower speeds and more resistance at higher speeds. This varying control of knee resistance is accomplished through channels in which resistance to the flow of air or oil increases with increasing cadence.[4] Pneumatic and hydraulic units are also closed systems, so debris does not interfere with function of the unit.

Pneumatic control units use compressed air to serve as a friction control. They are unaffected by drastic changes in air temperature. Knee friction resistance remains the same regardless of temperature. Energetic walkers frequently overpower the pneumatic resistance;

therefore these units are recommended for slow- to moderate-cadence walkers.[3]

Hydraulic

Hydraulic units are more commonly prescribed than pneumatic units because they allow ambulation at any speed from very slow to very fast. The knee resistance automatically compensates to change in walking speed. Hydraulic units use oil (typically silicone oil) for friction control.[3] Silicone oil minimizes viscosity fluctuations with temperature changes. Therefore, stiffness in cold weather and looseness in hot weather are avoided.

Indications for Hydraulic Units

Hydraulic units are indicated for those who

- Walk at varying cadences
- Walk on uneven ground
- Are unhappy with the lack of cadence responsiveness or the lack of stability of mechanical-friction knees
- Take small steps in their occupation

Disadvantages of Hydraulic Units

Disadvantages of hydraulic units include

- Increased expense
- Increased weight (although newer hydraulic units add only a few ounces)[3]

Types of Hydraulic Units

There are many different types of hydraulic units. Two of the most common units, the Modular Ergonomically Balanced Stride (EBS) Polycentric Knee Joint and the Henschke-Mauch Stance and Swing Control (SNS) unit are described.

Modular Ergonomically Balanced Stride (EBS) Polycentric Knee

This EBS knee possesses a four-bar linkage that offers a stable knee under weight bearing up to a maximum of 15° of knee flexion. This feature enables a smooth transition from full knee ex-

tension at initial contact to 15° of knee flexion at midstance. The resistance provided by the EBS unit may be adjusted to suit the activity level and weight of the individual (Fig. 9-3).

Henschke-Mauch Stance and Swing Control (SNS)

Mauch and Henschke developed a hydraulically actuated stance-phase control unit under the direction of the U.S. Air Force in the late 1940s and early 1950s.[4] Since this time, the SNS has undergone several improvements (Fig. 9-4).

Features

- The SNS unit provides increasing resistance to flexion. As the knee nears maximum flexion, greater resistance to flexion is reinstated to prevent falling. This feature, called the stumble control, allows the individual to walk downstairs and downhill, step over step, in a normal manner.[4] While this in-

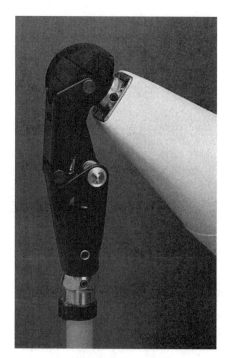

Figure 9-3. Modular EBS Polycentric Knee. (Reprinted with permission from Otto Bock Orthopedic Industry Inc.)

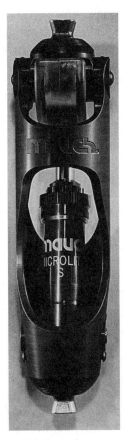

Figure 9-4. Henschke-Mauch Stance and Swing Control (SNS) Slimline Frame. (Reprinted with permission from Mauch Inc.)

creasing resistance to flexion helps to prevent falls, it poses a detriment to normal gait. However, this increasing resistance to flexion may be bypassed by the individual generating a hyperextension moment at the knee. This hyperextension moment occurs naturally in walking at preswing.

- The individual who wishes to sit down extends the affected hip, which decreases knee flexion resistance and allows sitting.
- The selector switch can allow a locked knee, useful when riding on a subway or being in a closed area. It also allows a free swing mode only, useful when bicycle riding or rowing.

- The SNS unit includes extension or forward bias. This bias occurs as the knee is flexed more than 20°. As a result, the foot is lifted from the floor, and the knee extends. This energy-saving feature is helpful in occupations requiring small steps such as a store clerk or teacher.

The SNS unit is reliable, durable, and widely used. A survey of 70 active, military-service-connected individuals with transfemoral amputations of traumatic etiology (mean age, 47 years) who were given a Mauch SNS unit between 1963 and 1980 found an overall success rate of 98.2%. Success was measured by subjective responses to questions regarding stability, smoother walking pattern, and the ability to change walking speed. Individuals reported increased activity, fewer falls, and less fatigue. This study concluded that the Mauch SNS unit was superior to the single-axis knee when appropriately prescribed. Its use was recommended for the active individual with a transfemoral amputation who has a strong, relatively long residual limb and desires a variable cadence gait and more stability in stance with increasing activity levels.[5]

Pediatric Hydraulic Units

Hydraulic knee joints have also been developed for children as shown in the Pediatric Perspective Box.

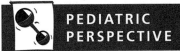

PEDIATRIC PERSPECTIVE

Many pediatric hydraulic protheses have a colorful appearance that may encourage initial acceptance. They are usually endoskeletal or modular so pylons and other components may be changed as the child grows. To avoid soiling, if the child is very active, no soft cosmetic covering is used (Fig. 9-5).

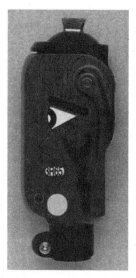

Figure 9-5. 3R65 Children's hydraulic knee joint. (Reprinted with permission from Otto Bock Orthopedic Industry Inc.)

Training Suggestions for the Hydraulic Unit

Individuals who have been mechanical friction users may need additional gait training to use a hydraulic knee unit successfully. Wearers should be taught to carry their body weight over the prosthesis in stance phase without hesitation. The body must move forward with the prosthetic limb and roll over the foot in terminal stance. During the early stages of ambulation training, the swing control on the hydraulic knee should be adjusted to allow minimum resistance. An individual who is used to a mechanical knee unit will often extend the hydraulic knee too forcibly in terminal swing to make sure the knee is extended for initial contact. This forcible knee extension is not necessary with a hydraulic unit and the individual must develop confidence that the prosthetic knee will extend. Forcible flexion and extension of the anatomic hip is energy fatiguing. An individual who is used to wearing a mechanical knee unit may vault (excessive plantarflexion on the sound side to permit the swing of the prosthesis) to clear the prosthetic toe.

The new hydraulic wearer should learn to walk at slow, medium, and fast speeds. It may be necessary to adjust the cadence-control knob on the hydraulic unit to find the ideal resistance for an individual. To check the extension bias of the hydraulic knee, the individual may stand at a counter and flex the knee up to 20°. When weight is taken off the prosthesis, the knee will automatically extend.[6]

Braking or Locking Mechanisms

Braking or locking mechanisms may exist in mechanical friction, pneumatic, or hydraulic units. A mechanical unit (stance- control knee) is described below.

Stance-Control Knee

The stance-control knee is sometimes called a weight-activated friction brake. This knee is often used for elderly or unstable individuals and those who walk on uneven surfaces. The stance-control knee is described in the Geriatric Perspective Box. A manual-lock knee is another stance-control knee used for individuals who need maximal stability because of poor coordination, poor vision, or muscular weakness. The manual-lock knee results in an uncosmetic gait, often characterized by an abduction or circumduction gait deviation. Therefore, it is rarely used.

Microprocessor Control

Microprocessor control units that work on strain and motion sensors have recently become available. These units sense whether a flexion or extension moment is occurring and the specific knee position that is present. Resistance is adjusted accordingly for ambulation on various types of walking surfaces such as sand or concrete. In addition, an on-board computer assists knee resistance, allowing a wide range of gait speeds from very slow to very fast. Case studies have shown an energy-saving feature of

GERIATRIC PERSPECTIVE

The stance-control knee is often used for an elderly patient or one who needs additional stability. When weight is put on the prosthesis during the first 15 to 20° of flexion, the friction brake is activated, and further knee flexion is resisted. An endoskeletal stance-control knee has been designed for individuals who weigh up to100 kg or 220 lb. Friction and swing- phase characteristics are adjustable. A spring extension assist aids in knee extension during the swing to initial contact phases of gait. A disadvantage of this knee is that when walking at a normal pace, the brake stability interferes with knee flexion during preswing. Therefore, this knee should be used only when the patient needs additional knee stability. A stance-control knee is suited for those with slow, limited ambulation capability.[3] An endoskeletal stance-control knee is shown in Figure 9-6.

microprocessor-controlled knees.[3] The 3C100 C leg is an example of a computer- controlled hydraulic unit (Fig. 9-7). Disadvantages of computer-controlled hydraulic units include increased cost, weight, and unknown durability.

Sockets

There are primarily two types of sockets used for individuals with transfemoral amputations, the quadrilateral and the ischial-containment socket. The transfemoral quadrilateral socket design was introduced by the University of California at Berkeley in 1950 to permit use of the remaining musculature.[4] In 1980, the ischial-containment socket was developed.[4] The ischial-containment socket is becoming the socket of choice in many areas of the country.

Quadrilateral Socket

The quadrilateral socket is named for the appearance of the socket when viewed in the transverse plane. It has four sides or walls (Fig. 9-8). The quadrilateral socket can be rigid or can have a flexible inner liner with an outer rigid socket (ISNY, Icelandic Swedish New York).

Functions

The functions of each of the walls are as follows.

Medial Wall

The medial wall functions to contain tissues medially and to provide counterpressure to the lateral wall. The proximal brim is horizontal and parallel to the floor, and the distal end is contoured for total contact. The height of the

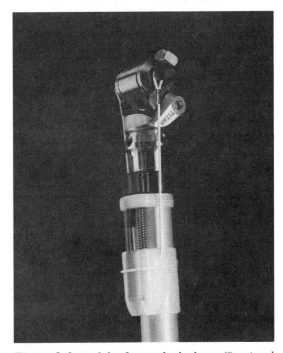

Figure 9-6. Modular friction-brake knee. (Reprinted with permission from Otto Bock Orthopedic Industry Inc.)

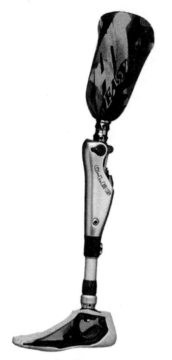

Figure 9-7. 3C100 C leg. (Reprinted with permission from Otto Bock Orthopedic Industry Inc.)

medial wall is usually the same as that of the posterior wall, to prevent an adductor roll. If an adductor roll occurs, the quadrilateral socket is enlarged below the top of the medial wall to accommodate the adductor roll.[7] The adductor roll is illustrated in Figure 6-15.

Lateral Wall

The lateral wall must provide adequate lateral support to the femur in midstance to prevent a Trendelenburg sign as the unamputated side is in swing. As reviewed in Chapter 5 on biomechanics, weakness of the amputated-side gluteus medius or an inadequately shaped lateral wall results in lateral trunk lean toward the prosthesis. This lateral lean brings the support line and ground reaction force vector (GRFV) closer to the joint axis, thereby decreasing the moment arm. (Fig. 5-46). In the nonamputated

limb, the gluteus medius does not abduct the limb because it is on the ground. In the amputated limb, the residual limb must be prevented from abducting. Therefore, the lateral wall is sloped so that the femur is in adduction to resist this abduction and stabilize the pelvis. Because of the small amount of counterforce provided by the socket, a short residual limb will often result in lateral trunk bend toward the prosthesis. Adduction of the socket also puts the gluteus medius and other hip abductors on stretch, which allows these muscles to function most effectively. The lateral wall rises $2\frac{1}{2}$ inches above the ischial shelf to stabilize the greater trochanter and prevent medial socket displacement.[7]

Anterior Wall

The anterior wall blocks forward motion of the residual limb. The anterior brim rises $2\frac{1}{2}$ inches above the ischial seat. If the anterior wall is too high, it impinges on the abdomen or the anterior superior iliac spine (ASIS).[7] The anterior medial corner contains a channel or relief for the adductor longus and gracilis tendons. An individual will frequently determine if the quadrilateral socket is donned properly by performing an isometric contraction of these adductor tendons to make sure they are contained in this anterior medial corner.

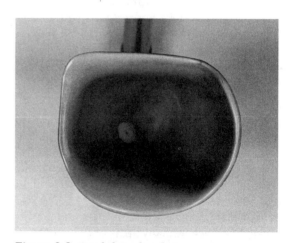

Figure 9-8. Quadrilateral socket.

Posterior Wall

The posterior wall provides a weight-bearing surface for the ischial tuberosity. Weight bearing in a quadrilateral socket is primarily through the ischial tuberosity and the gluteal muscles. The ischial tuberosity sits 1 inch lateral from the medial wall and $\frac{1}{2}$ inch posterior on the ischial shelf.[8] If the mediolateral dimension of the socket is too small, the ischium may be pushed too far medially and thus may crowd the adductors. In addition, excessive trochanteric pressure may result. The posterior wall slopes 5 to 7° to increase prosthetic function in two ways:

1. To permit easier access to the ischial tuberosity so that weight bearing may occur on the top edge of the posterior wall on and around the ischial tuberosity
2. To place the hip extensors in a stretched position enabling them to move powerfully to extend the hip and stabilize the pelvis and prosthesis during weight bearing[7,9]

Potential Problems with Quadrilateral Sockets

Potential problems with quadrilateral sockets include the following:

1. The femur of the residual limb abducts due to the wide mediolateral dimension and poor abductor restraining force. This femoral movement may result in lateral trunk bending toward the prosthetic side (compensated Trendelenburg) and increased perineal pressure. This poor abductor restraining force is due to loss of adductor strength weakened by the transfemoral amputation. Figure 5-42 illustrates this loss of adductor strength.
2. Wearers may complain of the socket being uncomfortable with pressure over the ischial tuberosity.[8]
3. Pressure is increased in the quadrilateral socket because a smaller portion of the residual limb is contained in the socket than in the ischial-containment socket. The shorter the residual limb, the more difficult the task of establishing and maintaining mediolateral pelvic and trunk stability and the higher the pressure concentration. Longer residual limbs have a greater ability to distribute pressure and forces.

Ischial-Containment Socket

As a result of the problems with a quadrilateral socket, the ischial-containment socket was developed with a wider anteroposterior (AP) dimension and a narrow mediolateral (ML) dimension.

Features

Features of the ischial-containment socket include

1. Maintenance of normal femoral adduction and a narrow-base gait. After a transfemoral amputation, the abductor muscles are more powerful than the adductor muscles because of the loss of the insertions of the adductor muscles. The shorter the residual limb, the more adductor strength is lost. Loss of the distal attachment of the adductor magnus muscle results in a loss of 70% of adductor strength.
2. Containment of the ischial tuberosity and pubic ramus.
3. More-optimal distribution of forces along the femoral shaft.[10]

Significantly more residual limb volume is contained within the ischial-containment socket than in the quadrilateral socket, and a larger residual limb volume may result in a wider distribution of forces.[11] The posterior brim of the ischial-containment socket is proximal to, and slightly posterior to, the ischium. The ischial tuberosity is contained in the socket, resulting in a bony lock between the ischium, trochanter, and lateral distal aspect of the femur. This containment may provide a stable mechanism to control mediolateral and rotational stability.[4]

Flexible Sockets

Ischial-containment sockets have been made of flexible thermoplastic materials contained within a rigid frame. They are considered more comfortable than the traditional hard plastic laminate socket.[10] These have been called several names including the Total Flexible Brim, the ISNY, and SFS (Scandinavian Flexible Socket). An example of this flexible socket is shown in Figure 9-9.

Research Studies

There have been few large studies comparing the ischial-containment socket with the quadrilateral socket. Research, to date, has been limited by small subject samples. One study analyzed five individuals with unilateral transfemoral amputations (mean age, 34.3 years) who initially used quadrilateral sockets and then converted to ischial-containment sockets. Results of this study showed that most gait deviations disappeared or improved, especially lateral trunk bending toward the prosthesis, with the use of the ischial-containment socket. In addition, the femoral shaft moved 6.5° toward adduction, and increased gait velocities resulted. Also, oxygen consumption was 50% lower with the ischial-containment socket than with the quadrilateral.[12] Another study used 20 healthy males between the ages of 18 and 55 with unilateral nonvascular transfemoral amputations and found that the ischial-containment socket design used less energy than the quadrilateral design in normal and fast-paced ambulation.[13] In contrast, one radiologic study of 50 individuals with transfemoral amputations demonstrated that the position of the residual femur could not be controlled by the prosthetic socket shape. This study found no benefit of the ischial-containment socket in controlling femoral adduction and decreasing lateral trunk bend.[14] The different results of these three studies may have been due to the different subject sample sizes as well as different measurement parameters.

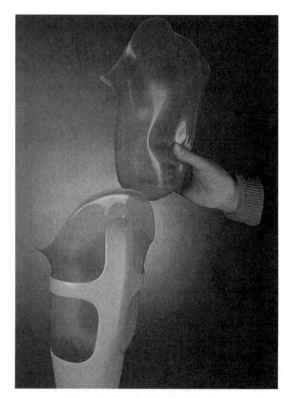

Figure 9-9. Flexible ischial-containment socket. (Reprinted with permission from Otto Bock Orthopedic Industry Inc.)

Summary

Deciding which socket to use can be confusing. However, these guidelines for socket appropriateness may be helpful:

1. Quadrilateral sockets are most successful on long residual limbs with firm adductor musculature. The more of the adductor magnus that is intact, the more successful the quadrilateral socket will be.
2. Ischial-containment sockets are more successful on short, fleshy residual limbs and are better suited for high-activity sports participation.[7]
3. Flexible brims of the ischial-containment socket are best for maximal ischial ramus containment.

4. No specific contraindications have been noted for any socket design.

5. Some clinicians advocate not changing successful quadrilateral socket wearers to ischial-containment sockets.[11]

An understanding of the biomechanical principles of each socket is indicated to optimally recommend a specific socket for a particular patient.[11]

Suspensions

Various types of suspensions may be used to secure a transfemoral prosthesis to the residual limb. Selection of the best suspension is critical to achieving a stable, efficient, cosmetic gait. An improperly fitting suspension may result in discomfort, skin breakdown, and falls.

Types of Suspensions

The most common types of suspensions include suction, hypobaric, soft belts, and pelvic belts.

Suction Suspension

Suction suspension is one of the most frequently used forms of suspension for the definitive transfemoral prosthesis.[14] The ideal wearer of suction suspension is an active, stable individual with a long muscular residual limb and no edema problems. However, with the advent of the ischial-containment socket, even very short residual limbs can often be fitted with this suction suspension. Additional auxiliary soft belt suspensions, such as a Silesian bandage or total elastic suspension (TES) belt (discussed below), may be used by a new suction suspension wearer. Suction plus a soft belt is often called *partial suction.*[4]

Types of Suction Suspension

There are two types of suction suspension, traditional and roll-on silicone liner.

Traditional Suction Suspension

Traditional suction suspension is accomplished by surface tension, negative pressure, and muscle contraction. The direct skin fit reduces pistoning between the residual limb and socket and increases proprioception.[15] If an individual with a transfemoral amputation is unable to apply a traditional suction suspension, the thigh and socket may be lubricated with lotion and the residual limb slid into the socket. This is commonly called *a wet-fit suction suspension.*[7]

Application of a Traditional Suction Suspension

Application of a traditional suction suspension is included in Practical Application Box 9-1

Roll-on Silicone Liner Suction Suspension

For patients who have difficulty applying a traditional suction suspension, a roll-on silicone liner may be used. The roll-on silicone liner is

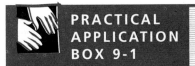

PRACTICAL APPLICATION BOX 9-1

Application of a Traditional Suction Suspension

While sitting, talcum powder is applied to reduce friction between the skin and the donning sock. The donning sock is applied to the residual limb, extending 2 inches above the groin. This extra length ensures that all soft tissues will be pulled into the socket. The valve is removed from the prosthesis, and the donning sock is threaded through the hole. The individual then stands and gently pumps the residual limb as the sock is pulled out of the valve hole. If the residual limb is seated properly in the socket, soft tissue should protrude slightly through the valve opening. Finally, the valve is screwed in place, and air is released to create negative pressure (Fig. 9-10).

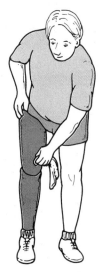

Figure 9-10. Application of traditional suction suspension.

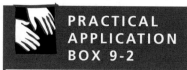

PRACTICAL APPLICATION BOX 9-2

Application of Roll-on Silicone Liner Suction Suspension

The silicone liner is turned inside out, and lotion is poured into the liner. The residual limb is slid into the liner, ensuring full contact between the distal end of the residual limb and the liner. After the liner is rolled on the residual limb, the outer surface of the liner is lubricated and pushed into the socket.[15] The socket valve is then screwed in place, and air is released to create a negative pressure. The locking mechanism may then be secured. The application of the roll-on silicone liner suction suspension is much less taxing on the individual than the traditional suction method. A recent study of 58 elderly individuals with new transfemoral amputations who wore an ischial-containment socket compared the use of the roll-on silicone suction suspension to use of an unlined socket. Results showed greater gains in distances ambulated and fewer prosthesis adjustments needed in the roll-on silicone suction suspension group.[16]

similar to the pin/shuttle suspension of the transtibial prosthesis (Fig. 9-11).

Application of Roll-on Silicone Liner Suction Suspension

The application of roll-on silicone liner suction suspension is included in Practical Application Box 9-2.

Advantages and Disadvantages of Suction Suspension

Advantages and disadvantages of suction suspension are listed in Table 9-1.[4,7]

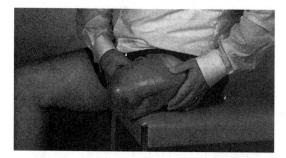

Figure 9-11. Application of roll-on silicone liner suction suspension. (Reprinted with permission from Otto Bock Orthopedic Industry Inc.)

Hypobaric Suspension

A hypobaric suspension involves use of a 1-inch fabric ring impregnated with silicone that is generally placed 5 cm below the ischial tuberosity. This ring is pushed into the socket and air is expelled through the valve in the distal socket. This suspension is contraindicated with short and conical residual limbs because of difficulty maintaining a seal. Due to its ease of application, it is frequently used for the elderly or less active patient.[7,15]

Soft Belts

Soft belts are typically of two types, TES and a Silesian bandage, described as follows.

Table 9-1. Transfemoral Suspensions

Suspension	Indication	Advantages	Disadvantages
Traditional suction suspension	Most patients who have stable volume residual limbs	Increased comfort and cosmetic appearance, since no belts are attached Increased proprioception, since the residual limb is against the socket Decreased piston action because of an intimate fit needed between the residual limb and socket	Fitting may be difficult, especially for an individual with a deep scar over the residual limb or volume fluctuations due to dialysis or weight changes May be unsuitable for individuals with balance problems, upper limb deficiencies, strength deficiencies, or cardiovascular problems because of the amount of effort associated with application An individual with a new amputation due to the presence of fluctuating edema and muscle atrophy may have fitting problems with this suspension Those with perspiration problems may develop rashes with the use of suction suspension
Roll-on silicone liner suction suspension	Those who cannot apply traditional suction	Same as traditional suction	Same as traditional suction Not durable Excessive perspiration and heat May not fit all sizes
Hypobaric Suspension	Those who cannot apply traditional suction	Ease of application	Same as traditional suction, difficult to maintain a seal with short and conical residual limbs
Soft belts	May be used with other suspensions when rotation control is needed	Keeps the prosthesis from coming off in sitting Good psychologic aid for those wearing suction suspension Adjusts to the size of the individual Controls rotation problems to some degree on initial contact	Body heat retention and hygiene May be uncomfortable because of constriction around the waist
Pelvic band and hip joint	Individuals with short, weak, poorly shaped residual limbs Activities including walking on uneven terrain where additional medial lateral stability is needed to control rotation between the residual limb and the socket	Permits satisfactory fit if suction cannot be used due to scarring or weakness The individual does not have to stoop over to pull the sock out of the socket Can be used by individuals who are allergic to socket finishes	Increased weight Restricted motion of hip in ambulation and sitting Increased maintenance due to the mechanical joint Poor cosmetic appearance

Total Elastic Suspension (TES)

A TES belt is made of elastic neoprene material lined with a smooth nylon material. This belt fits around the proximal end of the prosthetic socket and then around the waist, fastening anteriorly. The TES belt is comfortable since it spreads pressures over a greater surface area. It is an excellent auxiliary suspension that may be used with either suction suspension (Fig. 9-12).[15]

Silesian bandage

A Silesian bandage is a soft belt made of cotton webbing or Dacron materials. Attached to the prosthetic socket over the trochanter, the Sile-

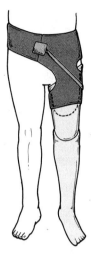

Figure 9-12. Total elastic suspension (TES).

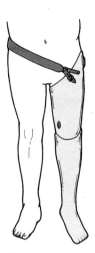

Figure 9-13. Silesian belt suspension.

sian bandage encircles the sound-side pelvis between the iliac crest and trochanter and terminates at the vertical midline of the anterior socket. It is most commonly used when the TES belt fails to provide adequate suspension or rotational control. Significant hip instability, weak musculature, or very short residual limbs are contraindications for use of the Silesian belt. Individuals with any of these conditions would be better served with a pelvic band and hip joint (Fig. 9-13).[15]

Advantages and Disadvantages of Soft Belts

Advantages and disadvantages of soft belts are listed in Table 9-1.

Pelvic Belt

The use of the pelvic belt for suspension occurred about the time of World War I. This suspension consists of a pelvic belt that passes between the iliac crest and the greater trochanter of each hip and a joint that is positioned slightly above and ahead of the greater trochanter. The joint of this suspension is made of metal or polypropylene and is placed over the anatomic hip joint. The pelvic band consists of a 2-inch-wide metal pelvic band attached to the joint,

which extends from the posterosuperior iliac spine to a point 1 inch medial to the anterosuperior iliac spine (Fig. 9-14).[15]

Indications, Advantages, and Disadvantages of the Pelvic Band and Hip Joint Suspension

Indications, advantages, and disadvantages of the pelvic band and hip joint suspension are listed in Table 9-1.

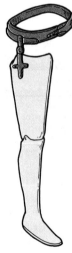

Figure 9-14. Pelvic band and hip joint suspension.

Application of the Pelvic Band Suspension

Application of the pelvic band suspension is included in Practical Application Box 9-3.

Other Prosthetic Features

Other prosthetic features include a knee disarticulation prosthesis and a torsion adapter unit.

Knee Disarticulation

A knee disarticulation amputation is infrequently used in adults due to functional and cosmetic reasons. In this amputation, the residual limb, due to its bulbous end containing the femoral condyles, is often considered unsightly. Most available prosthetic knee units are designed for transfemoral amputations. When these units are used for knee disarticulation, they protrude as much as 2 inches beyond the anatomic knee center. Therefore external hinge joints sometimes are used. These hinges are cumbersome, are somewhat unstable, and often damage overlying clothing. In traumatic cases when the residual length is too short to support a transtibial prosthesis, a knee disarticulation amputation may be indicated. This amputation may also be indicated in cases of severe knee flexion contracture. In children, a knee disarticulation has the advantage of preservation of distal femoral growth potential and the elimination of bony overgrowth. Phantom pain and residual limb pain are rare with this amputation.

Suspension of the knee disarticulation socket is provided by the intimate fit just

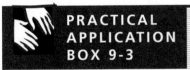

PRACTICAL APPLICATION BOX 9-3

Application of Pelvic Band Suspension

To apply a transfemoral pelvic band suspension prosthesis, the individual must apply a multiple-ply sock. This sock may be partially split down the side so it fits around the pelvic band suspension. The sock should be long enough to extend 4 to 5 inches above the socket brim. A new wearer may initially put a coin in the bottom of the sock and tie a string around the sock and coin. The coin and distal end of the sock can be put through the hole on the distal medial aspect of the socket and pulled downward. This will ensure that the residual limb can be pulled all the way into the socket.

There should be no wrinkles in the nylon sheath or prosthetic socks. Seams should not be over bony areas or directly across the scar. Wrinkles and seams over bony, sensitive areas may cause tissue breakdown. The pelvic band suspension may then be buckled loosely. The individual may stand and shift weight over the prosthesis while pulling the sock down further so that the distal end of the residual limb is pulled into the socket. The therapist can determine that the proper amount of toe-out (5–7°) is present and that the ischial tuberosity is positioned on the quadrilateral socket ischial shelf. Several factors may account for the ischial tuberosity being above the posterior shelf: the prosthesis may have been applied incorrectly, socks may be excessively thick, or the residual limb may not have been pulled all the way into the socket. The pelvic band can be tightened by placing the prosthesis behind the remaining foot. This placement will ensure that weight is borne on the prosthesis and that a slight amount of toe-out of the prosthesis can occur.[8]

proximal to the femoral condyles.[4] Fitting of a knee disarticulation prosthesis may be difficult with larger thighs. In these cases, an auxiliary suspension such as a TES belt may be required. A flexible liner and a flexible suction socket have been advocated for use with knee disarticulation prostheses.[16,17] A polycentric knee is often used with a knee disarticulation prosthesis and has advantages over the external hinge joints in that it shortens with increasing knee flexion, which helps avoid toe stubbing. In addition, the shank automatically decelerates late in stance, which adds to knee stability.[4] The knee disarticulation prosthesis is shown in Figure 9-15.

Torsion Adapter Unit

A torsion adapter allows up to 20° rotation. This rotation is advantageous for golfers and

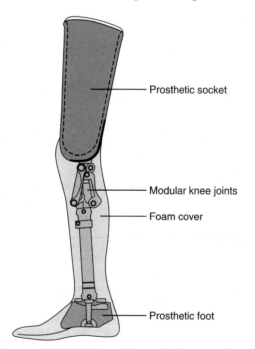

Figure 9-15. Knee disarticulation prosthesis. (Reprinted with permission from Otto Bock Orthopedic Industry Inc.)

- Prosthetic socket
- Modular knee joints
- Foam cover
- Prosthetic foot

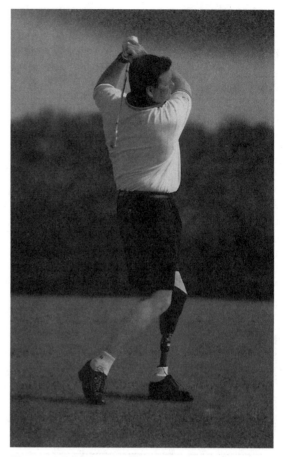

Figure 9-16. Torsion adapter unit being used by a golfer. Note the rotation of the prosthetic foot compared with the knee. (Reprinted with permission from College Park Industries Inc.)

those with skin breakdown. The torsion adapter unit absorbs ground reaction force to minimize friction between the socket and residual limb (Fig. 9-16).

Examination (Checkout)

The purpose and considerations of an examination or checkout procedure are reviewed in Chapter 8 on transtibial components. Specific steps to consider with a transfemoral prosthesis are described below.

Examination (Checkout) for a Transfemoral Prosthesis

Standing Position

1. The patient should be comfortable while standing with the midlines of the heels (heel seams) not more than 6 inches (15 cm) apart.[7] The fit of the adductor longus tendon into its channel in the anterior medial part of the quadrilateral socket is important, as it determines whether or not the socket is positioned correctly on the residual limb. If there is difficulty palpating the adductor longus tendon, ask the patient to adduct the residual limb against resistance. This will cause the tendon to become more prominent.[8] If the tendon is improperly located, the patient should be asked to remove the prosthesis and then put it on again with the adductor longus tendon properly located in its channel. In the ischial-containment socket, the position of the adductor longus tendon is not as critical.

2. The ischial tuberosity should rest approximately ½ inch behind the inner surface of the ischial shelf and ¾ to 1 inch lateral to the inner surface of the medial wall of the quadrilateral socket. To check the position of the ischial tuberosity on the ischial shelf, stand behind and ask the patient to bend forward and take most of the weight off the prosthesis. Probe for the ischial tuberosity with the palmar surface of the index and middle fingers. The spot in which the ischial tuberosity contacts the ischial shelf may be marked with a washable marker. When the prosthesis is removed, this location may be measured to determine if the ischial tuberosity is properly located on the ischial shelf. If the tuberosity is too posterior, there may be pressure on the hamstring tendons and the gluteal muscles. If the tuberosity is inside the quadrilateral socket, the patient may have discomfort in the adductor region where the pubic ramus contacts the medial wall. If the ischial tuberosity is above the posterior brim, the patient may need to readjust the application of the prosthesis or decrease the number of sock plies.[8] In an ischial-containment socket, the ischial tuberosity is seated within the socket.

3. The prosthesis should be the correct length so that the patient's iliac crests are even.[7] If too few ply socks are used, the ischial tuberosity may slip into the quadrilateral socket. This is a common occurrence as the residual limb becomes less edematous with further exercise and ambulation.

4. The knee should be stable on weight bearing. To check stability of the knee, the patient may stand near a support, bearing weight through the arms, with weight evenly distributed on both feet. The back of the knee should be struck with moderate force. The knee should give only slightly, but should return to full extension. The patient should be able to maintain stability of the knee.[7]

5. The patient wearing a quadrilateral socket should not experience pain at the ischial tuberosity. A brief period of burning may be noted initially at the beginning of weight bearing, but this should resolve. Burning may also result if the ischial shelf is not slanted forward slightly. In addition, if the medial anteroposterior dimension of the quadrilateral socket is too small, the ischium can be located too far posteriorly on the shelf, resulting in excessive compression of the hamstring tendons.[7]

6. The individual using a roll-on silicone liner suction suspension should be able to apply this suspension successfully and lock the shuttle pin in place.

Sitting Position

7. The socket should remain securely on the residual limb. Ask the patient while sitting to bend to touch the shoe and determine if

the socket remains on the residual limb. If the socket changes position, it may be due to a poorly placed pelvic joint or a loss of suction due to poor socket fit.

Kneeling Position

8. With the prosthesis in the kneeling position, the thigh piece should be vertical and the posteromedial and posterolateral parts of the shank should be equidistant from the thigh piece. If the thigh piece cannot be brought to the vertical position, the prosthesis may force the individual to lean forward when kneeling.[7] More than 90° of knee flexion is necessary for kneeling.

Walking

9. Suction should be maintained during walking, stairs, and inclines. There should be no piston action in a suction suspension prosthesis. The individual should be able to rise to a standing position without objectionable air noise. Failure to maintain suction may be due to:

- Accumulation of foreign material such as powder in the threads of the valve
- An inadequate seal around the edges of the valve
- Flesh obstructing the valve
- Air leakage between the residual limb and the anterior or lateral brim
- Escape of air through an invaginated scar or skin fold beneath the brim[7]

Prosthesis-Wearing Schedule

The prosthesis wearing schedule is reviewed in Chapter 8 on transtibial components.

Prosthetic Prescription

Medicare and approved prosthetic feet are reviewed in Table 8.3. Knees reimbursed by Medicare are listed in Table 9-2.[18,19]

Recommendation Guidelines

Recommendation guidelines are presented in Chapter 8. These also apply to recommendation of a transfemoral prosthesis.

Prosthetic Prescription Cases

It is helpful to consider cases in which prosthetic components may be ordered for a particular patient. Additional cases in a *Guide to Physical Therapist Practice* format are presented in the Appendix.[1] Answers to these cases are included at the end of the case. The reader should attempt to answer the case, considering which prosthetic component would be best for that particular patient. Use of the prescription guidelines discussed in Chapter 8 may be helpful. For each question, several components may be correct. It is important for the reader to be able to give a plausible rationale for the suggested prosthetic component.

Table 9-2. Approved Prosthetic Knees According to Medicare	
Medicare Level	*Approved Prosthetic Knees*
Level 0	Noncandidate
Levels 1 and 2	Single-axis/constant-friction, single-axis/stance-control, polycentric/stance-control
Levels 3 and 4	Hydraulic or pneumatic variable-cadence swing-control, with or without stance control

C A S E   1

PATIENT/CLIENT HISTORY

General Demographics

Jack Hall is a 27-year-old machinist who had a right transfemoral amputation 4 months ago due to trauma following a motorcycle accident.

Employment/Work

Jack plans to return to his job as a machinist, which involves some welding, and enjoys playing recreational basketball.

General Health

Jack describes himself as being otherwise healthy, with no chronic illnesses

TESTS AND MEASURES

Anthropometric Characteristics

Residual limb is 10 inches (22 cm) long. Shrinkage is adequate, the circumference of the residual limb has remained stable over the past 3 weeks. Jack weighs 160 lb.

Integumentary Integrity

The scar over the medial distal end of the residual limb is well healed.

Muscle Performance/Range of Motion

Strength in upper extremities and left lower extremity is graded on manual muscle testing as 5/5; strength in the right hip is 4/5. Range of motion is within normal limits.

Gait, Locomotion, and Balance

Jack is independent in ambulation with axillary crutches for more than 500 feet on level surfaces as well as uneven terrain, stairs, and inclines. Even though Jack does not have Medicare insurance reimbursement, he would be classified Medicare level 4 (Has the ability or potential for prosthetic ambulation that exceeds basic ambulation skills, exhibiting high impact, stress, or energy levels. Typical of the prosthetic demands of the child, active adult, or athlete).

a. **Which socket would you recommend? Why?**
b. **Which suspension would you recommend? Why?**
c. **Which knee assembly would you recommend? Why?**
d. **Which foot–ankle assembly would you recommend? Why?**

a. Jack Hall would benefit from either a quadrilateral or ischial-containment socket. Quadrilateral sockets are most successful on long, firm residual limbs with firm adductor musculature; ischial-containment sockets are more successful on short, fleshy residual limbs and are better suited for high activity sports participation. Since Jack has good strength and is young, a quadrilateral socket may be most indicated. An exoskeletal or endoskeletal titanium prosthesis without soft cover is needed because his occupation involves welding.

b. Since Jack is a young, active individual, traditional suction suspension is most indicated.

c. An active individual like Jack would benefit from a hydraulic unit, typically one that will give both stance and swing- phase control such as a Mauch SNS unit. The Total Knee polycentric axis is another option and would be lighter in weight than the Mauch SNS.

d. Any type of dynamic-response foot would be appropriate considering Jack's age and activity level. Considering this individual's young age, work, and recreational activities, a Flex Foot may be most indicated. The Flex Foot would permit vertical leaps.

C A S E   2

PATIENT/CLIENT HISTORY

General Demographics

Paula Rellinger is a 47-year-old who had a right transfemoral amputation 5 months secondary to a distal thigh soft tissue sarcoma. Unfortunately, even with radiation, her prognosis is poor, a life expectancy of less than 1 year. Paula lives with her husband and two children. She desires to be as independent as possible.

Employment/Work

Paula works as a book publisher and plans to continue to work at home by corresponding with her clients via computer.

TESTS AND MEASURES

Anthropometric Characteristics

Her residual limb is 5 inches (11 cm) long, shrinkage has been minimal due to the sarcoma and difficulty in obtaining a suitable shrinker. She weighs 105 lb.

Integumentary Integrity

The residual limb scar is well healed.

Muscle Performance/Range of Motion

Strength in upper extremities and left lower extremity is graded on manual muscle testing as 4/5, strength in the right hip is 3/5. Range of motion is within normal limits.

Gait, Locomotion, and Balance

Paula is independent in ambulation with a walker for 50 feet on level surfaces. She is unable to navigate uneven terrain, stairs, and inclines. Even though Paula does not have Medicare insurance reimbursement, she would be classified Medicare level 2 (Has the ability or potential for ambulation with the ability to transverse low level environmental barriers such as curbs, stairs, or uneven surfaces. The limited community ambulator is an example of this level).

a. Which socket would you recommend? Why?
b. Which suspension would you recommend? Why?
c. Which knee assembly would you recommend? Why?
d. Which foot–ankle assembly would you recommend? Why?

a. Due to the short residual limb, an ischial-containment socket with a flexible inner liner and rigid outer frame is advised. Titanium components in an endoskeletal prosthesis should be used because of their light weight advantage.

b. A roll-on silicone suction suspension with auxiliary suspension of a TES or Silesian belt is recommended for Paula. This suspension would be easier to apply than regular suction.

c. Considering her prognosis, a polycentric-axis knee would allow household and limited community ambulation. In addition, an individual with weak hip extensors and a consistent cadence would benefit from a polycentric-axis knee.

d. A SACH foot would allow household and limited community ambulation.

CASE 3

PATIENT/CLIENT HISTORY

General Demographics

Leona Hamilton is a 62-year-old who lives in a rural, small, two-story home. Her bedroom and bath are on the second floor. She has a history of obesity and underwent a left transfemoral amputation 3 months ago because of an infected total knee.

Employment/Work/Recreation

Leona is retired but plays competitive bridge 3 days a week. She also watches her grandchildren for 2 hours after school. She drives independently.

General Health

She describes herself as being otherwise healthy. She has worn a conventional ankle–foot orthosis (AFO) on her right foot because of a peripheral nerve injury encountered many years ago.

TESTS AND MEASURES

Anthropometric Characteristics

Her residual limb is 8 inches (17.6 cm) long, is edematous, and has a bulbous appearance due to an improperly fit shrinker and her inability to wrap the residual limb on her own. She weighs 260 lb.

Integumentary Integrity

The scar over the distal end of the residual limb is well healed.

Muscle Performance/Range of Motion

Strength in upper extremities and right lower extremity is graded on manual muscle testing as 5/5, strength in the left hip is 4/5. Range of motion is within normal limits.

Gait, Locomotion, and Balance

Leona ambulates with forearm crutches 100 feet independently on level and uneven surfaces. According to Medicare insurance reimbursement, she would be classified Medicare level 2.

a. Which socket would you recommend? Why?
b. Which suspension would you recommend? Why?
c. Which knee assembly would you recommend? Why?
d. Which foot–ankle assembly would you recommend? Why?

a. Because of the edematous residual limb, an ischial-containment socket would be best. Stainless-steel components in an endoskeletal prosthesis must be used since she weighs more than 225 pounds.

b. Because of her weight and living alone, a roll-on silicone liner suction suspension may be the easiest to apply. If rotation between the residual limb and the socket occurs, an auxiliary suspension such as a TES or Silesian may be indicated.

c. A polycentric-axis knee, such as a Total Knee, will give her stance control and will be approved under Medicare. She will need the stance-control support on stairs and uneven terrain. Polycentric knees are indicated for individuals who walk at the same speed and need greater toe clearance at midswing.

3d. A SACH foot with a dense heel for her increased weight is indicated

Gait Analysis of an Individual with a Transfemoral Amputation

It is helpful when analyzing gait to divide the gait cycle into various phases and analyze from above to below or below to above eg. the posi-

tion of foot, shank, knee, hip, pelvis, and trunk. Table 9-3 contains gait deviations that are commonly seen with the use of a transfemoral prosthesis, when they occur in the gait cycle, characteristics, and prosthetic and musculoskeletal causes.[2, 7, 14] Phases of the gait cycle and the biomechanical reasons of these gait deviations were reviewed in Chapter 5 on Biomechanics.

Gait Analysis Problems

Guidelines for analyzing gait problems are presented in Chapter 8 on transtibial components. Three cases involving gait deficiencies of individuals with transfemoral prostheses are as follows.

C A S E   1

The following deficiencies were found on initial examination of a patient with a right transfemoral prosthesis on an adjustable leg with a quadrilateral socket, traditional suction with TES suspension, polycentric knee axis, and Carbon Copy II foot–ankle assembly. This patient has had a 30-lb weight loss, resulting in a smaller residual limb.

a. Adductor longus tendon 3/4 inch back along the medial wall of the socket
b. Prosthesis is 1/2 inch short
c. Lateral bending of trunk to prosthetic side during stance
d. Medial whip during swing
e. Patient feels a falling sensation and premature knee flexion during stance

As a physical therapist, which of these deficiencies can you correct?

All of these deficiencies may be caused by the prosthesis being applied incorrectly. The prosthesis may have been put on with too much external rotation of the prosthetic socket.

a. The adductor longus tendon should fit into the anterior medial groove of the quadrilateral

Table 9-3. Common Gait Deviations Associated with a Transfemoral Prosthesis

Problem	Gait Cycle	Characteristics	Prosthetic Causes	Musculoskeletal Causes
Lateral bending of trunk (Fig. 9-17)	Initial contact to midstance	Excessive bending occurs laterally away from the midline, generally to the prosthetic side	Prosthesis may be too short An improperly shaped lateral wall, especially with a quadrilateral socket, may fail to provide adequate support for the femur A high medial wall may result in leaning away to minimize discomfort A prosthesis aligned in abduction may cause a wide-base gait, resulting in this deviation Lateral distal residual limb pain due to a poor prosthetic fit	Inadequate balance Hip abduction contracture Sensitive and painful residual limb A short residual limb may fail to provide a sufficient lever arm for the pelvis Habit pattern Weak hip abductors may cause a compensated Trendelenberg gait so the torso does not fall to the sound side
Abducted gait (Fig. 9-18)	Stance phase, during double support	There is a wide-base gait with the prosthesis held away from the midline at all times	Prosthesis may be too long Shank aligned in a valgus position in relation to the socket A high medial wall may cause the prosthesis to be held in abduction to avoid pubic ramus pressure	Hip abduction contracture Habit pattern due to insecurity

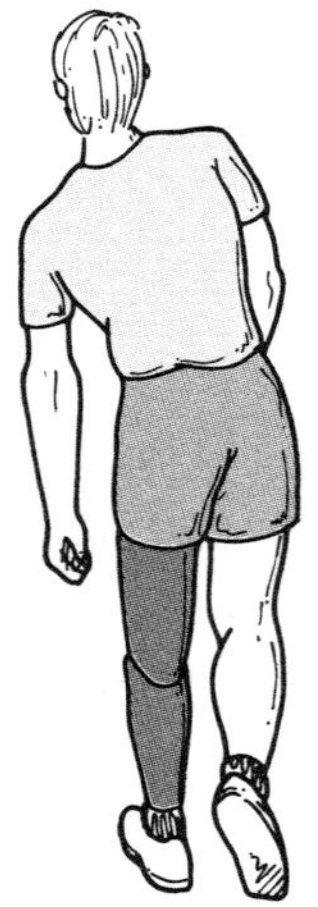

Figure 9-17. Lateral bending of the trunk.

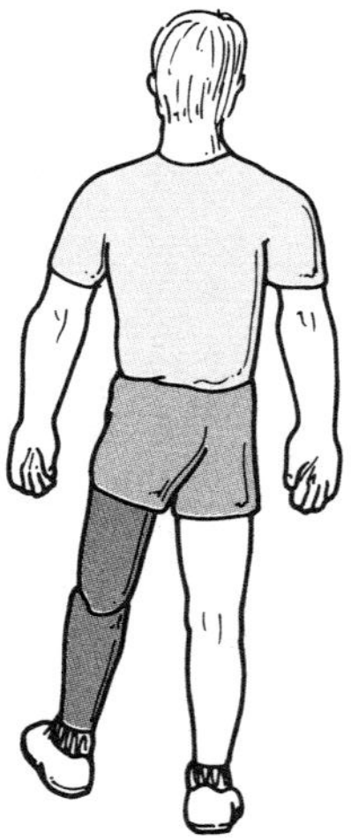

Figure 9-18. Abducted gait.

Deviation	Phase	Description	Prosthetic causes	Patient causes
Circumducted gait (Fig. 9-19)	Through swing phase	The prosthesis swings laterally in a wide area during swing phase	Prosthesis may be too long because the prosthetic foot is in too much plantarflexion or socket is too small Prosthesis may have too much alignment stability or friction in the knee, making it difficult to bend the knee in swing phase Loose suspension causing pistoning of the prosthesis	Hip abduction contracture Habit pattern due to insecurity and fear of stubbing toe Residual limb discomfort
Vaulting (Fig. 9-20)	Through swing phase	Excessive plantarflexion of the sound ankle and raising the entire body vertically permits the prosthesis to swing through	Prosthesis may be too long because prosthetic foot is in too much plantarflexion or socket is too small Prosthesis may have too much alignment stability or friction in the knee, making it difficult to bend the knee in swing phase Loose suspension causing pistoning Prosthetic foot may be in too much plantarflexion	Habit pattern due to insecurity
Rotation of the prosthetic foot on initial contact	At initial contact of stance phase (heel rocker)	Prosthetic foot externally rotates on initial contact	Too much resistance to plantarflexion Too much toe-out may have been built into the prosthesis (5–7° is normal) Socket fits too loosely	Short, fleshy limb with poor muscle tone

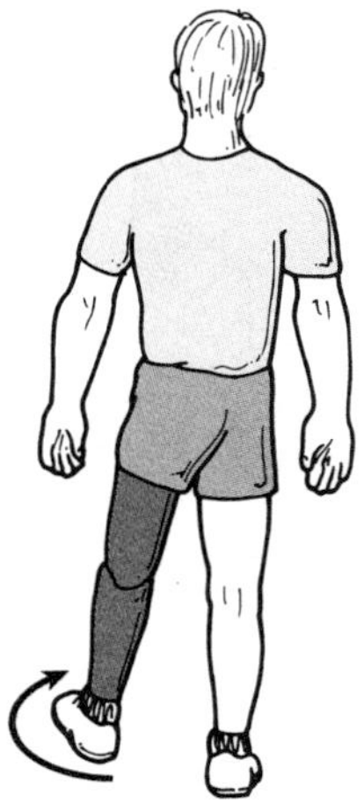

Figure 9-19. Circumducted gait.

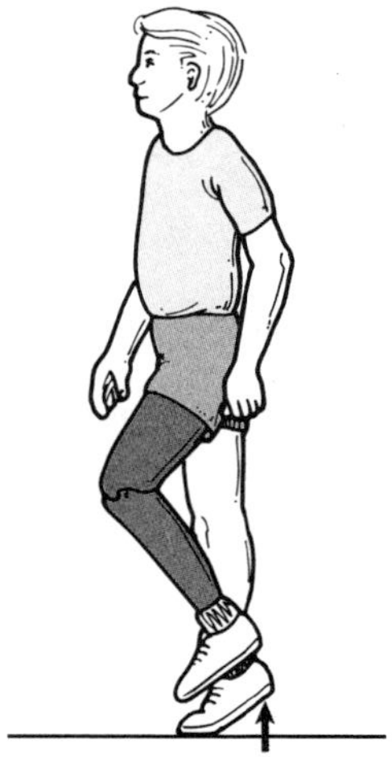

Figure 9-20. Vaulting.

(continued)

Table 9-3. Common Gait Deviations Associated with a Transfemoral Prosthesis *(Continued)*

Problem	Gait Cycle	Characteristics	Prosthetic Causes	Musculoskeletal Causes
Uneven arm swing	Throughout the gait cycle	Arm on the prosthetic side is held close to the body	Inadequate suspension	Poor balance Habit pattern due to insecurity
Uneven timing	Stance phase, during double support	The length of the step taken with the prosthesis is different (usually shorter) than that with the sound leg	Insufficient friction can cause excessive heel rise, resulting in a longer prosthetic step length than sound-leg step length Hip flexion contracture or insufficient socket flexion causes decreased hip extension, which results in a shorter step on the sound side	Habit pattern due to pain or insecurity Lack of pelvic rotation
Excessive heel rise (Fig. 9-21)	Beginning of swing phase	Prosthetic heel rises more than the sound heel	Knee joint has insufficient friction Inadequate extension aid	Forceful hip flexion to ensure knee extension at initial contact
Terminal impact (Fig. 9-22)	At the end of swing to initial contact	A sudden and audible stop as the prosthetic knee extends	Knee joint has insufficient friction Too strong an extension aid	Fear of prosthetic knee buckling causes excessive hip movement to lock the knee

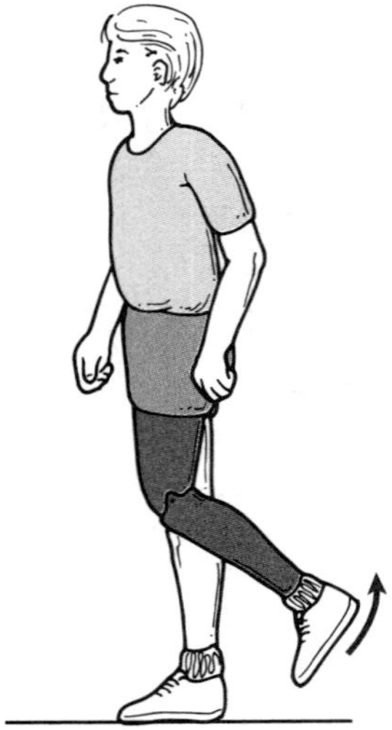

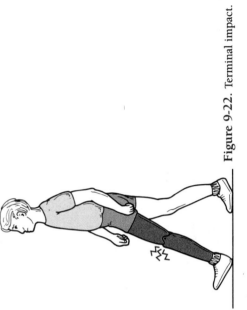

Figure 9-21. Excessive heel rise.

Figure 9-22. Terminal impact.

Instability of the knee (Fig. 9-23)	Initial contact to midstance (heel to ankle rocker)	Knee buckles during early stance phase	Knee joint may be too far ahead of the TKA line (TKA line is reviewed in Chapter 5 on biomechanics) Insufficient initial flexion may have been built into the socket Heel on shoe may be too high causing the knee joint to be too far ahead of the TKA line Plantarflexion resistance in the prosthetic foot may be too great at initial contact Malfunctioning stance-control knee unit	Hip extensor weakness Severe hip flexion contracture may cause instability Lack of gait training

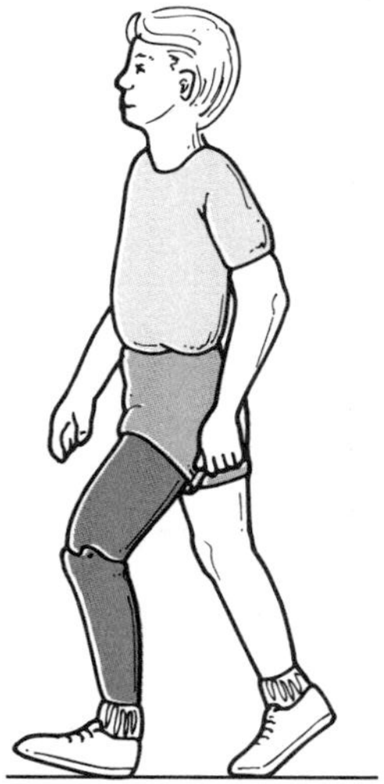

Figure 9-23. Instability of the knee.

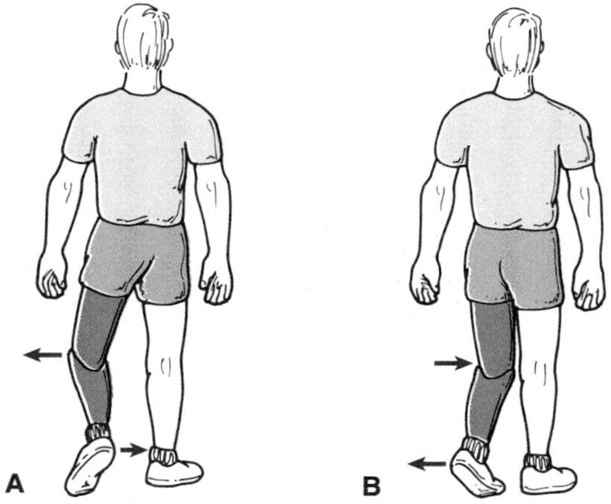

Figure 9-24. A. Medial whip B. Lateral whip.

Medial or lateral whips (Fig. 9-24)	During swing phase	A medial whip is present when the heel travels medially at the beginning of swing phase, almost hitting the sound malleolus; a lateral whip is just the opposite	Medial whips may result from excessive lateral rotation of the knee; lateral whips from excessive training medial rotation of the knee Socket may be too small or too large causing residual limb rotation	Prosthesis improperly applied, causing rotation

Table 9-3. Common Gait Deviations Associated with a Transfemoral Prosthesis *(Continued)*

Problem	Gait Cycle	Characteristics	Prosthetic Causes	Musculoskeletal Causes
Foot-slap (Fig. 9-25)	Initial contact to weight acceptance (heel rocker)	There is rapid descent of the front of the prosthetic foot often striking the floor with a slapping sound	Plantarflexion resistance inadequate	None
Drop-off at the end of stance phase (Fig. 9-26)	Terminal stance to preswing (forefoot rocker)	There is a downward movement of the trunk as the body moves forward over the prosthesis	Dorsiflexion resistance is inadequate The keel of the prosthetic foot may be too short or the toe break too far posterior The foot may be too posterior in relation to the socket	None
Excessive trunk extension (Fig. 9-27)	During stance, especially terminal stance to preswing	The lumbar lordosis is exaggerated, and the trunk is carried backward	Insufficient socket flexion Insufficient support from the anterior wall of the socket	Hip flexor tightness Weak hip extensors causing a posterior lean to get the center of gravity behind the hip joint Weak abdominals causing an anterior pelvic tilt and a compensatory posterior trunk lean

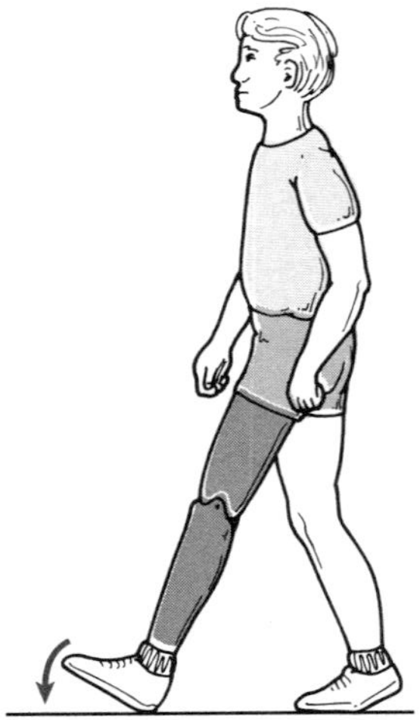

Figure 9-25. Foot slap.

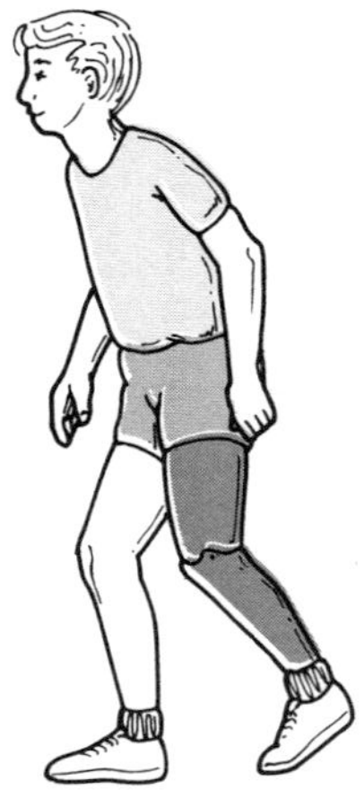

Figure 9-26. Drop-off at the end of stance phase.

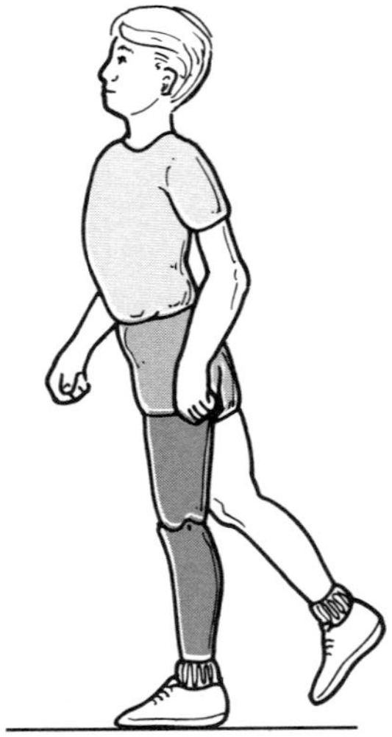

Figure 9-27. Excessive trunk extension.

socket as explained in the examination (check-out) procedure.

b. The prosthesis is too short compared with the sound extremity, possibly because the prosthesis was put on in too much external rotation. As a result, the wearer is falling into the quadrilateral socket.

c. Lateral bending of the trunk toward the prosthetic side may be due to a shortened prosthesis caused by improper application of the prosthesis.

d. A medial whip in which the prosthetic foot swings inward to almost touch the malleolus on the sound leg may also be caused by improper donning of the prosthesis.

e. The patient feels a falling sensation and premature knee flexion during stance because of the external rotation of the socket. The excessive external rotation causes the weight line to fall medial to the foot, resulting in knee instability

As a physical therapist, you could correct all of these problems by ensuring proper prosthesis application.

CASE 2

The following deficiencies were found on initial evaluation of a patient with a right transfemoral prosthesis on an adjustable leg with a quadrilateral socket, pelvic band suspension, hydraulic knee assembly, and SACH foot:

a. Ischial tuberosity slips inside ischial seat
b. Pain over the perineum on weight bearing
c. Prosthesis is $1/2$ inch short, compared with the sound limb
d. Abducted gait

As a physical therapist, which of these deficiencies can you correct?

a. Determining correct placement of the ischial tuberosity on the posterior shelf of a quadrilateral socket is reviewed in number 2 of the examination (checkout) procedure. The ischial tuberosity slipping off the ischial seat occurs commonly, since the residual limb will shrink with ambulation and exercise, causing the socket to become too large. The individual, when wearing a pelvic band suspension, can simply add more plies of socks. A general rule is that the individual can use up to 15 plies of socks. More than this is too bulky and promotes heat buildup. If the individual needs more than 15 plies, a prosthetist will often add a foam liner to the inside of the socket.[8]

b. Pain in the perineum can be caused by the residual limb slipping inside the quadrilateral socket.

c. Since the residual limb is slipping inside the socket, the prosthesis becomes shorter than the sound extremity

d. As a result of too much proximal medial pressure, the individual abducts the prosthesis to avoid weight bearing over this sensitive area.

In summary, all of these deficiencies are caused by the quadrilateral socket being too large, resulting in the residual limb slipping inside the socket. As a physical therapist, you could correct all of these problems by adding additional socks.

CASE 3

The following deficiencies were found on initial examination of a patient with a left transfemoral prosthesis on an adjustable leg with an ischial-containment socket, roll-on silicone liner suction suspension, stance-control knee, and SACH foot:

a. Terminal impact
b. Left prosthetic heel rises more than the right
c. Ischial tuberosity is inside the socket

As a physical therapist which of these deficiencies can you correct?

a and **b** may be corrected by increasing the friction in the knee. Too little friction results in terminal impact or a banging noise as the individual extends the knee from midswing to initial contact. Too little friction also results in excessive heel rise.

c. The ischial tuberosity should be inside the ischial-containment socket.

The prosthetist would most likely correct problems **a** and **b.**

KEY POINTS

- The single and the polycentric are two types of knee axes that are commonly used.
- There are three types of friction that are commonly used: mechanical, pneumatic, and hydraulic.
- Braking or locking mechanisms may exist in mechanical friction, pneumatic, or hydraulic units.
- Microprocessor units have a computer to assist knee resistance, allowing a wide range of gait speeds.
- Two types of sockets used with transfemoral amputations include the quadrilateral and the ischial-containment socket. The ischial-containment socket has wider anteroposterior, and narrower mediolateral, dimensions than the quadrilateral socket.
- The most common types of suspensions include suction, hypobaric, soft belts, and pelvic belts.
- An examination (checkout) procedure is a systematic method of examining the individual with an amputation and the prosthesis.

CRITICAL THINKING QUESTIONS

1. Working with a group of your classmates, differentiate the types of prosthetic knees, sockets, and suspensions. Indicate what type of patient may be a candidate for each.

2. Characterize which knees, according to Medicare reimbursement guidelines, would be approved for a household ambulator, for a limited community ambulator, for a community ambulator, and for a child, active adult, or athlete.

3. Review the prosthetic prescription cases. Which other prosthetic components could be used for these cases?

4. Review the gait analysis cases. What other causes could exist for these gait deviations?

5. Refer to case 2 in the Appendix for a comprehensive case in the *Guide to Physical Therapist Practice* format.

REFERENCES

1. American Physical Therapy Association. (2001). A guide to physical therapist practice. *Physical Therapy, 81.*
2. Michael, J. W. (1988). Component selection criteria: Lower limb disarticulations. *Clinics in Prosthetics and Orthotics, 12,* 99–108.
3. Michael, J. W. (1999). Modern prosthetic knee mechanisms. *Clinical Orthopaedics and Related Research, 361,* 39–47.
4. Bowker, J. H., & Michael, J. W. (1992). *Atlas of limb prosthetics.* St Louis: Mosby Year Book.
5. Whitesides, T. E., Jr., & Volatile, T. B. (1985). Mauch SNS hydraulic knee units in above knee amputees. A long term follow-up study. *Clinical Orthopaedics and Related Research, 194,* 264–268.
6. Erback, J. R. (1963). Hydraulic prostheses for above knee amputees. *Journal of the American Physical Therapy Association, 43,* 105–110.
7. Anon. (1990). *Lower limb prosthetics.* New York: Prosthetic Orthotic Publications.
8. Anon. (1977). *Beginning prosthetic training for the above knee amputee.* Chicago: Rehabilitation Institute of Chicago.
9. Shurr, D. G., & Cook, T. M. (1990). *Prosthetics & orthotics.* Norwalk, CT: Appleton & Lange.
10. Pritham, C. H. (1990). Biomechanics and shape of the above knee socket considered in light of the ischial containment concept. *Prosthetics Orthotics International, 14,* 9–21.
11. Schuch, C. M., & Pritham, C. H. (1999). Current transfemoral sockets. *Clinical Orthopaedics and Related Research, 361,* 48–54.
12. Flandry, F., Beskin, J., Chambers, R. B., et al. (1989). The effect of the CAT-CAM above knee prosthesis on functional rehabilitation. *Clinical Orthopaedics and Related Research, 239,* 249–262.
13. Gailey, R. S., Lawrence, D., Burditt, C., Spyropoulos, P., Newell, C., & Nash, M. S. (1993). The CAT-CAM socket and quadrilateral socket: A comparison of energy cost during ambulation. *Prosthetics Orthotics International, 17,* 95–100.

14. Gottschalk, F., Kourosh, S., Stills, M., McClellan, B., & Roberts, J. (1989). Does socket configuration influence the position of the femur in above-knee amputation? *Journal Prosthetics Orthotics 2*, 94–102.

15. Kapp, S. (1999). Suspension systems for prostheses. *Clinical Orthopaedics and Related Research, 361*, 55–62.

16. Trieb, K., Lang, T., Stulnig, T., & Kickinger, W. (1999). Silicone soft socket system: Its effect on the rehabilitation of geriatric amputees with transfemoral amputations. *Archives of Physical Medicine and Rehabilitation, 80*, 522–525.

17. Yack, H. J., Nielsen, D. H., & Shurr, D. G. (1999). Kinetic patterns during stair ascent in patients with transtibial amputations using three different prostheses. *Journal of Prosthetics and Orthotics, 11*, 57–62.

18. Toburn, L., Schweiger, G. P., Perry, J., & Powers, C. M. (1994). Below knee amputee gait in stair ambulation. A comparison of stride characteristics using five different prosthetic feet. *Clinical Orthopaedics and Related Research, 303*, 185–192.

19. Marshall Labs LTD. (1996, February). Reference for prosthetic prescription.

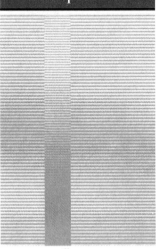

Chapter 10

THE PATIENT WITH A BILATERAL AMPUTATION—CLINICAL DECISION MAKING

Objectives

1. Describe the causes and functional outcomes associated with bilateral amputations
2. Describe interventions including exercises and functional activities that are appropriate for an individual with a bilateral lower limb amputation
3. Differentiate among the type of sockets and suspensions that are often used with an individual with bilateral lower limb amputation

This chapter is divided into the following sections:

This chapter consists of information concerning the physical therapy examination, evaluation, and intervention for patients with bilateral amputations. The *Guide to Physical Therapist Practice* in the practice pattern "Impaired Motor Function, Muscle Performance, Range of Motion, Gait, Locomotion, and Balance Associated with Amputation" (4J) refers to interventions with prosthetic devices.[1] Regional differences and philosophies may alter the prosthetic components that are recommended. This chapter is not intended to be an inclusive list but representative of commonly used components for bilateral amputations.

Fortunately, the number of bilateral amputations is lower than the number of unilateral transtibial or transfemoral amputations. However, bilateral amputations are becoming more frequent because of an aging population with diabetes and peripheral vascular disease (PVD). Of those individuals with a single amputation due to PVD, 30% will have another amputation within 3 years.[2]

♦ ♦ ♦

Characteristics of Bilateral Amputations

Bilateral amputation may be of the same level such as foot, ankle, transtibial, knee disarticulation, transfemoral, and hip disarticulation, or any combination of these. Retention of maximum limb length by amputation at the distal, most suitable level is particularly important. If the patient has been previously trained with a prosthesis for the first amputation, the success rate of successful prosthetic ambulation is improved. Rapid prosthetic rehabilitation ensures the best results in returning to an independent lifestyle.

Prosthetic candidates should be able to transfer independently, otherwise they are unlikely to use a prosthesis. Individuals with bilateral amputations require good trunk and upper body strength, sense of balance, and muscle control for successful prosthetic use. Weight bearing has physiologic advantages, including increased bone density and prevention of complications such as pneumonia or urinary stasis. The advantage of weight bearing was illustrated in a radiographic study of the hips of 20 non–weight-bearing individuals with either amputation or femoral nonunion that showed joint space narrowing of 10–30%.[3] Therefore, to avoid narrowing of the hip joint space, if possible, individuals with bilateral amputation should weight bear through the lower extremities.

Most individuals with bilateral transtibial amputations become functional ambulators with prostheses. However, energy and balance requirements prevent many patients with bilateral transfemoral amputations from successful prosthetic ambulation except the very young. Some patients with bilateral transfemoral amputations find it easier to move around the house on their knees, buttocks, or ends of residual limbs. These individuals may benefit from use of heavy foam knee pads to prevent skin breakdown.[4] A view of the elderly patient with bilateral lower extremity amputation is contained in the Geriatric Perspective Box.

GERIATRIC PERSPECTIVE

In a retrospective study of 18 elderly patients (mean age, 65.9 years) who underwent bilateral lower-extremity amputation, the most frequent reason for rejection of prosthetic rehabilitation immediately after amputation of the second leg was poor endurance. This poor endurance was associated with congestive heart failure or neurologic or joint disorders.[5] Deciding which prosthetic components to prescribe and the type of rehabilitation for the elderly patient with bilateral amputations is difficult. Age alone is not a factor in success or failure of prosthetic rehabilitation. Careful evaluation by a multidisciplinary team is paramount for the correct intervention decision and successful rehabilitation.

Use of Prostheses

The physical and psychologic adaptation of individuals with bilateral amputations and the use of prostheses have been investigated in numerous studies.[5] Successful use of prostheses has been found in two studies done in the United States and one done in India. High indexes of life satisfaction were found in a study from the Netherlands.

A long-term follow-up study of 30 individuals in the United States with bilateral transfemoral amputations from the Vietnam War found that 22% still used their prostheses for walking an average of 7.7 hours per day. An additional 43%, although not using their prostheses at the time of the study, reported using their prostheses after military discharge, with an average prosthesis use of 12.9 years (range, 0.5–29 years). The use of a wheelchair as the primary means of moving from one place to another was reported by 78% of the respondents. Seventy percent were or had been employed outside the home. Ninety-one percent were married, and 87% had children. As expected, the physical functional score on the Short Form-36 (SF-36) Health Survey showed significantly lower physical functioning scores for the amputation group than for a group of age- and gender-matched controls. However, no significant differences were detected between the groups with regard to physical role functioning, bodily pain, general health, vitality, social functioning, emotional role functioning, or mental health. This study concluded that contrary to the portrayal in the popular media, respondents with bilateral transfemoral amputations have led relatively normal, productive lives within the context of their physical limitations.[6]

A United States study of 61 individuals (mean age. 61.5 years) with bilateral lower limb amputations investigated ambulation ability and length of rehabilitation center stay.[7] Most of the patients at the time of discharge, with the exception of those with bilateral transfemoral amputations, achieved a level of limited household walking (use of a prosthesis only in the home to ambulate independently at a distance less than 37 m or 120 feet and independent performance of all activities of daily living (ADLs)). A significant improvement in ambulation ability was noted for all patients 3 months after discharge. Some 82% of the individuals with bilateral transtibial and 50% of the transfemoral/transtibial amputations achieved a household ambulation level (use of a prosthesis to ambulate more than 37 m or 120 feet and independent performance of all ADLs). Ten percent of the patients used a wheelchair for full-time mobility. This study found that the average length of rehabilitation center stay for all levels of amputation was 24.2 days.[7]

An investigation of 41 patients in India showed that individuals with bilateral transtibial amputations did well with prosthetic mobility (not defined), but those with bilateral transfemoral amputations had mostly abandoned

their prostheses at a minimum 21-month follow-up survey.[8]

Life satisfaction indexes were studied in a group of 31 individuals with bilateral lower limb amputations in the Netherlands. A follow-up survey ranged from 2 to 12 years after the second amputation. Mean age at second amputation was 66.3 years. Despite high levels of impairment for ambulation, work, and home management, the Life Satisfaction Questionnaire demonstrated that respondents were rather satisfied to very satisfied with life. Only two individuals used their prosthesis at the time of follow up.[9] Thus, this study showed that life satisfaction and functioning is not necessarily proportional to the use of prostheses.

Interventions

Preprosthetic management involves intensive strengthening of the upper and lower extremities. Individuals with bilateral amputations spend considerable time sitting and are therefore more prone to develop hip flexion contractures. If possible, these individuals should sleep prone or at least spend some time during the day in the prone position. In addition, hip-extension flexibility exercises, in either the prone or side-lying position, should be stressed. Balance activities, such as weight shifting, playing ball, rotation in sitting and, if possible, kneeling are also important aspects of preprosthetic rehabilitation.[10] Residual lower extremity and upper extremity resistive exercises may be performed using isometric, isotonic, proprioceptive neuromuscular facilitation (PNF), or isokinetic techniques as described in Chapter 7.

Individuals with bilateral amputations who will not be functional ambulators should be taught basic mobility and advanced wheelchair skills similar to those taught to individuals with paraplegia. Basic mobility skills may include how to move in bed avoiding shear forces on the skin, rolling, coming to sit, weight shifts and scooting in sitting, transfers, and wheelchair propulsion. Advanced wheelchair skills may include independent wheelchair propulsion on level and uneven surfaces and navigation in tight spaces.

Prosthetic Components

The immediate postoperative prosthesis (IPOP) may be an excellent choice with traumatic amputations in younger individuals. Prosthetic components for the individual with bilateral amputations often differ from those used for individuals with a unilateral amputation.

Transtibial Components

Individuals with bilateral transtibial amputations are often fit with patellar tendon bearing (PTB) sockets with supracondylar cuff suspension or a total surface bearing (TSB) socket with roll-on silicone liner suction suspension. Often wider feet, which will increase medial lateral stability, and two feet of the same style are needed.[11] Bilateral endoskeletal prostheses rather than exoskeletal prostheses are common with both transfemoral and transtibial amputations, because of lighter weight, more easily interchanged components, and better cosmetic appearance.

Transfemoral Components

With a bilateral transfemoral amputation, some advocate shorter prosthetic legs measuring 2–3 inches, also called *stubbies*. Stubbies allow the center of gravity to be close to the base of support. This advantage makes stubbies a good introductory prosthesis as an interim step to full-length prostheses. They consist of rocker bottoms modified to prevent backward falls and have no articulated knee joints (Fig. 10-1). Stubbies require much less energy output and are less cumbersome; also, wearers have less fear of falling than with the regular full-length prostheses. Stubbies also have the

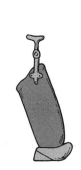
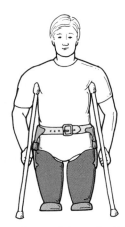

Figure 10-1. Stubbies may be used by individuals with bilateral transfemoral amputations. They are more stable than regular prostheses since the center of gravity is lowered. (Adapted from O'Sullivan, S. B., & Schmitz, T. J. (1994). *Physical rehabilitation: Assessment and treatment* (3rd ed.). Philadelphia: F. A. Davis.)

advantage of decreasing hip flexion contractures and allowing the physiologic effects of being upright. However, stubbies result in slower ambulation. One case study of a 37-year-old individual with bilateral transfemoral amputations of traumatic cause found that treadmill ambulation lasted 27% longer with stubbies than with regular transfemoral prostheses.[12] However, the acceptance of stubbies varies. This shortening of stature must be balanced with psychologic problems that may result. Some individuals like to use stubbies at home and a wheelchair outside the home.[13]

Definitive prostheses that are 2–3 inches (5–7 cm) shorter than the preamputation legs often result in improved balance by lowering the center of gravity.[11]

Many individuals with bilateral transfemoral amputations prefer ischial-containment sockets to quadrilateral sockets. Ischial-containment sockets provide enhanced stability and perineal comfort.[14] Individuals with bilateral transfemoral amputations may be able to use a wet fit or roll-on silicone liner suction suspension. This suspension is much easier to use than the traditional suction suspension and provides an excellent fit. A pelvic band suspension may also be used if suction suspension is not viable.[15] These suspensions are described in Chapter 9.

There are several prosthetic knee options indicated for individuals with bilateral transfemoral amputations. Bilateral polycentric (four-bar linkage) knees offer maximum stance-phase stability. This knee has the advantage of shortening during swing phase, thus helping to improve toe clearance. Bilateral hydraulic knees may be ideal for optimal efficiency, but the cost is higher.

It would be impossible for a transfemoral amputee to unload both artificial knees simultaneously; therefore, sitting with two stance-control knees is almost impossible.[16] If an individual with bilateral transfemoral amputations were to use one stance-control knee and one manual-lock knee, stair climbing would be nearly impossible. Likewise, bilateral manual-lock knees should not be used, since these result in a swing-through gait. In effect, bilateral manual-lock knees result in a gait similar to that used by an individual with paraplegia. The indications, advantages, and disadvantages of these knees are reviewed in Chapter 9.

Functional Activities

For an individual with bilateral amputation, functional activities may consist of dressing, transfers, ambulation, and wheelchair use.

Dressing Activities

Individuals with bilateral lower-extremity amputations may require clothing adaptations such as Velcro closures or a reaching device. Individuals with bilateral amputations should master rolling to pull trousers up over their hips. The prosthesis should be dressed first, since it is very difficult to first put on the prosthesis and then put on trousers. Bilateral prostheses may be applied in bed or, if the patient

uses a wheelchair, may be applied from the wheelchair. Applying bilateral prostheses is similar to applying a unilateral transtibial or transfemoral prosthesis as described in Chapters 8 and 9, respectively. Dressing activities may involve the need for occupational therapy services.

Transfers may be done directly using a front-in or back-in approach (Fig. 10-2). If good trunk stability and upper-extremity strength is present, a lateral transfer using a transfer board may be performed (Fig. 10-3).

Ambulation Activities

Many individuals with bilateral transfemoral amputations need a cane or crutch for successful ambulation, especially on unlevel surfaces. To move from a seated to a standing position, the patient with bilateral transfemoral amputations may do the following as illustrated in Figure 10-4:

1. Place one foot in front and straighten the knee (Fig. 10-4A).

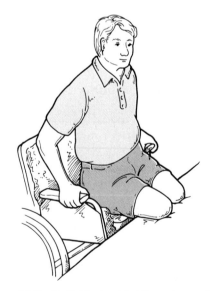

Figure 10-2. Individual with bilateral transfemoral amputations performing a backward/forward transfer.

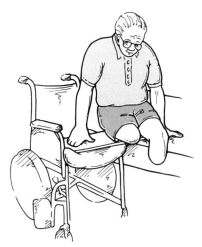

Figure 10-3. Individual with bilateral transfemoral/transtibial amputations performing a transfer board transfer

2. Twist the trunk on the seat of the chair toward the flexed knee and ease the trunk forward so that the foot of the flexed knee is in total contact with the floor (Fig. 10-4B).
3. Push up on the arms of the chair, leaning slightly toward the flexed knee.
4. Extend the hip on the side of the flexed knee as a cane or assistive device is used on the side of the extended knee (Fig. 10-4C).
5. If needed, additional support may be had with another cane (Fig. 10-4D).[2]

To sit, these steps are reversed. The patient with bilateral amputations must *not* sit at an angle grabbing only one arm rest. This maneuver may tip the chair and makes the procedure unsafe.

Stairs, Ramps, and Curbs

Ascending or descending stairs is often done with a wide arc of movement of each prosthesis and lateral trunk bending to clear the prosthesis. If one residual limb is longer than the other, such as a transtibial/transfemoral bilateral amputation, the longer residual limb should ascend the stairs first. The shorter residual limb should descend the stairs first. Railings *must* be secure and should be constantly monitored for safety. The amount of force the individual with a bilateral amputation puts on these railings may be considerable (Fig. 10-5).[2] For individuals who are more unstable, one railing may be used with the individual descending or ascending sideways. This method of stair ascent and descent requires much hip flexion to clear the prosthesis (Fig. 10-6).

Ascending and descending ramps require much trunk flexion, otherwise a backward fall may result. Consequently, ramps may be difficult for the individual with bilateral transfemoral amputations. Again, if one residual

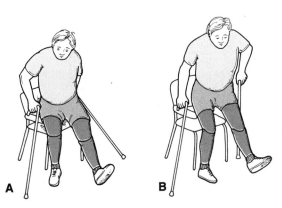
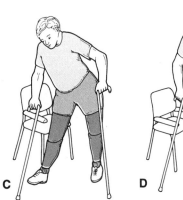
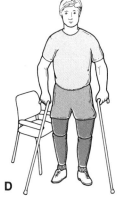

Figure 10-4. Sit to stand transfer.

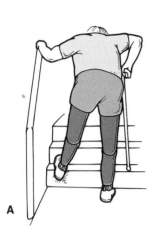

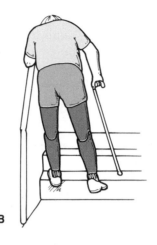

A

B

Figure 10-5. Individual with bilateral transfemoral amputations ascending stairs, front approach.

limb is longer than the other, such as a transtibial/transfemoral bilateral amputation, the longer limb should ascend the ramp first. The shorter residual limb should descend the ramp first (Fig. 10-7). A sideways or lateral ap-

proach is also an option in ascending and descending ramps.

Curbs or a small step may be approached with the curb in front as shown in Figure 10-8 or a sideways approach as shown in Figure 10-9. Both methods require much hip flexion, good balance, ability to transfer weight, and arm strength. These methods are best achieved with low curbs or steps.

Getting up from the floor requires much trunk and hip mobility as well as increased upper extremity strength. This activity is not possible for most individuals with bilateral transfemoral amputations. A method of getting up

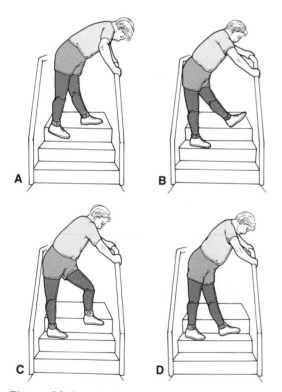

A

B

C

D

Figure 10-6. Individual with bilateral transfemoral amputations descending stairs, side approach.

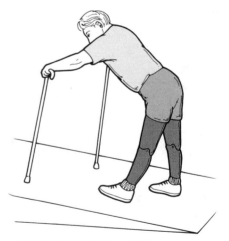

Figure 10-7. Individual with bilateral transfemoral amputations ascending a ramp, front approach.

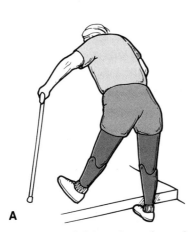 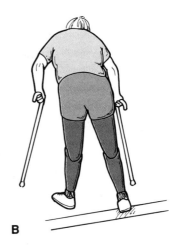

Figure 10-8. Individual with bilateral transfemoral amputations ascending a curb, front approach.

from the floor for an individual with bilateral transfemoral amputations is illustrated in Figure 10-10. Alternately, individuals with bilateral transtibial amputations may be able to get to a kneeling position, a half-kneel, and finally a standing position.

Wheelchair Use

Patients with bilateral amputations often use a specialized wheelchair, sometimes called an *amputee wheelchair.* This wheelchair has a wheel axis posterior to the center support to al-

low better balance and is illustrated in Figure 7-37. This wheelchair should also have removable armrests and swing-away legrests. An individual with bilateral transtibial prostheses should use two inserts as shown in Figure 7-4, to prevent knee flexion contractures.

Energy Requirements

Reports of extraordinary individuals who have become independent in ADLs and ambulation are found in the literature. These include a 20-year-old individual with a bilateral amputation

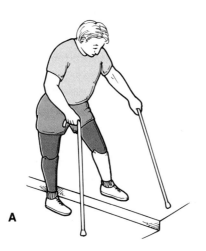 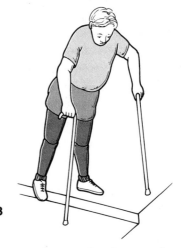

Figure 10-9. Individual with bilateral transfemoral amputations ascending a curb, side approach.

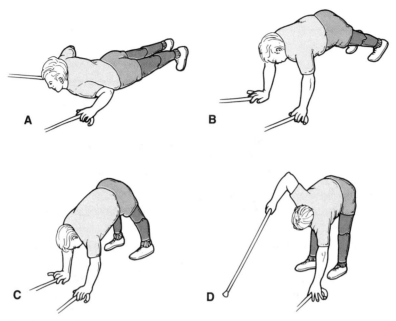

Figure 10-10. Individual with bilateral transfemoral amputations getting up from the floor.

of transfemoral and hip disarticulation and another 37- year-old individual with a transtibial, transhumeral and hip disarticulation.[16,17] These cases show that even individuals with devastating bilateral amputations can accomplish independent ADLs.

The energy requirements of ambulation for those with bilateral amputations are high. The oxygen cost of ambulation in six individuals with bilateral transtibial amputations was 123% higher than that of able-bodied, age-matched controls and 157% higher than with wheelchair propulsion.[18] The energy demands of ambulation for an individual with bilateral transfemoral amputations is 280% higher than that of unimpaired subjects.[19] As can be seen from the higher energy costs for individuals with bilateral transfemoral compared with those for individuals with bilateral transtibial amputations, the knee joint is a major determinant in energy cost of ambulation. Successful rehabilitation of an individual with a bilateral amputation requires much strength, balance, improved cardiovascular status, and determination.

KEY POINTS

- Bilateral amputations are more frequent now than in the past because of an aging population with diabetes and peripheral vascular disease.

- Retention of maximum limb length by amputation at the distal most suitable level is particularly important.

- If the patient has been previously trained with a prosthesis for the first amputation, the success rate for successful prosthetic ambulation is improved.

- Prosthetic candidates should be able to transfer independently; otherwise, they are unlikely to use a prosthesis.

- Individuals with bilateral amputations require good trunk and upper body strength, sense of balance, and muscle control to use a prosthesis successfully.

- Shorter prostheses called "stubbies" may be appropriate temporary prostheses in the early ambulation training of an individual with bilateral transfemoral amputations.

- Bilateral endoskeletal prostheses are common with both transfemoral and transtibial amputees because of their lighter weight, more-easily interchangeable components, and better cosmetic appearance.

- Ischial-containment sockets are preferred over quadrilateral sockets by many individuals with bilateral transfemoral amputations.

- Most individuals with bilateral transfemoral amputations need a cane or crutch for successful ambulation, especially on unstable surfaces.

- Successful rehabilitation of an individual with a bilateral amputation requires much strength, balance, and determination.

CRITICAL THINKING QUESTIONS

1. Using the information in Chapter 7 on exercise and functional activities, characterize positioning, flexibility, and strengthening exercises that may be appropriate for a patient with bilateral lower-extremity amputations.

2. Describe how an individual with bilateral lower-extremity amputations may attempt functional activities such as lower-extremity dressing; transfers; getting to stand; ascending and descending stairs, ramps, and curbs; and getting up from the floor.

3. Differentiate prosthetic components including feet, sockets, suspensions, and knees that would be appropriate for individuals with either bilateral transtibial or bilateral transfemoral amputations.

4. Contrast the energy expenditure of ambulation activities for individuals with either bilateral transtibial or transfemoral amputations.

REFERENCES

1. American Physical Therapy Association. (2001). A guide to physical therapist practice. *Physical Therapy, 81.*
2. Engstrom, B. & Van Deven, C. (1985). *Physiotherapy for amputees: The Roehampton approach* (p. 201). New York: Churchill Livingstone.
3. Teshima, R., Otsuka, T., & Yamamoto, K. (1992). Effects of nonweight bearing on the hip. *Clinical Orthopedics and Related Research, 279,* 149–156.
4. Pandain, G., & Kowalske, K. (1999). Daily functioning of patients with an amputated lower extremity. *Clinical Orthopedics and Related Research, 361,* 91–97.
5. Wolf, E., Linning, M., & Ferber, I. (1989). Prosthetic rehabilitation of elderly bilateral amputees. *International Journal Rehabilitation Research, 12,* 271–278.
6. Dougherty, P. J. (1999). Long-term follow-up study of bilateral above-the-knee amputees from the Vietnam War. *Journal Bone Joint Surgery Am, 81,* 1384–1390.
7. Torres, M. M., & Esquenazi, A. (1991). Bilateral lower limb amputee rehabilitation. A retrospective review. *Western Journal of Medicine, 154,* 583–586.
8. Datta, D., Nair, P. N., & Payne, J. (1992). Outcome of prosthetic management of bilateral lower-limb amputees. *Disability and Rehabilitation, 14,* 98–102.
9. DeFretes, A., Boonstra, A. M., & Vos, L. D. W. (1994). Functional outcome of rehabilitated bilateral lower limb amputees. *Prosthetics and Orthotics International, 18,* 18–24.
10. Gailey, R. S., & Gailey, A. M. (1994). *Stretching and strengthening for lower extremity amputees.* Miami: Advanced Rehabilitation Therapy.
11. Berger, N., & Fishman, S. (1998). *Lower limb prosthetics.* New York: Prosthetic Orthotic Publications.
12. Crouse, S. F., Lessard, C. S., Rhodes, J., & Lowe, R. C. (1990). Oxygen consumption and cardiac response of short leg and long leg prosthetic ambulation in a patient with bilateral above knee amputation: Comparisons with able bodied men. *Archives of Physical Medicine and Rehabilitation, 71,* 313–317.
13. O'Sullivan, S. B., & Schmitz, T. J. (1994). *Physical rehabilitation: Assessment and treatment* (3rd ed.). Philadelphia: F. A. Davis.

14. Michel, J. W. (1999). Modern prosthetic knee mechanisms. *Clinical Orthopedics and Related Research, 361,* 39–47.

15. Bowker, J. H., & Michael, J. W. (1992). *Atlas of limb prosthetics.* St Louis: Mosby Year Book.

16. Dunlap, S. W. (1969). Bilateral amputation: Above knee and hip disarticulation. *Physical Therapy, 49,* 500–502.

17. Shin, J. C., Park, C. I., Kim, Y. C., Jang, S. H., Bang, I. K., & Shin, J. S. (1998). Rehabilitation of a triple amputee including a hip disarticulation. *Prosthetics and Orthotics International, 22,* 251–253.

18. Dubow, L. L., Witt, P. L., Kadaba, M. P., Reyes, R., & Cochran, G. V. (1983). Oxygen consumption of elderly persons with bilateral below knee amputations: Ambulation vs wheelchair propulsion. *Archives of Physical Medicine and Rehabilitation, 64,* 255–259.

19. Huang, C. T., Jackson, J. R., Moore, N. B., Fine, P. R., Kuhlemeier, K. V., Truahg, G. H., & Saunders, P. T. (1979). Amputation: Energy cost of ambulation. *Archives of Physical Medicine and Rehabilitation, 60,* 18–24.

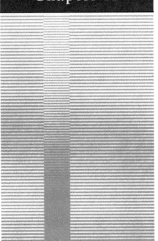

Chapter 11

THE PATIENT WITH A TRANSPELVIC/HIP DISARTICULATION AMPUTATION— CLINICAL DECISION MAKING

Objectives

1. Describe the history and etiology associated with transpelvic/hip disarticulation amputations

2. Characterize physical therapy interventions that may be used with a patient with a transpelvic/hip disarticulation amputation

3. Differentiate among components that may be used with transpelvic/hip disarticulation prostheses

4. Perform an examination (checkout) procedure on a transpelvic/hip disarticulation prosthesis

5. Demonstrate how you would instruct a patient to apply a transpelvic/hip disarticulation prosthesis

This chapter is divided into the following sections:

This chapter consists of information concerning the physical therapy examination, evaluation, and interventions for patients with transpelvic (formerly called hemipelvectomy) and hip disarticulation amputations. These amputations are fortunately rare. A physical therapist knowledgeable in the care of individuals with these amputations is critically important for the patient to attain maximum use of the prosthesis.[1]

History and Incidence of Transpelvic and Hip Disarticulation Amputations

The transpelvic amputation is a relatively recent operative technique. Sir Gordon Gordon-Taylor first developed this successful technique and reported 21 cases in Great Britain in 1946.[2] The first hip disarticulation recorded in the United States was performed in 1806 to remove a severely open, comminuted fracture in a 17-year-old boy. The procedure was done without anesthesia or antiseptic techniques. Two other accounts of hip disarticulations were described in Great Britain in 1824. Analgesia consisted of alcohol and powdered opium. These disarticulations were done with much speed to minimize blood loss. At the time, violent controversy regarding the necessity and propriety of these procedures resulted.[3]

Many transpelvic and hip disarticulation amputations are done because of malignant lower-extremity bone tumors.[4–6] One study found that the most common causes of amputation at the hip disarticulation level were tumor (48%), infection (20%), vascular disease (20%), trauma (10%), and congenital abnormalities (2%).[4] Patients undergoing hip disarticulation have a 2:1 male to female ratio.

The medical management and subsequent rehabilitation of many of these patients may be prolonged. Patients undergoing chemotherapy or radiation may become debilitated, resulting in slow wound healing. In addition, complications of infection due to altered immune status may occur. Cardiac disease or limb ischemia has great influence on postoperative mortality.[6] Infection is a common complication of these amputations. The mortality rate tripled when a hip disarticulation was performed in the presence of preoperative infection.[6] In a study of 53 patients who underwent hip disarticulation, the incidence of wound infection and necrosis was 60%. Wound infection ranged from 47% with an etiology of tumor to 83% with an etiology of ischemia. Surprisingly, age and the presence of diabetes did not influence mortality rates.[6]

Bilateral hip disarticulation has been reported in individuals with paraplegia and severe decubitus ulcers.[2] However, this procedure has been criticized for its substantial blood loss, potential for developing perineal pressure ulcers, and marked disfigurement.[6]

Interventions

Physical therapy interventions directed to the patient with a transpelvic or hip disarticulation amputation require adaptation of the flexibility, strengthening, and balance principles discussed in Chapter 7. Patients with either of these amputations need to maximize strength of the upper extremities, abdominals, and sound lower-extremity musculature. As discussed further in this chapter, patients with a hip disarticulation amputation need to perform a posterior pelvic tilt to initiate swing phase. Therefore, good abdominal control is necessary to initiate this posterior pelvic tilt. Balance training, as described in Chapter 7, is important to enable the patient to transfer independently, apply and remove the prosthesis, and ambulate safely.

Prosthetic Components

To be an effective advocate for the patient and to converse effectively with a prosthetist, the physical therapist should have a sound knowledge of transpelvic and hip disarticulation prosthetic components including sockets, hip, knee, and feet.

Sockets

The transpelvic socket encases the abdominal cavity and provides hard walls that protect and compress the abdominal viscera so these areas can accept weight-bearing pressures.[6] The transpelvic socket extends superior to the tenth rib, allowing additional vertical loading.

In the transpelvic socket, the patient's weight is transferred to the ischial tuberosity and buttock of the remaining leg.[5] The hip disarticulation socket encloses the ischial tuberosity and gluteal muscles for weight bearing and extends over the ilium to provide suspension. The socket also encases the opposite pelvis, which assists in mediolateral trunk stability. Reliefs are built into the socket for the anterior and posterior iliac spines and the spinous processes of vertebrae.

A plaster cast is often taken of the patient's pelvis as soon as 3–4 weeks after surgery. Stockinette is stretched over the patient's pelvis and iliac crests and trim lines are marked (Fig. 11-1). There is very little edema with either a transpelvic or a hip disarticulation amputation so little or no bandaging is required.[3] Commercially made shrinkers for transpelvic/hip disarticulation patients are available (Fig. 11-2). Although the transpelvic socket is larger, prosthetic components for transpelvic and hip disarticulation amputations are similar.

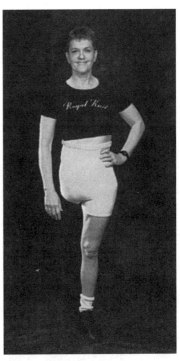

Figure 11-2. Shrinker for a transpelvic or hip disarticulation amputation. (Reprinted with permission from Royal Knit Inc.)

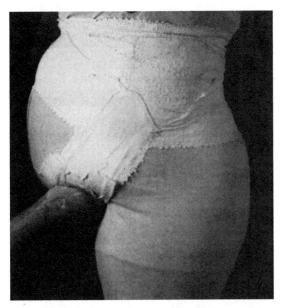

Figure 11-1. Casting for a transpelvic or hip disarticulation prosthesis. (Reprinted with permission from Jeffries, G. E. (1999). Fitting for hip disarticulation and hemipelvectomy level amputations. *InMotion, 9,* 38-45.)

The Canadian, the diagonal, and the total-contact suction socket designs are the primary three hip disarticulation prostheses in use today. The Canadian hip disarticulation prosthesis was introduced in 1954.[7] The diagonal socket, smaller than the Canadian, is suitable for short transfemoral amputations at the level of the lesser trochanter.[8] Today, an endoskeletal or modular prosthesis is preferred over the exoskeletal prosthesis because of its light weight, interchangeable adjustable features, and better cosmetic appearance (Fig. 11-3). An exoskeletal hip disarticulation prosthesis is shown in Figure 11-4. It is now more common for individuals with a transpelvic or hip disarticulation amputation to wear a total-contact suction-socket-design containment system that allows better stabilization of the prosthesis.[1]

The basket-shaped socket of the Canadian hip disarticulation prosthesis often results in discomfort and poor cosmesis, leading to prosthetic rejection by some patients. As a result, a newer total-contact suction socket

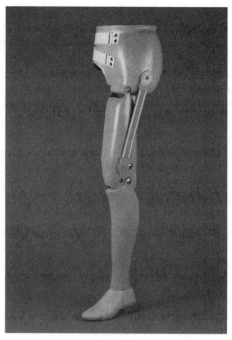

Figure 11-4. Exoskeletal hip disarticulation prosthesis. (Reprinted with permission from Otto Bock Orthopedic Industry Inc.)

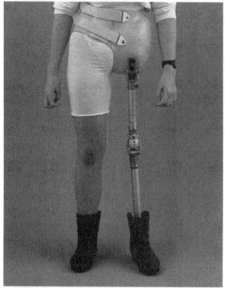

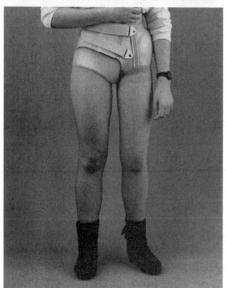

Figure 11-3. Endoskeletal hip disarticulation prosthesis (**A**) without cosmetic cover, (**B**) with cosmetic cover. (Reprinted with permission from Otto Bock Orthopedic Industry Inc.)

design has been introduced (Fig. 11-5). In one case study, two patients reported that the total-contact suction socket design, compared with the Canadian prosthesis, enhanced proprioception and significantly decreased piston action.[8]

Hip and Knee Components

The prosthetic hip joint is attached to the socket anteriorly in both the total-contact suction and Canadian hip disarticulation socket design prostheses. This anteriorly placed hip joint causes the weight line to fall behind the hip and in front of the knee to assist with extension. The anteriorly placed hip joint and weight line are shown in Figure 11-6. The hip joint can be placed directly under the transpelvic socket, since the wearer has no ischium.[1] If the prosthetic hip joint was placed under the hip disarticulation socket, sitting

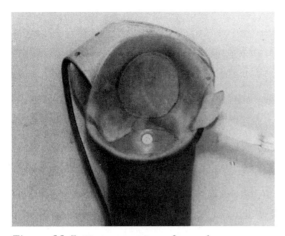

Figure 11-5. Transverse view of a total-contact suction ischial containment socket with custom-shaped pelvic belt. (Reprinted with permission from Zaffer, S. M., Braddom, R. L., Conti, A., Goff, J., & Bokma, D. (1999). Total hip disarticulation prosthesis with suction socket. Report of two cases. *American Journal of Physical Medicine and Rehabilitation, 78,* 160-162.)

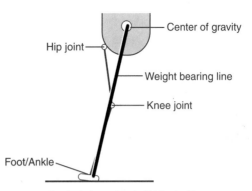

Sagittal view of an individual with a transpelvic or hip disarticulation prosthesis

Figure 11-6. Standing alignment of the hip disarticulation prosthesis *(hashed line).* (Adapted from Berger, N., & Fishman, S. (1998). *Lower limb prosthetics.* New York: Prosthetic Orthotic Publications, and Jeffries, G. E. (1999). Fitting for hip disarticulation and hemipelvectomy level amputations. *InMotion, 9,* 38-45.)

would be difficult because the prosthetic hip joint would elevate the socket too much to allow level sitting.[9]

A hip-flexion bias system is frequently used for transpelvic and hip disarticulation prostheses. This system consists of a spring-loaded hip joint that shortens the effective length of the leg, allowing the wearer to swing the limb forward without having to assume the gait deviation of vaulting. The hip-flexion bias system may be locked for increased stability (Fig. 11-7).

The transpelvic or hip disarticulation socket may possess an elastic stride-length-control strap that passes behind the hip and in front of the knee. This strap limits hip flexion and may assist with knee extension.[6]

Individuals with a transpelvic or hip disarticulation prosthesis often use a stance-control knee or a polycentric axis (four-bar) knee. The stance-control knee resists knee flexion in excess of 15°. However, a disadvantage of this knee is that the limb must be non-weight bearing for more than 15° of

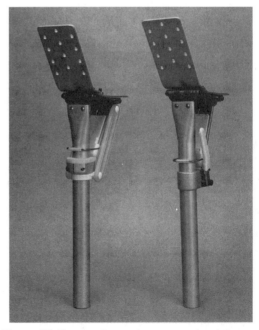

Figure 11-7. A hip-flexion bias system (Modular Hip Joint 7E4). (Reprinted with permission from Otto Bock Orthopedic Industry Inc.)

knee flexion to occur. Individuals frequently have difficulty mastering the weight shift necessary for sitting. The polycentric knee has a center of rotation that changes or adapts to the degree of knee flexion. This knee has the advantage of shortening during swing phase to aid toe clearance. The polycentric knee with pneumatic control prevents excessive heel rise and terminal swing impact in swing phase. The polycentric knee is depicted in Figure 9-2. In the future, a computer-controlled hydraulic unit, such as the C leg, illustrated in Figure 9-7, may be used with transpelvic or hip disarticulation amputations.

Another useful component of the transpelvic or hip disarticulation sockets is a rotator adapter. The rotation adapter allows the knee and shin to be rotated in relation to the hip. This feature enables the prosthetic leg to be crossed over the sound leg and assists in getting in and out of an automobile. A locking mechanism prevents the unit from rotating unless a button is depressed (Fig. 11-8).[1]

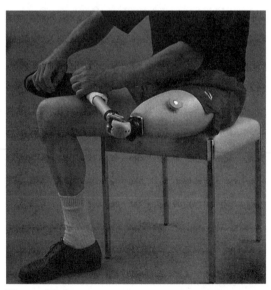

Figure 11-8. Rotation adapter. (Reprinted with permission from Otto Bock Orthopedic Industry Inc.)

Feet

Little has been written about prosthetic feet for the individual with a transpelvic or hip disarticulation amputation. Choice of feet ranges from the conventional to the dynamic-response feet. Conventional feet may not allow an efficient gait. Conversely, a dynamic-response foot may result in too much spring and instability. The type of foot chosen should match the activity level of the individual with amputation.[1]

Gait Characteristics

Gait characteristics of the transpelvic and hip disarticulation prostheses are as follows:

1. At initial contact, the stride-length-control strap (if used) limits hip flexion to about 15°. The prosthetic heel should be planted firmly on the ground.
2. At loading response, a soft heel allows a quicker transition from initial contact to weight acceptance. This quick transition aids in stability.
3. At preswing, the wearer "sits hard" by performing a posterior pelvic tilt to initiate knee flexion.
4. At initial swing, the stride-length-control strap resists excessive heel rise and assists knee extension. If inadequate prosthetic toe clearance occurs, the individual may need to "hip hike" on the amputated side, do a more forceful posterior pelvic tilt, or vault on the sound side.

The transpelvic/hip disarticulation prostheses are often made 1.25 cm shorter for easier foot clearance. Therefore, lateral trunk bending toward the prosthetic side may be normal.

Examination (Checkout) Procedure

The purposes and procedures of an examination (checkout) procedure are reviewed in Chapters 8 and 9. They are described in relation to a transpelvic or hip disarticulation prosthesis as follows.

Socket (Standing Position)

1. The iliac crests should be accommodated within the socket, with no excessive flesh over the brim of the socket. Likewise, no large gaps should exist between the socket walls and the patient.
2. The individual with a transpelvic amputation weight bears on the ischium and buttock of the sound side. The individual with a hip disarticulation weight bears on the ischium of the amputated side. If the socket is too small, weight-bearing areas will be above these bony landmarks.
3. The uppermost brim of the socket should not contact the lower ribs; rather, the area below the uppermost socket brim contacts the lower ribs to assist with vertical loading.[5]
4. If skin irritation and general discomfort occur because of socket pressure, a rubberized socket may be an option.[10]
5. The alignment of the prosthesis should enable the wearer to be stable during stance and allow swing phase. If the alignment is not correct, socket fit, adequate suspension, and prosthesis length should be checked.[5]

Suspension

The suspension should be adequate to avoid excessive pistoning between the patient and the socket during swing phase. The patient can be asked to shift weight to the sound leg and lift the prosthesis. There should be only minimal drop of the prosthesis.

Length

Depending on the knee unit used, the prosthesis may be between 1 and 2.5 cm shorter than the remaining leg to facilitate toe clearance in swing phase. Prosthesis length may be determined by checking the bilateral iliac crest heights of an individual with a hip disarticulation amputation and the lower rib height in those with transpelvic amputation.

Application of the Prosthesis

Practical Application Box 11-1 contains a description of application of the prosthesis.

Research Studies

The use of transpelvic and hip disarticulation prostheses varies in different studies. In a survey of 60 patients at the University of Iowa

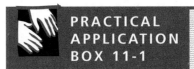

PRACTICAL APPLICATION BOX 11-1

The prosthesis may be applied in a standing position as illustrated in Figure 11-9. Specific steps in the application of the prosthesis are as follows:

1. Stand, with the trunk supported against a wall or sturdy object, wearing suitable underwear or a body sock (Fig. 11-9A and B).
2. Place the pelvis laterally into the socket with the prosthesis slightly rotated laterally. The pelvis should be in contact with all of the socket (Fig. 11-9C).
3. Fasten the strap of the prosthesis, which will slightly medially rotate the prosthesis (Fig. 11-9D).[5]

The prosthesis may also be applied in a sitting position at the edge of the bed. The prosthesis is taken off in reverse order. The patient's skin *must* be checked for areas of irritation. This is especially important for patients receiving chemotherapy or radiation or those with burns. A mirror may be needed to view inaccessible skin areas.

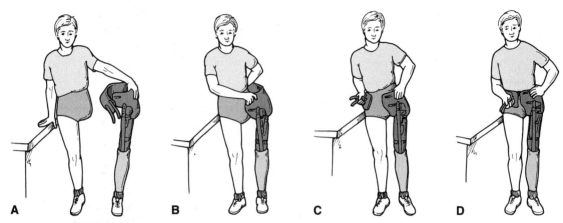

Figure 11-9. Application of the hip disarticulation prosthesis

who underwent transpelvic or hip disarticulation amputations, 15 (25%) were fitted with a prosthesis. Twelve of the 15 (80%) were still using their prostheses at the time of the survey (amount of time between prosthetic fitting and the survey was not specified). An average of 20 visits was needed to attain independent gait.[4] Conversely, in a survey of 38 individuals (age range, 20–95 years) with hip disarticulation at the University of Texas, no patient was able to use a prosthesis. However, most were independent in wheelchair use. This study found 60% mortality in patients with ischemia and preoperative infection, 20% in patients with ischemia without preoperative infection, 100% in patients with trauma and preoperative infection, and 33% in patients with trauma without preoperative infection.[11]

One investigation found that the reason for hip disarticulation determines successful rehabilitation. In a study of 63 individuals with hip disarticulations in Hungary, the 24 patients with disarticulation for a tumor were able to ambulate; only 2 of the 37 patients cases with vascular cause were able to ambulate with a prosthesis.[12]

One 1974 study investigated the use of the hip disarticulation prosthesis with children and concluded that children with congenital defects were more likely to wear a hip disarticulation prosthesis successfully than those with acquired amputations.[13]

One author has noted that the rejection rates for lower-limb prostheses are the highest at these proximal levels of amputation.[14] This rejection is due in large part to the increased energy demand of using a prosthesis. In a study of two patients, ages 31 and 46, using Canadian hip disarticulation prostheses, energy consumption was 2.3 times the resting metabolic rate and 1.7 times greater than that of patients with transfemoral amputations, at a speed only 28% as fast.[15] In a study of eight patients using a hip disarticulation prosthesis, comfortable walking speed was 37% slower than that of able-bodied subjects, and the wearers expended 82% more energy.[16] A study of 10 patients with transpelvic prostheses found that they walked at a comfortable speed 47% slower than, and expended 125% more energy than, able-bodied subjects. In contrast, walking with crutches and without the prosthesis expended 45% more energy than was expended by able-bodied subjects. This difference in energy expenditure explains why some individuals with these high-level amputations prefer ambulation with crutches and without a prosthesis.[16]

KEY POINTS

- Many transpelvic and hip disarticulation amputations are done because of malignant lower-extremity bone tumors.

- Patients undergoing hip disarticulation have a 2:1 male to female ratio.

- Infection is a frequent complication of these amputations and can greatly affect mortality and morbidity.

- Physical therapy interventions for a patient with a transpelvic or hip disarticulation amputation require adaptation of flexibility, strengthening, and balance principles described in Chapter 7.

- Although the transpelvic socket is larger, prosthetic components for hemipelvectomy and hip disarticulation amputations are similar.

- Three hip disarticulation prostheses used today include the total-contact suction socket, the Canadian, and the Diagonal design systems.

- A hip-flexion bias system and a stance-control or polycentric knee are often used with transpelvic and hip disarticulation prostheses.

- Gait characteristics and examination (checkout) procedures for transpelvic and hip disarticulation prostheses are discussed.

- The use of transpelvic and hip disarticulation prostheses varies in different studies. The rejection of these prostheses is due in large part to the increased energy expenditure necessary for their use.

CRITICAL THINKING QUESTIONS

1. With a group of your classmates, design flexibility, strengthening, and balance activities that would be appropriate for a patient with a transpelvic or hip disarticulation amputation.

2. Discuss common sockets, hip, knees, and feet associated with these prostheses.

3. Describe gait-training principles that you would adopt with a patient with a transpelvic or hip disarticulation prosthesis.

4. Explain examination (checkout) procedures that you would use with these prostheses.

5. Instruct a patient in application of transpelvic or hip disarticulation prostheses.

REFERENCES

1. Jeffries, G. E. (1999). Fitting for hip disarticulation and hemipelvectomy level amputations. *In-Motion, 9,* 38–45.
2. Lawton, R. L., & De Pinto, V. (1987). Bilateral hip disarticulation in paraplegics with decubitus ulcers. *Archives of Surgery, 122,* 1040–1043.
3. Walden, J. D., & Davis, B. C. (1979). Prosthetic fitting and points of rehabilitation for hindquarter and hip disarticulation patients. *Physiotherapy, 65,* 4–6.
4. Shurr, D. G., Cook, T. M., Buckwalter, J. A., & Cooper, R. R. (1984). Hip disarticulation: A prosthetic follow-up. *Orthotics and Prosthetics, 37,* 50-57.
5. Engstrom, B., & Van Deven, C. (1985). *Physiotherapy for amputees: The Roehampton approach* (p. 98). New York: Churchill Livingstone.
6. Berger, N., & Fishman, S. (1998). *Lower limb prosthetics.* New York: Prosthetic Orthotic Publications.
7. McLaurin, C. A. (1957). The evolution of the Canadian-type hip disarticulation prosthesis. *Artificial Limbs, 4,* 22–28.
8. Zaffer, S. M., Braddom, R. L., Conti, A., Goff, J., & Bokma, D. (1999). Total hip disarticulation prosthesis with suction socket. Report of two cases. *American Journal of Physical Medicine and Rehabilitation, 78,* 160–162.
9. Nietert, M., Englisch, N., & Kriel, P. (1998). Loads in hip disarticulation prostheses during normal daily use. *Prosthetics and Orthotics International, 22,* 199–215.
10. Van Der Waarde, T. (1984). Ottawa experience with hip disarticulation prostheses. *Orthotics and Prosthetics, 38,* 29–35.
11. Unruh, T., Fisher, D. F., Unruh, T. A., Gottschalk, F., Fry, R. E., Clagett, G. P., & Fry, W. J. (1990). Hip disarticulation: An 11 year experience. *Archives of Surgery, 125,* 791–793.

12. Denes, Z., & Till, A. (1997). Rehabilitation of patients after hip disarticulation. *Archives of Orthopaedic and Traumatic Surgery, 116,* 498–499.

13. Raiford, R. L., & Epps, Ch, Jr. (1974). Experiences with the Canadian hip disarticulation prosthesis in the juvenile. *Journal of the National Medical Association, 66,* 71–75.

14. Bowker, J. H., & Michael, J. W. (1992). *Atlas of limb prosthetics.* St Louis: Mosby YearBook.

15. Huang, C. T. (1983). Energy cost of ambulation with Canadian hip disarticulation prosthesis. *Journal of the Medical Association of the State of Alabama, 52,* 47–48.

16. Nowroozi, F., & Salvanelli, M. L. (1983). Energy expenditure in hip disarticulation and hemipelvectomy amputees. *Archives of Physical Medicine and Rehabilitation, 64,* 300–303.

Chapter 12

Pediatric Patients with Lower-Extremity Amputations— Clinical Decision Making

Mary Evans, PT

Objectives

1. Differentiate the types of congenital amputations
2. Explain the causes of acquired amputations
3. Describe the surgical and prosthetic-fitting implications of postoperative terminal overgrowth
4. Differentiate the most common limb salvage procedures
5. Compare prosthetic components and training that may be used for children of various ages
6. Characterize the principles of parent–child interaction and its effect on rehabilitation outcomes
7. Differentiate examination and intervention of pediatric patients and adults with amputations
8. Analyze the psychologic factors of an amputation on the child and parents

This chapter is divided into the following sections:

Causes of childhood amputations are 60% congenital and 40% acquired.[1] Congenital amputation is the most common cause of limb deficiency in children under 10 years of age.[2] Both of these amputation causes, congenital and acquired, are discussed in detail.

◆ ◆ ◆

Congenital Disorders

Congenital disorders include an absence of one or more limbs, a deformity of one or more extremities, and/or loss of muscles and ligaments with no skeletal deficits. Congenital musculoskeletal disorders or birth defects may evolve from multiple factors. Skeletal limb deficiencies are due to primary intrauterine growth inhibition or secondary intrauterine destruction of normal embryonic tissue.[3]

Congenital amputation, which occur in utero, may result from drug toxicity, the use of illegal drugs, malformation, or strangulation of limb **buds** by the umbilical cord.[4] Congenital amputations are associated with **annular constricting bands**, which represent failure of circumferential growth of the skin and soft tissue at a specific level during intrauterine development. Shallow constrictions may be seen without any abnormality distally; deeper constrictions result in distal losses of the limb at some time during intrauterine life.

The International Society for Prosthetics and Orthotics (ISPO) and the International Organization for Standardization (ISO) have adopted international terminology and classifications based on anatomic and radiologic features to classify the two major types of congenital skeletal limb deficiencies.[5] These deficiencies involve partial or complete loss of bone segments. Congenital deficiencies may be classified as **transverse** or **longitudinal**. For example, if a child is missing all bones below the right acetabulum, this condition is termed a *complete transverse deficiency of the right thigh.* The limb essentially ends at the location of the deficit, although sometimes digital buds or

nubbins may be present. Function and appearance proximal to the deficit are normal. Transverse deficiencies, whether partial or total, do not usually require revisional surgery.

When there is total or partial absence of a structure along the long axis of a segment of bone, a longitudinal deficiency exists. Distally, beyond this deficient segment, normal skeletal structures may exist. An example of a longitudinal deficiency is the complete or partial absence of the tibia or fibula, with an essentially normal foot. **Hemimelias** are longitudinal deficiencies in which all or part of one bone is missing. Fibular hemimelia results in bowing of the tibia, producing a leg length difference. The congenital absence of part or all of the femur, referred to as **proximal femoral focal deficiency (PFFD)**, is another example of a longitudinal deficiency. Despite a defective femur, the tibia, fibula, and foot are intact.[6] Longitudinal deficiencies became common in the early 1960s with the use of the drug thalidomide. Thalidomide, which was used to counteract nausea in the first trimester, resulted in fetal longitudinal deficiencies or **phocomelia**.[7] Phocomelia is a developmental anomaly characterized by the absence of the proximal section of a limb or limbs. The hand or foot can be attached to the trunk of the body by a single small, irregularly shaped bone.

Infants with either transverse or longitudinal limb deficiencies may also have **hypoplastic bones**, **bifid bones**, **synostoses**, duplications, dislocations, joint instability, range-of-motion deficits, and angulation deformities. Any or all limbs may be affected, and defects may be of a different type in each limb. Many variations of the deformities may be encountered, especially when more than one limb is involved.

Longitudinal defects often present a major challenge for prosthetic design. Limb deficiencies tend to require nonstandard prostheses. Surgery or conversion is often necessary to achieve an ideal level for prosthetic fitting.[8] Conversion may consist of amputation at a recommended level or may be associated with proximal joint **fusion** to increase the residual-limb skeletal length and stability. A child's current functional capacity for mobility and future potential must be carefully assessed before a prosthesis or any surgical procedure is recommended. Therapeutic amputation of any limb or even a portion of a limb should be avoided unless essential for optimal fitting of a prosthetic device. Any amputation should only be considered after estimating the functional implication of the loss.

Types of Transverse and Longitudinal Deficiencies

Transverse and longitudinal deficiencies are introduced in Chapter 1. A classification of limb deficiencies is shown in Table 12-1.[5]

Transverse Deficiencies

Transverse deficiencies may involve lower and/or upper extremities (Fig. 12-1). Transverse deficiencies of the phalanges usually do not require surgical intervention. Revisional surgery is also usually unnecessary for partial

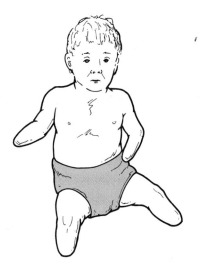

Figure 12-1. Child with transverse deficiencies. (Adapted from Kalamchi, A. (Ed.). (1989). *Congenital lower limb deficiencies*. New York: Springer-Verlag.)

or complete metatarsal deficiencies, unless it is necessary to remove **vestigial phalanges** that may become irritated, ulcerated, or pose a problem with shoe fitting.[9]

A partial or complete tarsal deficiency or congenital ankle disarticulation may be managed by a prosthesis, with no surgical interven-

Table 12-1. Classifications of Transverse and Longitudinal Deficiencies

Transverse Deficiencies	Longitudinal Deficiencies
Pelvis	Ilium (total or partial)
Thigh (total, upper third, middle third, or lower third)	Ischium (total or partial)
Leg (total, upper third, middle third, or lower third)	Pubis (total or partial)
Tarsal (total or partial)	Metatarsal (total or partial)
Phalangeal (total or partial)	Femur (total or partial)
	Tibia (total or partial)
	Fibula (total or partial)
	Tarsals (total or partial)
	Metatarsals (total or partial)
	Phalanges (total or partial)

Adapted from Day, H. J. B. (1992). The ISO/IPSO classification of congenital limb deficiency. In J. H. Bowker (Ed.), *Atlas of limb prosthetics: Surgical, prosthetic, and rehabilitation principles* (2nd ed., pp. 743-746). St. Louis: Mosby.

tion. Partial tarsal deficiencies with a normal distal tibial **epiphysis** and no leg length discrepancy may require conversion surgery. Proximal revisions may provide better function and cosmetic appearance through the use of a **Syme** ankle disarticulation. The Syme amputation offers a long end-bearing residual limb, free from the problems of overgrowth.[7] Overgrowth is described in more detail later in this chapter. The Boyd amputation, first described in 1939, involves removal of bone from the superior and anterior aspects of the calcaneus. The remaining calcaneus is then placed under the tibia to form a calcaneotibial fusion. Both the Syme and Boyd amputations preserve the distal tibial growth plates; however, the Boyd amputation results in a longer residual limb.[7]

Transfemoral deficiencies occur less frequently than transtibial deficiencies. Surgical intervention is seldom indicated with transfemoral deficiencies; however, prosthetic restoration is common. Children with total transverse deficiency of the thigh, or **amelia**, can be fitted with a prosthesis when standing and balancing begins on the contralateral leg. Any vestige can be incorporated into the prosthetic socket (Fig. 12-2).

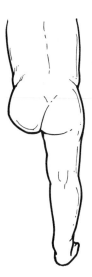

Figure 12-2. Total transverse deficiency of the left thigh (amelia). (Adapted from Kalamchi, A. (Ed.). (1989). *Congenital lower limb deficiencies*. New York: Springer-Verlag.)

Longitudinal Deficiencies

Longitudinal deficiencies may be unilateral or bilateral, and either partial or complete. Fibular deficiency is an example of a true limb deficiency with associated problems in addition to the absent bone. For example, with a fibular deficiency, the tibia may be bowed and the femur shortened. Deficiencies may also exist in the muscles, tendons, nerves, and skin. Dimpling is frequently noted over the deformed tibia. A longitudinal deficiency of the fibula presents as a foreshortened limb with an equinovalgus foot, tarsal anomalies, and possible absence of the metatarsal rays.[10] A Syme amputation may be performed in cases of severe foot deformity.

Longitudinal deficiency of the tibia is much less frequent than fibular deficiency. If the involved tibial segment is shorter than one-third the length of the normal tibia, the procedure of choice is synostosis of the fibula to the tibia and disarticulation of the foot. This procedure produces a long transtibial residual limb. If the proximal segment of the tibia is long, synostosis is generally not necessary, and a Syme amputation is generally performed. Prosthetic fitting is accomplished with a transtibial-type prosthesis.[7,10] In cases of complete longitudinal deficiency of the tibia, to avoid recurrent surgeries to construct a knee joint, the surgical treatment of choice is disarticulation of the knee.

Longitudinal deficiency of the femur is primarily identified as PFFD of the hip. The clinical picture is that of a short femoral segment, positioned in flexion, abduction, and external rotation (Fig. 12-3). Four classifications of PFFD are described in Table 12-2.[10–13] Many intervention options are available, depending upon the length of the femoral segment. Unilateral PFFD may be divided into three groups:

1. Femoral segment is less than 20% of the sound-side femur
2. Femoral segment is between 20 and 70% of the sound-side femur
3. Femoral segment is more than 70% of the sound-side femur[10]

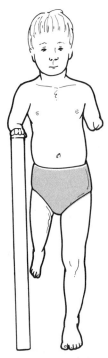

Figure 12-3. Example of proximal femoral focal deficiency (PFFD). (Adapted from Kalamchi, A. (Ed.). (1989). *Congenital lower limb deficiencies.* New York: Springer-Verlag.)

The inequality in leg length necessitates some type of intervention. For example if more than 70% of the normal length of the femur is present, various options exist. These options include lengthening the shortened femur, arrest of bone growth at the epiphysis of the nor-

mal knee, shortening the normal femur, or a combination of these options. If the femoral segment is between 20 and 70% of the sound-side femur and there is resistance to amputation, then a platform orthosis would be a viable solution. If less than 20% of the femoral length is present, a Syme amputation or a **rotationplasty** (described later in this chapter) may be indicated. In cases of bilateral PFFD, ambulation may be possible without prostheses if the limbs are the same height.[11] To achieve normal height, modified transfemoral prostheses, such as those used in a rotationplasty may be an option.

Acquired Amputations

Acquired amputations may be necessary in the following conditions:

- Trauma
- Peripheral vascular disease
- Malignant tumors
- Infections
- Paralysis
- Diabetes
- Thermal, chemical, or electrical injuries
- Therapeutic reasons such as intractable pain[7,14]

Trauma causes roughly twice as many pediatric limb losses as disease. Motor vehicle accidents, power tool and machinery injuries, gunshot wounds, and explosions are common examples of trauma. In the 1- to 4-year-old age

Table 12-2. Classifications of Proximal Femoral Focal Deficiency (PFFD)	
Class A	Femoral head is present; the acetabulum is normal; the head of the femur is within the acetabulum; a short femoral segment with subtrochanteric varus angulation is present
Class B	Femoral head is present; acetabulum is adequate but defective; capital fragment is within the acetabulum
Class C	Femoral head is absent or represented by **ossicle;** acetabulum is not present; short femoral fragment; no articular relation between femur and acetabulum
Class D	Femoral head is absent; acetabulum is not present; no relationship exists between the femur and the acetabulum

Adapted from Kruger, L. M. (1992). Lower limb deficiencies: Surgical management. In J. H. Bowker (Ed.), *Atlas of limb prosthetics: Surgical, prosthetic, and rehabilitation principles* (2nd ed., pp. 795–838). St. Louis: Mosby.

group, power tools such as lawn mowers and farm machinery and household accidents account for most amputations.[15] Partial or complete removal of the limb may be necessary after the traumatic event.

Malignant tumors are responsible for more than half of the disease processes necessitating amputations in children. The highest incidence of tumors occurs in the 12- to 21-year-old group, with males outnumbering females 3:2. Bone tumors tend to occur in the proximal aspect of the limb, making high-level limb amputation necessary. **Osteogenic sarcoma** and **Ewing's sarcoma** are examples of commonly seen bone tumors. In many cases, irradiation, chemotherapy, or resection with limb-sparing techniques have been used successfully instead of amputation.[15]

Amputation may be indicated when the blood supply is destroyed and/or the muscle tissue is so damaged that necrosis or gangrene is inevitable or reconstruction is impossible.[16] Occasionally, amputation is indicated when permanent, irreparable loss of nerve supply is present. Extensive, severe tissue damage from excessive heat or cold, chemicals, or electricity may cause mutilating loss of muscle or bone, painful scars, or deforming contractures that make amputation preferable.

Postoperative Terminal Overgrowth Complications

Terminal overgrowth is one of the most common complications in the skeletally immature individual who has undergone amputation surgery (Fig. 12-4). Terminal overgrowth is a sharp protrusion of bone from the end of the residual limb. Terminal overgrowth is more common in individuals with acquired amputations and is caused by bone growing at a faster rate than the overlying soft tissues. Due to the sharp bony overgrowth, the residual limb often becomes inflamed and tender. Bony overgrowth is especially common with long bone

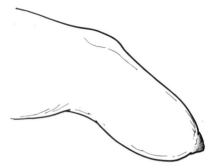

Figure 12-4. Bony overgrowth at the distal end of a transtibial amputation. (Adapted from Kalamchi, A. (Ed.). (1989). *Congenital lower limb deficiencies.* New York: Springer-Verlag.)

involvement such as humeral, fibular, tibial, and femoral amputations.[17]

Bony overgrowth generally ceases when the epiphyseal line closes. An intervention commonly used with bony overgrowth is a revision of the residual limb with sufficient resection of the bony overgrowth to allow coverage of terminal bone with an adequate soft tissue envelope. Surgeons generally perform an ankle or knee disarticulation whenever possible, thereby preserving the epiphyseal growth plates and eliminating overgrowth.[17] The disadvantage of a disarticulation is that fewer prosthetic components are available to accommodate the long residual limb for young patients.

Retention of the longitudinal growth centers at the distal femur and proximal and distal tibia in the infant or young child is essential to promote continued growth of the residual limb for optimal prosthetic fitting at an older age. Because of epiphyseal plate involvement, the residual limb generally grows at a slower rate than the sound side. A long amputated transfemoral or transtibial residual limb of a young child can become a short residual limb by maturity.[10] If normal growth does occur in the residual limb during childhood, the slightly shortened, slower growing limb will be ideal for prosthetic fitting in adulthood.

Limb Salvage

Limb salvage procedures are more complex than amputations in terms of operative procedures, potential complications, and postoperative management.[11,18] Survival rates for patients with tumors have improved with advancements in surgical approaches in addition to preoperative and postoperative chemotherapy, radiotherapy and antibiotic therapy. The goals of limb-sparing surgery are total eradication of the tumor and preservation of a functional limb. The decision to spare a limb is made after ensuring that the neurovascular structures are not compromised by tumor and that the expected function following reconstruction would be superior to that with amputation.

Limb-Salvage Procedures

Limb salvage may consist of an arthrodesis, arthroplasty, skeletal substitutes, use of the **Ilizarov** method, or a rotationplasty procedure.

Some methods of skeletal reconstruction may consist of **arthrodesis** (surgical fusion of a joint) or **arthroplasty** (surgical fabrication of an artificial joint). Skeletal substitutes used in combination or singularly include **autografts** (a graft derived from one's own body), **allografts** (a graft from a cadaver), and metallic endoprostheses. These skeletal substitutes do not disturb growth centers and allow for full growth.

Endoprosthetic devices are an extension of the joint arthroplasty procedure. Devices are implanted in the area of the excised bone and function as a joint or straight bone. Expandable, customized metallic implants are being used successfully in children with tumors of long bones of the limbs. Expandable prostheses at the proximal and distal ends of the femur and proximal parts of the tibia allow periodic lengthening of the device if the epiphyseal growth plates had to be destroyed during the resection. An endoprosthetic device is illustrated in Figure 1-9B. Complications of expandable prostheses include infection, loosening of the device due to poor durability, and the need for periodic surgical procedures to accommodate growth.[19] In trauma cases, improved methods of fracture fixation, neurovascular repair, and new techniques for myofascial transplantation and tissue expansion provide opportunities for limb salvage with improved function and cosmesis.

The Ilizarov Method

Dr. Gavriil Abramovich Ilizarov, a physician in Siberia after World War II, developed a technique to lengthen bone. This technique uses modular-ring external fixators and transosseous wires attached to circular rings.[20] This is commonly called the Ilizarov Method (Fig. 12-5). Ilizarov used a distraction rate of 1 mm per day to facilitate bone formation. In North America, his limb-salvage techniques have been adopted primarily for limb lengthening, correction of limb deformities, and treatment of bone loss secondary to trauma, infection, and tumors. The Ilizarov method allows the surgeon to perform complex, extended lengthening of both congenital and acquired short limbs. Advantages of this method include simultaneous lengthening of limbs at several sites, protection of adjacent joints in a frame, and healing without bone grafting or internal fixation. Complications include infection, temporary or permanent stretch paralysis of an adjacent nerve, joint stiffness, and ischemia. In certain congenital conditions, such as PFFD or fibular hemimelia, amputation may still be the best option.[20]

Rotationplasty

Van Nes popularized the rotationplasty technique in England during the 1950s, when he used the technique for children with PFFD.

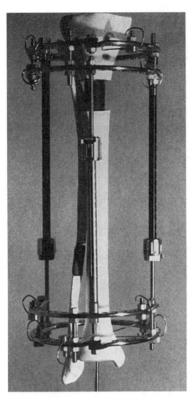

Figure 12-5. Ilizarov (circular frame) used for limb lengthening. (Reprinted with permission from Dr. Christopher Geel, Department of Orthopedics, Upstate Medical University, Syracuse, NY.)

joint, and a long lever arm for better prosthesis control (Fig. 12-7).[21,22] A rotationplasty can be used for lesions of the femur and proximal third of the tibia; however, the ankle–foot must be disease free, with adequate blood/nerve supply and muscle power.[23]

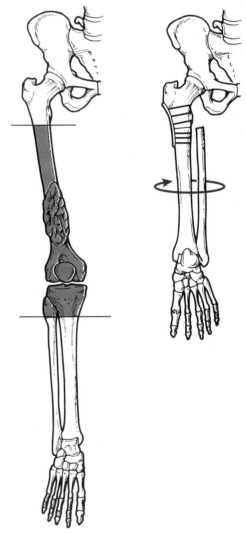

Figure 12-6. Procedure for a rotationplasty used in cases of a tumor in the middle distal femur. (Adapted from Hillmann, A., Rosenbaum, D., Schroter, J., et al. (2000). Electromyographic and gait analysis of forty three patients after rotationplasty. *Journal of Bone and Joint Surgery (Am) 82,* 187–196.)

Rotationplasty is sometimes done for patients who have a malignant tumor in the middle or distal femur. An osteotomy is performed in the proximal third of the femur, distal to the lesser trochanter, and in the proximal part of the tibia, distal to the tibial tuberosity. The rotationplasty procedure is illustrated in Figure 12-6. The foot is rotated 180°, and the tibia reattached to the remaining femur. The foot is fit into the prosthesis. The talocrural (ankle) joint acts as a knee joint. Ankle plantarflexion is used to extend the knee. Ankle dorsiflexion is used to flex the knee. Prosthetically, this amputation has the advantages of preservation of the anatomic ankle joint, which acts as a knee

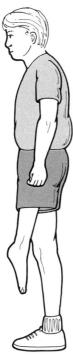

Figure 12-7. Final result of rotationplasty showing the foot rotated 180° and the tibia reattached to the remaining femur. The ankle acts as a knee joint. (Adapted from Hillmann, A., Rosenbaum, D., Schroter, J., et al. (2000). Electromyographic and gait analysis of forty three patients after rotationplasty. *Journal of Bone and Joint Surgery (Am) 82,* 187–196.)

Prosthetic Components

Prosthetic care for a child with a limb deficiency is an on-going process from infancy into adulthood. The longevity of a prosthesis for a child can range from 3 months to 2 years, depending upon the feasibility of repairs and the capacity to accommodate modifications for growth. Regularly scheduled appointments with a prosthetist every 3–4 months are essential until the child becomes a young adult. If the child experiences a rapid growth spurt, more-frequent appointments may be needed. Many localities have limb disorder clinics that provide prosthetic consultations with a team of

health professionals who specialize in the care of patients with amputations. The roles of various members of these health-care teams are reviewed in Chapter 3.[24]

The following section of this chapter discusses principles and characteristics of lower-limb prostheses that are relevant to infants, children, adolescents, and young adults. Preceding chapters on transtibial, transfemoral, bilateral, transpelvic, and hip disarticulation amputations (Chapters 8–11) should be reviewed for more-detailed information and descriptions of components that may be similar in style and function for both the pediatric and adult patient.

Infants are being fitted at an earlier age for the purposes of improved cosmetic appearance or the enhancement of functional mobility. However, manufactured prosthetic components are often limited for infants. Therefore, the prosthetist must be creative and often custom-fabricate appliances. Parents should be advised of the rationale for the decision regarding the selection and development of the prosthetic prescription. Their views and concerns should be acknowledged and addressed. Children are encouraged to maximize their functional potential by participating in age-appropriate developmental play and physical recreational activities. As a result, heavy physical demands are placed on their prosthetic devices. A prosthetic prescription for a child should consider two important factors in the design of the prosthesis: durability and simplicity. Prosthetic devices must meet the needs and match the functional abilities of each patient without being too complex or frustrating for the child to operate.[2]

Transfemoral Components

The choice between a lightweight exoskeletal design or an endoskeletal device depends upon what is appropriate for the child and what is acceptable by the parents. For infants, plastic tubing can be used with an endoskeletal design for a lightweight cosmetic appliance. Thermoplastic sockets mounted inside rigid frames can allow socket replacement due to growth without constantly remolding the entire prosthesis.[25]

In many cases, the durable exoskeletal components are preferred, since the endoskeletal units with their soft foam covers can quickly become worn and dirty. However, some parents may accept the need to replace the soft outside covers at frequent intervals in exchange for the benefit of increased cosmetic appearance and the lighter weight of the endoskeletal unit.[24] An endoskeletal device without soft covering would be appropriate for individuals with bladder and bowel incontinence. Endoskeletal systems were initially thought to be too fragile to endure heavy wear. However, titanium and carbon graphite materials are now being used to make lighter but durable units. Parts from the endoskeletal systems may be recycled into the child's next prosthesis. Aluminum tubing may telescope to allow length adjustments for growth.

For the child with a transfemoral amputation, the quadrilateral and ischial-containment sockets have both worked well. Each of these sockets is described in Chapter 9.

Any suspension system for the pediatric patient must be moisture resistant and washable.[24] Suspensions may consist of a Silesian bandage or total elastic suspension (TES). Parents need instruction in techniques for applying and removing the prosthesis. Compliance in monitoring the residual limb for any skin irritation or a child's expressions of pain or discomfort is essential.

Transfemoral knee components were reviewed in Chapter 9. Parents should be informed that knee components are usually omitted from the prosthesis for infants until their standing balance has developed and dynamic balance can be challenged. However, a constant-friction polycentric knee with a manual lock can be incorporated for short sitting in highchairs, strollers, and car seats. In a study of seven children, ranging in age from 1 year 5 months to 6 years 1 month with amputations, mobile knees were used. Investigators found that gait deviations such as circumduction, posterior pelvic tilt, excessive internal rotation, and hip hiking were avoided. In addition, normal childhood activities such as crawling, squatting, and kneeling were facilitated. Young children are often not tall enough to allow a knee joint to be placed into the prosthesis. However, this study concluded that a child should be fitted with an articulated knee as soon as height allows.[26]

One transfemoral component, the polycentric Otto Bock 3R66 knee joint, allows 165° of knee flexion and an integrated foot rotation unit that facilitates typical postures of children, such as kneeling and floor sitting (Fig. 12-8). When the child stands up and unloads the prosthesis, the prosthetic foot automatically returns to the original position. Among some of the newer prosthetic knee components are the Century XXII Innovations Child's Play Small Wonder Knee (Fig. 12-9) and the DAW Industries pediatric knee used for knee disarticulations. The Otto Bock 3R65 children's hydraulic knee offers dynamic swing-phase control and promotes natural movements through a broad range of adjustable gait speeds. It also has a colorful appearance.

Transtibial Components

Comfort and control of the prosthesis is directly related to good socket retention on the residual limb. A child with a transtibial amputation will often use a supracondylar cuff suspension. However this suspension may stress the knee ligaments if not adjusted regularly as the child grows. Since the medial and lateral walls of the transtibial prosthesis with supracondylar suspension extend above the femoral epicondyles, mediolateral stability of the prosthesis is enhanced.[5] Sleeve suspensions are more suitable for the less-active child.[24] Sleeves and the roll-on silicone-liner suction suspensions work well with active transfemoral and

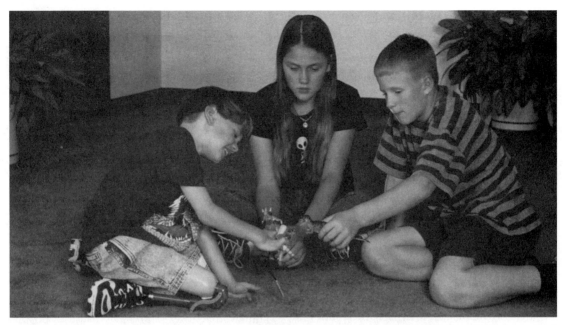

Figure 12-8. Polycentric 3R66 Knee Joint. (Reprinted with permission from Otto Bock Orthopedic Industry Inc.)

transtibial prosthetic wearers.[27] The roll-on silicone-liner suction suspensions are easier to apply than traditional suction suspensions, are less demanding on the residual-limb tissue, and can accommodate volumetric changes in the residual limb.[28]

Dynamic-response feet and ankle components also affect the socket comfort and functional capabilities of all lower-limb prosthesis users. Most children previously received a solid-ankle cushion-heel (SACH) foot, which is adequate for low-level activities but not suitable or durable enough for dynamic activities. Many dynamic-response feet are now available in pediatric sizes to meet the needs of active children. Dynamic-response feet may give children the ability to jump. Prosthetic feet are discussed in Chapter 8. The Pediatric Springlite II is designed to be very durable for a child's high activity level. It is adjustable in length to match the child's growth (Fig. 12-10).[29]

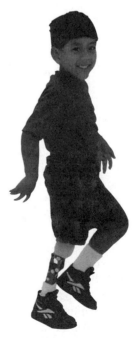

Figure 12-9. Century XXII Innovations Child's Play Small Wonder Knee. (Reprinted with permission from OSSUR.)

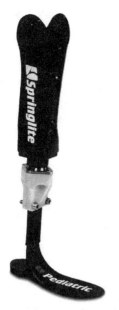

Figure 12-10. Pediatric Springlite II. (Reprinted with permission of Springlite Inc.)

Parent–Child Interaction

The prosthetic team's approach to intervention including a listing of the members, their function, and the team's purpose and procedures is described in Chapter 3. In Chapter 4, the young child's and the adolescent's psychologic reactions to their amputation are discussed. Parents must be considered vital members of the prosthetic team. Their interest and attitudes can make the difference between whether a child accepts or rejects the prosthesis. Children can easily adopt the attitudes of others, especially those of their parents.

The manner in which parents respond reflects their acceptance of their child's disability. With parental support, development of self worth, and good body image, the child accepts the prosthesis.[2,30] The parents must become educated and involved in the prosthetic management of the child. Parents and child need reassurance and understanding from the entire prosthetic clinic team. They should feel comfortable addressing their concerns on various

topics regarding the design, fit, and function of the prosthetic device, specific training procedures, emotional adjustments, and anticipation of future problems. A well-fitting, functional prosthesis can help to keep the child and family focused on positive adaptations. Members of the prosthetic team can help facilitate a child's adjustment and integration within the school environment by arranging get-acquainted conferences for school personnel to meet the child and family. A show-and-tell discussion may be arranged with the child's classmates regarding prosthetic devices.

A support network can be helpful for a child with a newly acquired amputation and the parents. A support network can provide empathy, acceptance, and an understanding of the disability. The family and child may find it helpful to meet peers and their families who have similar diagnoses and have made a positive transition toward acceptance of their disability.[2] Important resources for children with amputation, family members, and health professionals are contained in Practical Application Box 12-1.

Parents have the potential to influence public opinion regarding children with physical disabilities. Parents can educate and foster positive encounters for their child. The way parents respond and answer questions reflects their acceptance of, and attitude toward, their child's limb deficit.[30]

Young children with congenital limb deficiencies do not experience a sense of loss of a body part. The prosthesis is viewed as an assistive device or helper, not as a replacement. In contrast, children with acquired amputations experience adjustment reactions similar to those of adults. The child can be expected to go through the stages of grief before accepting the disability. A child's initial adjustment reaction to the loss of a limb may include feelings of disbelief, anger, rejection, and loneliness. Some may mourn, in addition to the loss of a limb, their possible inability to participate in a favorite sport or other activity.[31] Early fitting of the prosthesis may minimize some psychologic

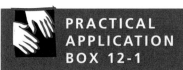

PRACTICAL APPLICATION BOX 12-1

Resources for Children with Amputations

National Limb Loss Information Center (NLLIC)
900 East Hill Avenue Suite 285
Knoxville, TN 37915-2568
(888)-267-5669
(888)-AMP-KNOW
www.nllicinfo@amputee-coalition.org

Amputee Resource Foundation of America
6480 Wayzata Blvd.
Golden Valley, MN 55426
www.amputeeresource.org

National Rehabilitation Information Center (NARIC)
1010 Wayne Avenue Suite 800
Silver Spring, MD 20910-3319
(800)-346-2742
www.naric.com

Association of Children's Prosthetic and Orthotic Clinics (ACPOC)
222 South Prospect Avenue
Park Ridge, IL 60068
(708)-698-1632
www.acpoc.org

Government resources regarding prosthetics and orthotics are available at web site: http://www.pubmedcentral.nih.gov

difficulties. The use of an immediate postoperative prosthesis (IPOP) will enable early ambulation and may lessen psychologic difficulties.

Children with limb deficiencies have special psychosocial issues dealing with parents, peers, and society. They also have concerns regarding the acquisition of new skills. Parents must be aware of some of the issues that the child may encounter at different age levels. Erikson has provided a framework for recognizing dominant psychosocial issues within four age groupings.[32] Infants from birth through age 2 years establish trust and security through a relationship with their parents. They learn through the sensorimotor experiences of touching, tasting, pulling, reaching, and crawling. As toddlers, a sense of self-worth and independence is developed. School-age children have to deal with peer curiosity and teasing. Adolescents form their own identities and values regarding body image, sexuality, and career. Peer acceptance and a pleasing cosmetic appearance are a very high priority at this age. Finally, family support and encouragement from friends, teachers, and classmates can have a positive effect on the child's adaptation.[2,33]

Physical Therapy Examination and Interventions

Ideally, infants with congenital limb deficiencies should be examined by a physical therapist within the first 4 weeks of life to establish a baseline record for future reference. The examination should document range of motion, strength, skin condition, dimensions of extremities, skin sensitivity, postural assessment including the effect of head and trunk positions on structural malalignment, and developmental progression on a monthly basis. Examination then may occur on a 3- to 6-month basis.[29] Examination forms are presented in Chapter 2.

Gait training should begin as soon as is medically feasible in patients with acquired lower-extremity amputations. An IPOP, described in Chapter 6, may be an option. Preprosthetic strengthening exercises and gait-training procedures for children with transfemoral amputations and rotationplasty procedures will require more training for knee control.[2] Prosthetic training is essential for guiding the child toward the achievement and resumption of age-appropriate developmental milestones. Parents should be active participants in their child's pre-prosthetic and prosthetic training sessions. Initially, physical therapy outcomes should focus on preprosthetic care and preparation of the residual limb, including healing, shaping of the residual limb, and strength training.

Parents and adolescent individuals with acquired amputations should be instructed in skin hygiene including the daily inspection and washing of the residual limb and massage techniques to mobilize scar tissue. The rationale and procedures for the reduction of edema and shaping of the residual limb should be explained and demonstrated. Elastic bandages or shrinkers are used to minimize and control edema. Controlling edema contours the residual limb in preparation for maximizing the fit of the prosthesis. Exercises should consist of positioning, range of motion, strengthening, functional activities, and age-appropriate mobility skills.[34] These activities are reviewed in Chapter 7. Prosthetic training should begin with instruction in applying and removing the prosthesis, wearing time schedule, skin assessment, determining the fit of the prosthesis, transitional activities such as sit-to-stand, and ambulation activities. Training also involves care of the prosthesis, including when to contact the prosthetist for adjustments or modifications. Based on a particular family's learning style, written and demonstrated instructions including diagrams and videotapes may be provided. Physical therapy interventions may range from home program suggestions with periodic scheduled examinations to direct treatment interventions.

Principles of Lower-Extremity Prosthetic Training from Birth through 18 Years

Prosthetic training interventions may consist of prevention of deformities and enhancement of function. Activities that have been suggested in this chapter support learning for infants and toddlers through sensorimotor experiences described by Piaget.[35] However, newer theories such as motor learning and dynamic systems may further augment intervention effectiveness. The principles of motor learning may optimize retention of learned tasks and their transfer to other settings. Larin provides an excellent review of motor learning applicable for children of all ages. Principles of lower-extremity prosthetic training are discussed below for the ages of birth to 6 months, 7–14 months, 15–36 months, 3–6 years, 7–12 years, and 13–18 years.[36]

From Birth to Six Months of Age

A child with a limb deficiency is similar to an able-bodied child in most aspects of growth and development. Children need to master lower developmental tasks, enhance weight shifting, and balance reactions. Mastery of these tasks aids the transition from quadruped to kneeling to standing and, finally, to ambulation.[2] Children with multiple limb deficiencies may present with delayed motor development due to deficits in crawling, pulling-to-stand, etc. A child with PFFD may need range-of-motion activities to correct hip flexion, abduction, and external rotation tightness that are present at birth.[29] Mastery of tasks such as head control, crawling to explore the environment, and supported and unsupported sitting should be emphasized as part of a preprosthetic training program. Usually a prosthetic limb is not provided before 6 months of age.

It is important to assess how the child manipulates the residual limb and incorporates the limb into purposeful movement patterns. The use of a prosthetic limb at this stage enables the infant to develop an awareness of the prosthesis as part of the body from the beginning of movement. The parents may request a light-weight prosthetic device for their infant for cosmetic purposes. However, the device also addresses the child's perception of body symmetry, body weight and size, positive and negative sensations of neurologic input, and mechanical aspects of its use. The child should incorporate the residual limb and prosthetic devices into early movements to allow self-organization to occur.

Seven to Fourteen Months

Achievement of developmental milestones between the ages of 7 and 14 months should reflect the following:

- Refinement of sitting and crawling skills
- Transitions through kneeling to half-kneeling to pull-to-stand
- Standing momentarily alone
- Stepping movements holding onto furniture
- Walking with two hands held, then one hand, and subsequently walking alone

For an infant with a unilateral amputation, a functional knee component is initially omitted from a prosthesis. Therefore, an infant with a congenital transfemoral deficiency must learn to modify movement patterns to achieve developmental milestones that require knee flexion. Developmental skills such as combat crawling can be achieved with symmetry in posture, but creeping and kneeling skills would be asymmetric.

Children usually begin to pull to stand between the ages of 8 and 10 months and walk between the ages of 9 and 15 months. A child with a congenital lower-limb deficiency will use the residual limb and the normal lower extremity to pull to stand. When this occurs, fitting with a prosthesis with appropriate components is indicated. When motivated, a child will start to walk during training activities if provided with a prosthesis that is light weight, appropriate in length, and stable at the knee. Initially, gait training may be done with an assistive device such as a walker to promote controlled weight bearing, balance, proper trunk alignment, and reciprocal gait pattern. Once more control over the prosthesis is achieved, the child can be weaned from the assistive device.

When fabricating a pediatric prosthesis, components that are appropriate for a child's specific developmental stage should be provided. The prosthetic socket should accommodate rapid linear growth. The suspension system should not encumber the child.[37] Prosthetic training should focus on lower developmental skills such as rolling, crawling, transitions into and out of sitting, kneeling, and pulling to stand. The infant should be comfortable wearing the prosthesis for progressively increased time spans throughout the day. Symmetry in posture and movement, promoting increased emergence of balance reactions, and protective extension of the arms and legs are useful activities at this stage. Controlled weight-shifting activities from one leg to the other ensure weight bearing on the prosthetic side.

Activities at this stage that may be incorporated into an intervention plan may include the following:

- Standing alone with two hands on a surface
- Squatting or reaching for objects while holding with one hand for support
- Crawling then creeping on all fours while incorporating trunk rotation and weight shifting for alternating side sitting
- Pulling-to-stand through half-kneeling

To prevent acetabular problems, children should be discouraged from kneeling and sitting back between their knees with the legs excessively internally rotated.

Therapeutic exercise balls provide an enjoyable way to promote sensory motor skills and improve balance, equilibrium, and trunk stability. Heavy duty spring balls simulate bouncing and other vestibular activities. Transparent balls with objects inside can help stimulate audio senses and develop eye-tracking skills. Tactile input can be enhanced by small bumps on the outer surfaces of objects. Rocker balance boards can also provide vestibular stimulation, balance, and coordination responses in different developmental positions such as sitting, kneeling, half-kneeling, and standing. Weighted push strollers can be used for support during ambulation; child-sized basketball hoops, bean bag toss games, and activities at an easel board may be used to enhance standing.

Fifteen to Thirty-Six Months

Developmental skills at the lower end of this age range should demonstrate the emergence of equilibrium reactions for walking without support, stand to sit by falling on buttocks, creeping up stairs, and pulling toys while walking. At about 30 months of age, children start to jump, stand on one foot for 1 to 5 seconds, climb up ladders on slides, pedal tricycles, and initiate a running pattern. A child with an amputation will demonstrate modifications in movement patterns to accomplish these tasks. The therapist may train the child to use more-efficient patterns with less expenditure of energy.

Three to Six Years

During these ages, the prosthesis is subjected to rigorous activity levels; therefore, it should be simple, rugged, and repairable.[38] At this time, developmental skills for ball handling, balancing, and advanced movement patterns such as those needed for stairs are becoming more refined. Children are involved in kicking, jumping, hopping, and running activities. Children with congenital transtibial deficiencies should be functional ambulators at this age. They should be expected to wear the prosthesis for most of the day and engage in age-appropriate activities with their peers. Equal weight bearing on the amputated and sound sides as well as symmetric stride length, progressing to galloping, and eventual running should be emphasized. Parents of preschool and kindergarten children will have increased

anxiety about the child's appearance and acceptance by others. The preschool years should emphasize development of independence in self-care skills, mobility, acquisition of school skills, and organized play activities. Functional outcomes should focus on the child learning age-appropriate skills.

During these ages, the child with a transfemoral amputation is ready for the first functional knee. Children usually cannot control an articulating knee joint until 3 to 4 years of age. A knee is often introduced with a manual locking option. The knee can be unlocked as the child gains more balance and control with specific activities. Controversy exists among clinicians and third-party payers about the appropriateness of sophisticated technology and expensive devices for toddlers and infants. Objective evaluations of change in functional status as a result of prosthetic fitting may be useful information for the clinician as well as third-party payers.

The Child Amputee Prosthetics Project–Functional Status Inventory (Capp-Fsit) was developed to objectively evaluate the change in functional status as a result of prosthetic fitting. The Capp-Fsit is a standardized instrument design of 37 developmentally appropriate behaviors to assess functional status in toddlers aged 1 to 4 years who have either upper- or lower-limb acquired or congenital limb deficiencies. Parents rate their child's performance on 37 developmental behaviors on a scale of whether the use of a prosthesis enables the child to perform an activity. The instrument may provide the answers to whether functional gains are made as a result of prosthetic fittings. The assessment of the functional status as an outcome of the prosthetic prescription for preschool children is one strategy to determine the effectiveness of the rehabilitation approach.[38] Table 12-3 outlines some of the lower-extremity behaviors assessed in the Capp-Fsit inventory.

Table 12-3. Selected Lower Extremity Items from the Child Amputee Prosthetics Project–Functional Status Inventory (CAPP-FSIT)

Task	Performance
Stands	Does activity
	Uses prosthesis
Walks on even ground	Does activity
	Uses prosthesis
Steps up and down a street curb	Does activity
	Uses prosthesis
Jumps	Does activity
	Uses prosthesis
Jumps over an object	Does activity
	Uses prosthesis
Runs	Does activity
	Uses prosthesis

Adapted from Pruitt, S. D., Varni, J. W., & Setoguchi, Y. (1999). Toddlers with limb deficiency: conceptual basis and initial application of a functional status outcome measure. *Archives of Physical Medicine and Rehabilitation*, 80, 819–824.

Seven to Twelve Years

Children demonstrate continuous growth changes as the preteen years approach and new interest and activities evolve. The fit, design, and componentry of the prosthesis must gradually be adapted to address growth and increasing function. Dynamic-response feet for children can improve their chances for successful sports competition.[37] Athletic children will begin to participate in complex low-level organized games then progress to regulated sports with adult rules. At school, when a child with an amputation does not appear secure during gym activities, an adapted physical educator may need to provide supplemental activities for balance and coordination training. Numerous recreational rehabilitative programs have been developed through hospital facilities, rehabilitation centers, or community-based organizations. The primary focus of these programs is to promote physical challenges and achievement of skills within a peer group framework. Participation in these programs has also proved to enhance the child's self-image and promote confidence in physical and social abilities. Recreational and sport activities for the individual with an amputation are presented in Chapter 13.

Thirteen to Eighteen Years

Physiologic changes and psychologic issues are intensified during the transition into adulthood for this age group. Cosmetic appearance and acceptance by one's peers become increasing important concerns for adolescent boys and girls. The older teenager must resolve issues regarding independence and career decisions.[11]

In this age group, advanced adult componentry, fitting, and training principles become more applicable. The prosthetic training program for this age group is contained in Chapter 7. The training program should be individually designed and include strengthening, balance drills, and coordination skills. Specific tasks to be achieved should include rising to standing from sitting; stationary upright balancing; challenged balancing; weight shifting forward, backward, and to the side; instructions in falling and how to rise from the floor; reciprocal gait patterns; distance walking on level surfaces; and walking on raised surfaces such as stairs, ramps, and curbs.[4] Advanced physical activities can be incorporated into an aerobic physical fitness program with the use of stationary bicycles, treadmills, and stair steppers. These young adults can also be challenged with climbing, jumping, and running activities within the capabilities of their prosthesis. Special adaptations can be provided to facilitate involvement in competitive sports, outdoor endeavors, and water activities.

Teenagers with a high unilateral or bilateral transfemoral amputation may opt to ambulate with the prosthesis only for special social occasions. Ambulation energy expenditure of individuals with lower-extremity amputations is presented in Table 7-1. The use of a wheelchair may become more practical for the individual with bilateral amputations. Ideally, these individuals should be self-sufficient and independent in transfers and mobility for community travel.[37]

Children with high-level residual limb amputations and complex prosthetic componentry will eventually decide whether to be prosthesis wearers when they reach adulthood. The decision of whether to make use of the prosthesis full-time may be influenced by the individual's commitment to be a household or community ambulator and the efficiency of ambulation with a prosthesis for work, school, or social events.

Financial Issues

The costs of a prosthesis or orthosis vary widely, depending on the degree of disability, the activity needs of the wearer, and the types of components and materials used. Financial issues are discussed in Chapter 3. For those who cannot afford the cost of a prosthesis or orthosis, there are various options for payment. An individual may apply for Medicaid funding. Medicaid approval for the device will be granted on the basis of need and income level. Local or national organizations such as the American Cancer Society may be of assistance. The Barr Foundation is a tax-deductible nonprofit national organization that often pays for prostheses (Resource Box 3-4).

CASE STUDY

PATIENT/CLIENT HISTORY

General Demographics/History of Current Condition

Mike Carnevale is a 1½-year-old toddler who developed a *Staphylococcus aureus* infection 3 months ago. Gangrene in the distal segments of all four extremities

and multiple organ system failure developed subsequently. He required multiple amputations consisting of a right knee disarticulation, left partial foot (five toes and half of the heel), and bilateral distal finger amputations. His acute hospital course was complicated by multiple skin grafts and residual limb revisions. He is currently medically stable. Mike also developed severe contractures of his fingers, wrists, and left heel cord. Two months ago, the right knee disarticulation was revised to a transfemoral amputation because of bone protrusion and lack of skin and muscle for coverage of the residual limb. Also, at this time, Mike underwent a left heel cord release to be appropriately fitted with an elevated wedged shoe for the left foot. Mike is scheduled for hand surgery to initiate releases of flexor contractures. His parents would like Mike to walk and develop skills that are age appropriate.

Social History

Mike lives with both parents in a first-floor apartment with two steps at the entrance. His mother is the primary care giver. He has no siblings.

Growth and Development

Mike was born full term, was healthy at birth, and reportedly met all developmental milestones on time prior to this infection and subsequent hospitalization. These milestones include fine and gross motor activities, cognitive, language, and social skills. He is right hand dominant.

Cognitive and Psychosocial Status

Mike is alert, is oriented to people and place, and demonstrates age-appropriate moods. He is beginning to express himself with one- to two-word phrases and understands short instructions such as "give me the toy."

TESTS AND MEASURES

Neuromotor Development/Sensorimotor Integration/Reflex Integrity

Mike demonstrates a scattering of gross motor skills, up to the 12-month level. He rolls independently in all directions, pushes up into sitting, combat crawls, creeps, pulls to stand with furniture and manual support, and sits back down by falling. He is revealing more motivation to be mobile in an upright standing position and to initiate gait training. Upper- extremity protective reactions are reemerging. Mike demonstrates functional reactions in all directions when sitting. However, these are delayed more posteriorly. Head and trunk righting and equilibrium reactions are reemerging in lower developmental positions. Balance reactions are nonfunctional in standing.

Anthropometric Characteristics

Mike's right residual limb is conical and measures 6 inches (15 cm) long from the ischial tuberosity.

Integumentary Integrity

Intact with all surgical incisions closed. Skin over the transfemoral incision is tender.

Range of Motion (ROM)

Bilateral upper-extremity ROM is significant for contractures of wrists, thumbs, and metacarpophalangeal and proximal interphalangeal joints. He holds his left hip in external rotation and has no internal rotation past neutral. Left plantarflexion ROM is 20–50° with an equinus contracture present. In a Thomas test position, left hip extension is missing 15° from neutral.

Muscle Performance

Muscle strength was graded in developmental activities. Strength, within available ranges, is graded as follows: bilateral hip flexion, 4/5; right hip extension, 2/5; left hip extension and knee extension and flexion, 3/5; left foot dorsiflexion and plantarflexion, 1/5.

Posture

The head and spine are held in proper alignment. Mike has a tendency to bear weight on the lateral aspects of the forearm and wrists. In standing, the left leg is externally rotated, and weight is on the ball of the foot.

Orthotic, Protective, and Supportive Devices

Mike wears an elevated wedged shoe for the left foot.

Functional Status

Mike is ready for upright standing and gait training.

a. Which socket would you recommend? Why?
b. Which suspension would you recommend? Why?
c. Which knee component would you recommend? Why?
d. Which foot–ankle assembly would you recommend? Why?

a. A quadrilateral socket allows weight bearing to be achieved by the ischium resting on the posterior brim. In a quadrilateral socket, the residual femur is allowed to drift more into abduction, which facilitates a wide-base gait that is appropriate for a toddler's gait pattern. The narrow medial lateral dimensions of the ischial-containment socket may be too confining and uncomfortable for the initial prosthesis.

b. A roll-on silicone suction suspension is recommended for Mike. This suspension will protect the tender skin over the incision. However, a disadvantage of this suspension is that frequent changes may be necessary as he grows.

c. Children younger than 2 years of age usually receive a prosthesis without a knee. This prosthesis allows the child to begin early weight bearing and gain confidence during ambulation activities before beginning to learn to control the knee component. If a knee is used, a hydraulic knee such as the Century XXII Innovations Child's Play Small Wonder Knee may be used.

d. A SACH foot is the traditional foot of choice for a child. It is stable, durable, and inexpensive. The SACH foot provides shock absorption through the heel cushion.

KEY POINTS

- Childhood amputations can be classified as congenital or acquired.

- Congenital deficiencies are identified as transverse or longitudinal; most transverse deficiencies do not usually require revisional surgery; longitudinal deficiencies present the most challenge in accommodating the deformity into a prosthetic device.

- Longitudinal and transverse deficiencies are identified according to the anatomic location of the defect.
- Trauma is the primary cause for acquired amputations, and malignant tumors are responsible for more than half of the amputations from disease processes.
- Terminal bony overgrowth is one of the most common complications affecting a residual limb from an acquired amputation.
- Retention of growth centers at the distal femur and proximal and distal tibia promotes growth of the residual limb for optimal prosthetic fit as an adult.
- The Ilizarov method and rotationplasty are two types of surgical procedures for limb salvage.
- Manufactured prosthetic components for infants are limited; manufacturers are beginning to address the need for more attractive, durable, simplistic, modular components for children.
- Parents and children must be considered vital contributing members of the prosthetic team. A parent's attitude can determine whether a child accepts or rejects the prosthesis.
- Children with congenital amputations do not usually experience a sense of loss of a body part at a young age. Children with acquired amputations experience grief and adjustment reactions similar to those of an adult.
- Physical therapy outcomes for prosthetic training should focus initially on preprosthetic care and preparation of the residual limb, total body strengthening and endurance training, and functional mobility with and without ambulation aids.
- Prosthetic training should be geared toward the acquisition of developmental milestones for infants and the achievement

of functional gait patterns with the least-restrictive walking aid for children and young adults; they should promote more-challenging experiences through sports and recreational activities.

CRITICAL THINKING QUESTIONS

1. Describe the different causes for, and types of, congenital and acquired amputations.

2. Differentiate among the types of limb salvage.

3. Assess the different types of sockets, suspensions, knees, and feet that may be used for pediatric patients with an amputation.

4. Describe ways in which the physical therapist may initially interact effectively with a child with an amputation and the parents.

5. Explain the developmental milestones that are present at different ages and the physical therapy and prosthetic implications for each of these age groups.

6. Review the prosthetic prescription case. Which other prosthetic components may be used for this case?

REFERENCES

1. Kay, H. W., & Fishman, S. (1967). *1018 Children with skeletal limb deficiencies.* New York: New York University Post Graduate Medical School, Prosthetic and Orthotics.
2. Jain, S. (1996). Rehabilitation in limb deficiency. The pediatric amputee. *Archives of Physical Medicine and Rehabilitation, 77,* S9–13.
3. Cotran, R. S., Kumar, V., & Robbins, S. L. (Eds.) (1994). *Robins pathologic basis of disease* (5th ed.). Philadelphia: W. B. Saunders.
4. O'Sullivan, S., & Schmitz, T. (1994). *Physical rehabilitation: Assessment and treatment* (3rd ed.). Philadelphia: F. A. Davis.
5. Day, H. B. (1991). The ISO/ISPO classification of congenital limb deficiency. *Prosthetics Orthotics International, 15,* 67–69.
6. Tecklin, J. S. (1999). Pediatric physical therapy (3rd ed., p. 391). Philadelphia: J. B. Lippincott.

7. Duthie, R., & Bentley, G. (Eds.) (1983). *Mercer's orthopaedic surgery* (8th ed., pp. 118–200). Baltimore: University Park Press, 1983.

8. Shurr, D. G., & Cook, T. M. (1990). *Prosthetics & orthotics* (pp. 183–193). East Norwalk, CT: Appleton & Lange.

9. Mueller, M. J., & Sinacore, D. R. (1994). Rehabilitation factors following transmetatarsal amputation. *Physical Therapy, 74*, 1027–1033.

10. Kruger, L. M. (1992). Lower limb deficiencies: Surgical management. In J. H. Bowker (Ed.), *Atlas of limb prosthetics: Surgical, prosthetic, and rehabilitation principles* (2nd ed., pp. 795–838). St. Louis: Mosby.

11. Bowker, J. H. (Ed.). (1992). *Atlas of limb prosthetics: Surgical, prosthetic, and rehabilitation principles* (2nd ed.). St. Louis: Mosby.

12. Aiken, G. T. (1969). Proximal femoral focal deficiency: Definition, classification, and management. In *Proximal femoral focal deficiency: A congenital anomaly*. Washington, DC: National Academy of Sciences.

13. Tachdjian, M. O. (1990). Congenital deformities. In M. O. Tachdjian (Ed.), *Pediatric orthopedics* (2nd ed.). Philadelphia: W. B. Saunders.

14. Stern, P. H. (1991). The epidemiology of amputations. *Physical Medicine and Rehabilitation Clinics of North America, 2*, 253–261.

15. Tooms, R. E. (1992). Acquired amputations in children. In J. H. Bowker (Ed.), *Atlas of limb prosthetics: Surgical, prosthetics, and rehabilitation principles* (2nd ed., pp. 735–741). St Louis: Mosby.

16. Shands, A. R., & Raney, B. (1971). Amputations, prostheses, and braces. In *Handbook of Orthopaedic Surgery* (7th ed., 268–298). St. Louis: Mosby.

17. Aiken, G. T. (1963). Surgical amputations in children. *Journal of Bone and Joint Surgery (Am), 45*, 1735–1741.

18. Tornetta, P., & Olson, S. A. (1997). Amputations versus limb salvage. *Instructional Course Lectures, 46*, 511–518.

19. Kenan, S., & Lewis, M. M. (1991). Limb salvage in pediatric surgery: The use of the expandable prosthesis. *Orthopedic Clinics of North America, 22*, 121–131.

20. Aronson, J. (1997). Limb lengthening, skeletal reconstruction, and bone transport with the Ilizarov method. *Journal of Bone and Joint Surgery (Am), 79A*, 1243–1258.

21. Krajbick, J. L., & Bochmann, D. (1992). Van Nes rotationplasty in tumor surgery. In J. H. Bowker (Ed.), *Atlas of limb prosthetics: Surgical, prosthetic, and rehabilitation principles* (2nd ed., pp. 855–899). St. Louis: Mosby.

22. Herzenberg, J. E. (1991). Congenital limb deficiency and limb length discrepancy. In S. T. Canale & J. H. Beatty (Eds.), *Operative pediatric orthopedics*. St. Louis: Mosby.

23. Gillespie, R. (1990). Principles of amputation surgery in children with longitudinal limb deficiencies of the femur. *Clinical Orthopaedics and Related Research, 256*, 29–38.

24. Smith, D. G., Burgess, E. M., & Zettl, J. H. (1992). Special considerations: Fitting and training the bilateral lower limb amputee. In J. H. Bowker (Ed.), *Atlas of limb prosthetics: Surgical, prosthetic, and rehabilitation principles* (2nd ed., pp. 599–622). St. Louis: Mosby.

25. Edelstein, J. E. (1996). Prosthetic assessment and management. In *Amputations and prosthetics* (pp. 397–422). Philadelphia: F. A. Davis.

26. Wilk, B., Karol, L., Halliday, S., Cummings, D., Haideri, N., & Stephenson, J. (1999). Transition to an articulating knee prosthesis in pediatric amputees. *Journal of Prosthetics and Orthotics, 11*, 69–74.

27. Madigan, R., & Fillauer, K. (1991). 3-S prosthesis: A preliminary report. *Journal of Pediatric Orthopedics, 11*, 112–117.

28. Nelson, (2000, Spring). Prosthetic and orthotic laboratory. Transfemoral socket and suspension. In *Your physical challenge*. Publication No. 14.

29. Stanger, M. (2000). Limb deficiencies and amputations. In S. K. Campbell (Ed.), *Physical therapy for children* (2nd ed., pp. 370–397). Philadelphia: W. B. Saunders.

30. Cliff, S., Gray, J., & Nymann, C. (1974). *Mothers can help: A therapist's guide*. El Paso, TX: El Paso Rehabilitation Center.

31. May, B. (1996). Assessment and treatment of individuals following lower extremity amputations. In *Amputations and prosthetics* (pp. 375–395). Philadelphia: F. A. Davis.

32. Erikson, E. H. (1968). *Identity: Youth and crisis*. New York: W. W. Norton.

33. Varni, J. W., & Setoguchi , Y. (1993). Effects of parental adjustment on the adaptation of children with congenital or acquired limb deficiencies. *Journal of Developmental and Behavioral Pediatrics, 14*, 13–20.

34. Friedmann, L. W. (1990). Rehabilitation of the lower extremity amputee. In F. J. Kottke & J. F. Lehmann (Eds.), *Krusen's handbook of physical medicine and rehabilitation* (4th ed.). Philadelphia: W. B. Saunders.

35. Berger, K. S. (1998). *The developing person through the life span* (4th ed.). New York: Worth Publishers.

36. Larin, H. (2000). Motor learning: Theories and strategies for the practitioner. In S. K. Campbell (Ed.), *Physical therapy for children* (2nd ed., pp. 173–197). Philadelphia: W. B. Saunders.

37. Oglesby, D. G., & Tablada, C. (1992). The child amputee: Prosthetic and orthotic management. In J. H. Bowker (Ed.), *Atlas of limb prosthetics: Surgical, prosthetic, and rehabilitation principles* (2nd ed., pp. 835–838). St. Louis: Mosby.

38. Pruitt, S. D., Varni, J. W., & Setoguchi, Y. (1999). Toddlers with limb deficiency: Conceptual basis and initial application of a functional status outcome measure. *Archives of Physical Medicine and Rehabilitation, 80,* 819–824.

Chapter 13

Sports Implications for the Individual with a Lower Extremity Prosthesis

Kendra Miller, PT

Objectives

1. Describe the value of sports for people with physical disabilities
2. Review the psychologic and physiologic benefits of exercise
3. Describe the categories of limb disablement
4. Differentiate among specific adaptations of various sport/prosthetic componentry to the individual with an amputation including swimming, cycling, golf, skiing, and running
5. Explain how physical therapists can be involved in training individuals with amputation to participate in sports
6. Describe obstacles to training or competition in sports for the individual with a lower-extremity amputation

This chapter is divided into the following sections:

The ultimate goal of physical therapy for the individual with a lower-extremity amputation is to restore safe ambulation with a prosthesis. For most people with lower-extremity amputation, who have comorbidities such as vascular disease, safe ambulation is the highest expected functional outcome. However, one must realize that it is possible for some individuals with lower-extremity amputations to engage in more-dynamic activities than walking. Over the past several decades, the desires of individuals with amputations to be more active have driven the advances in the prosthetic industry. As a result of enhanced componentry, the capability of this population to engage in competitive sporting events is becoming more and more impressive. Endoskeletal components make it easier to accommodate the specialized needs of almost any individual with an amputation. For example, with the use of a coupling device, an individual with a lower-extremity amputation can quickly change a prosthetic foot used for walking to one used for running or to one designed especially for swimming.

Physical therapists who are training individuals with lower-extremity amputation must be aware that the loss of a limb certainly does not preclude participation in sports. Patients, who are devastated after losing a limb, may initially focus on the things they will not be able to do. The rehabilitation team must present the opposite point of view and encourage them to achieve the highest level of activity and fitness possible. Physical therapists need to address the issue of sports and recreational activities in their initial subjective interview with patients. Knowing the specific activities a patient finds enjoyable or new activities he or she might want to pursue, allows the physical therapist to target training at the preprosthetic level toward a particular activity. For example, if an individual with a transfemoral amputation was a runner and wants to return to running, then it is important to specifically train the hamstrings and gluteal muscles for better knee control.

Physical therapists can encourage involvement in sports as a new activity for the individual who is seeking ways to stay physically fit. In addition to establishing new interests, sports involvement can also be an effective means of readjustment and community reentry for an individual with limb loss. Individuals with lower-extremity amputation may find great value in a variety of sport activities, whether for occasional leisure or for the challenges of Paralympic-level competition. A multitude of resources and community programs on an international level offer information and training for a wide variety of sports for the disabled (Resource Box 13-1).

Psychosocial and Physiologic Benefits of Exercise

Perhaps the greatest challenge the individual with an amputation must face is the psychologic one.[1] An individual who has undergone amputation will most likely experience a disturbance in body image, which can have a direct negative impact on well-being.[2] Involvement in sports and exercise can improve a person's physical and psychological well-being, whether disabled or not.[3–5] Recreation for individuals with an amputation not only promotes cardiovascular endurance but also enhances self-esteem.[6,7] Individuals who have undergone amputation of a limb may experience anxiety, sadness, depression, and anger as they grieve the loss of their limb. Sports participation is a positive way to rechannel or sublimate negative emotions.[6,8] A study of runners revealed that the most powerful motivator was the self-esteem created by overcoming the athletic challenge of running. The second and third top motivators were health, fitness, and mental well-being, respectively.[9] Getting the community of disabled individuals involved in sports can demonstrate their ability to achieve success and recognition to a sometimes skeptical society.[10]

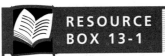

Sports Organizations and Suppliers for Persons with Limb Loss

Disabled Sports USA
451 Hungerford Drive; Suite 100
Rockville, MD 20850
Ph: (301)-217-0960
Fax: (301)-217-0968
e-mail: dsusa@dsusa.org
Web address: www.dsusa.org

O&P Athletic Fund
1650 King Street; Suite 500
Alexandria, VA 22314
Ph: (703)-836-7114
e-mail: opaaf@aol.com

Challenged Athletes Foundation
2148-B Jimmy Durante Blvd
Del Mar, CA 92014
Ph: (858)-793-9293
web address: www.challengedathletes.org

Wheelchair Sports USA
3595 East Fountain Blvd
Suite L-1
Colorado Springs, CO 80910
e-mail: wsusa@aol.com

Achilles Track Club
9 East 89th Street
New York, NY 10128
Ph: (212)-967-9300

Amputee Coalition of America
900 East Hill Road; Suite 285
Knoxville, TN 37915
Ph: (423)-524-8772
e-mail: acainfo@amputee-coalition.org
web address: www.amputee-coalition.org

American Amputee Soccer Association
web address: www.ampsoccer.org

Online Sports Links
web address: www.activeamp.org

Sled Hockey
web address: www.sledhockey.com

Zerosock Pro Pump
(877)-227-5195
web address: www.waterproof-cast-cover.com

Ski Eze USA Inc
4401 Devonshire
Lansing, MI 48910
Ph: (517)-487-0924

Sport for Disabled Ontario
web address: www.disabledsports.org

National Amputee Golf Association
P.O. Box 23285
Milwaukee, WI 53223
Ph: (800)-633-6242
Fax: (414)-376-1268
e-mail: naga@execpc.com

Eastern Amputee Golf Association
e-mail: info@eaga.org
web address: www.eaga.org

Amputee Golfer Magazine
web address: www.amputee-golf.org

US National Sports Center
P.O. Box 1290
Winter Park, CO 80482
Ph: (970)-726-1540
Fax: (858)-793-9291
e-mail: info@nscd.org
web address: www.nscd.org

Canadian Association of Disabled Skiers
(CADS)
P.O. Box 307 Kimberley, BC, Canada
web address: www.canuck.com

Canadian Amputee Soccer
web address: www.amputee-online.com/casa

Inline Skating
web address: www.pieretti.com

U.S. Wheelchair Basketball Association
web address: www.nwba.org

Alberta Amputee Sport and Recreation
Association
web address: www.aasra.ab.ca

Natural Access (Landeez Beach Chair)
Ph: (800)-411-7789
web address: www.natural-access.com

Patients sometimes feel isolated and alone following an amputation. It is often valuable to have individuals living with amputation who are already involved in sports activities provide peer visitation to those who have had a recent amputation. Sports participation is an excellent way to promote social integration and community reentry.[11] In addition, it encourages healthy competition, which gives the individual with an amputation a sense of accomplishment and the ability to overcome the feeling of being "disabled." Furthermore, competitiveness is goal oriented, which may assist the individual with an amputation in setting and achieving goals in other aspects of life.

Involvement in sports is instrumental as a therapeutic way to stay physically fit. In general, sports can serve as a way to improve range of motion, strength, endurance, coordination, and balance. Studies show that sedentary, able-bodied adults exercising their lower limbs can increase their cardiovascular fitness levels and muscle strength by 15 to 25%.[11-13] Muscular strength and cardiovascular endurance are extremely important to meet the extra demands of using a prosthesis. There is a direct relationship between energy expenditure for ambulation with a prosthesis and level of amputation. Patients with higher-level amputations have a less-efficient gait and higher oxygen cost than individuals with lower-level amputations.[14] Specific energy requirements for different amputation levels are reviewed in Chapter 7.

Physical therapists often provide their patients with an individualized, but basic, home exercise program to maintain or improve flexibility and strength. However, the addition of specific sports or sports-related activities can help to achieve additional fitness goals. For example, the individual with an amputation who wants to improve overall cardiovascular endurance and has good tolerance for higher-impact activities may benefit from learning to run. On the other hand, an individual with an amputation who also wants to improve overall cardiovascular endurance but cannot tolerate

high impacts may be better suited to pursuing walking or cycling instead. For an individual whose vascular system is moderately compromised, which is a common cause of amputation, a modified version of golf might be more appropriate. Many sports can be modified to facilitate an individual's level of comfort and success. Physical therapists can help their patients make informed decisions about which activities to pursue.

Categories of Limb Disablement

Individuals with lower-extremity amputations of all levels can participate in sports. From partial toe amputation, which requires no adaptation, to a transpelvic amputation, where extensive modifications may be likely, it is possible to enjoy many of the benefits of exercise and sports. The major categories of limb disablement include unilateral transtibial, unilateral transfemoral, unilateral hip disarticulation, and bilateral amputation of similar or combined levels. In general, the individual with a unilateral amputation can perform sports with or without the prosthesis; sports involvement for the individual with a bilateral amputation is more likely to require an adapted wheelchair or sitting apparatus. For most amputation categories, prosthetic advances and adaptive devices allow the sport to be played as true to form as possible. Successful competition is possible because of improvements in prosthetic componentry.[15] The modifications available to the sport or prosthetic componentry for the various amputation categories are presented as each particular sport is described in this chapter.

Sport-Specific Adaptations

Virtually any sport or activity imaginable can be performed with a little creativity on the part of the individual with an amputation, prosthetist, and therapist. Motivation and ingenuity of the patient and the rehabilitation team continue to drive the fabrication of many new special devices that enable an individual with an amputation to perform an infinite number of recreational activities.[16] The advent of endoskeletal componentry and more-flexible, lighter-weight and more-durable materials used to fabricate prostheses have further enabled athletes with amputation to participate in recreational activities. The use of a wide array of new materials has provided the improved socket suspension, fit, and comfort necessary for participation in sports. These materials include plastics such as polypropylene and polyethylene, synthetic rubbers, carbon, and other materials adopted from the aerospace industry. In addition, titanium has replaced heavier metals to create more-dynamic pylons and prosthetic feet. Fluid-controlled knee components allow smoother transitions and varying cadences. These prosthetic components are discussed in Chapters 8 and 9.

However, even with the most sophisticated prosthetic components, the individual often requires skilled training to resume or begin a particular sport with a specific prosthesis. It is the role of the physical therapist not only to understand what specialized components and adaptations exist, but also to know how to assist an individual in the use of them. Although the list of potential sports seems endless, the following description of prosthetic adaptations and training aspects relates to the more popular sports activities of swimming, cycling, golf, skiing, and running.

Swimming

Swimming is one of the best forms of physical conditioning and full-body strengthening, which minimizes impact stresses on the residual limb.[17] One detailed questionnaire study of 100 individuals with lower-extremity amputation showed that 76% of the active individuals with an amputation went swimming at least once per week.[18] This was one of the most common recreational activities performed, and nearly 100% of those who swam before the amputation were able to return to this activity postamputation. The backstroke is often the easiest stroke to accomplish[7,19] and the butterfly the most difficult to master.[18] Of consideration is not only whether to swim with or without a prosthesis, but also the method of getting in and out of different water sources.

Many individuals with an amputation can swim well without using a prosthesis. In fact, competitive swimmers at the Paralympic level are not permitted to wear a prosthesis while competing.[15,19] However, there are advantages to wearing a prosthesis. These include getting in and out of the water with greater ease and safety, increased balance and stability when standing in the water, and the provision of added propulsion. Some individuals report feeling unbalanced when kicking without a prosthesis, because they tend to drift toward the sound side.[15,17,20] This drift is due to differences in relative density and buoyancy between the two sides of the body. Side-bending the head and breathing toward the sound side may help a person with amputation to swim straight. Swimming without a prosthesis may cause the residual limb to swell somewhat in the water, making it difficult to put on the prosthesis afterward.[19] Without using any modifications to the individual's everyday prosthesis, getting to and from the water source is often more challenging than the act of swimming itself. One option is to walk to a swimming pool's edge and then remove the prosthesis and jump into the water. Some pools have stairs or ladders that the individual can negotiate without a prosthesis. Other individuals choose to take the prosthesis off away from the water to prevent any damage and then hop to the water, with or without an assistive device.[18] A nonskid shoe should be worn when hopping on a wet pool deck.

Water-resistant prostheses may be used for walking to and from the water source, for swimming, or for showering (Fig. 13-1). These

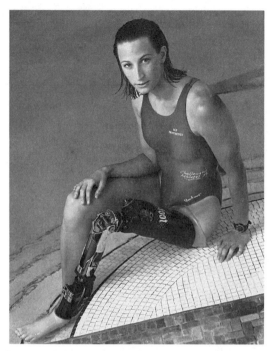

Figure 13-1. Individual wearing the prosthesis to the waters edge. (Photo by Tim Montoani, Reprinted with permission from Challenged Athletes Foundation.)

special prostheses allow water to flow in and out of the shank. Water enters a hole drilled through the ankle block and then flows into a hollow shank. This helps to equalize the specific gravity of the prosthesis to the surrounding water while swimming and decreases buoyancy, thereby minimizing the tendency of the prosthesis to float. Likewise, when the swimmer exits the pool, the water flows out of the prosthesis, making it lighter, for more-efficient gait.[16] The typical design of this waterproof transtibial prosthesis is a hard socket with rubber supracondylar cuff suspension and a SACH foot.[21] In addition, a removable heel lift can accommodate for the change in heel height from bare foot to shoe.[16] A similar device can be used as a diving limb.[22]

Another option is an adjustable foot–ankle unit, which tends to be used by more-proficient swimmers. This system has an ankle unit that locks in two positions, 90° for walking and 120° for swimming. The plantarflexed position helps to eliminate drag in the water when swimming.[16] Positions may be easily switched by activating a ring located in the posterior calf area. This unit, also called the *swim/walk leg,* is constructed of waterproof and corrosion-resistant polypropylene and stainless steel, which is especially important when exercising in salt water.[15,19]

A swimming flipper is another excellent modification to provide more-efficient swimming. A flipper is fitted to foam on the distal end of the socket, and a sleeve suspension secures the socket on the limb. The overall length of the flipper device is made to be equal to the other leg. The flipper should be offset laterally just enough to avoid repeated contact with the contralateral leg.[20] Individuals with transfemoral or bilateral transtibial amputations may find it more practical to swim without the added lever arm resistance of a prosthesis. For those with transfemoral amputations, the flipper replaces an easily detachable knee–pylon unit, allowing one to walk to the swimming area, change to the flipper, and then reattach the walking components afterward, without having to make a socket change.[16] Swimming flippers or fins are also nice modifications for snorkeling or scuba diving.[15,21]

A socket device is available for individuals with bilateral transtibial amputations. It consists of a supracondylar fiberglass-reinforced socket with a rubber rocker laminated to the distal end. This system is beneficial because it allows ambulation to the water source and use in the water.[20] Prostheses may also be used to enable surfing (Fig. 13-2). Persons with amputations can use the water as a medium to exercise if not to swim. With or without a prosthesis the individual can work on strength, weight shifting and balance in a variety of positions.

For those who enjoy the beach, one must consider maneuvering on the sand. Walking may be more difficult due to the soft, giving nature of the sand. Extra assistive devices may be necessary for safe walking on the beach, re-

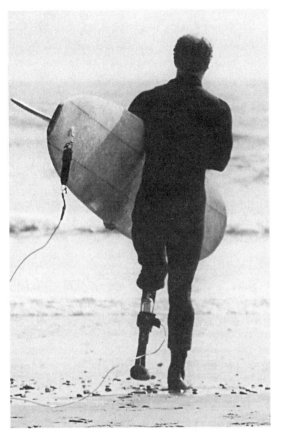

Figure 13-2. Individual wearing a waterproof transfemoral prosthesis for surfing. (Reprinted with permission from NextStep Orthotics and Prosthetics Inc.)

gardless of the prosthetic componentry used. Vacuum sealed covers can be worn over the everyday prosthesis to protect from sand and water. Standard wheelchairs are also difficult to maneuver in the sand and may not be fully protected from the effects of sand and water. Aquatic wheelchairs are designed for use both on the beach and in the water. The Landeez all terrain vehicle is shown in Figure 13-3. The aquatic chair has hand-operated flippers for propulsion in the water, and an anchor to stabilize the chair. The backrest may be used as a life vest. A 20-foot tethering cord is also available to allow the individual with an amputation to swim safely out of the chair.[19]

Cycling

Cycling is an activity that can be done at recreational or competitive levels, on a stationary bike, or outdoors by the more proficient cyclist. Many individuals with an amputation choose cycling as a mode of exercise to increase aerobic conditioning without high-impact weight bearing and stresses to the residual limb. Another advantage of cycling as a primary exercise or recreational activity is that riding a bicycle is familiar to most people, even if from one's youth. Riding can be done with or without a prosthesis, but generally individuals with a transtibial amputation wear a prosthesis, and cyclists with transfemoral amputations do not.[15,17,19]

Individuals with a transtibial amputation more commonly choose to use their everyday prosthesis for cycling (Fig. 13-4). Generally, little modification is needed. The posterior rim of the socket may need to be lowered to decrease the friction from the repeated knee flexion of cycling. Additional suspension may also be required for more rigorous cycling. One

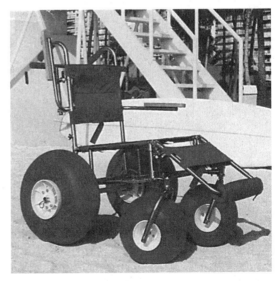

Figure 13-3. The Landeez all terrain wheelchair which can be used on the beach, in snow, or on grass. It can be folded for traveling. (Reprinted with permission from Natural Access)

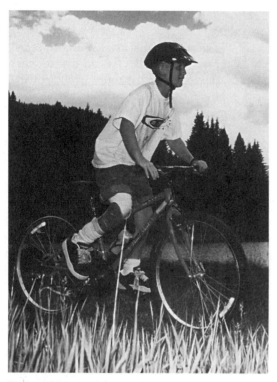

Figure 13-4. Individual with a transtibial prosthesis cycling. (Photo by Darcy Kiefel, Reprinted with permission from National Sports Center for the Disabled.)

must consider the consequences of not using a prosthesis, which include decreased overall cycling power, the residual limb being in a dependent position, and the danger that the residual limb may be struck and injured by the pedal. Before riding outdoors, an individual should practice on a stationary bike to ensure proper socket fit and comfort.[15,17,21] An individual may wear a cycling prosthesis, which is a custom socket without a foot, that clips directly into the pedal (Fig. 13-5).

An individual with a transfemoral amputation often chooses not to wear a prosthesis for biking for several reasons. The increased, repeated hip flexion may cause irritation at the site where the proximal anterior socket meets the anterior pelvic area. Sitting on a bicycle seat can be uncomfortable when wearing a transfemoral socket. It is often difficult to

power the prosthetic side when cycling, because of either lack of inherent knee control or increased prosthetic knee resistance. When cycling without a prosthesis, it is common to remove the pedal on that side. To maintain balance, one must keep both hands on the handlebars, as the upper body must compensate for the imbalance of single-legged cycling. Setting the handlebars slightly higher than usual may also help to maintain balance.[23]

The safety of mounting and dismounting the bicycle without a prosthesis is a concern. The individual should stand with the amputated side closer to the bike to swing the residual limb over the seat more easily. Another option is to walk to the bike and remove the prosthesis once securely on the seat. This should be done with the sound side closer to the bicycle so one can stabilize on the prosthetic side while more freely swinging the sound limb over the seat. It is especially easier for the person with a transfemoral amputation to swing the sound side over the seat and then use it for leverage to lift the rest of the body up onto the bike.

Should an individual with a transfemoral amputation choose to cycle with a prosthesis, there are several factors to consider. A comfortable seating saddle must be wide enough to provide balance without pinching the residual thigh between the seat and the socket. A racing saddle is generally used, but a woman's saddle may be preferable for its wider posterior aspect and subsequent added balance.[15] A flexible, brimmed socket with lower trim lines anteriorly may limit the irritation with repetitive hip flexion. To increase the ease of the cycling motion, a hydraulic knee in the free-swinging mode is ideal.[17,19] Figure 13-6 depicts two individuals, one with a transtibial prosthesis and one with a transfemoral prosthesis, enjoying cycling.

Toe clips or straps may be used to help keep the foot on the pedal. Toe clips render a more-effective circular motion, giving the individual more power in both the upward and downward movements of the pedal. However, toe clips

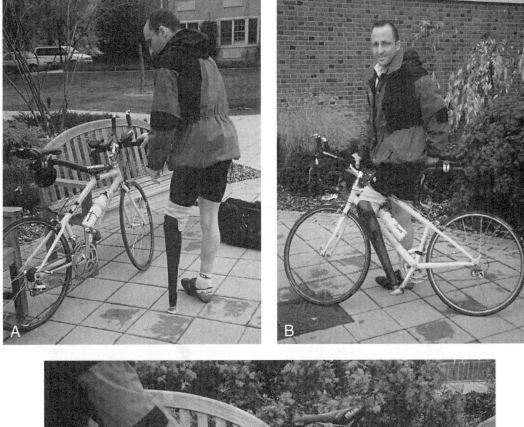

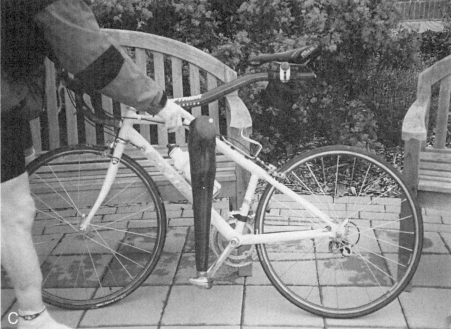

Figure 13-5. Individual with a transtibial cycling prosthesis with pin suspension that clips directly into the bicycle pedal. (Photo by Kendra Miller, PT.)

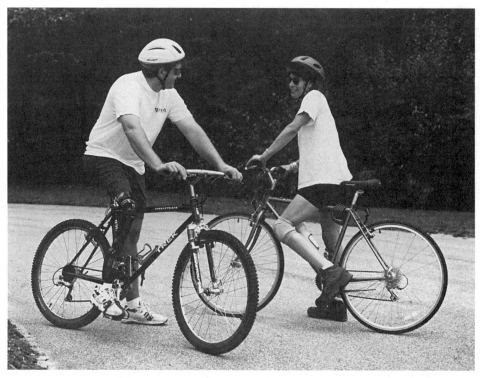

Figure 13-6. Two individuals, one with a transtibial and one with a transfemoral prosthesis, enjoying cycling. (Reprinted with permission from NextStep Orthotics and Prosthetics Inc.)

should be used with caution, because the foot may be trapped in the clip during a fall. An individual may achieve powerful pedal motion without the use of a toe clip by positioning the prosthetic heel directly over the pedal, rather than using the more conventional placement of the metatarsal heads over the pedal.[15,17,19,21] Another suggestion with regard to the pedal on the prosthetic side is to extend it laterally away from the bike approximately 2 inches to allow greater heel clearance, as the prosthetic heel tends to strike the frame of the bike.[23]

Individuals with hip disarticulation amputations face additional challenges in bicycling because of the greater imbalance between the two sides of the body. These individuals or those with bilateral lower-extremity amputations often choose to ride a hand-cranked cycle device which can be a separate road racing cycle. For less active individuals, a stationary upper extremity ergometer may be used.[19]

Stationary bicycles offer additional variations that may be desirable. One type of stationary bicycle has a recumbent seat that is much broader than a bicycle saddle and has a backrest. Many stationary bicycles have stirrups attached to the pedals for improved foot positioning and stability (Fig. 13-7). Some stationary bikes come with reciprocating arm attachments to provide a full-body workout, with the arms and legs moving together or separately. A lower extremity ergometer that may be attached to a standard wheelchair is another option.[19]

Golf

In one study, 28% of the 100 survey responders played golf prior to their amputation, while

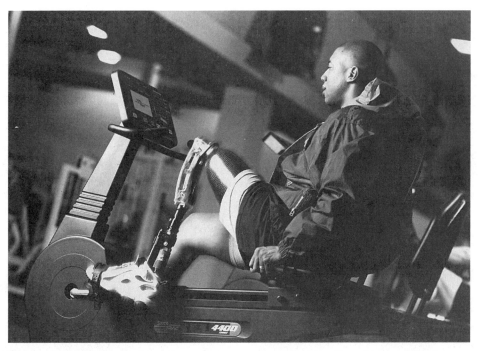

Figure 13-7. Individual with transfemoral prosthesis on a recumbent bike. Does this prosthetic foot appear to be optimally positioned? (Reprinted with permission from Ohio Willow Wood.)

35% said they played golf postamputation.[18] This statistic indicates that golf is a reasonable activity for individuals with amputation to learn for the first time if they are not returning to the sport. Individuals of many ages with any level of amputation can enjoy playing golf. More modifications may be warranted for those with higher-level amputations and bilateral amputations.

Golf course terrain and distance may be too challenging for some individuals with an amputation, especially if there is vascular insufficiency in the nonamputated leg. Walking 18 holes can total 5 miles; therefore, the golfer with an amputation may benefit from using an electric golf cart.[19,21] Individuals who choose to play golf without wearing a prosthesis can play standing while leaning against the golf cart or wheelchair for support. Golf can also be played in the sitting position, usually in an electric cart with a swivel seat. Another option for the indi-

vidual with bilateral transfemoral amputations is an elevated seat placed in a wheelchair (Fig. 13-8). One investigator described a method of increasing stability, especially helpful for the individual with bilateral transfemoral amputations.[19] This method involves mounting a bicycle seat on top of a standard camera tripod, enabling the golfer to sit on the seat while weight bearing through the prostheses.[19]

Golfers who play while standing independently on their prosthesis usually have a rotator adapter unit attached to the pylon. This permits rotation over a fixed foot and reduces the shear at the residual limb socket interface.[16,21] If a right-handed golfer has a left lower-extremity amputation, the prosthesis can have the rotator device to allow smoother inward rotation of that forward leg during backswing (Figs. 13-9 and 13-10). The right-handed golfer with a right-sided amputation is at a disadvantage and may need to modify the swing

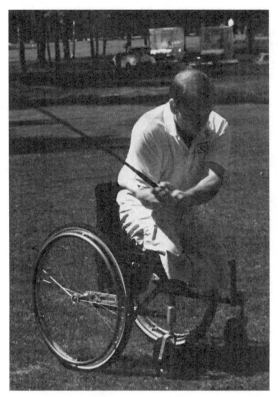

Figure 13-8. Individual with bilateral transfemoral amputations playing golf from a wheelchair. (Reprinted with permission from NextStep Orthotics and Prosthetics Inc.)

Skiing

Individuals with amputations at any level can enjoy alpine or downhill skiing. As with golf, there are a number of national organized classes to teach individuals to ski using a variety of methods and adaptive equipment. The concept of skiing for individuals with amputation originated in Austria and Germany in 1948. The National Amputee Ski Association was formed in 1967, helping those with limb loss learn to ski both recreationally and competitively.[19] Today snow skiing is a popular competitive sport for individuals with an am-

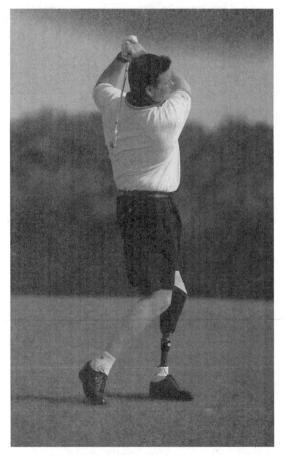

Figure 13-9. Individual displaying rotating pylon. Note that the prosthetic foot and knee are pointing in opposite directions. (Reprinted with permission from College Park Industries Inc.)

by maintaining the weight over the sound limb. Another option is to play left-handed. One disadvantage of a rotator unit is that it adds weight to the prosthesis. Some golfers remove the spikes from golf shoes to permit greater rotation on the ground through the shoe.[15,19] A swivel golf shoe has an adaptive device that attaches directly to the golf shoe to allow greater rotation on the prosthetic side.[19]

There are several organizations that teach adaptive golf to individuals with an amputation or the general population with disability and host national tournaments. One such group is the National Amputee Golf Association, incorporated in 1954, from which the First Swing Clinics began.[24]

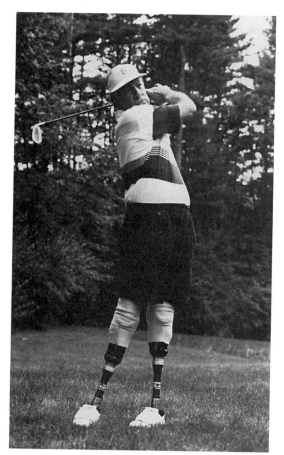

Figure 13-10. Individual with bilateral transtibial amputations with rotating and tilting pylons playing golf. (Reprinted with permission from NextStep Orthotics and Prosthetics Inc.)

putation. Two national organizations that currently offer adaptive skiing programs are Disabled Sports USA[25] and the National Sports Center for the Disabled.[26]

Those with unilateral transtibial amputations can ski with or without a prosthesis (Fig. 13-11).The major concern when skiing with a prosthesis is simulating the increased ankle dorsiflexion needed to bring the skier's center of gravity far enough forward for proper balance and control. This can be done to some degree with a heel wedge. More-avid skiers benefit from a specialized ski prosthesis. This

specialized prosthesis consists of a socket that is aligned with the anterior brim approximately 1 inch posterior to the prosthetic toes. The overall length of this prosthesis is shortened to equal the length of the opposite leg with maximum dorsiflexion. The foot and ankle unit used can be solid, single axis, or multiaxial, depending on the individual's skill level. The distal portion of the socket may need to be reinforced with carbon fiber to counteract the strong forward lean of the skier. Additional suspension, such as a belt, band, or sleeve, is often required with the ski prosthesis to avoid any pistoning of the residual limb. The bulging caused by the anterior socket alignment decreases the ski legs cosmesis and may make it difficult to wear ski pants. This prosthesis is not recommended for ambulation, so the individual must have the everyday prosthesis for use before and after skiing.[19]

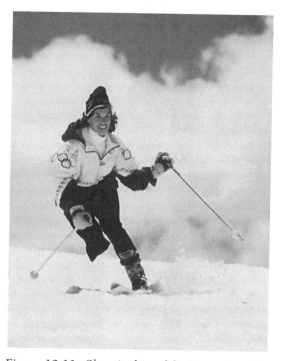

Figure 13-11. Olympic ski medalist Bonnie St. John Deane skis without a prosthesis, using regular ski poles. (Reprinted with permission from Bonnie St. John Deane.)

For those with unilateral amputations who elect to ski without a prosthesis, the three-track skiing method is used. The technique is called *three-track skiing* because the skier uses one ski and two outriggers, leaving tracks from three skis in the snow. Outriggers, devised by the West Germans after World War II, are forearm crutches with ski tips mounted on a rocker base (Fig 13-12).[27] In contrast to regular ski poles, outriggers offer increased balance to the single-legged skier. An adjustable pull cord allows the ski tips to be locked horizontally when skiing and locked vertically for use as regular crutches when walking on flat surfaces.[15] A more advanced skier can use regular ski poles instead of outriggers.

Those with bilateral amputations can learn four-track skiing, using two skis and two outriggers. This is the method of skiing taught to individuals with a variety of physical disabilities. A metal ski handle device may be clamped to the ski tips to maintain the skis in a consistent parallel or wedge position as the person is skiing downhill. This provides great lateral stability (Fig. 13-13).[15,26,27]

If one cannot ski in a standing position, either a sit-ski device or the more sophisticated monoski may be used. The sit ski is a kayaklike sled consisting of a lightweight fiberglass shell

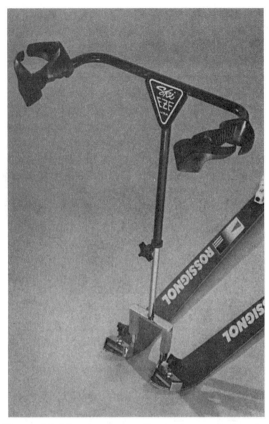

Figure 13-13. The Ski Handle may be attached to the ski tips for increased stability. (Reprinted with permission from Ski Eze USA Inc.)

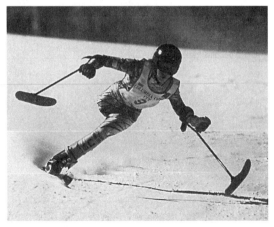

Figure 13-12. Downhill skiing with outriggers. (Photo by Byron Stetzler, Reprinted with permission from National Sports Center for the Disabled.)

with metal edges. The sit skier turns the sled by weight shifting and trunk leaning in conjunction with using short ski poles. Otherwise, gravity does the work of pulling the sit ski down the hill, and the more challenging task may be stopping the sled. It is common to have an assistant behind the sit ski, attached by a tether, to help control turning and stopping. This partner, or "tetherer," also gives better visibility to the person in the sled as well as to surrounding skiers, as the sit ski rests close to the ground.[15,19,27] The monoski, introduced in the United States in 1985, offers much faster motion than the sit ski. It has a bucket seat that is suspended over a single ski. For greater balance and stability, it can be mounted over two skis, referred to as a *bi-ski* (Fig. 13-14), A tether may be used with a bi-ski for controlled descent (Fig. 13-15). The monoski has a hydraulic lift that allows the seat to be raised for easier transfer in and out of the device. The monoski is locked in the lowered position while skiing. Shortened outriggers are used to control and steer the monoski. Successful use of the monoski requires great strength and balance.[15,19,25–27]

Nordic, or cross-country, skiing provides an excellent full-body strengthening and cardiovascular workout without causing impact stresses to the residual limb. Like downhill skiing, this sport can be done in standing or in a sit ski with regular short poles or outriggers. Many hand cyclists and wheelchair racers train with a cross-country sit ski during the winter. In standing, the skiing movement is comparable to the gliding motion of skating, and therefore, good mediolateral stability is required. A slightly inset prosthetic foot helps maintain the foot underneath the skier's body for improved side-to-side weight shifting. Bindings and

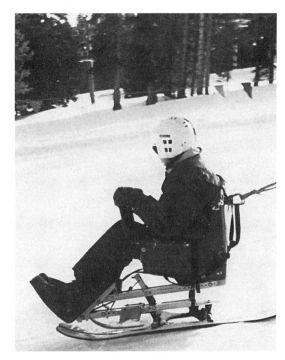

Figure 13-15. Use of a tether for controlled descent on a monoski (Reprinted with permission from Mountain Man Inc.)

boots attach the toes, but not the heels, to the ski. Straps placed behind the heel plate are available to prevent excessive backsliding during push-off of the ski. Cross-country skis are longer and narrower than downhill skis, for an even greater challenge to balance.[17,19,26,27]

Running

Most individuals with amputation agree that one of the hardest activities to master is running. One study of 100 individuals with amputation found that 28% of respondents jogged regularly prior to amputation, whereas, only 5% did so after amputation.[18] Those with amputation can learn to jog or run for the recreational benefits of the task itself or to incorporate it into other sports such as basketball or baseball. However, running is one basic skill that can be considered a safety tool, for example, to avoid a moving vehicle or to chase after

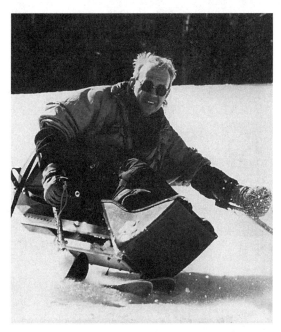

Figure 13-14. Skier using a bi-ski device and outriggers. (Reprinted with permission from Mountain Man Inc.)

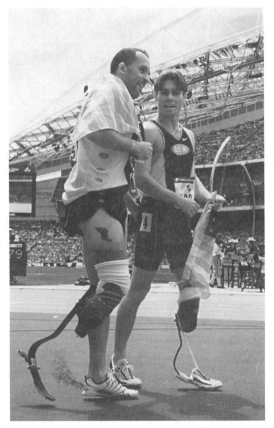

Figure 13-16. Two individuals with transtibial amputations at a track competition event. (Reprinted with permission from Flex Foot and Jim Rae.)

shock absorption, the natural knee flexion during early stance provides additional forward momentum. This allows smoother, faster, and more-efficient motion throughout the running cycle. It is recommended that the individual with a transtibial amputation with adequate quadriceps strength land closer to the ball of the prosthetic foot than to the heel during initial ground contact to further reduce the stresses transmitted to the spine. [15,17] Figure 13-16 shows two individuals with transtibial amputa-

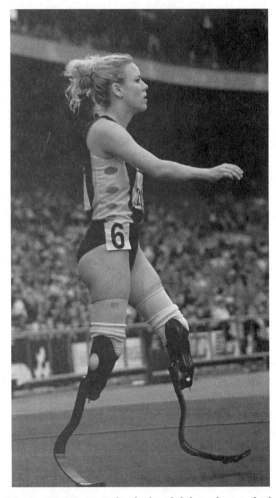

Figure 13-17. An individual with bilateral transtibial amputations ready for competition. (Reprinted with permission from Flex Foot and Jim Rae.)

one's child. [28-30] Unlike the sports discussed above, running absolutely requires the use of a prosthesis and can cause musculoskeletal stress to the residual limb and other joints from the impact of vertical landing.

Those with transtibial amputations can run with biomechanics similar to those of the able-bodied runner and can learn to run considerably more easily than individuals with a transfemoral amputation. The intact quadriceps muscles provide eccentrically controlled knee flexion to dampen the vertical load at initial contact and midstance for the individual with a transtibial amputation. Along with greater

tion at a track competition event. Figure 13-17 depicts an individual with bilateral transtibial amputations ready for competition. (Note specialized shock-absorbing prostheses in which the keel extends directly to the socket.)

Individuals with a transfemoral amputation require excellent balance and prosthetic knee control to be able to run leg over leg. Traditionally, these individuals learn to run with a hop-skip pattern that provides a double period of support on the sound limb. Although this method is not performed with both legs off the ground simultaneously as with true running, it does yield a faster speed than walking. The hop-skip running cycle is described in Practical Application Box 13-1. The need for double time on the sound limb exists to allow the prosthetic foot proper time to clear the ground and land. This takes more time due to the excessive heel rise caused by some prosthetic knees. Individuals with transfemoral amputation who can run leg over leg do so less efficiently than persons with an intact knee extensor mechanism. This decreased efficiency is due to the residual limb having to absorb more of the ground reaction force during initial contact. The prosthetic industry has played a significant role in improving the running capabilities of individuals with amputation in recent years. A special transtibial running prosthesis can weigh less than 3 lb.[17] Those with lower-extremity amputations experience a more comfortable and normal running stride with shock-absorbing pylons, which help dampen the impact at initial contact. In the early 1980s dynamic-response feet appeared, starting with the Seattle foot. This foot and the many other dynamic-response prototypes that followed provide a varying amount of push-off in the late stance phase. The use of lighter-weight, flexible materials such as Delrin plastic, carbon fiber, and graphite composite give these feet a springlike quality. Dynamic-response feet are especially effective for higher-impact activities such as running because they reduce the vertical ground reaction force, which can exceed two to three times a person's body

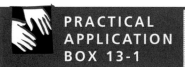

PRACTICAL APPLICATION BOX 13-1

The Hop-Skip Running Cycle

The hop-skip running cycle begins with a long stride with the prosthetic leg, landing and rolling over an extended knee, followed by a short-stride hop with the sound leg. Then, the double-stance phase occurs as the individual hops on the sound limb again. This gives sufficient time to clear the prosthetic foot in swing phase and safely achieve full knee extension again at or before initial contact to complete the gait cycle.[15,17,30]

weight.[5,19,30,31] Dynamic-response feet are described in Chapter 8.

The type of socket used can affect the stability and comfort of individuals with an amputation while running. Proper socket fit is crucial for any activity that involves running or jumping. A solid outer socket with a flexible liner with cutouts for bony, sensitive, or muscle-bulging areas is preferred. For individuals with a transtibial amputation, a total-surface bearing (TSB) socket is better for high-impact sports because of its increased surface area for weight bearing. This is in contrast to the patellar tendon bearing socket, which concentrates the weight-bearing load and stress mostly onto the patellar tendon. The transfemoral socket should be an ischial containment design to provide optimal alignment stability and control of the femur in the frontal plane.[17] Transfemoral sockets are discussed in Chapter 9.

The evolution of new knee components has also had a great positive impact on the quality of running for the individual with a transfemoral amputation. In the mid-1980s, John Sabolich introduced the O.K.C. running system. This system consists of a cable-housing arrangement that runs from the posterior hip joint to the proximal anterior shank of an exoskeletal prosthesis. At preswing, when the hip first starts to flex, tension in the cable causes a dynamic extension moment at the knee. The tension is at its maximum when the hip is fully flexed. This reduces the excessive heel rise otherwise seen during swing, and allows quicker movement into knee extension before initial contact. The O.K.C. system permits more efficient, true running in a leg-over-leg pattern.[19,32]

The ideal prosthetic knee for running and other vertical-impact sports is the hydraulic unit. Adjustable hydraulic resistance during knee flexion and extension allows varying cadences. When running, faster prosthetic knee extension is achieved with decreased resistance to extension, while increasing the flexion resistance decreases the amount of heel rise. This combination of adjustments lowers the amount of time needed for the prosthetic swing phase, thus eliminating the need for a double-stance phase. Therefore, hydraulically controlled knees are the units of choice for individuals with a transfemoral amputation who wish to run quickly, leg over leg.[17,33] Figure 13-18 shows a young individual with bilateral transfemoral prostheses using hydraulic knee units.

Microprocessor-controlled knee units, recently introduced, take prosthetic technology one step further. An onboard computer adjusts the pneumatic or hydraulic resistance of the knee, permitting a broadened range of cadence, from very slow to very fast. Based on adjustments that the prosthetist selects and inputs, the onboard sensors control the swing-phase timing in response to ambulation cadence. This microprocessor knee unit is shown in Figure 13-19. This feature is very beneficial for runners with an amputation.[33]

In addition to optimizing the prosthetic components used, one must consider the surface on which the individual is running. Grass is relatively soft and decreases impact, causing

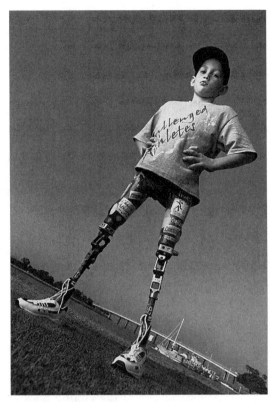

Figure 13-18. Young individual with bilateral transfemoral prostheses using multiaxial and hydraulic knee units. (Photo by Tim Montoani, competition. Reprinted with permission from Challenged Athletes Foundation.)

less traumatic stress to the residual limb. However, increased balance and caution are required because of the uneven nature of this terrain. Concrete, on the other hand, provides a better platform for dynamic-response feet, but it can cause greater impact stresses to the body. Hard rubber tracks seem to offer the best combination of a flat, but slightly forgiving surface. Treadmills with shock-absorbing platforms are a good choice for indoor training.[17] However, treadmills are not as good for faster-pace running because they do not allow true forward motion.

For those who cannot tolerate the stresses and impact of running, especially the geriatric population, a good alternative is walking for exercise or recreation. Walking does not require the same dynamic prosthetic componentry that running does. However, those with a transfemoral amputation benefit from a hydraulic or pneumatic knee unit for varying cadences. Maintaining a consistent walking pace is necessary to elevate the heart rate for a cardiovascular training effect. Another option for endurance training is negotiating upward elevations; however, the person with transfemoral amputation must take caution to sidestep up a steep incline. Because no current ankle unit can flex in the open-chain swing-through cycle of gait if an incline is too steep, the prosthetic foot will not clear the incline. This makes it unsafe to negotiate leg over leg. Persons with transtibial amputation can compensate for this by flexing their hip and knee at a greater angle to clear the foot. Walking on a treadmill can be an excellent source of exercise. Many treadmills have objective speed and distance readings, an option to incline the tread to a varying

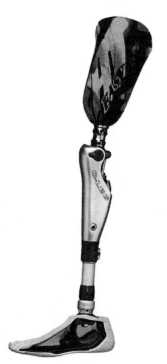

Figure 13-19. Otto Bock 3C100 leg. (Reprinted with permission from Otto Bock Industries Inc.)

degree, and safety features to stop the machine quickly.

Physical Therapy Involvement in Training

Physical therapists can be involved in training individuals with limb loss either during the patient's rehabilitation process or at the community level. The patient needs to understand that wearing a prosthesis does not limit participation in recreational or competitive activities. Intervention plans and outcomes should extend beyond the basic functional activities of daily living to some degree, especially if the individual identifies a particular activity to resume or pursue. The physical therapist can be instrumental in helping the patient, based on medical and physical status, select a suitable activity to learn. The emphasis should be placed on enjoying the activity, without pressure to participate. Training can begin in the preprosthetic phase of rehabilitation. Although a basic strength and endurance program is essential for the sake of performing functional tasks, with or without a prosthesis, greater strength, balance, and control may be required to do certain activities. For example, if the patient wants to return to playing golf, it will be necessary to focus considerably on the patient's static standing balance and trunk mobility. On the other hand, if the individual wishes to return to playing tennis, interventions must focus on overall strength, endurance, and dynamic stability.

It is unrealistic to expect a new prosthetic wearer to be proficient in a particular sport by the time of discharge from early physical therapy. It is unsafe and detrimental to do too much too soon, as the patient's soft tissues must develop a tolerance to the constant pressure and new weight bearing surfaces of the prosthesis.[17] During initial rehabilitation, higher-level activities may seem unimportant to the patient who just wants to be able to walk first. However, eventually new recreational outlets are needed.[6] What the physical therapist should do during the course of rehabilitation is encourage and prepare the patient, both physically and mentally, for involvement in recreational or competitive sports, as appropriate. In addition, the earlier stage of rehabilitation is a good time to introduce the patient to other, more-seasoned individuals with amputation in the community. This not only allows peer exchange of information that the rehabilitation team may not be able to provide, but also helps to bridge a gap between the hospital and community settings. Likewise, the physical therapist should keep the patient with an amputation informed of any organized events such as support groups or sports clinics. Observation of a sporting event (e.g., a triathlon) involving individuals with prostheses may be a good motivating influence (Figs. 13-20, 13-21).

Many individuals with amputation who pursue different sports are no longer receiving skilled physical therapy. Physical therapists, with their knowledge of biomechanics and prosthetics and an awareness of how comorbidities and medications may affect a person's exercise tolerance, can act as educators and consultants to coaches in the community who are providing the training. Remember that safety is *always* paramount. For example, swimming should be performed in a supervised swimming pool initially rather than a lake or other large body of water. Golfing on a full course should be preceded by practice runs at the golf range. A cart should be used the first time on a golf course, as the individual may not anticipate the possible fatigue of repeated walking and standing. These are only some examples; one must use common sense and think ahead in all situations. As with any organized sports program, one must keep certain supplies on hand.[6] A list of first aid supplies is contained in Practical Application Box 13-2.

Individuals with amputation who participate in organized sports need to be well adapted to their prosthesis if they are to use the prosthesis for the activity. Soft tissues of the residual limb must be intact and have accommodated to the changes in pressure from the socket. The individual must learn to trust the prosthesis when weight bearing. One outcome of skilled therapy intervention may be to in-

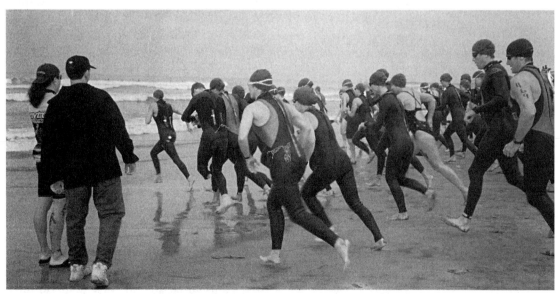

Figure 13-20. Can you find the individual with a transtibial amputation entering the water to begin this triathlon?

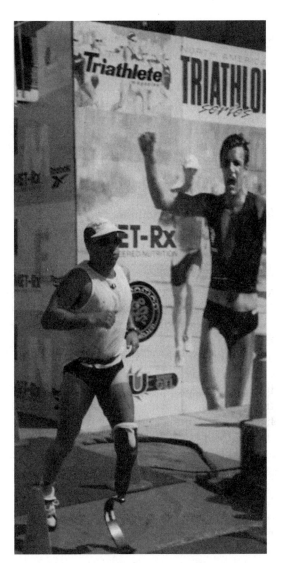

Figure 13-21. Individual with a transtibial amputation crossing the finish line in a triathlon competition. (Reprinted with permission from Ray Viscome.)

crease the weight bearing, balance, and stability over the prosthesis with dynamic activities. The therapist may want to recommend a specific prosthetic adaptation for a particular sport. In general, the participant's prosthetist should be aware of what sports an individual with an amputation is pursuing. The indi-

vidual who wears the prosthesis for more-dynamic activities should be taught proper hygiene procedures to prevent pressure sores or other residual limb problems. Individuals who choose not to wear the prosthesis during a sporting activity should be forewarned that increased activity may cause edema of the residual limb, making it difficult to apply the prosthesis afterward.[34]

There are a number of national organizations that offer community recreational clinics. These clinics provide stretching and strengthening exercise instruction and basic maneuvers to begin running.[35] Some of these clinics are designed for the population with disability as a whole, while others are limited to persons with limb loss. Some are free, and others charge a nominal fee to cover the costs of supplies, food, and/or transportation. Physical therapists

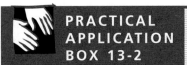

PRACTICAL
APPLICATION
BOX 13-2

First Aid Supplies for the Athlete with a Lower-Extremity Amputation

Spare/backup prosthesis
Spare ply socks or gel liner
Location/phone number of nearby prosthetist
Elastic bandages or shrinker sock
Screwdriver or Allen wrench
Donning creams or devices
Antibiotic cream
Gauze bandages
Medical/sports tape
Skin lotion
Crutches
Towels
Aspirin
Saline

are usually welcomed participants or assistants in these community recreational clinics.

Physical Therapy Intervention in Training to Run

Physical therapists are often involved in teaching individuals with an amputation how to run. The ability to run gives an individual with an amputation greater safety in emergency situations. Running is fundamental to many other sports, such as baseball and basketball. Therefore, it can be a needed or desired skill at varying levels of basic function or competition.[36] In general, the physical therapist can initiate running training when an individual with an amputation can ambulate safely without the use of an assistive device.[29] However, it is possible to learn to run with an assistive device when needed in urgent situations. Prerunning activities include balance activities to challenge pelvic and hip control specifically and jumping to increase residual limb tolerance.[29] Those with transfemoral amputations particularly need to practice the portion of prosthetic initial contact to ensure that they can spring off the sound side and land safely on an extended prosthetic knee.

Several studies analyzing running mechanics render helpful training tips for physical therapists to use during the rehabilitation process.[36,37] For example, in the stance phase of running, the prosthetic limb does only about half of the total muscle work as that of the non-amputated limb. Furthermore, the muscular distribution and contribution to the total work differ in the prosthetic and anatomic limbs. Normally, the knee does four to five times the mechanical work of the hip. However, on the prosthetic side, the hip musculature does one to one-and-a-half times more work than the knee. Therefore, the hip extensor muscles become the primary energy source in the amputated lower extremity.

When running is a rehabilitation goal, physical therapists should focus on the hip and knee extension musculature on the amputated side.[37] One investigator concluded that individuals with transtibial amputation tended to maintain the knee on the amputated side in excessive extension during the stance phase. This excessive extension reduces shock absorption at the knee, forcing unnatural stress upon the more proximal structures. This tendency may be attributed to weak quadriceps and/or attempts to increase stability to prevent buckling. Therefore, quadriceps strengthening, with an emphasis on eccentric control, is necessary for optimal running training.[36]

Obstacles to Training or Competition

Many factors limit individuals with amputation from participating in sports activities. Many of these limitations can be overcome with proper education and training. Considering that most amputations occur because of vascular insufficiency, many patients may be limited by comorbid medical conditions. It is not reasonable to think that all patients with amputation will have sports training in their rehabilitation or in their futures at all. The overall number of persons with amputation who can take part in competitive sports is relatively small. It is logical to assume that the younger, healthier population is better suited to pursuing sports seriously than the geriatric population, which is more likely to have comorbidities such as diabetes or vascular disease. However, these comorbid conditions do not preclude engagement in recreational activities. These can include some of the above-mentioned activities such as walking, indoor cycling, swimming or water exercises, and golfing.

The process of acceptance of loss varies with the individual. However, this process must be completed before one is both psychologically and physically ready to take part in sports. An amputation can, in itself, become an excuse to lead a sedentary lifestyle. Physical therapists play an integral role in health promotion by advising patients about what activities are appropriate. Fear is also a common reason for nonparticipation in sports programs and is often the most difficult obstacle to overcome. The pros and cons of sports participation are included in the pros and cons box.

Fear of failure and embarrassment about being "different" create anxiety and distress, obviating enjoyment of the activity. This prevents individuals from experiencing any success, even if very small, in overcoming the disability or improving well-being.[3,6,11,18] Physical therapists need to communicate that sports programs are a way to maintain or improve overall fitness and reinforce the noncompetitive nature of activity.

Another legitimate fear is that of injury. Risk of injury is inherent in all sports, whether the participant is disabled or not.[11] For example, long-distance runners often develop blisters on their toes and feet, skiers occasionally fall, and many other athletes strain muscles. An individual with amputation should be comfortable with falling and getting up from the floor. Proper skin care and protection must be reinforced. There are a large number of skin care products and protective and cushioning residual limb liners on the market to make sports participation more comfortable, with less risk of injury to the soft tissues.[17] Obviously, injuries do happen, but with proper supervision and training they can be minimized. One must reassure an individual with an amputation that the physical and psychologic rewards of activity may outweigh any risks to the body when the proper precautions are taken.[3]

Studies reveal that many individuals with amputation do not know that special adaptive equipment or prosthetic modifications exist to enable them to fully enjoy the activities they used to do. The physical therapist and the prosthetist are responsible for educating and informing their patients about what is available. Thus therapists and prosthetists must maintain continual open communication. In many cases, clients are aware of the adaptive devices and prostheses but cannot afford them.[18,28] Unfortunately, most insurance companies do not pay for recreational items. However, with a creative effort, the patient and prosthetist can often find a way to modify a walking prosthesis at little cost. The temporary, or training socket can sometimes be used to fabricate a sport-specific prosthesis once the definitive prosthesis is made. There may also be another way to perform the desired activity without modifying or using the prosthesis at all. Having specific componentry is certainly not essential for a person with amputation to engage in any particular activity. The physical therapist and prosthetist can help with problem solving in these situations.

Pain or mechanical difficulties may also dissuade a person from participating in sports.[18] If pain is a limiting factor, adaptations such as socket modification or the use of a liner may be necessary. Better suspension may be required

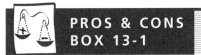

PROS & CONS BOX 13-1

Sports Participation for the Individual with a Lower-Extremity Amputation

Pros	Cons
Promotes general fitness	Not appropriate for many individuals with comorbidities
Promotes psychologic well-being	Risk of injury
Promotes goal-oriented tasks	Prosthetic adaptations or equipment can be costly
May promote social involvement & sense of teamwork	

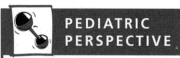

PEDIATRIC PERSPECTIVE

Sports Involvement Considerations for the Pediatric Population with Lower-Limb Amputation

Promotes general fitness while having fun

Promotes psychologic well-being by instilling sense of belonging and accomplishment

Teaches goal-oriented behavior

Promotes social interaction and importance of teamwork with peers and typically developing children

Recreational or competitive level of involvement

May require frequent prosthetic adjustments

Prosthetic adaptations or equipment may be costly

Risk of injury

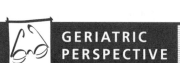

GERIATRIC PERSPECTIVE

Sports Involvement Considerations for the Geriatric Population with Lower-Limb Amputation

Promotes general fitness through recreational activities

Promotes psychological well-being via accomplishments and increased fitness level

Promotes social interaction/peer support

Need to monitor vital signs and be aware of comorbidities

Prosthetic adaptations or equipment may be costly but is not as necessary because involvement is less competitive

Risk of injury

for improved socket fit, comfort, and reliability. If an individual cannot tolerate high-impact sports regardless of repeated changes or liners, there may be a less stressful activity that he or she could enjoy without pain or risk of injury. Many activities do not require the use of a prosthesis. Mechanical difficulties such as poor balance, decreased endurance, or poor coordination may warrant more individualized training or therapy prior to participating in the desired activity but do not automatically preclude the activity. Like anything else that someone is learning, either for the first time or with modifications, there is a process that must occur for the learning to be successful. Most of these possible obstacles can be overcome with proper education and training.[15] Pediatric and geriatric perspectives of sports involvement for individuals with lower-extremity amputation are presented in the Pediatric and Geriatric Perspective Boxes.

C A S E   S T U D I E S

Four case studies are presented that summarize important features regarding sports implications for individuals with lower- extremity amputations. The suggested answers are given at the end of all of the cases.

C A S E   1

PATIENT/CLIENT HISTORY

General Demographics

A 76-year-old male who had a left transtibial amputation 6 days ago due to a gangrenous diabetic ulcer expresses an interest in returning to playing golf. This patient states that over the past year, he could not tolerate standing long enough to play golf since his foot was so painful. He states that he misses playing golf but cannot imagine how he could play with only one leg. He fears that his residual limb would be too painful. He has type 2 diabetes mellitus, well controlled by oral agents. He had a myocardial infarction at age 68 and bypass surgery involving two vessels at age 73.

TESTS AND MEASURES

Pain

The patient reports phantom sensation and pain consistent with surgical healing. He rates his pain as 2/10 at best and 8/10 at worst on the visual analog scale (VAS).

Integumentary Inspection

Incision line is healing well with staples in place. Surrounding skin is intact and dry, with positive hair growth. There is considerable edema in the residual limb, which is wrapped with an elastic bandage.

Muscle Performance

Manual muscle testing is 5/5 except left hip extension, right hip extension, and bilateral hip abduction, which are all graded 4/5.

Balance

Patient can stand at standard walker independently for 3 minutes.

Locomotion

Patient is independent with all bed mobility and sit-to-stand transfers. Patient is independent with wheelchair propulsion for 200 feet in 1 minute. Patient can hop 50 feet with standard walker with supervision and verbal cues for posture.

PROSTHETICS PRESCRIPTION/ MANAGEMENT

Patient does not have any prosthetic knowledge and has not been seen by a prosthetist at this time. He is a good candidate for prosthetic rehabilitation.

a. How would you respond to this patient's concerns?

b. What activities could be emphasized in this patient's intervention plan?

c. What types of prosthetic componentry would you recommend?

d. What national organizations might be helpful for this patient?

a. The patient should be reassured that many individuals with amputation can play golf without difficulty or with some adaptation. He should be informed that his foot was painful from the lack of blood to the gangrenous area and that he should no longer experience that kind of pain. The prosthesis will be made to fit as comfortably as possible. It may be too early to know what his functional outcomes will be with regard to playing golf.

b. Initially, focus on self-care, strengthening, functional training, and endurance. Standing tolerance, trunk rotation, and shoulder strengthening are important activities in preparation for playing golf. Once he has a prosthesis, progressive lower extremity weight-shifting exercises should be emphasized. These strengthening and functional activities are reviewed in Chapter 7.

c. Assuming that his medical status is stable, a total-surface bearing (TSB) socket with sleeve suspension may be indicated. A TSB socket would provide a greater surface area for weight bearing. The sleeve suspension has the advantage of being light weight and results in minimal pistoning between the socket and residual limb. A torsion adapter unit will help with rotation necessary in a golf swing. A foot such as a multiaxial, SAFE, or College Park will adapt to uneven terrain. More basic componentry may be chosen for initial training. Higher-level componentry may be chosen for the definitive prosthesis, based on the patient's functional progress.

d. The National Amputee Golf Association and the Eastern Amputee Golf Association are national organizations that will serve as resources.

CASE 2

PATIENT/CLIENT HISTORY

A 63-year-old female who has had a recent right transfemoral amputation expresses concern about watching her 3-year-old grandchild several days a week. She feels helpless because she cannot chase after him. She had an amputation due to a thrombosis caused by a rare blood disorder that is controlled pharmacologically. She also has hypothyroidism.

TESTS AND MEASURES

Pain

Patient experiences occasional phantom sensation, but it does not interfere with her functional abilities. She states she is comfortable with her present prosthesis.

Integumentary Inspection

Her incision line is well healed, with good scar mobility.

Muscle Performance

Manual muscle testing shows 5/5 strength throughout bilateral upper extremities, left lower extremity, and right hip.

Balance

Patient is able to stand unsupported independently with the prosthesis and sustain moderate perturbations without loss of balance.

PROSTHETICS PRESCRIPTION/ MANAGEMENT

Patient has an ischial-containment socket, roll-on silicone suction suspension, modular ergonomically balanced stride (EBS) polycentric hydraulic knee, and Carbon Copy II foot. She is independent applying and removing the prosthesis, and currently wears one 3-ply sock

Gait

She ambulates independently with a straight cane and has good gait quality except for slightly decreased right weight- bearing in stance. She is able to vary her cadence, and she negotiates a full flight of steps with one rail independently with a step-to-step pattern.

a. What specific muscles need to be strengthened intensively to enable this patient to run?

b. What exercises could you give this patient as a home program to strengthen these specific muscles?

c. Do you think her current prosthetic componentry is sufficient for teaching her to run safely?

d. What other information would you want to know before training this patient to run?

e. What method would you use to train this patient to run?

a. Gluteal and hamstring muscles are needed to help control and stabilize the prosthetic knee in extension during stance phase on the prosthetic side.

b. Various exercises are reviewed in Chapter 7 to strengthen the gluteals and hamstrings. These include prone hip extension and knee flexion; standing hip extension and knee flexion, wearing and not wearing the prosthesis; progression to prone activities while on an unstable surfaces such as a ball, bolster, or foam roll; and resistance in the form of rubber tubing or ankle weights. Neuromuscular control exercises while standing over the prosthesis would be warranted.

c. The hydraulic knee allows for cadence changes. The prosthetic foot is a dynamic-response one that will also be suitable for cadence changes and running. She may benefit from the additional suspension of a Silesian bandage or TES belt.

d. Important information to know would be any comorbidities, range of motion, strength, and cardiovascular status.

e. Training to run should first include the hop-skip method. She may need to learn to run with the cane for improved safety unless she becomes proficient in ambulating without an assistive device.

C A S E   3

PATIENT/CLIENT HISTORY

A 32-year-old female had a right transfemoral amputation 6 days ago due to a motor vehicle accident. She also sustained a fracture to her left tibial plateau, which was internally fixated. The patient reports that she is a triathlete. She states that she intends to return quickly to vigorous swimming, cycling, and running despite her present status. She says she needs to be ready to compete in a race that is coming up in a month. She has no chronic diseases such as diabetes or cardiac disease. She is married, with one young child, and works part time as a retail clerk.

TESTS AND MEASURES

Pain

She reports intermittent distal residual-limb pain, phantom limb pain, and phantom limb sensation. She has pain at end ranges of left knee flexion and extension.

Integumentary Inspection

Residual-limb surgical incision line is closed with sutures. There is minimal drainage coming from the wound. There is marked edema of the residual limb. The residual limb is 12 cm in length, measured from the greater trochanter. The surrounding skin has areas of ecchymosis but is intact and otherwise unremarkable. The left incision line is also closed with sutures, with moderate drainage noted. Surrounding skin is bruised and dry, with localized areas of edema.

Range of Motion

All joints are within normal limits except the left knee, which measures 10–90° actively and 5–95° passively.

Muscle Performance

Manual muscle testing is within normal limits in both upper extremities. Right hip muscles are 4/5, although pain is noted upon resistance to all motions of the residual limb. Left knee strength was not assessed because of pain from the internally fixated left tibial plateau fracture. Strength is 4/5 in the left hip and ankle musculature.

Balance

Patient has good sitting balance. She can stand at the edge of the bed for 10 minutes and lean against the bathroom counter at the sink to perform self-hygiene tasks.

Locomotion

She is independent with all bed mobility and transfers in the hospital room. She has propelled her wheelchair up and down the hall approximately 500 feet several times since the surgery.

PROSTHETICS PRESCRIPTION/ MANAGEMENT

She has not been seen by the prosthetist because it is too early in her healing process. She is a good candidate for prosthetic training.

a. **What can you determine about the patient's psychosocial status that may influence her rehabilitation?**
b. **What educational needs does this patient have with regard to her expectations to return to sports so soon?**
c. **What activities would you include in her initial plan of care that would be appropriate for her current functional level?**
d. **What kind of functional outcomes would you expect to see within the next month? Will she be ready to compete in the race?**

a. This patient has unrealistic expectations regarding a fast return to vigorous sporting activities. She may benefit from peer support through a support group or counseling. Psychosocial issues are reviewed in Chapter 4. The prosthetic clinic team should be informed about these expectations so all team members can help the patient make sound decisions.

b. She needs to receive education about

Functional limitations of non–weight-bearing status on the left lower extremity
The need for time to heal the surgical sites
The need to increase prosthetic wearing time tolerance gradually, to prevent undue stresses to the soft tissues
Potential dangers of doing high-impact activities too soon
Specialized componentry and/or adaptations for specific sporting activities

c. The patient's initial plan of care should include

Proper skin care and edema management for both lower extremities. This patient may be an ideal candidate for an immediate postoperative prosthesis (IPOP). The IPOP is discussed in Chapter 6.

Shaping of the residual limb

Restoring left knee range of motion and bilateral lower-extremity strength

Restoring optimal functional and cardiovascular endurance levels with upper- and lower-extremity ergometry

Locomotion at a wheelchair level, with progression to ambulation with left lower-extremity weight bearing as tolerated or when the prosthesis is fitted and delivered. Many of these strengthening, endurance, and flexibility activities are reviewed in Chapter 7.

d. Within the next month, physical therapy interventions will include the above plan of care. The patient may not yet be able to fully weight bear through the left leg. Her residual limb may be well healed and shaped for prosthetic casting within a month. However, it is unlikely that she will have the finished prosthesis in a month. Once she does have the prosthesis for training, it will take at least several weeks to achieve an independent functional status. Dynamic skills such as running and cycling will take even longer, especially considering her other orthopedic limitations. It is highly improbable that she will be ready for competition in a month, even if her range of motion, strength, and endurance are sufficient at that time.

C A S E   4

PATIENT/CLIENT HISTORY

You have met an individual who underwent bilateral transtibial amputations due to a motorcycle accident a year ago. He was discharged from physical therapy several months ago, but he is now motivated to return to skiing again. You note that he walked into the room with an unassisted, normal-appearing gait. He has returned to work full time without difficulty. He states that he was an avid recreational skier during the winter months. He wishes to return to skiing and is looking for some guidance.

a. What information about skiing could you give to him?

b. What activities would you recommend he do in the off season to enhance his ability to ski?

a. Inform him about organized ski clubs around the country such as Disabled Sports USA and National Sports for the Disabled. Knowledge of the ski adaptations and sit ski devices described above in this chapter will be helpful.

b. If he plans on skiing with prostheses, he could work on trunk mobility and strength, eccentric quadriceps strengthening, and mediolateral hip and knee balance and coordination. Encourage him to train on therapeutic devices made to simulate the motions of skiing. If he plans to sit ski, he could focus on trunk mobility and strength and upper body conditioning, including rotator cuff, latissimus dorsi, triceps, and deltoid musculature. Cardiovascular endurance training is important.

KEY POINTS

- Physical therapists should encourage the patient with an amputation to pursue recreational or sporting activities that provide pleasure, accomplishment, or purpose.

- Activities in the form of physical exercise can help promote emotional well-being in addition to physical health. Physical therapists should be advocates for an active lifestyle and, when appropriate, introduce recreational or competitive sports to their patients.

- The benefits of recreational or sporting activities are plentiful and include increased overall fitness, increased energy, greater social interaction, improved coping and adaptation to physical loss, and increased acceptance of self through acceptance of others with limb loss.

- The prosthetic industry continues to provide more specific and efficient components and adaptive equipment to enable the motivated individual to participate in sporting activities.

- Community resources continue to grow, providing many opportunities for individuals with amputation to learn new sports. The sooner the common fears of pain, nonaccomplishment, and injury are alleviated, the sooner the individual realizes that recreation focuses on one's ability rather than disability. Physical therapists play a pivotal role in guiding their patients to accept new challenges.

REFERENCES

1. Myers, C. (1998). The future of amputee rehabilitation. *Rehabilitation Management, 11*, 50–53.
2. Breakey, J. W. (1997). Body image: The inner mirror. *Journal of Prosthetics and Orthotics, 9*, 107–112.
3. Subotnick, S. (1999). *Sports medicine of the lower extremity* (2nd ed.). Philadelphia: Churchill Livingstone.
4. Kent, R., & Fyfe, N. (1999). Effectiveness of rehabilitation following amputation. *Clinical Rehabilitation, 13*, 43–50.
5. Dodds, J. (1992). Sports and amputees. In L. Karacoloff, C. S. Hammersley, & F. J. Schneider (Eds.), *Lower extremity amputation* (2nd Ed). Gaithersburg, MD: Aspen Publishers.
6. Winchell, E. (1995). *Coping with limb loss.* Garden City Park, NY: Avery Publishing Group.
7. Pandian, G., & Kowalske, K. (1999). Daily functioning of patients with an amputated lower extremity. *Clinical Orthopedics and Related Research, 361*, 91–97.
8. Ewart, A. (1985). Why people climb: The relationship of participant motives and experience level to mountaineering. *Journal of Leisure Research, 17*, 241.
9. Cough, P., Shepherd, J., & Maughan, R. (1989). Motives for participation in recreational running. *Journal of Leisure Research, 21*, 297.
10. Shearer, J. D., Buckner, M., & Bowker, J. H., (1981). Prostheses and assistive devices for special activities. In J. H. Bowker & J. W. Micheal, *Atlas of limb prosthetics: Surgical and prosthetic principles.* St. Louis: C. V. Mosby.
11. Jackson, R. W., & Davis, G. M. (1983). The value of sports and recreation for the physically disabled. *Orthopedic Clinics of North America, 14*, 301–315.
12. Pollock, M. L. (1973). The quantification of endurance training. *Exercise and Sports Science Reviews, 1*, 155–188.
13. Shepherd, R. J. (1977). *Endurance fitness* (2nd ed.). Toronto: University of Toronto Press.
14. Waters, R. (1992). The energy expenditure of amputee gait. In J. H. Bowker, & J. W. Micheal (Eds.), *Atlas of limb prosthetics: Surgical, prosthetic, and rehabilitation principles* (2nd ed.). St. Louis: Mosby Year Book.
15. Michael, J. W., Gailey, R. S., & Bowker, J. H. (1990). New developments in recreational prostheses and adaptive devices for the amputee. *Clinical Orthopaedics and Related Research, 256*, 64–75.
16. Rubin, G., & Fleiss, D. (1983). Devices to enable persons with amputation to participate in sports. *Archives of Physical Medicine and Rehabilitation, 64*, 37–40.
17. Burgess, E. M. (1993). *Physical fitness: A guide for individuals with lower limb loss.* Baltimore: Department of Veterans Affairs.
18. Kegel, B., Webster, J. C., & Burgess, E. M. (1980). Recreational activities of lower extremity amputees: A survey. *Archives of Physical Medicine and Rehabilitation, 61*, 258–264.
19. Kegel, B. (1992). Adaptations for sports and recreation. In J. H. Bowker, & J. W. Micheal (Eds.), *Atlas of limb prosthetics: Surgical, prosthetic, and rehabilitation principles* (2nd ed.). St. Louis: Mosby Year Book.
20. Saadah, E. S. M. (1992). Swimming devices for below-knee amputees. *Prosthetics and Orthotics International, 16*, 140–141.
21. Engstrom, B., & VandeVen, C. (1985). *Physiotherapy for amputees: The Roehampton approach.* New York: Churchill Livingstone.
22. Saadah E. S. M. (1989). Rehabilitation of a below-knee amputee with a diving limb. *Clinical Rehabilitation, 3*, 249–251.
23. Cycling Amputees Support. Amputee Life and Support Area. Available at: http://amp-domain.com/cycling.html. Accessed June 23, 2000.
24. The History of NAGA. National Amputee Golf Association. Available at: http://www.amputee-golf.org/history.html. Accessed May 22, 2000.
25. Adaptive Equipment. Disabled Sports USA. Available at: http://www.dsuafw.org/equip.html. Accessed July 17, 2000.

26. What is adaptive skiing? National Sports Center for the Disabled. Available at: http://www.nscd.org/adski/index.html. Accessed July 17, 2000.

27. Pringle, D. (1987). Winter sports for the amputee athlete. *Clinical Prosthetics and Orthotics, 11,* 114–117.

28. Kegel, B., Carpenter, M. L., & Burgess, E. M. (1978). Functional capabilities of lower extremity amputees. *Archives of Physical Medicine and Rehabilitation, 59,* 109–120.

29. Esquenazi, A., Wikoff, E., & Lucas, M. (2000). Amputation rehabilitation. In M. Grabois, S. Garrison, K. Hart, & L. D. Lehmkuhl (Eds.), *Physical medicine and rehabilitation.* Houston, TX: Blackwell Science.

30. Gailey, R. (1992). Physical therapy management of adult lower limb amputees. In J. H. Bowker, & J. W. Micheal (Eds.), *Atlas of limb prosthetics: Surgical, prosthetic, and rehabilitation principles* (2nd ed.). St. Louis: Mosby Year Book.

31. Romo, H. D. (1999). Specialized prostheses for activities. *Clinical Orthopaedics and Related Research, 361,* 63–70.

32. Sabolich, J. (1987). The O.K.C. above-knee running system. *Clinical Prosthetics and Orthotics, 11,* 169–172.

33. Michael, J. (1999). Modern prosthetic knee mechanisms. *Clinical Orthopaedics and Related Research, 361,* 39–47.

34. Gaydos, J. (1997, July). Fit for life. *O&P Almanac,* pp. 73–76.

35. Bassett, J. (2000). Chasing a dream. *Advance for Physical Therapists and PT Assistants, 11,* 6–7.

36. Enoka, R. M., Miller, D. I., & Burgess, E. M. (1982). Below knee amputee running gait. *American Journal of Physical Medicine, 61,* 66–84.

37. Czerniecki, J. M., & Gitter, A. (1992). Insights into amputee running: A muscle work analysis. *American Journal of Physical Medicine and Rehabilitation, 71,* 209–218.

Orthoses

Examination of Foot Biomechanics in Relation to Sporting Injuries and Foot Orthotic Intervention

Gabriel Yankowitz, PT

Objectives

1. Differentiate among the most common causes of running injuries including training errors, improper footwear, and abnormal biomechanics
2. Describe the kinematics of normal running
3. Differentiate common injuries that may occur due to pathomechanical gait
4. Describe the most common causes of abnormal pronation
5. Explain components of the clinical assessment of lower extremity posture and muscle balance
6. Compare and contrast the different types and fabrication methods of orthotics
7. Describe the contraindications to the use of foot orthotics

This chapter is divided into the following sections:

This chapter begins with a definition of terms that are often confusing. Chapters 14–17 use these definitions as a frame of reference. The term **orthotics** describes the practice and manufacture of orthoses. The term *orthotics* also refers to a shoe insert. An *orthosis* is an externally applied device used to modify the characteristics of the neuromuscular system. An *orthotist* is a person skilled in the profession of orthosis or orthotic manufacture. The use of the word *orthosis* rather than *brace, splint,* or *caliper* is encouraged. Health-care practitioners, in an effort to address biomechanical imbalances of the foot and lower extremity, have used foot orthotics for years. Such imbalances are thought by many to lead to a number of overuse or repetitive strain injuries in many athletes, particularly in running athletes. Orthotic devices are fabricated from a variety of materials, which may be classified as rigid, semirigid, or soft. Orthotic devices are cast or molded in a variety of ways and may include a variety of additions and adjustments to address specific problems.

Foot orthotics are designed to provide an external correction for structural imbalances in the foot that may cause abnormal gait mechanics, affecting musculotendinous and ligamentous structures in the lower extremities, pelvis, and low back. Various authors have defined these devices in the following manner:

"a type of shim placed between the foot and
   shoe to position the foot near its neutral position so it can function more effectively"[1]

"a means of aligning an improperly balanced
   foot by controlling the subtalar joint"[2]

"to reduce or eliminate compensatory motion
   by allowing the foot to function as nearly as
   possible around the neutral position"[3]

Clearly, the common underlying theme throughout these definitions is the use of orthotics to correct abnormal movement patterns, or pathomechanics, associated with gait.

Running Injuries

The "running boom" that began in the mid-1970s has maintained its popularity into the new millennium. Estimates range from 20–40 million regular runners in the United States,[4–6] with many engaging in races from 5 km (3.1 miles) up to the marathon (43 km, or 26.2 miles) on a regular basis. According to several investigators, most of these runners will suffer one or more injuries from this activity at some point in their "career."[5–8]

Most injuries sustained by runners affect the structures of the foot/ankle and knee,[7] although they are by no means limited to those areas. The most frequently seen injuries include

Plantar fasciitis
Shin splints (pretibial stress syndrome)
Metatarsalgia
Achilles tendinitis
Morton's neuroma
Patellofemoral pain syndrome (PFPS)
Hamstring strains
Iliotibial band friction syndrome
Trochanteric bursitis
Sacroiliac and lumbar joint sprains

Most experts agree that the bulk of running injuries (>60%) are caused by what are termed *training errors.*[1,5,6,9,10] The simplest explanation of this is the "too much, too soon" concept. Runners who increase their daily or weekly mileage too rapidly (generally considered to be more than 10% per week) or who initiate an overly ambitious program of track speedwork (interval training) or hill workouts appear to increase their risk for developing overuse injuries. Even the most perfectly built runner with optimal gait mechanics may become susceptible to injury. This injury often occurs if the soft tissue or bony structures of the lower extremity are stressed beyond the level of strain that has been previously adapted to through training.

Another 20–30% of injuries may be traced to the effects of improper footwear.[6,8,11] Athletic shoes with improper fit, poor construction, or a shape that may be inappropriate for a particular individual's foot type can alter the gait mechanics enough to cause excessive strain on muscles, tendons, or ligaments. For example, runners who exhibit a pes planus foot structure will suffer adverse effects from a shoe constructed on a "curved" last (shape) rather than a "straight" last (Fig. 14-1). A shoe built on a curved last will promote pronatory movements of the foot that may lead to injuries.[8] Shoes built on semicurved or straight lasts result in less pronation (Fig. 14-2). Shoes that are over-

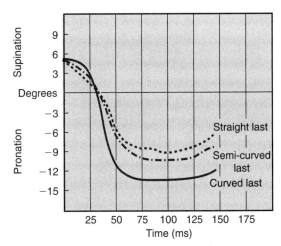

Figure 14-2. Comparison of subtalar motion with different shoe lasts.

worn may also alter gait mechanics enough to lead to injury.

The remainder of running injuries (~10–20%) may be traced exclusively to abnormal biomechanics, or pathomechanics, of gait.[1] The excessive forces that occur with improper gait patterns (particularly rotational movements on a longitudinal axis) can cause disproportionate strain and eventual failure of soft tissue and osseous structures.[12,13]

(The reader should note that while much of this chapter describes injuries that occur with running activities, individuals who engage in walking may experience many if not all of the same types of problems, though perhaps with less frequency and/or severity).

Normal Running Mechanics

The normal mechanics involved in human walking are covered in Chapter 5. While abnormal walking patterns may lead to injuries similar to those most often associated with running activities (and may consequently be treated similarly), the mechanics of running offer enough variation to explain the increased incidence of injury from this activity. Like walking, running involves the reciprocal move-

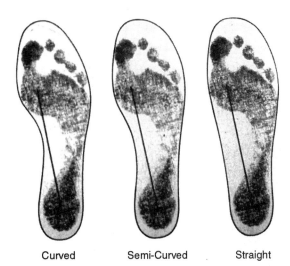

Figure 14-1. Curved, semicurved, straight, and shoe lasts.

ment of the lower limbs in a controlled, symmetric manner. Running, however, differs from walking in several respects. During walking, at least one limb is in contact with the supporting surface at all times. Additionally, there is a period of double-support during which both limbs are in contact with the ground.

With running, there is no period of double support, and there is also a period when neither limb is in contact with the surface. This period is called the *float* phase. In addition, the vertical displacement of the center of gravity (COG) is generally greater with running. These two factors combine to make the ground reaction forces at initial contact during running larger than those during walking by a factor of 2 to 3.[14] This increase is one of the primary reasons for the higher incidence of injuries with running.

Joint kinematics also change when one moves from walking to running, leading to increased stresses on muscle groups. In the sagittal plane, the joints of the ankle, knee, and hip all traverse a greater degree of motion during running. Angular velocity is also increased pro-portionate to the increase in forward speed of the body. Both factors increase the load on muscles initiating or controlling joint movements.

A critical component of kinematic activity in the lower limb during locomotion occurs as rotational movement in the transverse plane. The degree of internal and external rotation of the thigh and leg, in conjunction with triplanar movements of the foot, appears to play a significant role in the development of injuries throughout the lower extremity. Numerous studies have shown a correlation between excessive or deficient pronation movements of the subtalar (STJ) and midtarsal joints (MTJs) of the foot and most of the injuries of the lower extremity associated with running.[1,10,12,13,15,16]

The movements of pronation and supination are normally occurring movements of the subtalar joint that impart an enormous influence on movements throughout the lower limb and pelvis. These movements are triplanar, as they do not occur exclusively in any one of the cardinal planes because of the oblique axis of that joint (Fig. 14-3). Consequently, pronation

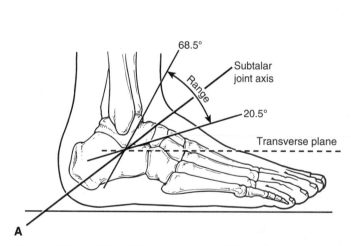

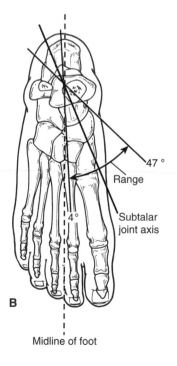

Figure 14-3. A. STJ axis has a range upward from the transverse plane between 20.5 and 68.5°. B. STJ axis has a range from the longitudinal reference of the foot when viewed superiorly between 4 and 47°. (Adapted from Hunt, G. C., & McPoil, T. G. (1995). Physical therapy of the foot and ankle (2nd ed.). New York: Churchill Livingstone.)

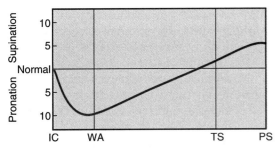

Figure 14-4. Normal STJ motion in the neutral foot. At initial contact, the STJ is slightly supinated. Pronation occurs between initial contact and weight acceptance. Supination then occurs so that just before terminal stance, a neutral position of the STJ occurs. Supination continues through preswing. (Adapted from Brown, L. P., & Yavorsky, P. (1987). Locomotor biomechanics and pathomechanics: A review. *Journal of Orthopaedic and Sports Physical Therapy, 9,* 3-10.)

at the STJ consists of the movements of dorsiflexion (sagittal plane), eversion (transverse), and abduction (frontal), while supination combines the opposite movements in each respective plane.[17-20]

Examination of the timing of these movements through the stance phase of gait reveals and confirms their functional nature (Fig. 14-4). As the foot strikes the ground at initial contact, the STJ is normally supinated to a very slight degree (~2°). Within the first 25% of stance phase, as the center of gravity drops and the metatarsal heads contact the surface, the STJ pronates to its maximum degree (8–12°). Two events occur during this period that benefit from the kinesiologic and kinematic effects derived from this movement. First, the rolling motion contributed primarily by the eversion component of pronation provides a shock-absorbing mechanism for dampening the ground reaction forces incurred at initial contact. This is accomplished in concert with the flexion movements at the ankle, knee, and hip. Second, as the foot makes full contact with the supporting surface, early man and woman not privy to the benefits of paved roads and shoes, needed a foot that could adapt to uneven surfaces. This objective is achieved as the pronatory movement of the STJ "unlocks"

the joints of the midfoot, resulting in a loose-packed condition with maximum passive range of motion at these joints.[17]

As the tibia moves forward over the STJ in preparation for propulsion, the STJ reverses movement via mostly active muscle action and begins to supinate, which then "locks" the joints of the midfoot, providing a rigid lever for efficient push-off. Again, this coincides with extension of the knee and hip, which also provide more stability throughout the lower extremity. The foot reaches maximum supination (~6°) at the end-stage of stance or preswing.

These pronating and supinating movements occurring at the STJ are crucial not just to the foot, but also to the normal function of the entire lower extremity. This is due to the principle of obligatory motion that mandates a direct relationship between the movements of the STJ and the rotational movements of the leg and, more indirectly, the thigh. During closed-chain (weight-bearing) pronation movement of the STJ, the talus rotates medially as a result of the lateral movement of the sustentaculum tali support as the calcaneus everts. Because the dome of the talus is enclosed tightly within the talocrural joint, forming the so-called ankle mortise, there is virtually no independent movement available to the talus in the frontal plane. Consequently, any rotational movement on the part of the talus must be transferred to the leg via the ankle mortise. Thus, medial rotation of the talus must be accompanied by internal rotation of the leg. Conversely, supinating movements of the STJ cause external rotation of the leg. Additionally, the limited rotation range available at the knee joint necessitates a certain amount of similar rotational force to the thigh (Fig. 14-5).[11,21]

One must also realize that the principle of obligatory motion applies equally to rotational influences of proximal structures on the movement patterns of the STJ. Therefore, the amount of pronation and supination at the STJ may be determined to some degree not only by foot structure, but also by forces imparted by the rotator muscles of the hip that are trans-

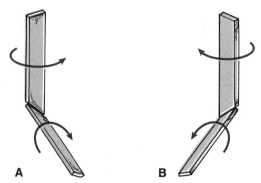

Figure 14-5. Ankle mortise "mitered" hinge necessitating obligatory motion. Therefore **A.** internal rotation of the leg occurs with subtalar pronation. Conversely, **B.** external rotation of the leg occurs with subtalar supination. (Adapted from Mann, R. A. (Ed.) (1986). Surgery of the foot (5th ed.). St. Louis: C. V. Mosby.)

ferred through the ankle mortise to the talus.[11] An understanding of this reciprocating relationship is critical in determining the underlying pathomechanical cause for a specific running injury, which in turn guides the appropriate course of intervention.

Pathomechanical Gait and Running Injuries

Although several investigators have established a correlative link between certain abnormal gait patterns and the incidence of running injuries, acceptance of a cause-and-effect relationship by clinicians has been largely intuitive. (The truth of this observation is supported by the work of several investigators in recent years[22,23] that has challenged some of the fundamental assumptions described in this and the previous section pertaining to the concepts of STN, normal gait, and injury etiology.) Logic dictates that improper movement patterns will place undue stress on bone, joint, ligament, and musculotendinous structures of the lower extremities, leading to structural failure that is classified as an overuse injury. Identifying and

correcting a pathomechanical gait pattern is accordingly the cornerstone of successful management of these types of injuries.

Abnormal gait patterns can occur in any one of the cardinal planes of movement or in combination. The most obvious are those that involve some asymmetry of the lower extremities. These can be the result of a leg length differential, an osseous malformation (either congenital or acquired), or posturally mediated muscle imbalance. Symmetric, as well as asymmetric, movement faults may be seen in the sagittal plane as restricted range of the hip, knee, and/or ankle joints. Less often seen are improper movements exclusive to the frontal plane. (A crossover gait pattern is the most common example).

Pathomechanical movements in the transverse plane are often cited as the most likely to cause overuse injuries in runners. Both investigators and clinicians point to the effects of excessive or deficient foot pronation and lower-extremity rotatory movements as critical in the genesis of a number of common injuries. Among the most often listed are

- Patellofemoral pain syndrome—The correct degree of hip and thigh rotation occurring during stance phase of gait is critical to maintaining proper tracking of the patella in the femoral trochlea during the flexion (initial contact to midstance) and extension (midstance to preswing) movements of the knee joint during stance. The eccentric and concentric loading forces of the quadriceps muscles during this period create significant compressive force at the patellofemoral joint. An excessive amount of internal hip rotation may result in the patella riding more along the lateral crest of the femoral groove, with a subsequent lessening of the total contact area of the retropatellar surface. The end result may be an overload failure of the articular cartilage, resulting in the painful condition commonly known as "runner's knee."[12,15,24]

- Posterior tibial stress syndrome—Excessive or prolonged pronatory movements occurring in the STJ and MTJs can place excessive strain on the muscles of the leg (tibialis posterior, gastrocsoleus) that eccentrically decelerate and concentrically reverse this movement, resulting in the tendinitis condition commonly referred to as "shin splints."[16]
- Plantar fasciitis—Excessive foot pronation places a strain on the plantar aponeurosis as the medial longitudinal arch flattens due to the talus and navicular moving inferiorly. Pronation movement that is prolonged past midstance creates an unstable midfoot, placing more strain on the plantar fascia.[25,26]
- Metatarsalgia—Excessive or deficient pronation alters the weight-bearing patterns on the plantar surface of the foot, particularly the metatarsal heads. Disproportionate weight-bearing on the 2nd and 3rd metatarsal (MT) heads, induced by excessive pronation, leads to bruising and inflammation; the same occurs at the 5th and 1st MT heads with deficient pronation.[3]
- Iliotibial band friction syndrome (ITBFS)—The iliotibial band may be affected by improper timing of femoral rotation secondary to excessive or prolonged foot pronation. Medial rotation of the femur may place the lateral femoral epicondyle in the wrong position as the knee is flexing and extending during stance phase of gait, causing the iliotibial band (ITB) to rub excessively and become irritated and inflamed. Inflexibility of the ITB caused by other factors, such as hip muscle imbalance, will compound this problem.[1,3,13]
- Sacroiliac joint sprain—Deficient foot pronation, or excessive supination, will diminish the ability of the foot–ankle complex to dissipate ground reaction forces during early stance, as described above. Such forces may then be transmitted via the lower limb to more superior structures, such as the sacroiliac joint, causing repetitive overload to the ligamentous supports for that joint. In run-

ners, the problem is often unilateral because of contributing factors that result in asymmetric distribution of forces, such as the curve on a track or the slant of the road.[4,27]
- Stress fractures—Excessive forces on various structures of the body may eventually cause failure of bone integrity. The most commonly injured areas in runners include the metatarsals and tibia. Pelvic stress fractures are also found in high-mileage runners.[1,4]

While most of the blame for these and other running injuries is usually assigned to the excessively pronating foot and/or medially rotating lower limb, less-than-normal pronation movement and/or excessive external thigh and leg rotation can cause problems. The rigid, pes cavus foot that has limited pronation movement will not provide the shock-absorbing or surface-accommodating qualities of the normal foot. Sprains of the foot and sacroiliac joints are some of the injuries associated with this type of foot.[27]

Movement faults in the sagittal and frontal planes may be corrected or minimized via appropriate stretching and strengthening exercises if the underlying cause for these faults involved soft tissue structures. Obviously, osseous abnormalities have limited potential for this type of management. Pathomechanical movements, such as abnormal pronation/supination in the transverse plane, may also be managed successfully with exercise but have the potential as well to be managed with appropriate orthotic devices. To determine the appropriate strategy, a complete understanding of the causes for these pathomechanics is necessary.

Etiology of Lower-Extremity Transverse-Plane Pathomechanics

The focus of this section is on the causes of abnormal pronation/supination movements at the STJ; by controlling these movements, we can often manage running injuries effectively. These causes can be assigned to one of two categories that refer to factors outside of (extrinsic) and within (intrinsic) the structure of the foot itself. The most common causes for these pathomechanical patterns are listed in Table 14-1. Obligatory influences have a superscript a, while compensatory movements have a superscript b.

Extrinsic Causes

Osseous and soft tissue conditions of the lower limb proximal to the STJ can cause movement patterns that result in changes in pronation/ supination movements of the foot. Some of these conditions will correspond, respectively, to factors that cause an increase in medial and lateral rotation of the lower limb which will then, via the principle of obligatory motion, re-

Table 14-1. Common Causes for Effective or Deficient Pronation

Excessive pronation	Femoral anteversion[a]
	Dominant, tight hip internal rotators[a]
	Internal femoral torsion[a]
	Internal tibial torsion[a]
	Genu valgum[b]
	Tibial varum[b]
	Dominant, tight foot evertors[b]
	"Long" leg[b]
	Restricted ankle dorsiflexion range[b]
Deficient pronation	
	Femoral retroversion[a]
	Dominant, tight hip external rotators[a]
	External femoral torsion[a]
	External tibial torsion[a]
	Dominant, tight foot invertors[b]
	"Short" leg[b]

[a]Obligatory influence.
[b]Compensatory influence.

sult in movement changes at the STJ. Other conditions will cause STJ pathomechanical changes that are compensatory in nature.

The reasons for increased or decreased pronation movements at the STJ secondary to obligatory motion should be evident; those that are compensatory may not be so apparent. Examination of the impairments caused by a particular condition will help explain the functional compensation achieved by the change seen in STJ movement. For example, a restriction in ankle dorsiflexion range, whether caused by shortening of the gastrocsoleus complex or talocrural joint hypomobility, will create a problem at the midstance phase of gait as the tibia moves forward over the ankle. One possible compensation would be early heel rise, but this would place significant stress on the calf muscles as well as disrupt normal foot mechanics. Another method of compensation would be for the foot to increase its pronation range, since one of the components of pronatory motion is dorsiflexion at both the STJ and MTJs, as described earlier in this chapter. The extra few degrees of sagittal plane dorsiflexion gained by increasing the overall pronation movement will allow the tibia to move through its normal range over the planted foot.

A leg length discrepancy may also alter STJ mechanics.[28] A "long" leg, whether actual or functional, may cause an increase in ipsilateral STJ pronation as a mechanism to "shorten" the extremity by lowering the height of the medial longitudinal arch. Conversely, the contralateral STJ will limit pronation movement to keep that limb "longer." Care should be taken when evaluating apparent leg length discrepancies to determine their true nature. Some investigators have questioned the tendency of clinicians to assume that discrepancies are due to actual bone length differences. Evidence suggests otherwise;[29] most discrepancies are attributable to hip and pelvic muscle imbalances in the frontal plane. Most of these can be addressed quickly and effectively with appropriate strengthening/

stretching exercises and patient education with respect to postural habits.

It is left to the reader as an exercise to discern the reasons behind compensatory STJ motions in response to the remaining conditions listed earlier. The critical concept for all of these extrinsic causes of faulty STJ movement patterns remains consistent: to normalize STJ motion in these cases. The focus of intervention should be on correcting these precipitating factors before attempting to control the STJ via external means such as orthotic devices.

Intrinsic Causes

Abnormal pronatory movements at the STJ can also be attributed to structural malalignments of the foot itself. In this case, the pathomechanics are due to compensatory movements occurring at the STJ and MTJs.[14,19] These compensations are best understood if it is assumed that there is a tendency for the human body to fulfill a requirement dictating that all five MT heads as well as the medial and lateral calcaneal tubercles contact the supporting surface at some point during stance. A failure to follow this pattern would inflict disproportionate forces on various foot structures, leading to injuries that could include stress fractures.

The malalignment conditions of the foot that lead to compensatory movements are generally assumed to be osseous. Classifications of foot structure are based on the subtalar-neutral concept that defines the relationships of the rearfoot to the distal leg and the forefoot to the rearfoot.

Subtalar neutral (STN) is defined as the position of the foot in which the talonavicular joint (TNJ) is palpated at maximum congruency of the medial and lateral joint lines.[1,3,17] With the midfoot then locked at full pronation, the clinician sights the vertical bisection of the calcaneus in relation to the bisection of the distal one-third of the leg. A normal alignment would be parallel or have less than 2° angulation. The bisection of the calcaneus is then sighted in relation to a line "drawn" through

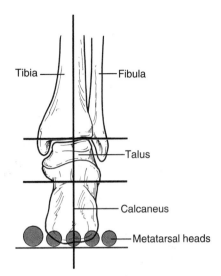

Figure 14-6. Normal rearfoot alignment showing a perpendicular relationship between the calcaneus and the MT heads.

the MT heads. A normal alignment would be indicated by a perpendicular relationship (Fig. 14-6). Abnormal alignment conditions, and the implications of each for pathomechanical movements of the STJ, are described as follows.

Rearfoot (Calcaneal) Varus

A position of more than 2° of inversion of the calcaneus in relation to the lower leg (in STN) indicates a condition of rearfoot varus (Fig. 14-7). In cases of rearfoot varus, the STJ must pronate to a greater degree than normal during the initial 25% of stance phase and remain pronated throughout stance phase. This is necessary to achieve contact of the medial calcaneal tubercle with the ground (Fig. 14-8).

Forefoot Varus

In STN, the line bisecting the MT heads is angulated in an inverted position in relation to the vertical bisection of the calcaneus (Fig. 14-9). To achieve contact of all MT heads with the ground at the point of midstance, the STJ must pronate to a greater degree and, more sig-

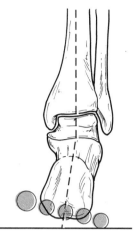

Figure 14-7. Rearfoot varus.

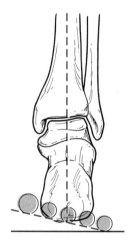

Figure 14-9. Forefoot varus.

nificantly, remain in a pronated position for a longer portion of the stance phase (Fig. 14-10). This pronation occurs at a point at which the foot would normally have achieved a supinated position at terminal stance to preswing, creating locking of the MTJs for stability as the foot is propelled from the ground. Therefore, greater muscle activity is required for push-off.

Forefoot Valgus

As the term implies, this condition is the opposite of forefoot varus, with the line bisecting the MT heads forming an everted position relative to the vertical bisection of the calcaneus (Fig.

14-11). Because contact of the medial MT heads occurs prematurely during the weight-acceptance phase of stance, the STJ does not have the opportunity to pronate to its normal extent (Fig. 14-12). At midstance then, the MTJs fail to unlock to provide a mobile, adaptive foot. The normal shock-absorption function of the pronatory movement is also attenuated.

Rigid Plantarflexed First Ray

A foot exhibiting a rigid plantarflexed first ray functions in much the same manner as the forefoot valgus condition (Fig. 14-13). Because the rigid first ray cannot move superiorly in re-

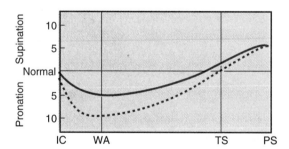

Figure 14-8. STJ motion with rearfoot varus (*dashed line*) and normal STJ motion (*solid line*). (Adapted from Brown, L. P., & Yavorsky, P. (1987). Locomotor biomechanics and pathomechanics: A review. *Journal of Orthopaedic and Sports Physical Therapy, 9,* 3-10.)

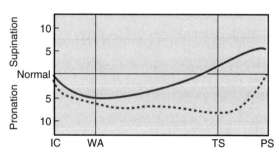

Figure 14-10. STJ motion with forefoot varus (*dashed line*) and normal STJ motion (*solid line*). (Adapted from Brown, L. P., & Yavorsky, P. (1987). Locomotor biomechanics and pathomechanics: A review. *Journal of Orthopaedic and Sports Physical Therapy, 9,* 3-10.)

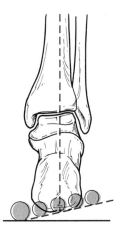

Figure 14-11. Forefoot valgus.

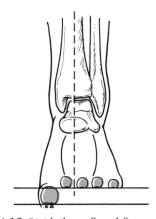

Figure 14-13. Rigid plantarflexed first ray.

sponse to ground reaction forces when the first MT head contacts the ground, it effectively acts independently of the other MT heads to limit the degree of pronation occurring at the STJ and MTJs. The effects on the midfoot as well as the entire closed kinetic lower-extremity chain are analogous to those described in the forefoot valgus condition above.

Clinical Assessment of Running Mechanics

The initial step in determining the underlying causes for running-related injuries requires examination of the subject's gait mechanics. The

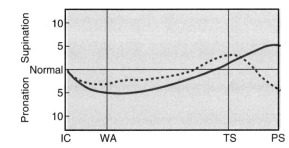

Figure 14-12. Forefoot valgus STJ (dashed line) and normal STJ motion (solid line). (Adapted from Brown, L. P., & Yavorsky, P. (1987). Locomotor biomechanics and pathomechanics: A review. Journal of Orthopaedic and Sports Physical Therapy, 9, 3-10.)

clinician is specifically looking for signs of abnormal movement patterns, particularly during the stance phase of gait, because during this phase the greatest forces are at work on the joints, ligaments, bones, and muscles.

One of the simplest and most cost-effective methods available is the use of a video camera with slow-motion and stop-action replay capabilities. Videotaping the subject on a treadmill from front, side, and rear angles can be especially helpful to the inexperienced clinician in assessing a variety of parameters pertaining to lower-extremity movement. More sophisticated, but costly, methods include the use of force plates, electrogoniometers, computerized biomechanical gait programs, and high-speed cinematography. This equipment is used in a well-equipped research motion-analysis laboratory.

A thorough gait examination should, first and foremost, look for any obvious asymmetry in frontal-plane movements at all the joints of the lower extremities, from the hips to the feet. The subject should be viewed from both front and back to accomplish this. Viewing from the side should examine for proper angular range of the hips, knees, and ankles during the various stages of stance phase.

The movements of the ankle and foot should be viewed carefully from the rear and front and analyzed for abnormal pronation/supination movements. Because these movements occur in an oblique plane, an assessment is made by extrapolating from pure calcaneal eversion/inversion motion, respectively, to determine excessive or deficient STJ and MTJ movements (Fig. 14-14). A normal value for calcaneal eversion at weight acceptance is 5–8°.[17] The clinician should consider the possibility that STJ range limitations may make it appear that pronation movement is within normal limits during early stance, despite forces such as forefoot or rearfoot varus, hip internal rotation, or side dominance that would dictate abnormal STJ movements. In such instances, these forces may consist of compensatory motions at other sites, such as the MTJ (talar bulge) or knee (valgus position) joint (Fig. 14-15).

Observation of abnormal lower-extremity movement patterns may be an important piece of the puzzle in the evaluation of running in-

juries, but only if the faulty mechanics correlate with the previously diagnosed pathology. If this is not the case, the clinician should consider other causes for the injury and address those in the most appropriate manner.

In summary, the assessment of the underlying causes for running injuries is an intuitive, logical process that incorporates the physical therapist's basic knowledge of kinesiology, muscle function, and pathologic processes associated with repetitive strain of bone and soft tissue structures. Combining that knowledge with the findings of the above-described gait and postural analysis should lead to a working hypothesis of the underlying causes for the overuse pattern that will guide the clinician's rationale for treatment of the injury.

Clinical Assessment of Lower-Extremity Posture and Muscle Balance

Once a dynamic examination of gait is performed, the next step is to examine the patient for postural and/or muscle imbalances. This would be the case even if the subject's gait pattern appeared perfectly normal, as certain injuries, such as PFPS, may be caused solely by unbalanced muscle action on a joint. If gait pathomechanics were observed, the primary goal of the static examination is then to discover the cause for the abnormal movement patterns.

A general posture examination should be performed from front, side, and rear, with particular attention paid to the following areas:

Foot and ankle
    Subtalar alignment with knee extended and
        flexed (pes planus/cavus)
    Toe-out/toe-in position
    Asymmetry of foot alignment
Knee
    "Squinting" or "frog eyes" patellas
    Genu valgum/varum/recurvatum
    Unlocked, flexed knees

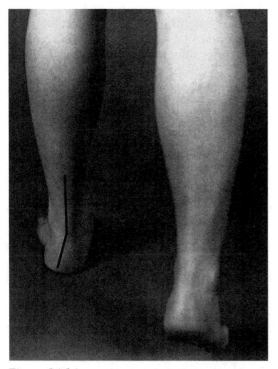

Figure 14-14. Calcaneal eversion at midstance.

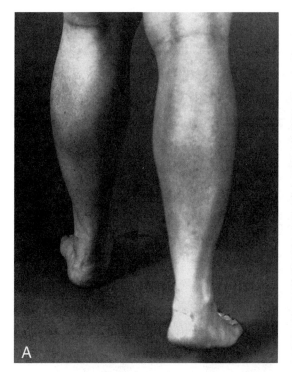
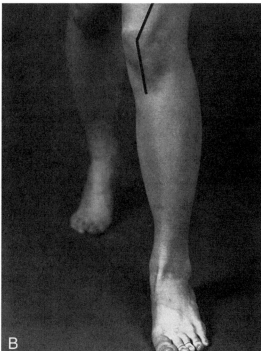

Figure 14-15. A. Midtarsal bulge at midstance. B. Genu valgum at midstance.

Hip/pelvis/lumbar spine
  Unequal pelvic heights
  Innominate rotation
  Coxa vara/valga
  Anterior/posterior pelvic tilt
  Sway-back/lordotic/flat-back lumbar spine

Perhaps the most critical element in the evaluation of the relationship between abnormal gait mechanics and postural deviations is the determination of forefoot, rearfoot, and distal leg alignment in the STN position. As described above in this chapter, malalignments such as forefoot and rearfoot varus/valgus can lead to an increase or decrease in normal pronatory movements of the foot during early stance phase that may be the underlying cause of overuse running injuries. The clinician therefore must be practiced in the technique of finding STN and then evaluating the alignment pattern of each foot. A "positive" finding may

be critical in solving the puzzle of the underlying reason for the increased stress and strain on various structures that result in injury. The accurate capture of STN is also critical for the casting of the foot when fabricating orthotics. (Casting is described later in this chapter.)

Rationale for Use of Orthotics in Management of Running Injuries

Many running injuries can be traced to abnormal movement patterns of the foot. As described earlier in this chapter, excessive, prolonged, or deficient pronatory motions can cause increased stress on numerous structures of the lower extremities leading to repetitive strain injuries. These abnormal movements may be the result of various muscle imbalances or joint malalignments proximal to the foot and, in these cases, the clinician will want to focus on addressing those problems as a means of eliminating the offending condition.

On the other hand, when abnormal foot motions are caused by inherent malalignments of the foot that cannot be altered via stretching or strengthening exercises and/or joint mobilization, the most effective alternative is to "correct" this malalignment by use of an external correction. This is essentially the function of the foot orthotics. As defined at the beginning of this chapter, the purpose of the orthotic is to enable the foot to function around the STN position. It does so by, in effect, altering the ground surface on which the foot rests so that the amount of pronatory/supinatory movement is controlled within normal limits. In so doing, it reduces the stress placed on muscles, tendons, ligaments, and other structures.[5,24,30–34]

Types of Orthotics

Foot orthotics are generally categorized by the characteristics of the materials used in their fabrication. Rigid orthotics are manufactured using acrylic plastics and, as the name implies, exhibit very little "give" in response to pressure from body weight and ground reaction forces. They therefore offer the most motion control during the stance phase of gait. Semirigid devices are made with thermoplastic materials, leather, or cork. These orthotics allow greater movement around the STN position and accordingly provide less-precise motion control (Fig. 14-16, A & B). Soft, or accommodating, orthotics provide minimal motion control and are most often used by patients whose feet cannot adjust well to the more stringent devices. They are also used with conditions such as diabetes.

There is no consensus in the literature as to the merits or disadvantages of each type of orthotic in the management of running injuries.[8,35–40] The advantages of the most commonly used orthotics are described in Resource Box 14-1.

Commercially fabricated orthotics are also available in a variety of styles and forms designed to meet special needs of patients. Many companies offer different devices specific to particular activities, such as marathon running, sprinting, walking, and biking, to particular age groups, and to footwear such as women's high heels and sandals (Fig. 14-17, A–C).

Fabrication and Casting

The key to successful management of running injuries via orthotic devices is the accurate capture and reproduction of the STN position of

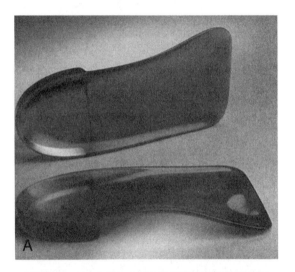

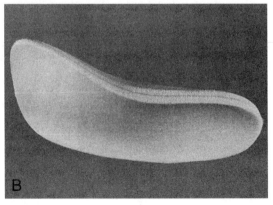

Figure 14-16. A. Rigid orthotic. B. Semirigid orthotic.

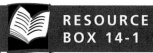

RESOURCE BOX 14-1

Advantages of Rigid Orthotics
- Precise control of subtalar movements
- Accurate reproduction of STN position
- More durable
- Assistance from laboratory fabricating orthotics in designing and prescribing device

Advantages of Semirigid Orthotics
- More accommodating to patient, especially athletes
- Quicker fabrication and delivery time to patient
- More accessible for in-house adjustments
- Less expensive

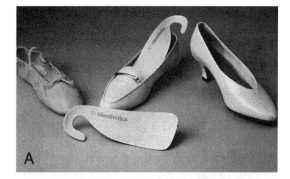

A

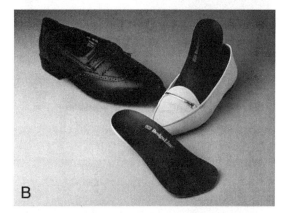

B

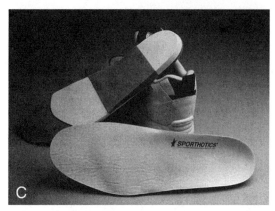

C

Figure 14-17. Varieties of orthotics. A. Slimthotics B. Dress shoe orthotics C. Sporthotics (Reproduced with permission from the Langer Biomechanics Group, Inc.)

the foot during both the casting and the fabrication of the orthotic. Failure to do so may potentially worsen the patient's condition, as improper foot motion is then transferred by the device. Therefore, the clinician casting or molding the material used in fabricating orthotics must be well versed in determining the STN position.

Detection of STN is most easily accomplished by placing the patient in a prone position on the examining table, with the foot extending beyond the end of the table. Care should be taken to ensure that the hip is in a neutrally rotated position (Fig. 14-18). The examiner places the thumb on the medial, and the index finger on the lateral, aspect of the TNJ. The fourth and fifth MT heads are grasped with the thumb and index fingers of the other hand, and the forefoot is then moved by that hand laterally and medially, thereby pronating and supinating the foot (Fig. 14-19). As the foot is pronated, the examiner should feel the head of the talus bulge into the thumb palpating the medial side of the TNJ. Likewise, when the foot is supinated, the index finger should feel the lateral side of the talus. The examiner then moves the foot in ever-smaller degrees of pronation/supination until there is no palpable bulge on either side. At that point, the thumb under the fourth to fifth MT heads

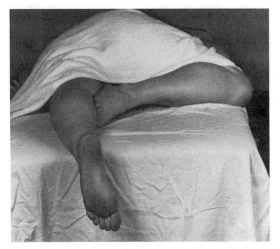

Figure 14-18. Patient in position to examine STN with opposite hip externally rotated and abducted.

pushes forward gently to dorsiflex the forefoot. This should only be done until resistance is felt (Fig. 14-20). At that point, the foot is in the STN position, and the examiner may assess the foot for normal or abnormal forefoot/rearfoot

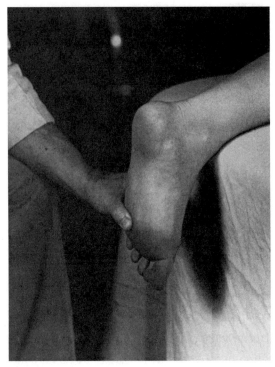

Figure 14-20. Examiner dorsiflexing patient's midfoot.

alignment. This is also the position in which the cast or mold will be taken for fabrication of the orthotic.

There are a variety of methods for taking an impression of the foot to send to a laboratory for fabrication of orthotics.[41] The most popular, and probably the most accurate, method remains the plaster cast. The procedure for this method is described below.

1. Have two extra-quick-drying splints (5 by 30 in.) folded in half lengthwise (Fig. 14-21).
2. Holding the splint at the ends, soak the first splint in warm water for a few seconds.
3. Squeeze out the extra water and pull the splint out lengthwise.
4. Fold the top edge over approximately $1/2$ to $3/4$ in. (Fig. 14-22).

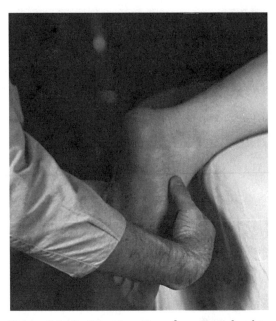

Figure 14-19. Correct position of examiner's hand to determine STN.

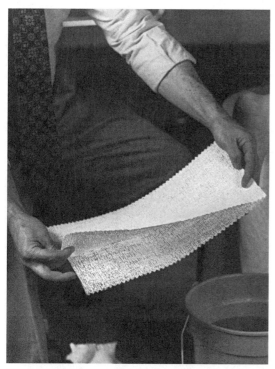

Figure 14-21. Plaster splints for casting.

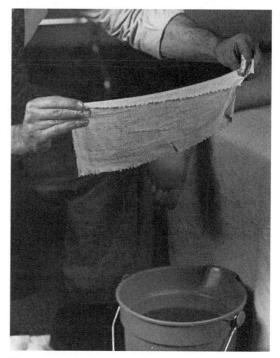

Figure 14-22. Top edge of splints folded ½ to ¾ in.

5. With the patient prone as described above, place the middle of the splint over the posterior heel and bring the top edge of the splint forward over the first and fifth metatarsals. The lower part of the splint is smoothed across the plantar surface of the foot, medial side then lateral (Fig. 14-23).

6. The excess "tab" at the heel should be pushed upward over the back of the heel (Fig. 14-24).

7. Follow steps 1–3 with the second splint.

8. Place the middle of the top of the splint approximately ½ in. above the toes, and bring the rest of the splint toward the back of the foot, covering the first and fifth metatarsals. Smooth the plantar surface as before, tucking the excess into the sulcus of the toes (Fig. 14-25, A & B).

9. When the foot is completely and smoothly covered by the splints, the examiner places

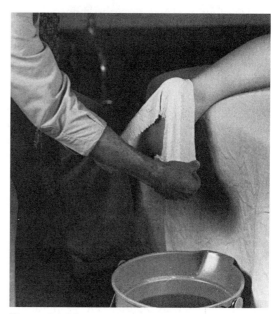

Figure 14-23. Placement of the first splint.

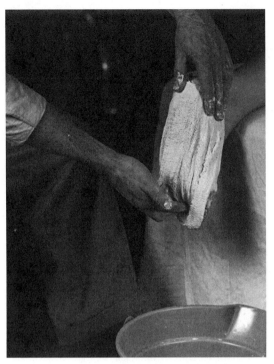

Figure 14-24. The "tab" position at the heel.

the foot in STN as described above. Do not worry about the indentation of the thumb under the fourth to fifth MT heads. The laboratory will fill this in.

10. When the cast has hardened (tapping it smartly with the fingers should produce a clicking sound), remove it by loosening the skin beneath the upper border and then pull downward from beneath the malleoli. As the cast clears the heel, slide it forward off the toes (Fig. 14-26).

11. The cast should be inspected and then stuffed with newspaper for mailing to the laboratory.

An alternative to laboratory fabrication of semirigid orthotics is in-house fabrication. This process is possible with a minimal investment in supplies and materials. Several companies offer precut forms that can be molded to capture the STN position via heat or water-

activated resin (Fig. 14-27 A & B). Other thermoplastic materials can be formed to the patient's foot and then cut and ground to custom requirements, with posting materials added that control foot motion more effectively. The process of fabricating semirigid orthotics is described below.

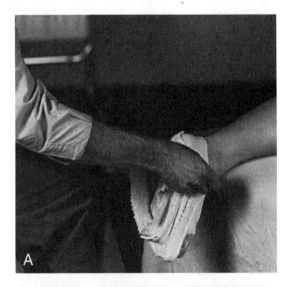

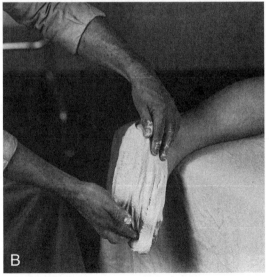

Figure 14-25. A and B. Placement of the second splint.

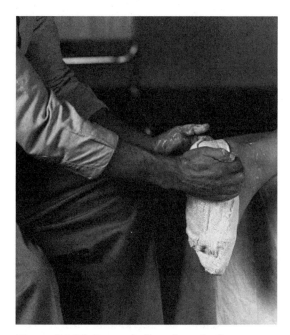

Figure 14-26. Removal of cast from the foot.

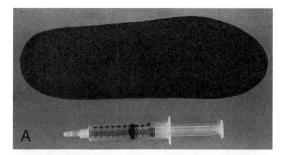

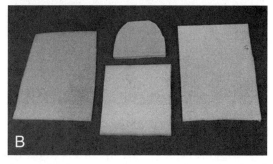

Figure 14-27. A. Biorthotic precut forms. **B.** Alimed precut forms.

Fabrication of Semirigid Orthotics

Required Materials

Two pieces of Aliplast XPE, 12 by 4 in.
Two pieces of Plastizote no. 2, 12 by 4 in.
Nickelplast material for posting
Contact cement
Convection oven (Fig. 14-28) Grinder (Fig. 14-29) Scissors

Procedure

1. Place one piece of Plastizote no. 2 beneath a piece of Aliplast XPE in an oven preheated to 300°F. After a few minutes, remove (with an oven mitt) after the Aliplast has curled and then flattened on the Plastizote.

2. Place the combined materials on a pillow or foam pad covered with a towel. Allow to cool to a temperature comfortable to the back of the hand.

3. Place the patient's socked foot on the materials, taking care to monitor the patient's reaction to the heat. (*Note:* the patient may be seated or standing with support.)

4. When the patient is comfortable, passively move the foot into a STN position. When stable, place a slight downward pressure

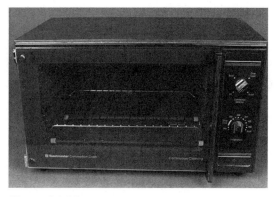

Figure 14-28. Convection oven.

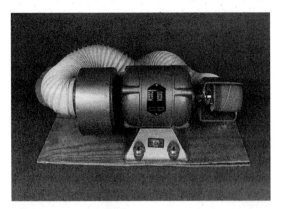

Figure 14-29. Grinder.

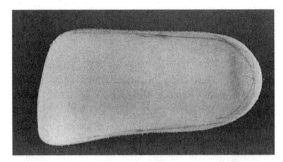

Figure 14-31. Sides and distal end of orthotic ground.

on the rearfoot to dorsiflex the forefoot. Hold this position for 3–5 minutes until the material hardens.

5. Draw an outline of the foot on the mold, with the front of the orthotic ending at the MTP joint (Fig. 14-30).

6. Grind the sides of the orthotic, with a slight angulation on the medial side, and taper the forefoot end so that the MTP joint will rest on a flat surface (Fig. 14-31).

7. Grind the bottom of the mold until the lateral side is almost down to the Aliplast layer (Fig. 14-32).

8. Cut out a piece of Nickelplast material in the form of a "cobra" pad that will cover the still remaining Plastizote material (Fig. 14-33).

9. Brush contact cement on the adjacent sides of the Nickelplast cutout and the surface of the orthotic mold to which it will be joined.

10. When the cement has thoroughly dried (~1 hour), place the Nickelplast piece in the oven for about a minute until it is pliable. Remove and join with the orthotic.

11. Grind the sides of the Nickelplast to conform to the orthotic and then grind the bottom until the lateral side of the distal section is flush with the orthotic. The rearfoot curve should be ground at the approximate angle of the rearfoot varus angle determined by the STN examination (Fig. 14-34).

12. Smooth the top edges of the orthotic.

Various covering materials may be applied to the upper surface of the orthotic for cushioning and/or cosmetic effect, but they are generally

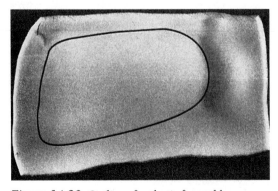

Figure 14-30. Outline of orthotic for mold.

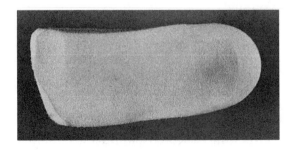

Figure 14-32. Bottom of orthotic ground.

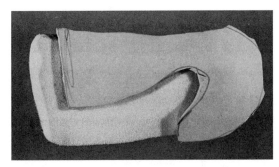

Figure 14-33. Nickelplast cutout in the form of a "cobra" pad.

not necessary and serve to add another layer that increases the height of the device. More functional additions may be added, such as MT pads or bars to address specific foot conditions that are beyond the scope of this chapter.

Contraindications

There are few definite contraindications in the use of foot orthotics, although there are many instances in which they will be of little, if any, value. Use of orthotic devices with the pes cavus foot is controversial, as the attempt to promote increased pronatory movement at the STJ through the use of a valgus forefoot posting has not been proven successful.[3] The most common misuse of orthotic devices is with the rigid pes planus foot (Fig. 14-35). Such feet appear to be ideal for orthotic intervention, at least when viewed with the subject weight

bearing. The problem arises, however, when the foot does not assume a more normal arch when non–weight bearing. Attempting to place a rigid or even semirigid device underneath a foot that lacks the flexibility to retain a normal arch height will usually only serve to irritate the midfoot joints. A more accommodating device, or at least one with the most minimal correction, may be more successful.

The prophylactic use of orthotics is also ill-advised. Runners often seek orthotic devices not because of injury, but because they have been told by "friends" and fellow athletes that they "pronate too much" and should see about getting a pair. In these cases, the clinician would be wise to adhere to the old adage, "If it ain't broke, don't fix it!" Despite the exhibition of the most pathomechanical gait pattern, if the subject has no injury or complaint it should be assumed that he or she has compensated for this in some other manner. Placing an orthotic in this individual's shoe may only result in iatrogenic injury.

The use of orthotics with children is described in the Pediatric Perspective Box.

Summary

Foot orthotics can play an important role in the management of selected injuries commonly found in the runner by helping to control abnormal movement patterns of the lower ex-

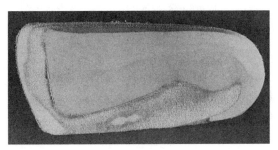

Figure 14-34. Posting material that has undergone grinding.

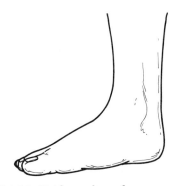

Figure 14-35. Rigid pes planus foot.

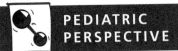

PEDIATRIC PERSPECTIVE

The use of orthotics with children should also be approached with caution. Clinicians should remember that children will normally display what appears to be a pronounced flatfoot in weight bearing up to at least 6 years of age. Wenger et. al.[42] demonstrated that early intervention with orthotics had no effect on eventual outcome of foot development in children, so it appears clear that there is no prophylactic role for orthotics in development. While some have flat feet that persist beyond 6 years of age, very few become significant in terms of causing injuries, at least until adolescence. Therefore, it is not necessary in most cases to prescribe orthotics preventatively.

- Excessive or deficient foot pronation and lower-extremity rotatory movements may cause a number of common injuries.

- Clinical assessment of lower-extremity posture and muscle imbalances may lead to the cause of pathomechanics.

- When abnormal foot motions are caused by inherent malalignments of the foot that cannot be altered by stretching or strengthening exercises and/or joint mobilization, an effective intervention is the use of foot orthotics.

- The most common orthotics are rigid, semirigid, or soft or accommodating.

- Semirigid orthotics are commonly fabricated in one of two ways: a plaster cast can be taken and sent to the laboratory or a semirigid orthotic may be fabricated inhouse with a minimal investment in supplies and materials.

tremities. They are successful, however, only when used with the appropriate patient and situation. Stan James, MD, a noted expert on running injuries noted:

"Orthotics are not a panacea but have added a new horizon to our treatment armamentarium for the overuse syndrome."[1]

KEY POINTS

- Most injuries sustained by runners affect the structures of the foot/ankle and knee, although they are by no means limited to those areas.

- Running injuries may be caused by training errors, improper footwear, and abnormal biomechanics.

- The movements of pronation and supination are normally occurring movements of the STJ that impart an enormous influence on movements throughout the lower limb and pelvis.

CRITICAL THINKING QUESTIONS

1. Differentiate among the terms *orthotics, orthosis,* and *orthotist.*

2. Differentiate among the causes of running injuries.

3. Describe the position of the STJ during the normal gait cycle.

4. Assess how deficient STJ pronation may result in commonly seen clinical conditions such as PFPS, posterior tibial stress syndrome, plantar fasciitis, metatarsalgia, ITBFS, sacroiliac joint sprain, and stress fractures.

5. Explain the extrinsic and intrinsic causes of abnormal STJ pronation and supination.

6. Describe the purpose of an orthotic in "correcting" malalignments.

7. Compare and contrast various types of orthotics.

8. Briefly describe the process of taking a plaster impression of the foot and fabrication of semirigid orthotics.

REFERENCES

1. James, S. L., Bates, B. T., & Osternig, L. R. (1978). Injuries to runners. *American Journal of Sports Medicine, 6,* 40–50.

2. Bates, B. T., Osternig, L. R., Mason, B., & James, L. S. (1979). Foot orthotic devices to modify selected aspects of lower extremity mechanics. *American Journal of Sports Medicine, 7,* 338–342.

3. D'Ambrosia, R. D. (1985). Orthotic devices in running injuries. *Clinics in Sports Medicine, 4,* 611–619.

4. Reid, D. C. (1992). Sports injury assessment and rehabilitation (1st ed.). New York: Churchill Livingstone.

5. Gross, M. L., Davlin, L. B., & Evanski, P. M. (1991). Effectiveness of orthotic shoe inserts in the long-distance runner. *American Journal of Sports Medicine, 19,* 409–412.

6. Cook, S. D., Brinker, M. R., & Poche, M. (1990). Running shoes: Their relationship to running injuries. *Sports Medicine, 19,* 1–8.

7. van Mechelen, W. (1992). Running injuries: A review of the epidemiological literature. *Sports Medicine, 21,* 320–335.

8. McKenzie, D. C., Clement, D. B., & Taunton, J. E. (1985). Running shoes, orthotics, and injuries. *Sports Medicine, 14,* 334–347.

9. Marti, B., Vader, J. P., Minder, C. E., & Abelin, T. (1988). On the epidemiology of running injuries: The 1984 Bern Grand-Prix Study. *American Journal of Sports Medicine, 16,* 285–293.

10. Messier, S. P., & Pittala, K. A. (1988). Etiologic factors associated with selected running injuries. *Medicine and Science in Sports and Exercise, 20,* 501–505.

11. Gross, M. T. (1995). Lower quarter screening for skeletal malalignment—Suggestions for orthotics and shoewear. *Journal of Orthopaedic and Sports Physical Therapy, 21,* 389–405.

12. Coplan, J. A. (1989). Rotational motion of the knee: A comparison of normal and pronating subjects. *Journal of Orthopaedic and Sports Physical Therapy, 10,* 366–369.

13. Hintermann, B., & Nigg, B. M. (1998). Pronation in runners: Implications for injuries. *Sports Medicine, 26,* 169–176.

14. Donatelli, R. (1987). Abnormal biomechanics of the foot and ankle. *Journal of Orthopaedic and Sports Physical Therapy, 9,* 11–16.

15. Powers, C. M., Maffucci, R., & Hampton, S. (1995). Rearfoot posture in subjects with patellofemoral pain. *Journal of Orthopaedic and Sports Physical Therapy, 22,* 155–160.

16. Viitsalso, J. T., & Kvist, M. (1983). Some biomechanical aspects of the foot and ankle in athletes with and without shin splints. *American Journal of Sports Medicine, 11,* 125–130.

17. Brown, L. P., & Yavorsky, P. (1987). Locomotor biomechanics and pathomechanics: A review. *Journal of Orthopaedic and Sports Physical Therapy, 9,* 3–10.

18. Donatelli, R. (1985). Normal biomechanics of the foot and ankle. *Journal of Orthopaedic and Sports Physical Therapy, 7,* 91–95.

19. Rockar, P. A. (1995). The subtalar joint: Anatomy and joint motion. *Journal of Orthopaedic and Sports Physical Therapy, 22,* 361–372.

20. Rogers, M. M. (1995). Dynamic foot biomechanics. *Journal of Orthopaedic and Sports Physical Therapy, 22,* 306–316.

21. Lundberg, A., Svensson, O. K., Bylund, C., Goldie, I., & Selvik, G. (1989). Kinematics of the ankle/foot complex—Part 2: Pronation and supination. *Foot and Ankle, 9,* 248–253.

22. Pierrynowski, M. R. (1996). Rear foot inversion/eversion during gait relative to the subtalar joint neutral position. *Foot and Ankle International, 17,* 406–412.

23. McPoil, T., & Cornwall, M. W. (1994) Relationship between neutral subtalar joint position and pattern of rearfoot motion during walking. *Foot and Ankle, 17,* 406–412.

24. Eng, J. J., & Pierrynowski, M. R. (1993). Evaluation of soft foot orthotics in the treatment of patellofemoral pain syndrome. *Physical Therapy, 73,* 62–70.

25. Campbell, J. W., & Inman, V. T. (1974). Treatment of plantar fasciitis and calcaneal spurs with the UC-BL shoe insert. *Clinical Orthopedics and Related Research, 103,* 57–62.

26. Sobel, E., Levitz, S., & Caselli, M. A. (1999). Orthoses in the treatment of rearfoot problems. *Journal of the American Podiatric Medical Association, 89,* 220–233.

27. Franco, A. H. (1987). Pes cavus and pes planus. *Physical Therapy, 67,* 688–693.

28. Subotnick, S. I. (1981). Limb length discrepancies of the lower extremity (the short leg syndrome). *Journal of Orthopaedic and Sports Physical Therapy, 3,* 11–16.

29. Friberg, O, Nurminen, M, Korhonen, K, Soininen, E, & Manttari T. (1988). Accuracy and precision of clinical estimation of leg length inequality and lumbar scoliosis: Comparison of clinical and radiological measurements. *International Disability Studies, 10,* 49–53.

30. Kitaoka, H. B., Zong, P. L., & Kai-Nan, A. (1997). Analysis of longitudinal arch supports in stabilizing the arch of the foot. *Clinical Orthopaedics and Related Research, 341,* 250–256.

31. McPoil, T. G., Adrian, M., & Pidcoe, P. (1989). Effects of foot orthoses on center-of-pressure patterns in women. *Physical Therapy 69,* 149–154.

32. Nawoczenski, D. A., & Ludewig, P. M. (1999). Electromyographic effects of foot orthotics on selected lower extremity muscles during running. *Archives of Physical Medicine and Rehabilitation, 80,* 540–544.

33. Nawoczenski, D. A., Cook, T. M., & Saltzman, C. L. (1995). The effect of foot orthotics on three dimensional kinematics of the leg and rearfoot during running. *Journal of Orthopaedic and Sports Physical Therapy, 22,* 317–327.

34. Novick, A., & Kelley, D. L. (1990). Position and movement changes of the foot with orthotic intervention during the loading response of gait. *Journal of Orthopaedic and Sports Physical Therapy, 12,* 301–311.

35. McPoil, T. G., & Cornwall, M. W. (1991). Rigid versus soft foot orthoses. *Journal of the American Podiatric Medical Association, 81,* 638–642.

36. Hannaford, D. R. (1986). Soft orthoses for athletes. *Journal of the American Podiatric Medical Association, 76,* 566–569.

37. Nigg, B. M., Khan, A., Fisher, V., & Stefanyshyn, D. (1998). Effect of shoe insert construction on foot and leg movement. *Medicine and Science in Sports and Exercise, 30,* 550–555.

38. Pfeffer, G., Bacchetti, P., Deland, J., Lewis, A., Anderson, R., Davis, W., Alvarez, R., et al. (1999). Comparison of custom and prefabricated orthoses in the initial treatment of proximal plantar fasciitis. *Foot and Ankle International, 20,* 214–221.

39. Smith, L. S., Clarke, T. E., Hamill, C. L., & Santopietro, F. (1986). The effects of soft and semirigid orthoses upon rearfoot movement in running. *Journal of the American Podiatric Medical Association, 76,* 227–233.

40. Weik, D. A., & Martin, W. (1993). Use of soft heat-molded orthoses in sports. *Journal of the American Podiatric Medical Association, 83,* 529–533.

41. McPoil, T. G., Schuit, D., & Knecht, H. G. (1989). Comparison of three methods used to obtain a neutral plaster foot impression. *Physical Therapy, 69,* 448–452.

42. Wenger, D. R., Mauldin, D., Speck, G., Morgan, D., & Lieber, R. L. (1989). Corrective shoes and inserts as treatment for flexible flatfoot in infants and children. *Journal of Bone and Joint Surgery, 71A,* 800–809.

Chapter 15

ORTHOSES FOR ORTHOPEDIC CONDITIONS

Carol A. Gambell, MSM, ATC, BOC

Objectives

1. Define common acronyms used in orthotics
2. Describe the functions of a lower-limb orthosis
3. Differentiate the classifications of ankle orthoses including stirrup orthoses, lace-up orthoses, elastic supports, prophylactic ankle orthoses, and controlled ankle motion (CAM) walkers
4. Compare and contrast the classifications of knee orthoses including prophylactic knee orthoses, postoperative rehabilitation knee orthoses, functional knee orthoses, orthoses for patellofemoral disorders, valgus control functional knee orthoses, and orthoses for osteoarthritis (unloader)
5. Describe orthoses that are used for hip muscle strains, dislocated hips, and Legg-Calvé-Perthes disease.

This chapter is divided into the following sections:

The word *orthosis* is derived from the Greek *ortho* meaning straight, upright, or correct. Perhaps the oldest known of all devices to splint the knee joint existed as early as the Fifth Dynasty (2730–2625 BC). Historically, several types of splints were used; bundles of straw bound together, bark strips, and mixtures of egg whites and solidifying pastes. Ambroise Paré (1509–1590) a pioneer in the art of orthosis making, commissioned armor makers who were proficient with metal, leather, and wood. However, these devices were heavy and cumbersome and had little functional assistance. The craft of orthosis making was often handed down from father to son, master to apprentice.[1] Over the last several years, a shift has occurred in the manufacturing of orthoses. Before the 1970s, orthoses such as those used for the knee or ankle, were fabricated by small orthotic shops on an individual-need basis. Due to the growing population and growing need, specialized manufacturing companies began to emerge. An increasingly more recreational lifestyle resulted in more athletic and industrial injuries that required, in many cases, orthoses to return to play or work. This lifestyle change hastened the need for commercially available orthoses. Manufacturing companies quickly developed ways to produce orthoses that are either sized to fit or can be quickly made from casts or measurements. These orthoses encompass the management of athletic injury, fracture, and neurologic and painful biomechanical abnormalities.[2]

The Committee on Prosthetics Orthotics Education (CPOE) has clarified terminology in orthotics.[3] Common acronyms used in orthotics are as follows:

FO   Foot orthosis
AFO   Ankle–foot orthosis
AO   Ankle orthosis
KAFO   Knee–ankle–foot orthosis
KO   Knee orthosis
HKAFO   Hip–knee–ankle–foot orthosis
THKAFO   Thoracic–hip–knee–ankle–foot orthosis

The CPOE also recommends that orthoses be described by the joints they encompass (e.g., the acronym KAFO for knee–ankle–foot orthosis) with elimination of terminology such as long leg brace. Additional terms are used to describe the function designed into an orthosis system such as "free," "assist," "stop," and "lock." These terms clearly present the nature of the controls in the planes of motion for all joints and limb segments.

A team approach to the prescription and evaluation of orthoses is often necessary, since the patient who needs an orthosis may present multiple deficits. The team approach is described in Chapter 3. Members of this orthotic team should include a physician interested in rehabilitation, an orthotist, a physical therapist, a social worker, and/or a vocational rehabilitation counselor. In some settings, an athletic trainer is a member of this team. To be an effective advocate for the patient and to converse effectively with an orthotist, the physical therapist should have a sound knowledge of orthosis components to be able to recommend or prescribe these components for a particular patient.

Orthotic intervention may change considerably with the same patient. The goal of orthotic intervention is based on the needs of the patient at a specific time. For example, a patient may need an orthosis for weight bearing and transfers in the early rehabilitation phases but a more functional orthosis for ambulation activities in later rehabilitation phases.[4]

Health professionals including physical therapists often measure patients for commercially available orthoses and have them custom fabricated within a few days. Prefabricated, or "off the shelf," orthoses can be fit immediately. These are sometimes called *custom-fitted orthoses*. Orthoses that are molded to the specific patient are called *custom-made orthoses*. Patients are taking part in their own injury management by choosing an orthosis on the basis of information made available to them by manufacturers, through the Internet, or in sport or health magazines. Clinical studies on the efficacy of different brands are ongoing, and health professionals should be aware of those manufacturers whose designs are biomechanically based.

Lower-limb orthoses have many functions. These are included in Box 15-1.[4]

This chapter first discusses ankle orthoses, then knee orthoses, and finally those used for hip and pelvic conditions.

BOX 15-1

Functions of Lower-Limb Orthoses

Correct deformity
Prevent deformity
Protect a weakened or painful musculoskeletal segment
Unload a joint or limb
Rest and immobilization
Assist movement
Provide feedback
Enhance gait
Alleviate pain
Promote osteogenesis

Ankle Orthoses

From an orthopedic standpoint, ankle orthoses are often used in interventions for injuries to the ankle and foot. AFOs for patients with a neurologic condition are discussed in Chapter 16. One of the most common ankle injuries is an inversion sprain. For example, 5000 ankle inversion injuries are treated per day in the United Kingdom. Sports such as basketball, volleyball, and soccer have a very high incidence of ankle injuries.[5] The ligamentous support of the lateral ankle is much weaker than its medial counterpart. As a result, an ankle inversion injury often results. The ankle inversion sprain is caused by excessive plantarflexion, supination, and adduction. It is common to see an athlete land unevenly from a jump, perform a cutting maneuver, or encounter uneven terrain. The anterior talofibular ligament is usually torn first, followed by the calcaneofibular ligament.[6] The posterior talofibular ligament is usually uninjured unless there is a dislocation of the ankle.[5] The mechanism of injury of an ankle inversion sprain is either (a) falling away to the opposite side with the foot firmly planted or (*b*) supinating the plantarflexed foot while weight bearing. This mechanism of injury is common with the basketball player who lands on another player's foot after grabbing a rebound.

Forty percent of individuals who have had inversion sprains are left with functional instability. Excessive motion, caused by the ligaments being stretched, reduces the ability of the foot to become a rigid lever. An external support, such as an ankle orthosis, may allow normal mechanics while restricting undesired motion.[7] The acute phase of treatment may include

1. Controlling inflammation
2. Limiting inversion and eversion
3. Promoting dorsiflexion by maintaining gastrocnemius/Achilles complex flexibility
4. Controlling forces to stimulate collagen alignment
5. Stimulating normal proprioceptive feedback[6]

If the treatment of ankle inversion sprains is based on biomechanical principles, recurrence will be lessened, and athletes will be able to return to competition at a faster rate.[8] An ankle orthosis is often part of the rehabilitation protocol for an ankle inversion sprain.

Ankle orthoses may be divided into several categories. These include

Stirrup orthoses
Lace-up orthoses
Elastic supports
Prophylactic ankle orthoses
Controlled ankle motion walkers

Each of these is discussed in detail as follows.

Stirrup Orthoses

Stirrup orthoses depend on the integrity of the footgear such as the heel counter to control the calcaneus. There are five commonly used stirrup orthoses. These include the following.

Aircast Air-Stirrup

The Aircast Air-Stirrup consists of rigid plastic molded medial and lateral sides, lined with preinflated air cells. The air cells provide comfortable uniform compression for reduction of edema. The rigid plastic sides resist inversion forces yet allow normal plantarflexion and dorsiflexion (Fig. 15-1).

Multi-Phase Ankle System

The Multi-Phase Ankle System also consists of rigid plastic molded medial and lateral sides in addition to an optional locked footplate that prevents plantarflexion. This plantarflexion restriction decreases tension in the torn anterior talofibular ligament and brings the ligament ends into close proximity for healing. The Multi-Phase Ankle System can be converted to a postacute functional orthosis that allows full

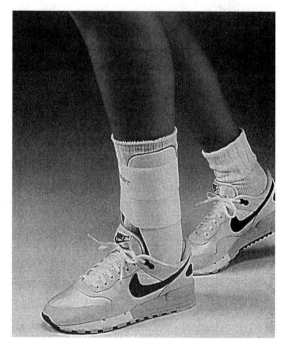

Figure 15-1. Aircast Air-Stirrup. (Reprinted with permission from Aircast Inc., Summit, NJ.)

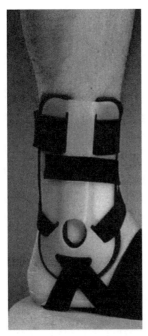

Figure 15-2. Multiphase ankle system. (Reprinted with permission from Omni Scientific, Concord, CA.)

dorsiflexion, plantarflexion, and compression, while continuing to resist inversion (Fig. 15-2).

Sure Step Ankle Support System

The Sure Step Ankle Support System possesses a rigid footplate that extends anterior to the proximal metatarsophalangeal joints to support the medial arch and midfoot. The foam-lined plastic medial and lateral sides may be fixed at first to reduce plantarflexion and then converted to free motion. The footplate of the Sure Step Ankle Support System helps to maintain the subtalar neutral position, allowing early weight bearing in proper alignment (Fig. 15-3).

Active Ankle System

The Active Ankle System is a variation of the original stirrup design. The hinge at the ankle allows plantarflexion and dorsiflexion while

discouraging inversion. The Active Ankle System is popular among athletes in jumping sports such as volleyball and basketball (Fig. 15-4).

Richie Brace

The Richie Brace is a combination of a biomechanical foot orthotic, deep heel cup, and a hinged stirrup. Foot problems, such as forefoot valgus, which may contribute to further ankle sprains, may be corrected in the footplate by extrinsic posting. A disadvantage of the Richie Brace is that casting is required (Fig. 15-5).

Lace-Up Orthoses

The functions of lace-up orthoses are similar to those of ankle taping. Lace-up orthoses are sized by shoe size and are available in right or left. Because of their similarity to taping, ath-

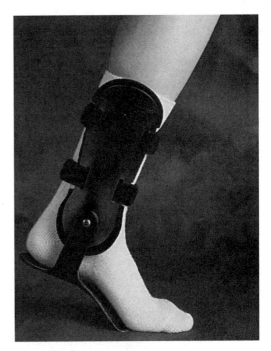

Figure 15-3. Sure Step Ankle Support System. (Reprinted with permission from USMC, Tustin, CA.)

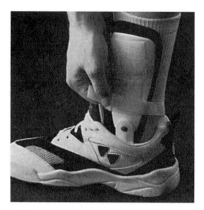

Figure 15-4. Active Ankle System. (Reprinted with permission from Active Ankle Systems Inc., Louisville, KY.)

letic organizations may use lace-up orthoses as preventive devices, especially in sports with high incidences of ankle inversion sprains, such as basketball. In lace-up orthoses, the midfoot, subtalar, and talocrural joints are encapsulated in a vinyl or nylon shell with a front lacing system. To add additional torque, most lace-up orthoses have Velcro straps that help to limit inversion. Velcro straps may also create a figure-8 cradle.[9] Two types of lace-up orthoses are described below.

Ankle Stabilizing Orthosis (ASO)

The Ankle Stabilizing Orthosis (ASO) is less bulky than stirrup orthoses, therefore wearing compliance is high. The ASO possesses a heel opening to allow easy foot placement. The laces and Velcro straps are secured at the top by a neoprene closure. The ASO is washable and will last for one to two athletic seasons (Fig. 15-6).

SwedeO Lightning Lok

The SwedeO Lightning Lok is a low-bulk, light-weight design that is constructed of a mesh material that allows improved air flow that keeps the wearer dry and cool. This orthosis fits either right or left ankles (Fig. 15-7).

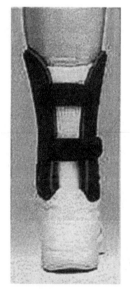

Figure 15-5. Richie brace. (Reprinted with permission from PAL Health Technology, Pekin, IL.)

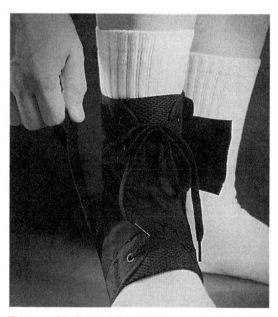

Figure 15-6. Ankle-stabilizing orthosis (ASO). (Reprinted with permission from Medical Specialties Inc., Charlotte, NC.)

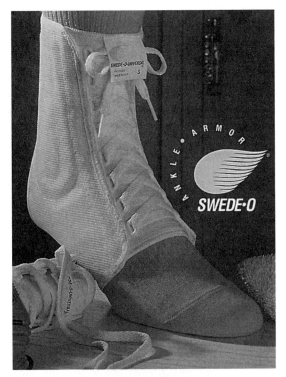

Figure 15-7. SwedeO Lightning Lok. (Reprinted with permission from SwedeO, North Branch, MN.)

Elastic Supports

Elastic supports may be used for specific ankle conditions such as a tendinitis. One elastic support is the Achillotrain.

The Achillotrain is an elastic pull-on sleeve with a silicone insert that extends parallel to the Achilles tendon for uniform compression. The Achillotrain is contoured to promote slight plantarflexion and has a viscoelastic heel wedge to raise the heel. The Achillotrain is available in right or left styles and is sized by ankle circumference (Fig. 15-8).

Prophylactic Ankle Orthoses

As injuries in athletics have risen over the past 30 years, prophylactic ankle taping and the use of prophylactic ankle orthoses have evolved to de-

crease the incidence of ankle injuries. However, taping often loses its control after a relatively short period of wear. Therefore, a prophylactic ankle orthosis is often used. Two prophylactic ankle orthoses are described as follows.

The Spatz

The Spatz is a combination ankle orthosis and elastic figure-8 support that is worn over the shoe. The Spatz is pulled over the sneaker or cleat and closed in front by Velcro. An elastic wrap is then applied that mimics taping. Finally, a sock made of Lycra is applied to protect the orthosis. All of these materials are washable (Fig. 15-9).

Arizona Ankle Orthosis

The Arizona Ankle Orthosis is similar to the ASO. This orthosis has two figure-8 lift straps for support and a cushioned neoprene tongue for comfort (Fig. 15-10).

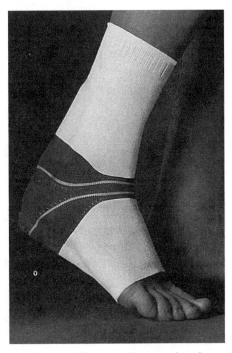

Figure 15-8. Achillotrain. (Reprinted with permission from Bauerfeind Inc, Kennesaw, GA.)

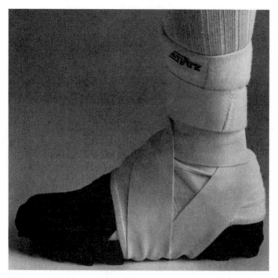

Figure 15-9. The Spatz. (Reprinted with permission from Brace International Inc. Atlanta, GA.)

Controlled Ankle Motion (CAM) Walkers

CAM Walkers are often used for the management of fractures, severe tendinitis, and tendon injuries and for postsurgical uses. CAM

Walkers are similar to a removable cast and have a rocker bottom that allows a more natural gait pattern. Many CAM walkers come disassembled and must be constructed for each patient. The medial and lateral hinges of the CAM Walker allow adjustable range of motion (ROM). In cases of fractures from the midtibia or fibula to the midfoot or in cases of third-degree ankle sprains, the CAM Walker may be extended higher up the leg (Fig. 15-11). A shorter CAM Walker may be used for midfoot sprains, metatarsal fractures, postsurgical incision protection, and immobilization for inflammatory conditions (Fig. 15-12). Patient compliance is high with the CAM Walkers because they are easily removed for bathing and sleeping if the physician allows.

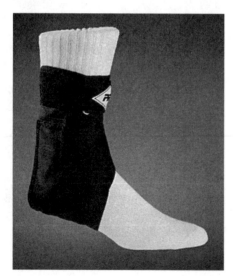

Figure 15-10. Arizona Ankle Orthosis. (Reprinted with permission from PRO Orthopedic Devices Inc, Tucson AZ.)

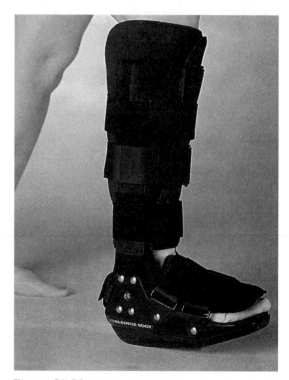

Figure 15-11. Hi-Top CAM Walker. (Reprinted with permission from Bledsoe Brace Systems, Grand Prairie, TX.)

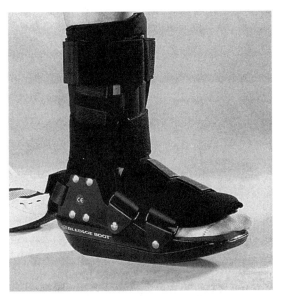

Figure 15-12. Mid-Calf CAM Walker. (Reprinted with permission from Bledsoe Brace Systems, Grand Prairie, TX.)

Research Studies

The beneficial effects of ankle orthoses are well documented. One study of 22 subjects compared passive ankle resistance of no orthosis, flexible orthoses, and semirigid orthoses. Results showed that the semirigid and flexible orthoses tolerated significantly greater torque forces as measured on a passive ankle resistance unit and less inversion range than the no-orthosis condition.[7] Another study found that prophylactic orthoses could prevent an estimated 30 ankle sprains per 1000 athletic exposures. Prophylactic orthoses were found to be cost-effective in a high-risk population.[9] One biomechanical investigation concluded that ankle orthoses increased ankle torque, counteracting inversion stresses. They also prevent the start of inversion movement by preloading and maintaining the ankle in a proper anatomic position.[10] In a meta-analysis design of 19 studies representing 253 cases, three methods of immobilization were compared: taping and lace-up and semirigid orthoses. Ex-

amples of a semirigid orthoses included stirrup orthoses such as the Aircast and Active Ankle. The semirigid support restricted inversion and eversion the most, while taping offered the most support for limiting dorsiflexion.[11] In a comparison of four common ankle orthoses, two lace-up and two semirigid, the semirigid orthoses provided more support in inversion and internal and external rotation ROM (measured by goniometry) than the lace-up orthoses.[11] The Active Ankle Orthosis provided the least interference with dorsiflexion and plantarflexion as measured by an instrumentation device with six degrees of freedom.[12]

One study of five cadaveric ankles and eight strap-on orthoses concluded that many of the orthoses functioned to resist inversion at a level that was comparable with, or exceeded, the capability of freshly applied athletic tape. Orthoses that were not as effective as freshly applied tape had the advantage of easy readjustability, whereas the support provided by the athletic tape decreased with usage. High-top athletic shoes significantly increased the passive resistance to inversion.[13] In one study of 66 patients with stage II lateral malleolar fractures, the effectiveness of a CAM Walker and an Aircast Air-Stirrup was compared. After 4 weeks, pain relief and inflammation control were higher in the CAM Walker group. However, 3 months after injury, no differences were observed in ambulation, pain, edema, ROM, or inflammation. Both groups were satisfied with comfort and ease of application.[14] A review article stated that the effect of ankle orthoses on athletic performance is usually studied by vertical jump, speed, and agility. Since some studies have found that plantarflexion may be restricted by ankle orthoses, athletic performance may be impaired. However, most studies indicate that ankle orthoses have no, or only a small, effect on vertical jump height, running speed, agility, and broad jumping.[15] In a comprehensive review of 113 studies of ankle injuries and their effective interventions, most studies showed that appropriately applied orthoses did not adversely affect performance.

These investigators recommended that athletes with a moderate or severe sprain should wear an appropriate ankle orthosis for at least 6 months during practice or competition.[16] In a review of five randomized trails with 3954 participants, evidence was found favoring the use of semirigid orthoses or Aircast braces to prevent ankle sprain during sport activities. These investigators concluded that in subjects with a history of ankle sprain, the use of such orthoses may reduce the incidence of future sprain.[5] Overall, the studies on ankle orthoses show beneficial effects and little interference with athletic performance.

One of the reasons for the effectiveness of ankle orthoses relates to their ability to increase proprioception. However, the question of the effectiveness of ankle orthoses in increasing proprioception is controversial. Some investigators have found that the application of ankle orthoses improved proprioception and neuromotor function.[17,18] Likewise, in a study of 11 healthy subjects, an increase in peroneal muscle motoneuron excitability as measured by the H-reflex was found with application of an ankle stirrup orthosis.[19] Conversely, one study compared 25 subjects with recurrent ankle sprains and 18 healthy controls. All subject ankles were measured, taped and untaped. Results showed no significant difference in the ability to perceive ankle movements between subjects with sprains and healthy controls at any velocity of movement tested. Also there were no significant differences between the taped and untaped conditions for either subject group at any velocity.[20] Further research is needed to determine whether ankle orthoses increase proprioception.

Knee Orthoses

Knee injuries are prevalent in sports, industrial accidents, and motor vehicle injuries. An estimated 989,000 people used knee orthoses in 1994, making it the second most popular anatomic assistive device, following spinal or-

thoses. Knee orthoses are the most popular anatomic assistive device used by younger patients. Seventy percent of all knee orthoses were used by persons 44 years and younger.[21]

Until the late 1960s, knee orthoses for instability were limited to cumbersome KAFOs that were designed for severe degenerative or paralytic knees.[1] The first modern functional knee orthosis was designed by Nicholas and Castiglia during the early 1970s. Many functional knee orthoses have been introduced since then. Unfortunately there are few studies that prove the efficacy of using knee orthoses during athletic performance. Many of these studies have been done at low forces that do not parallel the high forces seen in athletic competition.[22] No regulatory agency oversees the development and production of orthoses or investigates the claims made by manufacturers. Therefore, the recommendation of a particular orthosis is often empirical and not substantiated by well-controlled studies. Knee orthoses may be divided into seven categories. These are as follows:

1. Prophylactic
2. Postoperative or rehabilitative
3. Functional
4. Patellar
5. Valgus control
6. Orthoses for osteoarthritis (unloader)
7. Other

Prophylactic Knee Orthoses

Prophylactic knee orthoses are those designed to eliminate or reduce the severity of damage to the knee joint caused by contact and noncontact injuries.[23] These orthoses were first worn by football linemen to minimize an injury if one lineman should fall onto the lateral side of the knee of another lineman. Prophylactic orthoses were developed to dissipate the force of a lateral blow to the knee, diminishing the valgus force and resulting ligamentous damage.[1] One of the first prophylactic knee orthoses was the

Anderson Stabilizer, which is a prefabricated single lateral steel support secured to the thigh and leg with tape (Fig. 15-13).

Research Studies

The literature contains studies showing conflicting results regarding the efficacy of prophylactic orthoses. Prophylactic orthoses have fallen from favor as clinical studies have shown them to be less than effective in reducing injuries. One study found an increase in the number of knee injuries as well as an increase in ankle and foot injuries with the use of prophylactic knee orthoses.[24] Another study revealed no differences in football injury rates for players with and without the use of prophylactic knee orthoses.[25] Prophylactic orthoses have been thought to preload the knee and perhaps result in more knee injury.[26]

However, a positive effect of prophylactic knee orthoses was found in a study of 1396 cadets at the United States Military Academy at West Point, New York. In this study, the use of prophylactic knee orthoses significantly reduced the frequency of knee injuries, both in the total number of subjects injured and in the number of medial collateral ligament injuries. However, this reduction in the frequency of knee injuries depended on player position. Only football defensive players who wore prophylactic knee orthoses had statistically significant fewer knee injuries. Prophylactic knee orthoses did not significantly reduce the severity of medial collateral (MCL) and anterior cruciate ligament (ACL) knee injuries.[27] One investigator stated that currently available prophylactic knee orthoses can provide 20 to 39% more resistance to a lateral blow, with the possibility that the ACL is given even more protection than the MCL. The most effective prophylactic knee orthoses are those stiff enough to prevent an external force from causing orthosis hinge joint contact with knee tissues. The correct sizing and fitting of prophylactic knee orthoses is critical to their effectiveness. Improvements are needed in the ability of prophylactic knee orthoses to fit each individual's leg without the expense of custom-molding procedures.[28]

In conclusion, investigators have not been able to demonstrate the efficacy of these orthoses consistently.[4] The American Academy of Orthopaedic Surgeons (AAOS) states that the routine use of prophylactic orthoses currently available has not proven effective in reducing the number or severity of knee injuries. In some circumstances, such orthoses may even contribute to injury.[1]

Postoperative Rehabilitative Knee Orthoses

Postoperative rehabilitative knee orthoses are those designed to allow protected and controlled motion of the injured knee that has been treated operatively.[23] Rehabilitative knee orthoses are designed primarily to absorb direct or indirect stress and allow controlled motion. Rehabilitative knee orthoses, because of their long leverage, are often used after surgery and when knee motion needs to be restricted. For example, some postoperative protocols ini-

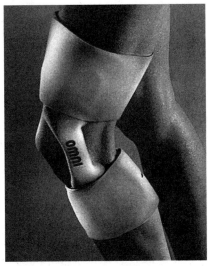

Figure 15-13. Anderson stabilizer. (Reprinted with permission from Omni Scientific Inc.)

tially allow only 30° of flexion to full extension. The knee may be unlocked to allow motion such as in sitting to prevent joint contracture and scarring in the intracondylar notch.[4] The medial and lateral uprights of the postoperative rehabilitative knee orthosis contain hinges that may limit ROM. Postoperative rehabilitative knee orthoses have soft foam liners that encapsulate the thigh and calf. These liners provide adjustability for edema and comfort over incision sites. These orthoses are prefabricated, usually come disassembled, and must be put together by a health professional. Once assembled, the patient may apply and remove the orthosis easily. One type of postoperative rehabilitative knee orthosis, the Bledsoe Post-operative Rehabilitative Knee Orthosis, is shown in Figure 15-14.

Research Studies

The effectiveness of postoperative rehabilitative knee orthoses is controversial. One study of subjects who wore postoperative and functional knee orthoses after ACL reconstruction found improved function at 3 months postoperatively using the Cincinnati Knee Score. However no difference between the orthosis and nonorthosis groups was found regarding knee joint laxity, ROM, muscle strength, functional tests, or pain.[29]Another study of 78 patients after patellar autograph ACL surgery found that the use of a postoperative rehabilitative orthosis did not influence either subjective function or objective stability (KT1000 test, one leg hop, Tegner and Lysholm scores) at 24-month follow-up. The investigators concluded that the use of a postoperative knee orthosis did not improve stability and function after arthroscopic ACL reconstruction and discontinued the use of these orthoses in their rehabilitation program.[30] Likewise, another study of 60 patients after patellar autograph ACL surgery found that the use of a postoperative rehabilitative orthosis did not result in any improvements in functional outcome, knee stability, or isokinetic muscle torque at 1–2 year follow-up. These investigators found that the straps of the

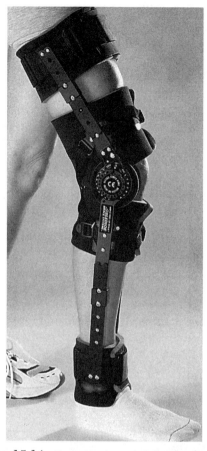

Figure 15-14. Postoperative rehabilitative knee orthosis. (Reprinted with permission from Bledsoe Brace Systems, Grand Prairie, TX.)

postoperative knee orthoses often produced a tourniquet effect resulting in patient discomfort.[31] Further research is necessary to prove whether postoperative rehabilitative knee orthoses are effective.

Functional Knee Orthoses

Functional knee orthoses are those worn by individuals who have returned to activity, especially a type of activity involving quick turns or cutting. Most functional knee orthoses control medial and lateral stability, anterior tibial translation, and recurvatum. The Lenox-Hill was the first derotational sports knee orthosis. It was popularized in 1972 by a quarterback for the New York Jets.[1] The DonJoy 4-Point Knee Orthosis was the first prefabricated, or "off the shelf," orthosis marketed for the athlete. Functional knee orthoses often use a four-point force system to restrict joint motion in unwanted directions comfortably. This motion control is accomplished by contacting and controlling the tibia and by use of a hinge that will not interfere with normal knee joint kinematics. The four-point force system is illustrated in Figure 5-23. The molded tibial shell is the anchor of the functional knee orthosis and reduces anterior tibial translation. The thigh straps stabilize the entire orthosis on the lower extremity. The most commonly used hinges are the polycentric and the single-axis. Practical Application Box 15-1 contains a description of hinges that may be used with orthoses.

Many types of functional knee orthoses are presently available. They are most commonly constructed of carbon-graphite, aluminum, or titanium materials. Functional knee orthoses, like AFOs, may be custom made to the patient's leg or prefabricated as an off-the-shelf item. Prefabricated orthoses meet a need for immediate application and low cost. Some manufacturers make both custom-made and prefabricated orthoses. Whether to prescribe a custom-made or prefabricated orthosis depends on the following factors:

1. Degree of instability
2. Level of sports competition
3. Length of time one is expected to wear the orthosis
4. Size and shape of the leg
5. Willingness to wear the orthosis for an extended period of time

Prefabricated Orthoses

One prefabricated knee orthosis, the DonJoy 4titude, is pictured in Figure 15-15. This orthosis is available in right or left, seven sizes, and three length options. The wearer should be instructed in proper application of the ortho-

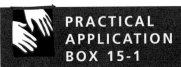

PRACTICAL APPLICATION BOX 15-1

Descriptions of Hinges

The anatomic knee joint is a modified hinge joint with a changing center of rotation. The center of rotation shifts posteriorly as the knee reaches full flexion. Most of the shift occurs during the first 30° of flexion. Different types of hinges built into an orthosis attempt to parallel this changing center of rotation. However, no mechanical hinge design can totally mimic anatomic knee-joint motion. The more the mechanical hinge and the anatomic joints parallel each other, the less the orthosis will migrate distally on the wearer. The most common hinges used in orthoses are as follows:

- Single axis: Circular motion around a fixed axis
- Posterior offset: Single axis point is located posterior to the uprights
- Polycentric: Two axes are engaged to one another by gears that allow a noncircular motion pattern
- Slotted cam: A noncircular motion is controlled by a slot pattern
- Geared tricentric: Geared polycentric hinge with three axes

The most popular hinges are the single axis and the polycentric.

sis, since application error accounts for slippage more than any other factor. Another prefabricated orthosis, the Lenox-Hill Precision Lite Orthosis, is shown in Figure 15-16.

Custom-Made Orthoses

The oldest custom-made functional knee orthosis is the Lenox-Hill. This functional knee orthosis is a double upright, monocentric-

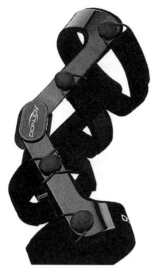

Figure 15-15. DonJoy 4titude prefabricated functional knee orthosis. (Reprinted with permission from DJ Orthopedics LLC, Vista, CA.)

hinge orthosis held in place with proximal thigh and distal calf elastic straps with Velcro closures. The derotation straps are narrow for comfort. It is available in standard, light weight, and spectralight weight. The latter weighs between 18 and 23 ounces. The Omni Icon XC (formerly the TS-7) Knee Orthosis was developed as a result of a physical therapist's masters degree research. The Omni Icon XC possesses an X-Cell design that accommodates the 4-cm posterior shift in the axis of knee rotation. This accommodation stops slippage that may occur due to thigh soft tissue deformation during flexion and extension (Fig. 15-17). Another custom-made functional knee orthosis is the Townsend. The Townsend Motion Hinge counteracts tibial shear with a 8- to 9-mm posterior tibial movement during the first 25° of knee flexion. The Townsend Motion Hinge is shown in Figure 15-18. Distal migration of the orthosis is decreased by the Synergistic Suspension Strap, which wraps inward between the lower shell of the orthosis and the sides of the calf (Fig. 15-19).

An unusual custom-made orthosis is the DonJoy Defiance, shown in Figure 15-20. This orthosis is popular because of its light weight

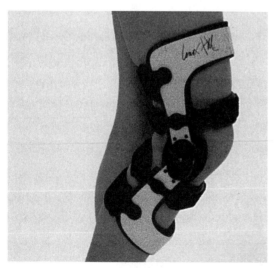

Figure 15-16. Lenox-Hill Precision Lite prefabricated functional knee orthosis. (Photo courtesy of Lenox Hill Brace Company, Long Island City, NY.)

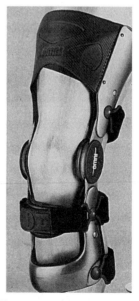

Figure 15-17. Omni Icon XC (formerly called the TS-7) functional knee orthosis. (Photo courtesy of Omni Life. Science, a division of Bodyworks Inc., North Springville, UT.)

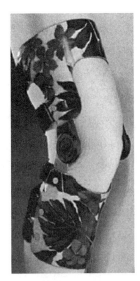

Figure 15-18. Townsend Motion Hinge functional knee orthosis. (Reprinted with permission from Townsend Design, Bakersfield, CA.)

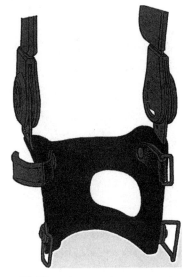

Figure 15-19. Synergistic suspension strap. (Reprinted with permission from Townsend Design, Bakersfield, CA.)

and low-profile look. It may be the only functional knee orthosis that uses a posterior calf frame instead of the usual molded anterior tibial shell. The first functional knee orthosis designed specifically for women is the Breg Women's Tradition. This orthosis is light weight and short to better fit the shape and angle of the female leg (Fig. 15-21).

Research Studies

The effectiveness of the use of functional knee orthoses is also controversial. The orthopedic literature lacks well-controlled prospective studies on specific uses of these knee orthoses. Orthoses fit around thigh and calf soft tissues. Since soft tissues are not rigid, it is difficult to develop a orthosis that rigidly controls rotational forces. Wearers of functional knee orthoses state that they are useful. One study found that of 47 patients with ACL deficient knees, 90% felt their symptoms were improved.[32] One study of cadaveric knees showed beneficial effects of functional knee orthoses that decreased anterior tibial displacement

(measured on a specialized testing apparatus) by 10 to 75%.[33] However, the applied loads used in this study were 125 newtons (28 lb), which are much lower than on-the-field loads.

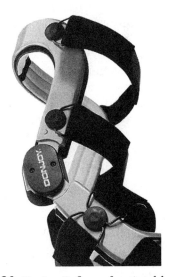

Figure 15-20. DonJoy Defiance functional knee orthosis. (Photo courtesy of DJ Orthopedics LLC, Vista, CA.)

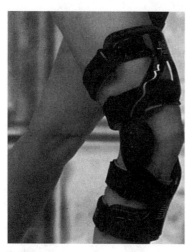

Figure 15-21. Breg Women's Tradition functional knee orthosis. (Reprinted with permission from Breg Inc, Vista, CA.)

Some feel there may be a proprioceptive protective component to functional knee orthoses. Since the wearer may pay more attention to the injured knee because of the proprioceptive protection offered by the knee orthosis, this may account for their effectiveness. In one study, researchers examined the effects of a sleeve-type knee orthosis on the proprioceptive ability of 20 subjects with no musculoskeletal or neurologic conditions. Subjects were blindfolded and one limb moved passively by a Kin-Com dynamometer. Subjects were instructed to duplicate the movement as closely as possible with the other limb. Results showed an 11% increase in the blindfolded tracking abilities of patients while wearing the knee orthosis. These investigators concluded that alterations in proprioception as a result of wearing of orthoses may be part of the reason for improved rehabilitation in knee injury patients.[34] Similarly, a study of subjects with chronic ACL disruption found that those wearing a functional knee orthosis or neoprene sleeve showed slight, but nonsignificant improvement in threshold to detect passive mo-

tion.[35] Conversely, a study of 20 post–ACL reconstruction and 10 control subjects found that the use of functional knee orthoses did not produce a statistically significant change in detection of passive motion with the knee at 15° of flexion.[36] This study also found no significant differences in proprioception between the ACL-reconstructed knee and the contralateral uninvolved knee 1 year or more after surgery. Likewise, another study, found that the use of functional knee orthoses did not alter electromyographic (EMG) activity in muscles surrounding the knee during a side-step cutting maneuver. The investigators concluded that the use of a functional knee orthosis did not enhance limb proprioception.[37]

ACL derotational orthoses appear to be effective in controlling rotation during stance phase in less-taxing athletic maneuvers such as walking and running. However, during activities such as side-step cutting, which stress the derotational properties of the orthosis to the greatest degree, the same support is not seen.[37] The use of orthoses after ACL reconstruction may be effective in reducing repetitive low loads encountered by the ACL during daily activity and thus may theoretically have an impact on graft creep.

The psychologic reaction that may occur from using a functional knee orthoses ranges from one extreme to the other. Patients may become either dependent on functional knee orthoses and fearful of any activity without the orthosis or conversely, increase risk taking because of a false sense of security that may lead to reinjury. Some patients report that use of functional knee orthoses results in both more stability and fewer episodes of knee buckling, while others say that there is annoying slipping of the orthoses and that performance is hindered.[38]

Differences among studies related to the effectiveness of functional knee orthoses may be due to the type (custom vs. prefabricated) and model of orthosis used.[39] Dissimilar results among studies may also be due to differences in nature of the injury, multiplanar motion, proprioception, and the design and fit of the orthosis among subjects. One investigator recommends that functional knee orthoses be prescribed to patients with moderate instability and that they be used during activities of moderate or low load potential.[37] Further research is needed to determine the situations in which a functional knee orthosis can be used most effectively.

Measurement

Measurement of prefabricated, or off-the-shelf knee orthoses, custom-made knee orthoses, and patellofemoral orthoses is described below.

Prefabricated, or Off-the-Shelf, Knee Orthoses

A typical measurement for prefabricated, or off-the-shelf, knee orthoses is a circumferential measurement 6 inches above the mid-patella, at the midpatella, and 6 inches below the midpatella. Some manufacturers provide special calipers to measure width or medial lateral (m-l) dimensions. These orthoses must be ordered in a right or left design. Some manufacturers also offer the option of a short or petite model for patients under 5 ft 2 in. (157 cm).

Custom-Made Knee Orthoses

Approximately half of the manufacturers require casting for fabrication of a custom-made knee orthosis. Casting requires that bony landmarks such as the patella, fibular head, and medial joint line be marked on stockinette with indelible ink. This ink then transfers to the inside of the cast. Carbon fiber composite materials are heated and vacuum formed over the positive mold to obtain the final knee orthosis. Many manufacturers have used meas-

urement systems to eliminate the need for a cast and the expense and the time delay in sending the cast mold to the manufacturer. The series of measurements can be faxed or phoned to the manufacturer. Normal fabrication time for a custom-made knee orthosis is approximately 5 days.

The pros and cons of prefabricated and custom-made orthoses are shown in Pros and Cons Box 15-1.

Patellofemoral Orthoses

Sizing for patellofemoral orthoses require measurements either at the mid-patella or 6 inches above the mid-patella. Static patellofemoral orthoses fit either a right or left leg. Dynamic patellofemoral orthoses, since they have medial pull straps, need to be ordered as a right or left. Proper fitting for patellar orthoses is accomplished when the anterior patella window is directly over the entire patella, with the knee in full extension. If popliteal pressure is a concern, such as in sports such as biking or rowing, a popliteal opening design is indicated. Many manufacturers design the orthoses on a curve in the popliteal area to decrease pressure and bunching. Even though thicker $\frac{1}{4}$" neoprene may be more supportive and durable, $\frac{1}{8}$" may be more comfortable for some patients. If skin rash or allergy to nylon occurs, a hypoallergenic orthosis is indicated.

Orthoses for Patellofemoral Disorders

The patellofemoral joint is a common source of knee pain, frequently due to contusion, subluxation, dislocation, extensor mechanism malalignment, lateral patellar compression syndrome, or patellofemoral chondrosis.[40] Patellar orthoses or taping attempts to centralize the patella within the trochlear groove through a mechanical buttress or by decreasing patellar

PROS & CONS
BOX 15-1

Comparison of Prefabricated and Custom-Made Orthoses

Type of Orthosis	Fit	Features	Cost	Advantages	Disadvantages
Prefabricated or off-the-shelf	Sized from xxsmall to xxlarge, right or left	Light-weight aircraft-grade aluminum, strong enough to provide a rigid frame for knee control	Lower cost, some insurance companies encourage their use	May be modified by the practitioner to enhance fit; delivery often in 1 day	If fit not optimal, distal migration on the calf may result
Custom-made	Made from a cast or series of measurements	Superior-grade materials, usually carbon fiber laminate; able to withstand contact-sport collisions.	Increased cost, about 50% more than prefabricated	Optimal fit provided; useful if patient will be wearing for a long time; ideal for hard-to-fit situations such as muscular or obese thighs; may include extended warranties such as no charge for remolding; numerous color and design choices	Increased cost, may take 10–12 days for delivery

excursion. Therefore, patellar tracking is improved. The taping used to control patellar motion, relieve patellar tendinitis, or unload the fat pad is described in other texts and is beyond the scope of this text. Three types of patellar orthoses are described below:

1. Static sleeve with silicone or felt buttress
2. Dynamic sleeve with lateral buttress and medial pull strap
3. Infrapatellar strap

Static Sleeve with Silicone or Felt Buttress

One example of the static sleeve with silicone or felt buttress is the Genutrain Active Knee Support shown in Figure 15-22. This orthosis consists of a three-dimensional compression knit with a silicone ring that circles the patella. There is a trapezoidal contour in the popliteal area to prevent bunching, and the patella is covered to avoid window edema. Patient com-

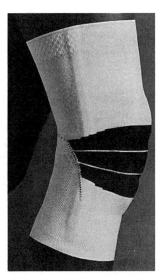

Figure 15-22. Genutrain patellar support. (Reprinted with permission from Bauerfind USA Inc, Kennesaw, GA.)

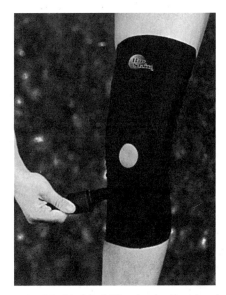

Figure 15-23. Bioskin "Q" orthosis. (Reprinted with permission from Cropper Medical, Ashland, OR.)

pliance is high because of the Genutrain's comfort and patellar silicone ring support.

Dynamic Sleeve with Lateral Buttress and Medial Pull Strap

The dynamic sleeve with lateral buttress and medial pull strap type of patellofemoral orthosis allows the wearer to position and apply appropriate tension to enhance proper patellar tracking. These orthoses are often used by patients with a history of patellar dislocation and chronic patellar subluxation. One example of this type of orthosis is the Bioskin "Q" Orthosis. This orthosis has a removable T-strap that attaches to the lateral side of the patella and is then pulled medially to be secured in a variety of positions (Fig. 15-23).

Infrapatellar Straps

Infrapatellar straps apply pressure to the patellar tendon, which causes the patella to be elevated. These straps are used for conditions such as patellar tendinitis and patellofemoral chondrosis. Infrapatellar straps have no effect on mediolateral alignment or tracking. Com-

mon infrapatellar straps include the Chopat and the Levine straps. One infrapatellar strap is the FLUK shown in Figure 15-24. The FLUK does not restrict knee function and can be adjusted quickly during competition. It is espe-

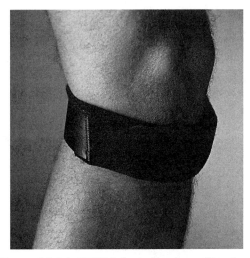

Figure 15-24. FLUK infrapatellar strap. (Reprinted with permission from Brace International, Atlanta, GA.)

cially popular in jumping sports such as basketball in which patellar tendinitis is common.

Research Studies

There are numerous patellar orthoses on the market today, but well-defined and controlled clinical studies of the use of these orthoses are lacking.[41] The exact function of patella orthoses is unclear. These orthoses may alleviate pain through increased sensory feedback, by warmth, or by applying a medial force to the lateral aspect of the patella in patients with tracking problems. Several studies have shown success of patellofemoral orthoses in alleviating pain. Patellofemoral orthoses by means of compression may increase the contact area between the patella and the trochlea. This increase in contact area could decrease stress, since forces are distributed over a greater surface area.[42] One study found that 76% of patients demonstrated a qualitative correction in patellar subluxation while wearing a patellofemoral orthosis.[43] The effectiveness of infrapatellar straps is questionable. One study reported that an infrapatellar strap offered relief from patellofemoral pain in 77% of 57 symptomatic knees studied. This investigation concluded that the infrapatella strap was an effective aid in the treatment of patellofemoral pain, possibly because of its ability to elevate the patella.[44] Conversely, another study found that only 24% of 37 patellofemoral pain patients among young military recruits showed symptom improvement at 1 week and 22% at 1 year following infrapatellar orthosis wearing.[45] In summary, based on the conflicting results of these studies, additional research is needed to determine the effectiveness of patellofemoral orthoses.

Valgus Control Functional Knee Orthoses

It is estimated that 6 to 22% of collegiate athletes will be injured each year. Of the injuries sustained, the MCL is one of the most common, with incidence as high as 73%.[1] Injuries to the MCL of the knee usually recover without surgery. If the MCL can heal in its normal position, without valgus stress, there will be no residual elongation and instability. A hinged MCL valgus control functional knee orthosis may allow an individual to function with less pain and return to work or competition in a shorter time. These orthoses are usually made of neoprene or Drytex material with heavy-duty hinges on the medial and lateral sides of the knee. Drytex is a good hypoallergenic option. Most hinges have extension and flexion stops that are easily adjusted for each individual patient. Various options exist such as popliteal opening, patellar opening, and wraparound. One valgus control functional knee orthosis, the Playmaker, is illustrated in Figure 15-25. This orthosis is prefabricated in seven sizes. The sleeves of the Playmaker can be replaced if worn, without repurchasing the entire orthosis.

Orthoses for Osteoarthritis (Unloader)

Orthoses for osteoarthritis (OA) were first developed in 1989 to unload the medial femoral and tibial condyles. It is estimated that 21 mil-

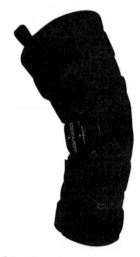

Figure 15-25. Playmaker valgus control functional knee orthosis. (Reprinted with permission from DJ Orthopedics LLC, Vista, CA.)

lion Americans have OA, and the incidence of OA will increase almost 50% in the next 20 years.[46] Other patients who may benefit from this orthosis are those who have a history of meniscectomy, ACL tears, genu varum or genu valgum, failed total knee, or high tibial osteotomy. Often in these conditions, joint surface pressures become unequal, leading to articular cartilage destruction. OA is most commonly present in the medial compartment, since the knee is often most subjected to varus loading during gait. Approximately 60 to 80% of the loads across the knee are transmitted to the medial compartment. These orthoses are designed to distract joint surfaces of either the medial or lateral compartments of the knee. Use of a three-point force system to create a varus or valgus correction unloads the joint. The three-point force system is illustrated in Figure 5-21. Two to 3 mm of distraction can result in considerable pain relief. In mild-to-moderate cases of OA, these orthoses may be effective and extend the patient's active lifestyle.

There are two types of unloader knee orthoses, thrust and prestressed. They are described below.

Thrust Unloader Orthoses

Thrust unloaders are single hinged and function in one of two ways; either pneumatic condyle pads are inflated or condyle pad thickness is increased until a bending moment is achieved. The first unloading orthosis, developed in 1989 by Generation II, is called the Generation II Unloader Orthosis. This 26-oz thrust unloader orthosis possesses a carbon Teflon–coated unilateral polyaxial hinge that joins the thigh and calf components. This orthosis is supported with a nylon force strap that wraps through the popliteal area and can place pressure over either the medial aspect of the joint to unload the medial compartment or over the lateral aspect to unload the lateral compartment. The unilateral joint of this orthosis is placed on the same side as the compartment being unloaded. For example, to un-

load the medial joint surfaces, the hinge is placed on the medial side (Fig. 15-26).

Prestressed Unloader Orthosis

Prestressed designs have bilateral hinges and incorporate angular corrections in the frame of the orthosis. The bilateral uprights of the prestressed unloader orthoses align the anatomic knee joint to a neutral alignment, helping to reduce the compression on the affected compartment. The joint stress-bearing forces are shared through the bilateral hinge and upright structures. One such prestressed unloader orthosis is the Omni Force XC Orthosis (formerly called the Align) (Fig. 15-27). A 3, 5, or 7° angular correction may be ordered from the manufacturer. Extension stops vary from 5, 10, 15, 20, to 25°.

Research Studies

Since the advent of orthoses for OA is relatively recent, there are few studies concerning their effectiveness. One study of 119 patients found that the unloader orthoses were more effective than the neoprene sleeve in improving func-

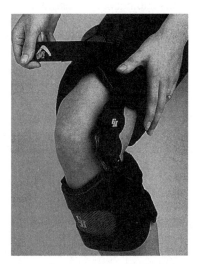

Figure 15-26. Generation II unloader knee orthosis. (Reprinted with permission from Generation II USA, Bothell, WA.)

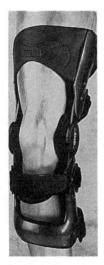

Figure 15-27. Icon Force XC. (Reprinted with permission from Omni Life Science, a division of Bodyworks Inc., North Springville, UT.)

tion and quality of life. These indices were measured by functional scales and the 6-minute walking and 30-second stair climbing tests.[48] Another study found that use of unloader orthoses resulted in knee condylar separation under fluoroscopy. At initial contact, 78% of the subjects demonstrated condylar separation; at midstance, 70% demonstrated condylar separation.[49] Heavier patients have more problems with the fit and function of orthoses for OA.[46] Besides unloader orthoses, lateral wedged insoles may also be used for OA. A study of 17 healthy subjects wearing a 5° lateral wedged insole showed reduction in knee varus moment and medial compartment load.[47] More research is needed to confirm the effectiveness of these orthoses.

Other Knee Orthoses (KOs)

There are many other knee orthoses available for a variety of conditions. Three of the most common knee orthoses—dynamic adjustable, positional, and hyperextension knee control or recurvatum—and their indications are described.

Dynamic Adjustable Orthoses

Dynamic adjustable orthoses are used to restore ROM of a joint surrounded by soft tissue tightness or contractures. These orthoses are most commonly used with knee contractures but are available for many other joints as well. They often use a spring mechanism to give a dynamic low-load force over a prolong period of time to stretch the elastic elements of a joint (Fig. 15-28). In a study of 13 subjects with nonosseous range-of-motion restrictions of either the elbow or knee, the use of a dynamic adjustable orthosis resulted in a 61% increase in ROM.[50] The effectiveness of a dynamic adjustable orthosis has also been shown in single-case study designs. One study of a 67-year-old with a total knee arthroplasty showed a 17° increase in active ROM using a progressive stretch–based protocol.[51] A study of a 22-year-old showed a 52 increase in elbow extension over 7½ months.[52] In contrast, in a study of 18 nursing home residents with 10° or more of

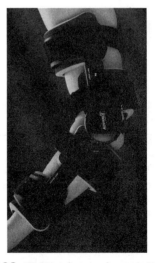

Figure 15-28. EMPI Advance dynamic ROM orthosis. (Reprinted with permission from EMPI, St. Paul, MN.)

knee flexion contracture bilaterally, no differences were found between the use of a dynamic adjustable orthosis and use of passive ROM and manual stretching. Residents wore the dynamic adjustable orthosis 3 hours a day, 5 days per week for 6 months on one knee while receiving passive ROM and manual stretching on the other knee. However, the investigators of this study cautioned generalization of results because of the low statistical power of this study.[53]

Positional Orthoses

A variety of orthoses such as the Multi-Podus System are available to correct foot-drop deformities and position the foot, ankle, knee, and hip. The heel design of this system is designed to eliminate friction or pressure on the heel. A spreader bar may be attached to two Multi-Podus systems to provide hip abduction and rotation. The Multi-Podus System is available in four adult and two pediatric sizes (Fig.

15-29). The Multi-Podus Phase II system provides a serial casting static stretch of the plantarflexors. The adjustment dial of the Multi-Podus Phase II system allows 1° adjustments ranging from 40° of plantarflexion to 10° of dorsiflexion. Straps may be added to reduce inversion and eversion positions (Fig. 15-30).

Hyperextension Knee Control or Recurvatum Orthoses

The hyperextension knee control or recurvatum orthoses are used to control hyperextension or genu recurvatum of the knee. Genu recurvatum is the most common stance-phase characteristic of postpolio syndrome.[54] One orthosis in this category is the Swedish knee cage. This orthosis uses a rigid three-point pressure to prevent mild recurvatum yet provides good mediolateral stability. The Swedish knee cage is available in a prefabricated or off-the-shelf form and is constructed of metal with

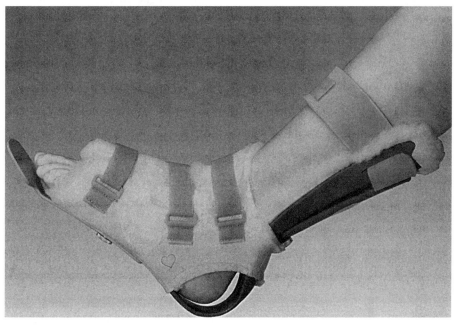

Figure 15-29. Multi-Podus System. (Reprinted with permission from Restorative Care of America Inc., Clearwater, FL.)

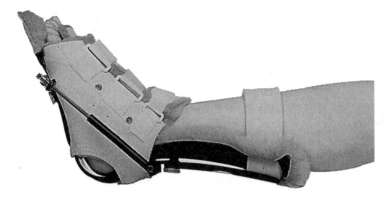

Figure 15-30. Multi-Podus Phase II. (Reprinted with permission from Restorative Care of America Inc., Clearwater, FL.)

a flexible U-shaped popliteal pad. The thigh and calf straps are constructed of heavy elastic. The advantage of this orthosis is its low cost and easy availability. However, its cosmesis is poor, mediolateral dimension is bulky, and the orthosis protrudes slightly when sitting (Fig. 15-31). Another commonly used orthosis in this category is the Townsend Polio Orthosis. This orthosis can control varus/valgus and ro-

tary instabilities that may accompany recurvatum. This orthosis has extension stops to prevent recurvatum (Fig. 15-32).

Orthoses Used for Hip Problems

There are a variety of orthoses used for hip problems. Hip orthoses may be divided into several categories. These include

1. Hip-compression orthoses
2. Orthoses used for hip dislocations
3. Orthoses used for Legg-Calvé-Perthes Disease

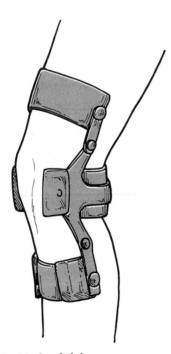

Figure 15-31. Swedish knee cage.

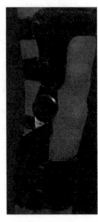

Figure 15-32. Townsend polio orthosis. (Reprinted with permission from Townsend Design, Bakersfield, CA.)

Hip-Compression Orthoses

Soft tissue injuries such as **hip pointers** and groin or hamstring pulls can be debilitating for the athlete. Compression and motion inhibition may make the acute stages of these injuries more comfortable. The BioSkin compression shorts, a commercially available orthosis for adductor and hamstring strains, are depicted in Figure 15-33. The BioSkin material is a trilaminate material that is breathable and one-third the thickness used of material used in other compression shorts. The groin cinch strap may be applied to provide compression over the groin or hamstring.

Orthoses Used for Hip Dislocations

There are two orthoses commonly used for hip dislocations. A hip-abduction orthosis is used for adults and a Pavlik Harness is used for congenital dislocations.

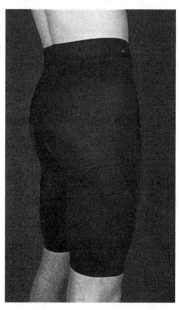

Figure 15-33. Bioskin compression shorts. (Reprinted with permission from Cropper Medical, Ashland, OR.)

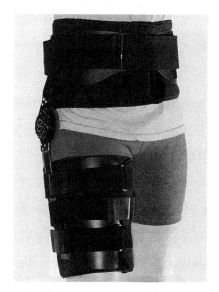

Figure 15-34. Post-op hip-abduction orthosis. (Reprinted with permission from Bledsoe Brace Systems, Grand Prairie, TX.)

Hip-Abduction Orthoses

Hip dislocations can occur in 1–3% of patients post–total hip arthroplasty.[55] The hip-abduction orthosis prevents extremes of rotation, flexion, and extension (Fig. 15-34). This orthosis is designed with a lateral hinge at the greater trochanter that attaches to the trunk by a Velcro waist section and to the thigh with a soft cuff with plastic flanges. ROM may be controlled to 30° of extension and 105° of flexion at 15° increments. This orthosis is lightweight and can be worn under normal clothing.

Pavlik Harness

The Pavlik Harness is used in the care of congenital dislocated hips. This harness was devised in 1944 by a Czechoslovakian orthopedic surgeon, Dr. Pavlik.[56] The Pavlik harness consists of washable materials for a shoulder harness, stirrups for the legs, and booties to hold the feet. The anterior leg strap allows hip flexion but limits extension. The posterior leg strap allows hip abduction but limits hip ad-

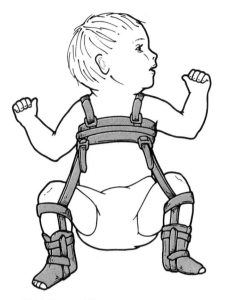

Figure 15-35. Pavlik harness.

duction. Both hip flexion and abduction are necessary to help relocate the femoral head and shape the acetabulum. The incidence of avascular necrosis with the use of this harness is nonexistent if it is used for correct indications. One study reported a success rate of 97% taking 1 to 4 weeks in reducing hip dislocations (Fig. 15-35).[57]

Orthoses used for Legg-Calvé-Perthes Disease

There are two orthoses often used for **Legg-Calvé-Perthes Disease**, the Scottish Rite and Newington orthoses. They are described below.

Scottish Rite Orthosis

The Scottish Rite orthosis holds the hips in 40–45° of abduction. A pelvic band is connected to two plastic thigh cuffs by a free-motion hip joint. The thigh cuffs are connected by a telescoping crossbar. The crossbar contains a swivel joint that allows reciprocal motion of the lower extremities. Advantages of this orthosis are ease of application, allowing ambulation without assistive devices, and better cosmesis than other orthoses (Fig. 15-36).[58]

Newington Orthosis

The Newington orthosis stabilizes the hips in 45° of abduction and 20° of internal rotation by two medial uprights connected by a horizontal bar. One study found good results in 63%, fair in 21%, and poor in 16% of patients using this orthosis (Fig. 15-37).[59]

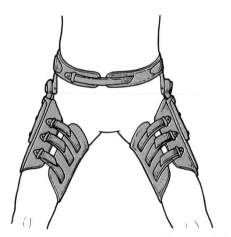

Figure 15-36. Scottish Rite orthosis for Legg-Calvé-Perthes disease

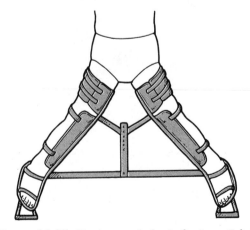

Figure 15-37. Newington Orthosis for Legg-Calvé-Perthes disease.

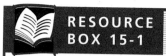

RESOURCE BOX 15-1

Addresses, Phone Numbers, and Web Sites of Various Orthosis Manufacturers

Innovation Sports
  19762 Pauling
  Foothill Ranch, CA 92610
  (800)-222-4284
  www.isports.com
DJ Orthopedics
  2985 Scott Street
  Vista, CA 92083
  (800)-336- 6569
  www.donjoy.com
Bledsoe Brace Systems
  2601 Pinewood Drive
  Grand Prairie, TX 75051
  (800)-253-3763
  www.bledsoebrace.com
Breg
  2611 Commerce Way
  Vista, CA 92083
  (800)-321-0607
  www.breg.com
Bauerfeind
  55 Chastain Rd
  Kennesaw, GA 30144
  (800)-423-3405
  www.bauerfeindusa.com
Restorative Care of America
  11236 47th Street North
  Clearwater, FL 33762
  (800)-627-1595
  www.rcai.com
Swede-O Inc
  6459 Ash Street
  North Branch, MN 55056
  (800)-525-9339
  www.swedeo.com

Townsend Design
  4615 Shepard Street
  Bakersfield, CA 93313
  (800)-700-2722
  www.townsenddesign.com
Generation II USA
  11818 North Creek Parkway Suite 102
  Bothell, WA 98011
  (800)-462-7252
  www.gen2.com
Pro Orthopedic Devices
  2884 E. Ganley Road
  Tucson, AZ 85706
  (800)-523-5611
  www.proorthopedic.com
Omni
  981 Park Center Drive
  Vista, CA 92083
  (800)-448-6664
  www.bw-omni.com
Aircast Inc.
  92 River Road
  Summit, NJ 07901
  (800)-526-8785
  www.aircast.com
PAL Health Technologies
  1805 Riverway Drive
  Pekin, IL 61554
  (800)-223-2957
  www.palhealthsystems.com
EMPI
  599 Cardigan Road
  St. Paul, MN 55126
  (888)-367-3674
  www.empi.com

Resources

Addresses, phone numbers, and websites of various orthosis manufacturers are contained in Resource Box 15-1.

KEY POINTS

- The CPOE recommends that orthoses be described by the joints they encompass, such as a KAFO.

- A variety of orthoses available today encompass the management of athletic injuries, fractures, and neurologic and painful biomechanical abnormalities.

- Ankle orthoses may be divided into five categories: stirrup orthoses, lace-up orthoses, elastic supports, prophylactic ankle orthoses, and controlled ankle motion walkers.

- Knee orthoses may be divided into seven categories: prophylactic, postoperative or rehabilitative, functional, patellar, valgus control, orthoses for OA (unloader), and others.

- Hip orthoses are designed for problems ranging from muscle strains and dislocated hips to Legg-Calvé-Perthes disease.

CRITICAL THINKING QUESTIONS

1. With a group of your classmates, describe which orthopedic conditions would need an ankle orthosis and which a CAM walker.

2. Describe the functions of a lower-limb orthosis.

3. With a group of your classmates, describe the orthopedic conditions that would need a prophylactic, rehabilitative, functional, patellar, valgus control or unloader knee orthosis.

4. Explain why the research concerning knee orthoses has yielded different conclusions.

5. Differentiate the advantages and disadvantages of prefabricated (off-the-shelf) and custom-made knee orthoses.

6. Describe the indications for hip compression, hip abduction, Scottish Rite, and Newington orthoses.

REFERENCES

1. Wirth, M. A., & DeLee, J. C. (1990). The history and classification of knee braces. *Clinics in Sports Medicine, 9,* 731–741.

2. Redford, J.B., Basmajian, J. V., & Trautman, P. (1995). *Orthotics clinical practice and rehabilitation technology.* New York: Churchill Livingstone.

3. Harris, E. E. (1973). A new orthotics terminology—A guide to its use for prescription and fee schedules. *Orthotics and Prosthetics, 27,* 6–19.

4. Nawoczenski, D. A., & Epler, M. E. (1997). *Orthotics in functional rehabilitation of the lower limb.* Philadelphia: W. B. Saunders.

5. Quinn, K., Parker, P., de Bie, R., Rowe, B., & Handoll, H. (2001). Interventions for preventing ankle ligament injuries (Cochrane Review). In the *Cochrane Library,* Issue 1. Oxford: Update Software.

6. Anderson, M. K., & Hall, S. J. (1995). *Sports injury management* (p. 243). Baltimore: Williams & Wilkins.

7. Hartsell, H. D., & Spaulding, S. (1997). Effectiveness of external orthotic support on passive tissue resistance of the chronically unstable ankle. *Foot and Ankle International, 18,* 144–150.

8. Vogelbach, D. (1993). Biomechanical approach to the treatment of ankle sprains. *Sports Medicine Update, 24,* 12–21.

9. Jerosch, J., Thorwesten, L., Bork, H., & Bischof, M. (1996). Is prophylactic bracing of the ankle cost effective? *Orthopedics 25,* 405–414.

10. Thonnard, J. L., Bragard, D., Willems, P. A., & Plaghki, L. (1996). Stability of the braced ankle. A biomechanical investigation. *American Journal of Sports Medicine, 24,* 356–361.

11. Cordova, M. L., Ingersoll, C. D., & LeBlanc, M. J. (2000). Influence of ankle support on joint range of motion before and after exercise: A meta-analysis. *Journal of Orthopedics and Sports Physical Therapy, 30,* 170–182.

12. Siegler, S., Liu, W., Sennett, B., Nobilini, R. J., & Dunbar, D. (1997). The three dimensional passive support characteristics of ankle braces. *Journal of Orthopedics and Sports Physical Therapy, 26,* 299–309.

13. Shapiro, M. S., Kabo, J. M., Mitchell, P. W., Loren, G., & Senter, M. (1994). Ankle sprain prophylaxis: An analysis of the stabilizing effects of braces and tape. *American Journal of Sports Medicine, 22,* 78–82.

14. Brink, O., Staunstrup, H., & Sommer, J. (1996). Stable lateral malleolar fractures treated with Aircast ankle brace and DonJoy R.O.M. Walker Brace: A prospective randomized study. *Foot and Ankle International, 17,* 679–684.

15. Bot, S., & van Mechelen, W. (1999). The effect of ankle bracing on athletic performance. *Sports Medicine, 27,* 171–178.

16. Thacker, S. B., Stroup, D. F., Branche, C. M., Gilchrist, J., Goodman, R. A., & Weitman, E. A. (1999). The prevention of ankle sprains in sports: A systematic review of the literature. *American Journal of Sports Medicine, 27,* 753–760.

17. Glencross, D., & Thornton, E. (1981). Position sense following joint injury. *Journal of Sports Medicine and Physical Fitness, 21,* 23–27.

18. Gross, M. T. (1987). Effects of recurrent lateral ankle sprains on active and passive judgments of joint position. *Physical Therapy, 67,* 1505–1509.

19. Nishikawa, T., & Grabiner, M. D. (1999). Peroneal motoneuron excitability increases immediately following application of a semirigid ankle brace. *Journal of Orthopedics and Sports Physical Therapy, 29,* 168–173.

20. Refshauge, K. M., & Kilbreath, S. L., Raymond, J. (2000). The effect of recurrent ankle inversion sprain and taping on proprioception at the ankle. *Medicine and Science in Sports and Exercise, 32,* 10–15.

21. Russell, J. N., Hendershot, G. E., LeClere, F., Howie, L. J., & Adler, M. (1997). Trends and differential use of assistive technology devices: United States 1994. *Advance Data, 292,* 3.

22. Zogby, R. G., Baker, B. E., Seymour, R. J., VanHanswyk, E., & Werner, F. W. (1989). A biomechanical evaluation of the effect of functional braces on anterior cruciate ligament instability, using the Genucom Knee Analysis System. *Transactions of the Orthopedic Research Society, 14,* 212.

23. Drez, D., DeHaven, K., D'Ambrosia, R., et al. (1984). *Knee braces seminar report.* Chicago: American Academy of Orthopaedic Surgeons.

24. Grace, T. G., Skipper, B. J., Newberry, J. C., Nelson, M. A., Sweetser, E. R., & Rothman, M. L. (1988). Prophylactic knee braces and injury to the lower extremity. *Journal of Bone and Joint Surgery, 70A,* 422–427.

25. Hewson, G. F., Mendini, R. A., & Wang, J. B. (1986). Prophylactic knee bracing in college football. *American Journal of Sports Medicine, 14,* 262–266.

26. Baker, B. E., VanHanswyk, E., Bogosian, S., Werner, F. W., & Murphy, D. (1987). A biomechanical study of the static stabilizing effect of knee braces on medial stability. *American Journal of Sports Medicine, 15,* 566–570.

27. Sitler, M., Ryan, J., Hopkinson, W., Wheeler, J., Santomier, J., Kolb, R., & Polley, D. (1990). The efficacy of a prophylactic knee brace to reduce knee injuries in football. *American Journal of Sports Medicine, 18,* 310–315.

28. Albright, J. P., Saterbak, A., & Stokes, J. (1995). Use of knee braces in sport. Current recommendations. *Sports Medicine, 20,* 281–301.

29. Risberg, M. A., Holm, I., Steen, H., Eriksson, J., & Ekland, A. (1999). The effect of knee bracing after anterior cruciate ligament reconstruction, a prospective randomized study with two years follow-up. *American Journal of Sports Medicine, 27,* 76–83.

30. Kartus, J., Stener, S., Kohler, K., et al. (1997). Is bracing after anterior cruciate ligament reconstruction necessary? A 2 year followup of 78 consecutive patients rehabilitated with or without a brace. *Knee Surgery Sports Traumatology Arthroscopy, 5,* 157–161.

31. Harilainen, A., Sandelin, J., Vanhanen, I., & Kivinen, A. (1997). Knee brace after bone-tendon-bone anterior cruciate ligament reconstruction. randomized, prospective study with 2 year follow-up. *Knee Surgery Sports Traumatology Arthroscopy, 5,* 10–13.

32. Colville, M. R., Lee, C. L., & Ciullo, J. V. (1986). The Lenox Hill brace: An evaluation of effectiveness in treating knee ligamentous instability. *American Journal of Sports Medicine, 7,* 257–261.

33. Wojtys, E. M., Loubert, P. V., Samson, S. Y., & Viviano, D. M. (1990). Use of a knee-brace for control of tibial translation and rotation. *Journal of Bone and Joint Surgery, 72A,* 1323–1329.

34. McNair, P. J., Stanley, S. N., & Strauss, G. R. (1996). Knee bracing: Effects of proprioception. *Archives of Physical Medicine and Rehabilitation, 77,* 287–289.

35. Beynnon, B. D., Ryder, S.H., Konradsen, L., Johnson, R. J., Johnson, K., & Renstrom, P. A. (1999). The effect of ACL trauma and bracing on knee proprioception. *American Journal of Sports Medicine, 27,* 150–155.

36. Risberg, M. A., Beynnon, B. D., Peura, G. D., & Uh, B. S. (1999). Proprioception after anterior cruciate ligament reconstruction with and without bracing. *Knee Surgery Sports Traumatology Arthroscopy, 7,* 303–309.

37. Branch, T. P., Hunter, R., & Donath, M. (1989). Dynamic EMG analysis of anterior cruciate deficient legs with and without bracing during cutting. *American Journal of Sports Medicine, 17,* 35–41.

38. Decoster, L. C., & Vailas, J. C. (1998). Braces: Post-reconstruction knee bracing practices vary. *BioMechanics, 5,* 31–33.

39. Orecchio, A. B. (2000). Rehabilitation effectiveness questions confound experts. *Biomechanics, 7,* 15–18.

40. Eifert-Mangine, M. A., & Bibo, J. T. (1995). Conservative management of patello-femoral chrondrosis. In R. E. Mangine (Ed.), *Physical therapy of the knee.* New York: Churchill Livingstone.

41. Cherf, J., & Paulos, L. E. (1990). Bracing for patellar instability. *Clinics in Sports Medicine, 9,* 813–821.

42. Powers, C. M. (1998). Rehabilitation of patellofemoral joint disorders: A critical review. *Journal of Orthopedics and Sports Physical Therapy, 28,* 345–354.

43. Shellock, F. G., Mink, J. H., Deutsch, A. L., Fox, J., Molnar, T., Kvitne, R., & Ferkel, R. (1994). Effect of a patellar realignment brace on patellofemoral relationships: evaluation with kinematic MR imaging. *Journal of Magnetic Research Imaging, 4,* 590–594.

44. Levine, J., & Splain, S. (1979). Use of the infrapatella strap in the treatment of patellofemoral pain. *Clinics in Orthopedics, 139,* 179–181.

45. Villar, R. N. (1980). Patellofemoral pain and the infrapatellar brace. A military view. *American Journal of Sports Medicine, 5,* 313–315.

46. Webber, P. T. (2001). Breakthroughs in bracing. *Rehabilitation Management, 14,* 20–22.

47. Crenshaw, S. J., Pollo, F. E., & Calton, E. F. (2000). Effects of lateral-wedged insoles on kinetics at the knee. *Clinical Orthopaedics and Related Research, 375,* 185–192.

48. Kirkley, A., Webster-Bogaert, S., Litshfield, R., Amendola, A., MacDonald, S., McCalden, R., & Fowler, P. (1999). The effect of bracing on varus gonarthrosis. *Journal of Bone and Joint Surgery, 81,* 539–548.

49. Komistek, R. D., Dennis, D. A., & Northcut, E. J. (1998). Fluoroscopic analyses support OA knee bracing. *BioMechanics, 5,* 61–67.

50. Hepburn, G. R. (1987). Case studies: Contracture and stiff joint management with Dynasplint. *Journal of Orthopedic and Sports Physical Therapy, 8,* 498–504.

51. Jansen, C. M., Windau, J. E., Bonutti, P. M., & Brillhart, M. V. (1996). Treatment of a knee contracture using a knee orthosis incorporating stress relaxation techniques. *Physical Therapy, 76,* 182–186.

52. MacKay-Lyons, M. (1989). Low-load prolonged stretch in treatment of elbow flexion contractures secondary to head trauma: A case report. *Physical Therapy, 69,* 292–296.

53. Steffen, T. M., & Mollinger, L. A. (1995). Low-load, prolonged stretch in the treatment of knee flexion contractures in nursing home residents. *Physical Therapy, 75,* 886–895.

54. Fish, D. J., & Kosta, C. S. (1997). Neuromuscular characteristic gait patterns influence therapy. *Biomechanics/O&P, 7–15.*

55. Clayton, M. L., & Thirupathis, R. F. (1983). Dislocation following total hip arthroplasty. management by special brace in selected patients. *Clinical Orthopedics, 177,* 154–159.

56. Agro, M. (1995). Orthotic and rehabilitation terminology. In J. B. Redford, J. V. Basmajian, & P. Trautman, (Eds.). *Orthotics clinical practice and rehabilitation technology.* New York: Churchill Livingstone.

57. Kalamchi, A., & MacFarlane, R. (1982). The Pavlik Harness: Results in patients over three months of age. *Journal of Pediatric Orthopedics, 2,* 3–8.

58. Tachdjian, M. O. (1990). *Pediatric orthopedics: vols. 1–4* (2nd ed.). Philadelphia: W. B. Saunders.

59. Curtis, B. H., Gunther, S. F., Gossling, H. R., & Paul, S. W. (1974). Treatment for Legg-Perthes disease with the Newington Abduction brace. *Journal of Bone and Joint Surgery 56A,* 1135–1146.

Chapter 16

Orthoses for Patients with Neurologic Disorders— Clinical Decision Making

Karen Kott PhD, PT

Objectives

1. Describe how common shoe and orthosis components may affect various impairments
2. Explain foot care principles you would use to instruct a patient to prevent complications with an insensitive foot
3. Describe the main purposes of lower-extremity orthoses
4. Differentiate the principles of design for lower-extremity orthoses
5. Given a particular patient problem, compare and contrast conventional and plastic orthoses as well as custom-made and custom-fit orthoses
6. Given a particular client, defend the choice of orthosis on the basis of examination findings, expected outcome, and application of evidence from the literature

This chapter is divided into the following sections:

The first goal of this chapter is to assist the reader in recognizing different shoe components and orthoses used with children and adults diagnosed with neurologic disorders. The reader will further develop an understanding of the principles for design of shoe components and orthoses. Indications and contraindications of the different types of shoes and orthoses are discussed in the section on types of orthoses. Advantages and limitations of these orthoses are considered through the review of the literature. The second goal of this chapter is learning to apply a clinical decision making model for prescribing an individualized orthosis that uses client examination information and the current literature. Examination techniques are discussed in Chapter 2. Deciding which orthosis to prescribe involves an awareness of the different types of orthoses, a familiarity with current research, and a team effort that includes the client, family, and health-care professionals. Each team member brings a unique view for the purpose of the orthosis. The team approach is discussed in Chapter 3.

The disablement model, as a frame of reference, forms the basis of the decision-making process necessary to evaluate the benefits and the limitations of orthosis use for each individual.[1,2] The disablement process emphasizes simultaneous examination and evaluation on multiple levels (i.e. impairment, functional limitations, and disability) to determine outcomes and effectiveness of an intervention. A review of literature provides the clinician with suggested ways to examine, document, and evaluate the link between intervention and outcome. Much of the literature reviewed in this chapter involves clinical trials, case reports, and case studies. This is the type of research currently available on orthosis use. In contrast, randomized, controlled studies are

the gold standard of research. However, many studies cited in this chapter use no randomization of interventions and no control groups. Therefore, due to lack of research design rigor, results should be generalized with caution.[3-5]

This chapter reviews the types of shoe modifications commonly used for the patient with a neuropathic or insensitive foot and orthoses commonly used for four different medical classifications: cerebral palsy, spina bifida, spinal cord injury, and cerebral vascular accident. These medical classifications, representing both pediatric and adult populations, were chosen because individuals with these diagnoses present with the most common clinical findings that suggest the need for orthoses. The principles of management for these individuals with orthoses may suggest applications for individuals with other disorders.

Purposes of Shoes

In the past, a major reason for shoes with corrections for children with severe ankle and foot deformities was the shoe's function as the attachment for metal uprights of a conventional orthosis. With the introduction of plastic orthoses, use of shoes for this purpose has become almost obsolete. In children, shoe corrections were widely used to correct flexible foot deformities. The shoe attempted to achieve correction by applying forces against these deformities. Shoes, however, are subject to distortion caused by the forces of the body and the ground. The more severe the deformity, the greater the distortion forces. Therefore, the effectiveness of many childhood shoe corrections for severe deformities has yet to be proven by long-term control studies. As a result, corrections for more severe flexible deformities are now designed into a plastic orthosis, such as an ankle–foot orthosis. The orthosis, in contrast to a shoe, can achieve a much closer fit for application of forces with no loss of shape or force.

The purposes of shoe modifications for children with mild-to-moderate deformities are to serve as a firm base for

- Sole modifications such as lasts, lifts, or flares, metatarsal bars or pads, and wedges
- Inserts for footplates and foot orthoses

The purposes of shoe modifications for adults are to

- Stabilize or accommodate the foot
- Provide a support surface for the foot for best mechanical advantage in walking
- Possibly serve as the attachment for a conventional orthosis

Understanding shoe components is helpful for prescribing them for use with both children and adults.

Shoe Components

Ill-fitting shoes may be responsible for various forefoot deformities including hallux valgus, hammer toes, bunions, neuromas, and metatarsalgia. One study found that more than 80% of women were wearing shoes that were at least one width narrower than their measured size.[6] Shoes should feel comfortable and fit well the first time they are worn. It is recommended that shoes be fit while standing at the end of the day, when feet tend to be at their largest. If the client has a size discrepancy between feet, shoes should be fit to accommodate the larger foot. Shoes should also display the following characteristics:

- There should be enough room for all toes to extend fully. Specifically, there should be a $1/2$-inch margin between the end of the longest toe and the end of the toe box to fa-

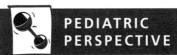

PEDIATRIC PERSPECTIVE

Children's shoes must include sufficient room for growth to allow $3/4$ inch between the end of the child's longest toe and the end of the toe box. Children may outgrow a shoe in 3 to 4 months.

cilitate foot movement from terminal stance to preswing in gait.[7] The Pediatric Perspective Box addresses shoe sizing for children.
- The width at the toe box should be comfortable both medially and laterally.
- The heel counter should be snug, yet comfortable.

Components of a good shoe are shown in Figure 16-1 and various shoe components are described as follows:

- Outer sole is the surface of the shoe that makes contact with the ground. Due to its durability, the most widely used outer-sole material is rubber. Highly compressed,

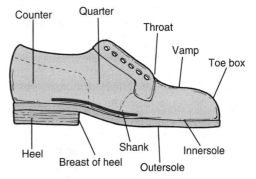

Figure 16-1. Shoe components. (Adapted from Nawoczenski, D. A., & Epler, M. E. (1997). *Orthotics in functional rehabilitation of the lower limb.* Philadelphia: W. B. Saunders.)

molded rubber or blown microcellular rubber are the most commonly used forms.

- Inner sole is the part of the shoe directly under the foot; it is often made of leather.
- Compressible filler is the material that lies between the inner and outer sole; its purpose is to separate them.
- Upper refers to all materials above the sole.
- Vamp is the anterior section of the upper, consisting of the soft area over the dorsum of toes and forefoot.
- Toe box is the most anterior aspect of the vamp, which overlies the toes. The toe box is constructed of a stiff material inserted between the shoe lining and the upper to prevent collapse and protect the toes.
- Goodyear welt is the stitching that holds the vamp onto the sole. A Goodyear welt allows the outer sole to be changed without replacing the entire shoe. Most athletic footwear lacks a Goodyear welt. Cement is used to anchor the vamp onto the sole.
- Ball is the area of the sole underneath the metatarsal heads.
- Shank is the portion of the sole between the ball and the anterior portion of the heel.
- Heel is the posterior, inferior aspect of the plantar surface of the shoe that attaches to the sole and makes contact with the ground. The function of the shoe is affected by the contours of the heel, and weight bearing by the foot is affected by the height of the heel.
- Quarters are the posterior portion of the upper. There are two types of quarters: a low quarter extends below the malleoli, as in a dress shoe, while a high quarter covers the malleoli, as in a boot. The high-quarter shoe reduces piston action and provides better ankle support. The shoe in Figure 16-1 is an example of a low-quarter shoe.
- Throat is the portion of the shoe that connects the rear part of the vamp and the front part of the quarters. The throat determines how wide the shoe can be opened. Two types of throats styles are

    Balmoral—the vamp is stitched to the forward edges of the quarter as one unit, making a "V" opening. This type of upper allows less space for the midfoot and thus is not indicated for foot deformity conditions.

    Blucher—the quarters lie over the vamp, allowing easier opening (Fig. 16-2).

- Heel counter is the firm cup incorporated into the rear posterior aspect of the shoe upper. Its purpose is to help hold the heel in position and control excessive motion. Most heel counters are made of durable plastic or polyvinyl.
- Last is the form, shaped in the general outline of the plantar aspect of the foot, over which the components of the shoe are molded. The last is the foundation for the shoe development. The shape of the shoe instep, the girth of the toe box, and foot curvature are determined by the last. There are four types of lasts: regular, straight, outflare, and inflare. The last three are made as shoe modifications and are discussed later. A regular last has a mild inward curve to the whole sole with the cutout of the medial curve at the instep of the foot. It is seen in a regular shoe and is not used to correct or accommodate a deformity. Most feet have this mild inward curve (Fig. 16-3A).

Practical Application Box 16-1 contains factors to consider when choosing a shoe.

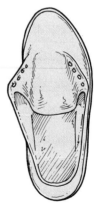

Figure 16-2. Blucher throat. (Adapted from Anon. (1975). *Atlas of orthotics. Biomechanical principles and application*, St. Louis: C. V. Mosby.)

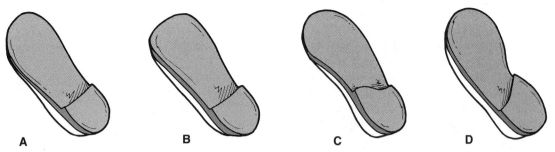

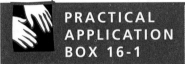

Figure 16-3. Four types of right shoe lasts. A. Regular last. B. Straight last. C. Outflare or reverse last. D. Inflare last.

Shoe Modifications

Modifications may be made to a shoe to help

- Transfer the weight or forces on the foot especially from insensitive areas
- Modify weight transfer patterns
- Accommodate fixed deformities or correct flexible deformities

The following are shoe modifications often used in clinical practice:

- Lift: A layer of firm material added to the heel or heel and sole to compensate for a leg length discrepancy.
- Metatarsal bar: A layer of firm material added across the sole, posterior to the metatarsal heads. The purpose of the metatarsal

---

PRACTICAL APPLICATION BOX 16-1

When choosing a shoe to fit with an orthosis, the following need to be considered:

1. What is the heel height?
   Heels are measured on the anterior aspect (called the *breast*) of the heel and are measured in 1/8-inch increments. The *pitch* of the heel is the slope of the posterior aspect of the heel. The higher the heel, the greater the pitch and the less surface for weight bearing. Even with the foot placed in a fixed position inside an orthosis, a shoe with a high heel puts the foot in an AFO into relative plantarflexion and decreases the weight-bearing surface. Conversely, a shoe with a low heel puts a foot in an AFO into relative dorsiflexion. Orthosis use necessitates wearing shoes that have approximately the same heel height.

2. What is the quarters height?
   Higher quarters height is more restrictive to ankle motion. What is the intent of the orthosis at the ankle in regards to active movement? Will the quarters add to the restriction of ankle motion or at least not hinder it?

3. What is the throat style of the shoe?
   The Blucher style provides a sizable opening to place either the foot after the orthosis or the foot in the orthosis into the shoe.

The best heel height, quarters height, and throat style should be discussed with the orthotic clinic team and the client. Factors such as optimal function of the orthosis and shoe, cosmesis, cost and funding sources, and growth (in cases of children) should be taken into account.

bar is to shift pressure from the heads to the shaft of the metatarsals.

- Metatarsal pad is the soft, dome-shaped pad that is placed inside the shoe. The purpose of the metatarsal pad is to shift pressure from one or more metatarsal heads to the metatarsal shaft. The size of the pad is dictated by the amount of relief needed for the metatarsal heads.

- Modified lasts are the variations of the form of the plantar aspect of the foot upon which the shoe is built.

  A straight last has the medial border of the sole form a straight line from the heel to the tip of the great toe. A straight last may be worn on either foot and can be bisected into equal left and right halves. A straight last is sometimes used for a mild valgus or varus deformity (Fig. 16-3B).

  An outflare or reverse last has the lateral border of the sole curving slightly outward. To achieve an outflare or reverse last, one essentially reverses wear, for example, placing a right shoe with a regular last on the left foot. The outflare or reverse last may be used to correct or control mild metatarsal adduction (Fig. 16-3C).

  An inflare last has an excessive form of the regular inwardly curved sole. Inflare lasts may be used to correct or control mild metatarsal abduction (Fig. 16-3D).

- Wedge is a firm material, such as leather, placed between the outer and inner soles to provide extra support or make correction. For example, a medial heel wedge places a flexible heel in a more varus position. A lateral heel wedge places the heel in a more valgus position. A wedge can also serve to accommodate a fixed deformity.

- Extra-depth shoe provides the foot with additional space to accommodate any orthotics (inserts) or orthoses that are necessary. An extra-depth shoe, as pictured in Figure 16-4, is less expensive and cosmeti-

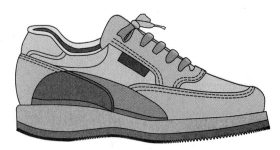

Figure 16-4. Extra-depth shoe. (Reprinted with permission from P. W. Minor.)

cally more acceptable than custom-molded shoes. A custom-molded shoe may be necessary to accommodate a fixed deformity, but it tends to be rather expensive. Extra-depth shoes are generally one size longer and two sizes wider than the regular foot size. Extra-depth shoes should possess the following features:

  The upper should be made of a flexible material, with a high toe box to avoid toe compression. For example, a high toe box is often used for toe deformities such as hammer toes.

  The length should be $\frac{1}{2}$-inch longer than the longest toe to aid foot movement in ambulation.[7]

  The heel counter should be firm to prevent movement during ambulation.

  The heel should be low and broad to provide maximal support.

  The insole should be resilient. Insoles made of microcellular neoprene bonded to a stretchable nylon fabric, foamed polyethylene with closed-cell construction, or viscoelastic polymer material can all significantly reduce high pedal pressure.

- Rocker sole is the firm material with skived anterior and posterior edges, placed across the sole. The rocker sole projects approximately $\frac{1}{4}$ to $\frac{1}{2}$ inch below the level of the sole and extends proximal to the metatarsal heads. Rather than concentrating the body weight at the metatarsal heads during termi-

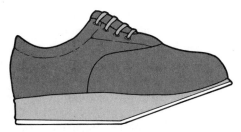

Figure 16-5. Rocker sole.

nal stance and preswing, a rocker sole allows wider distribution of weight. Therefore, body weight is shifted more from the metatarsal heads to the metatarsal shafts. A rocker sole is often used for an insensitive foot and may be helpful for those prone to skin breakdown over the metatarsal heads, forefoot fractures, or severe cases of turf toe (Fig. 16-5).[7] For the rocker sole to exert its maximal beneficial effect on the foot, a rigid sole can be fabricated by incorporating a full-length steel shank into the sole.[8] Because the design of a rocker sole can aid in a weight shift, it is added to the shoe plate of the hip guidance orthosis. This orthosis is discussed later in this chapter.

Shoes for the patient with a neuropathic or insensitive foot are discussed in Practical Application Box 16-2.

Care of the Insensitive Foot

In 1994, the annual cost of foot and leg amputation and ulcer care at the U.S. Veterans Administration alone was over $383 million.[9] Therefore, patients with insensitivity, such as those with diabetes, should be taught basic foot care principles. Prevention of serious foot complications from diabetes requires ongoing client education. Education in preventive care includes the following.

1. Daily skin inspection. The feet are usually the first to be impaired in a client with peripheral vascular disease (PVD) and neuropathy, because of their position of de-

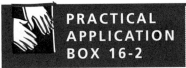

PRACTICAL APPLICATION BOX 16-2

Shoes for the Patient with a Neuropathic or Insensitive Foot

Patients with neuropathic or insensitive feet such as those with diabetes or PVD need shoes that protect, conform with, and do not compress the foot. A client with insensitivity should never go barefoot because skin would be exposed to damage that may not heal easily. Athletic footwear or regular shoes (possibly a half-size larger) that allow room for the toes to move freely may be worn by the patient with neuropathy. Extra-depth shoes are a common modification used for patients with neuropathy. Proper footwear is important because pressure ulcerations and foot deformities, such as hammer toes or bunions, may occur with improper footwear. When combined with poor circulation or neuropathy, pressures caused by common foot deformities may lead to pressure ulcerations. Once an ulceration has occurred, one must relieve pressure and distribute weight away from the area. A rocker sole can help remove pressure from an ulcerated metatarsal area, yet allow some mobility.[11] Other ways to relieve pressure are through the use of padding, frequent removal of shoes, and exposure to the air.

pendence related to body fluids and their weight-bearing role. When performing daily skin inspections, patients should pay attention to problem areas, such as between toes and bony prominences. Inspection of the feet is necessary to monitor blood flow and areas of pressure or skin damage. The foot examination should consist of checking for breaks in the skin, sores, redness, swelling, blisters, or fungal infections.[10] A mirror and/or magnifying glass can be used to inspect the feet. The patient can also be taught to inspect the feet by touch, checking for changes in foot topography or skin temperature and through smell, checking for changes in odors on socks or washcloths.

2. Skin cleaning. Skin cleaning should be done on a routine daily basis, when the feet are soiled, or after exercise. The feet should be washed in a basin of tepid, not hot, water. The water temperature should be tested with either a thermometer or a sensitized part of the body such as the elbow. The client can use a soft nailbrush to clean under the nails. Perfumed soaps and hot water should be avoided because they may cause skin irritations. A mild cleansing agent to minimize friction to the skin should be used to avoid damaging the skin through rough washing. The feet should be dried thoroughly by patting, not rubbing. Thorough drying prevents a moist environment conducive to bacterial growth. The skin can then be moisturized to prevent flaking and cracking, which can lead to ulcerations.

3. Skin lubrication. Proper care of the skin involves a balance between skin that is too dry or too moist. Lubrication occurs from a combination of internal and external factors. Negative environmental factors such as low humidity leading to dry skin, high humidity leading to damp skin, and extremes of hot and cold should be minimized. Lubricants such as cocoa butter should be applied daily; they will hydrate skin, help maintain tissue elasticity, and reduce friction. Reducing skin friction decreases the chance of skin damage from shearing forces. Lubricants should not be applied between the toes because this may set up a medium for infection. Finally, taking in the proper amount of fluids daily helps keep the skin hydrated.

4. Care of cold feet. Feet may become cold because of limitations in circulation. For cold feet, the client may wear loose-fitting socks to help maintain an external environment that will keep body temperature in balance. Feet should not be left wet or damp because of the effects on the skin and the overall temperature of the feet. High humidity situations necessitate carrying extra socks for changing. Use of heating pads, hot water bottles, and other external sources of heat should be avoided because they may increase the chances of perspiration and skin damage, including burns.

5. Use of shoes. New shoes should be worn initially for 2 hours/day, gradually increasing the time worn by 2 hours every week. Shoes should be constructed of soft leather or canvas, which allow the feet to breathe. Shoes with open toes or heels and straps at the ankle, foot, or between the toes (e.g., sandals) should be avoided because they may impair circulation and expose skin to damage more easily. It may be best to wear a fully closed shoe. Shoes should be inspected before wearing to make sure they have no sharp edges or objects in them. Shoe modifications may be needed as discussed previously.

6. Socks or stockings. The best socks are nonelastic, seamless, and made of cotton. Cotton is the best material because it is absorbent, which helps keep the foot dry, and has a soft texture for additional cushioning inside the shoe. All clients should be cautioned against knee-high or midcalf hose and any constricting elastic that restricts blood flow. Socks should be changed when they become wet or damp with perspiration.

7. Other precautions. Patients should not cut calluses or corns on their own. Chemical agents such as wart removers should not be used because they contain caustic substances that may lead to burns. Interventions for painful warts, calluses, and corns and nail trimming should be done by a podiatrist. Tobacco should be avoided because it causes blood vessels to narrow, which decreases cir-

culation and affects healing. Leg crossing when sitting should also be avoided because it puts additional pressure on structures. Obesity often compounds the problems of pressure and deformity on the feet. Proper nutrition should be considered for weight control as well as assistance with healing.[11]

Purpose of Orthoses

The purposes of orthoses are to

- Prevent and or correct deformity (impairment)
- Prevent worsening of, or provide support for, deformity (impairments)
- Improve function (functional limitation/disability)[12,13]

The primary function of an orthosis is to change or enhance the biomechanics of the lower extremity. Function may improve because of the biomechanical changes that occur. Functional improvements occur through many venues. One way orthoses may enhance function is to provide an opportunity to enhance learning of motor skills.[14] For example, if a foot is positioned in equinus, the weight-bearing surface for standing may be limited to the toes. Weight bearing on the toes of the foot limits the ability to shift weight throughout the whole foot while performing a standing transfer. As a result, the client may require assistance to transfer. If an orthosis can position the foot flat for weight bearing, the client is given the opportunity to learn to shift weight throughout the plantar surface of the foot, and he or she may perform a standing transfer more effectively and without assistance. Another way to improve function is to provide stability lost to impairments. For example, with a complete spinal cord injury, all motor function below the level of the lesion is lost. An orthosis can substitute for the loss of muscle function. As a result, moveable segments of the lower extremities, such as the hips, may still function, as in coming to stand and walking. The use of orthoses may also result in improvement and de-

velopment of physiologic and/or psychologic functions. The physiologic function of digestion may be improved through standing with the aid of orthoses. Feeling of well-being and control over one's life may be psychologic effects that are an indirect benefit of using orthoses.

The research section of this chapter reviews the evidence related to these purposes. To understand the literature, the reader must first be familiar with the different types of orthoses available. Remember that the types of devices prescribed may vary among facilities and geographic regions. Descriptions of some of the most common designs follows.

Terminology

The term *orthotics* describes the practice and manufacture of orthoses or a shoe insert. An orthosis or externally applied device is named for the joint(s) that it crosses, supports, or assists with motion.[15] Each orthosis is described by an acronym. For example, the acronym AFO describes the ankle–foot orthosis that encompasses the foot and ankle joint, extending to a point below the knee. The use of this acronym eliminates older terminology such as a short leg brace.[15] Compared with a splint, which may be used as a short-term intervention before fabrication of an orthosis, an orthosis is more durable and versatile. Therefore, in written and verbal communication, use of the term *orthosis* rather than *brace* or *splint* is encouraged.

Principles of Design

Optimal design of an orthosis results from the combined efforts of the team. A detailed prescription can only be developed after consideration of

- The client's identified outcome for intervention
- The client's examination and evaluation findings related to function/functional limitations, impairments, and desired outcome

- The principles of design related to function of the orthosis

The manufacturer (orthotist or therapist) decides upon the materials and components to meet the identified needs and suggested outcome. The team continues to provide input into the details of fitting or modifying an orthosis for the best possible outcome. Knowledge of the underlying rationale for design assists clinicians in measuring and evaluating orthosis use. Two major principles for design and use need to be considered.

The first principle is ground reaction force (GRF) control.[16] The GRF is the force exerted by the ground in response to the force that the body produces on the ground. This means that for every force downward that the body exerts when weight bearing, there is an equal and upward force that is exerted by the ground. If the line of the GRF does not pass directly through the center of the joint, there is a tendency for joint movement. This is called torque. Muscle activity at each joint is required to counteract this tendency for joint movement. The torque increases as the distance of the GRF line from the joint axes increases. The greater the moment, the greater the muscular activity needed to control it. Minimizing the torque that needs to be resisted results in greater energy efficiency.[17] In fabrication of an orthosis, design can influence the magnitude and direction of the GRF line. Proper location of the GRF line helps the body segment achieve optimum alignment and minimizes the force needed to maintain this alignment. The GRF is shown in Figure 16-6.

The second principle of orthosis design is three-point pressure control. The purpose of this control is to achieve joint stability by providing a point of pressure above the axis of rotation, a point below the axis of rotation, and a third, opposing point at or near the axis of rotation.[18] An example of this principle is seen in the application of an anterior strap to a conventional AFO. The calf band (above the axis

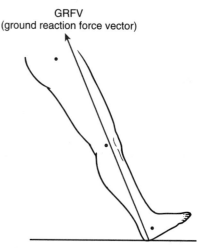

GRFV
(ground reaction force vector)

Figure 16-6. GRFV during gait. (Adapted from Levangie, P. K, & Norkin, C. C. (2001). *Joint structure and function, a comprehensive analysis* (3rd ed.). Philadelphia: F. A. Davis.)

of rotation) and stirrup of the heel (below the axis of rotation) apply anteriorly directed forces that oppose the posteriorly directed force of the anterior strap at the level of the talocrural joint. Other examples of the three-point pressure system are illustrated in Figure 16-7. Since applying pressure over a small area of the skin may be detrimental, pressure may be distributed over a large area by increasing the surface area that is in contact with the skin. The principles of GRF and three-point pressure control are discussed further in Chapter 5.

Fabrication and Materials

When plastic replaced metal in the fabrication of orthoses, orthoses became lighter and moldable. In addition, comfort and cosmetic appearance improved.[15] The increased ability to mold the orthosis afforded variability of purpose. For example, molding the orthosis around the foot allows buildup of support for the plantar aspect of the foot with a tighter overall fit. This buildup of support distributes the weight bearing more evenly on the surface of the foot, and the limited flexibility of the plastic helps to maintain the integrity of the fit. Prior to the use of plastic, the orthosis was attached to the shoe and distribution of weight on the foot was affected by the internal supports and flexibility of the shoe. A plastic orthosis worn within a shoe allows more options, such as use of athletic footwear. However, a limitation of wearing the orthosis in the sneaker or shoe is that shoe size must be larger. Therefore, shoes cannot be worn easily without the orthosis unless an added sock, thicker sock, or insole is used.

To fabricate a custom molded orthosis, a plaster cast impression of the limb is taken. A negative cast of the client's affected limb is made from a plaster of Paris or fiberglass bandage. This negative cast is filled with plaster, and a positive mold results. Vacuum-forming techniques are used over this positive mold. The most common plastics used in orthosis fabrication are polypropylene, polyethylene, and copolymer. Since these materials require high temperatures to mold, a positive mold is used. A premolded footplate may also be incorporated into this orthosis.

To construct a low-temperature plastic orthosis, materials are heated in warm water and molded directly to the individual.[19] These materials are often used in the fabrication of a temporary orthosis, which may be called a splint. In some cases, clients may wear an off-the-shelf or custom-fit plastic orthosis, which may be modified to the particular individual. A custom fit involves taking a prefabricated, or off-the-shelf, orthosis, such as an AFO, and adjusting it to fit the client. In contrast, a custom-molded orthosis is molded to a particular client and is more likely to be fit correctly with fewer complications. This fit may be critical for clients with insensitivity. Factors that may influence whether to order a custom-fit or custom-molded orthosis include

- Projected length of use: short-term use most often implies custom fit
- An insensitive limb: implies custom molded
- Support for existing deformities: implies custom molded
- How quickly the orthosis is required: implies custom fit

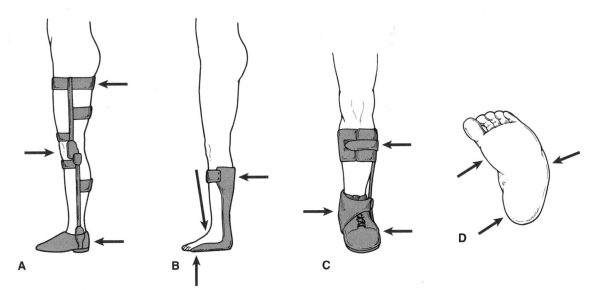

Figure 16-7. Three-point pressure system.

- Insurance/cost considerations: may imply custom fit, which is less expensive
- Age of individual: children almost always wear custom molded because of considerations of growth and development
- Height and weight of the individual: may require custom molded when extra-small or extra-large sizes are needed

Orthosis Components

The completed orthosis can include:

- Trim lines
- Footplates
- Joints
- Straps
- Posting[19]

Trim lines

The *trim lines*, or borders, of the orthosis delineate the height, width, length, and circumference of the orthosis. The trim lines adhere to the anthropometric characteristics of the individual's foot and the purpose of the orthosis. For example, trim lines posterior to the malleoli provide minimal resistance and increased ability to move the tibia forward. Trim lines through the malleoli offer moderate resistance. Trim lines anterior to the malleoli, extending the orthosis around the forefoot and over the ankle, provide increased support for mediolateral stability and maximal resistance to movement. By using proper alignment and pressure, trim lines stabilize a foot with minimal force production.

Footplates

The term *footplate* refers to the portion of the orthosis in contact with the plantar surface of the foot. Footplates may also extend to the dorsal, medial, and lateral surfaces of the foot. The term *footplate* may also refer to a premolded and/or custom-contoured plate that prepositions the foot for casting. This contouring may include depressions or recessed areas to hold the calcaneus and metatarsal heads, buildups to support extension of the toes, and medial and lateral longitudinal arches (Fig. 16-8).[20] The footplate may or may not extend all the way to the end of the toes to provide additional support. If it does, the term *toeplate* may be added to the description.

Joints

A *joint* in an orthosis aligns with the anatomic joint of the individual to allow motion to occur at that anatomic joint. The term *free* means a full range of motion in one plane. For example, a free ankle joint permits full plantarflexion and dorsiflexion but limits medial and lateral motion. If a joint is present, the terms *articulated* or *hinged* may be used instead of *free*. In the absence of a joint, the terms used to describe the orthosis are *fixed* or *solid*. Fixed or solid means no motion is allowed to occur, and often the ankle joint is fixed in a few degrees of dorsiflexion. The purpose of this position of

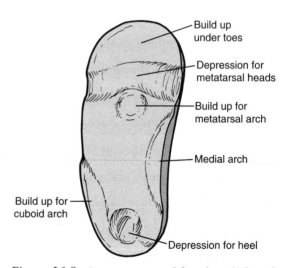

Figure 16-8. Custom-contoured footplate. (Adapted from Walker, J., Stanger, M. (1998). Orthotic management. In J. Dormans, & L. Pellegrino (Eds.), *Caring for children with cerebral palsy: A team approach* (pp. 391–426). Baltimore: Paul H. Brooks.)

dorsiflexion is discussed below. A *lock* is placed at a joint to prevent motion, provide added stability, and, when necessary, allow movement. For example, a lock at the knee joint will keep the knee in extension during standing and walking, but when the lock is lifted, the knee can flex for sitting. If some portion of the motion needs to be limited, a *stop* is built into the orthosis. This stopped motion can occur in one or both directions of a plane of movement. For example, an AFO with a single stop may allow free dorsiflexion but arrest plantarflexion at 90°. An AFO with a double stop or limited-motion stop allows controlled movement, for example, 5° of dorsiflexion and 10° of plantarflexion. Finally, an *assist* provides aid to a weakened muscle with active limited movement. For example, a dorsiflexion assist lifts the foot into dorsiflexion.

Straps

Straps, most often made of Velcro, attach the orthosis to the limb, enhance alignment, promote or limit motion, and provide additional stability. However, when an orthosis fits well, additional straps should not be needed.

Posting

Finally, the orthosis may include posting that is made of foam or thermoplastic materials. Posting is added to the external plantar surface of the orthosis. The purposes of posting are to provide extra support for any abnormal alignment, accommodate fixed deformities, and/or fine-tune the alignment once the foot is in weight bearing. Posting enhances the contact between the plantar surface of the orthosis and the floor.[21] Posting is described in Chapter 14.

Types of Orthoses

Orthoses may be constructed of metal, termed *conventional orthoses,* or, more commonly, of plastics or a combination of both materials.

Conventional Orthoses

Conventional orthoses contain uprights, typically made of aluminum, which attach to a shoe. A well-constructed shoe is necessary if uprights are used. Uprights attach to the shoe via a shoe plate or stirrup that is inserted between the sole of the shoe and upper end of the heel (Fig. 16-9). A conventional orthosis may be used if the lighter-weight plastics will not hold and support an individual. Conventional orthoses are also indicated in some cases of severe bony deformity and cases of fluctuating edema that may be present in patients undergoing renal dialysis, with congestive heart failure, on chemotherapy, or taking β-blockers for cardiac disease. The metal uprights serve to hold the limb in position and may have joints, assists, and stops. In summary, conventional orthoses are heavier, less close in fit, and less cosmetic than plastic orthoses, and they limit the ability to use other footwear. The rest of this

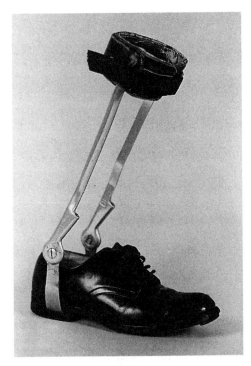

Figure 16-9. Conventional AFO.

section, therefore, is devoted to describing plastic orthoses, which are more commonly used.

Plastic Orthoses

A variety of plastic orthoses are in use today. This section of the chapter describes each type of plastic orthosis and provides general clinical indications and contraindications for use. More specific suggestions for applications of each orthosis are provided in the section of the chapter that reviews current literature. Caution should be used in applying any orthosis to an insensitive foot. The patient may not be able to indicate areas of pressure, tightness, or pain, which can lead to skin lesions. Extra care must be taken as indicated earlier in the section of this chapter on care of the insensitive foot.

In general, when patients use lower-extremity orthoses, most often a reciprocal gait pattern is used. Any level of assistive device (e.g., walkers, crutches, or canes) may be used to help maintain balance. For most children who are just learning to ambulate, walkers may be the support of choice. For frail and unsteady individuals, walkers may also be the support of choice. However, it may be desirable to use crutches (forearm or axilla) or canes (quad or straight) because their use enhances the ability to maintain a reciprocal gait pattern. Conversely, their use requires more stability and coordination than may be available. When using a hip–knee–ankle–foot orthosis (HKAFO), swing-to and swing-through gait patterns may initially be easier because the lower extremities are controlled as a unit. However, these gait patterns require good upper body strength and control to execute and may require more energy. All of these factors must be considered during examination.

Foot Orthoses

The least restrictive orthosis is a foot orthosis (FO), which extends below the ankle but surrounds the foot medially and laterally (Fig.

16-10). The clinical finding that indicates the need for a FO is excessive foot mobility, particularly in the hindfoot. However, for the FO to be effective, the client must have good muscular control and good dorsiflexion and plantarflexion range. With excessive hindfoot mobility there is a lack of support for the arches, and the foot collapses into pronation at midstance of gait. In many instances, a well-constructed shoe with an orthotic insert, as described in Chapter 14, may be substituted for a FO.

Supramalleolar Orthoses

In a supramalleolar orthosis (SMO), the trim lines extend above the malleoli and surround the foot, but the material does not encompass the calf (Fig. 16-11). The SMO can be designed to allow the tibia to move over the foot but can limit the range of dorsiflexion and plantarflexion available. This limitation is accomplished by changing the anterior trim lines, limiting forward tibial movement via a shin strap, and providing a narrow channel of space (posterior trim lines) between the malleoli.[22] For both the FO and SMO, a custom-contoured footplate may be incorporated into the construction.

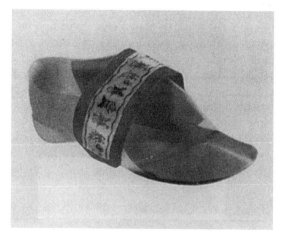

Figure 16-10. Foot orthosis (FO). (Reprinted with permission from Cascade Inc.)

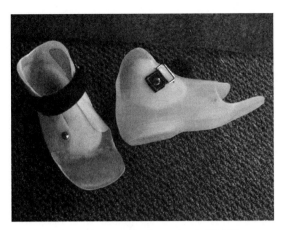

Figure 16-11. Supramalleolar orthosis (SMO).

The clinical findings that indicate the need for a SMO over a FO are

- Need for more mediolateral stability than is provided by a FO
- Some or all voluntary control of dorsiflexion and plantarflexion.

A clinical finding that contraindicates use of a SMO is a fixed deformity of the ankle.

Ankle-Foot Orthoses

An AFO is commonly worn by individuals with neurologic disorders. It may be the only orthosis worn or it may serve as the basic component to which more-extensive orthosis systems are added. Two general categories of AFOs are dynamic AFOs (DAFOs) and molded AFOs (MAFOs).[23] A major difference in these two types of AFOs is the custom-contoured footplate used in the construction of the DAFO.[20,22] The purpose of this footplate is to promote balance of muscle power and reduce the need to seek stability through compensatory balancing methods. Inhibitory casts and inhibitory orthoses are molded on this principle. In the literature, a reader may see such terms as *inhibitory AFO, tone-reducing AFO,* and *neurophysiologic AFO or DAFO* for an orthosis that is molded on this contoured footplate.[20]

In contrast, an MAFO does not include the custom-contoured footplate (Fig. 16-12). Therefore in most cases, an MAFO offers minimal support to the arches, offers no support to the toes, and is made from a less flexible plastic. However, it is possible to modify an MAFO to hold the subtalar joint and support the arch.

The versatility afforded by plastics has allowed the different styles of, and degrees of flexibility in, AFOs. Ideally, the construction of the orthosis should occur only after the results of a biomechanical analysis of the extremity(ies) and a discussion of the client's expected intervention outcomes, impairments, functional limitations, and disabilities are considered. The desired components should then be specified and incorporated into the orthosis.[15]

Whether the orthosis is a DAFO or MAFO, there are variations to be found. They vary in the amount of restriction or assistance to movement that they provide. The general indications and contraindications for use of an

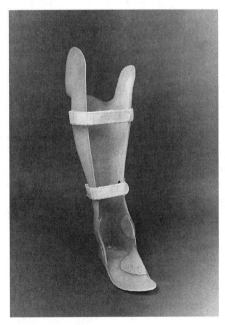

Figure 16-12. Molded ankle foot orthosis (MAFO).

PROS & CONS BOX 16-1

General indications for use of an AFO
• Flexible deformity of the foot and/or ankle
• Weakness or loss of the foot and ankle musculature, with possible weakness of knee musculature
• A need to stabilize the foot for the use of musculature above the foot

General contraindications for use of an AFO
• Fixed deformity of the ankle
• Open wound in contact with the orthosis

AFO are listed in Pros and Cons Box 16-1. The neurologic reasons for orthosis use are reviewed later in this chapter. Factors that influence this process of prescription writing are enumerated in Practical Application Box 16-3. For a format for examination of the patient requiring an orthosis see Figure 2-7.

Solid or Fixed AFO

A solid AFO, or fixed AFO (FAFO), derives its name from being fixed at the ankle. The purpose of a FAFO is to provide support and positioning for the ankle and possibly the subtalar joint. The amount of forward movement of the tibia that can occur in a FAFO is based upon the location of the trim lines, discussed above. The FAFO is usually set at 2–3° of dorsiflexion to limit the tendency for knee flexion at initial contact. However, setting the amount of dorsiflexion as high as 5–7° can also limit the tendency for genu recurvatum or knee hyperextension at stance (Fig. 16-13). Additional clinical findings that indicate the use of a FAFO are

• Little or no voluntary control of dorsiflexion
• Excessive knee extension during weight bearing

Some clinical findings that contraindicate use of a FAFO include

• A knee flexion contracture
• A need to use ankle motion in skill development

Articulated or Hinged AFO

An articulated (A) AFO or hinged (H) AFO allows dorsiflexion and/or plantarflexion at the ankle (Fig. 16-14). The range of those motions may be limited by a stop. Most often the AAFO or HAFO blocks ankle plantarflexion while al-

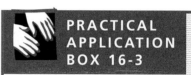

PRACTICAL APPLICATION BOX 16-3

Factors Related to Prescriptions for Orthoses

1. Identify impairments that require orthosis use
2. Gather data regarding the client/family such as
   Personal characteristics, e.g., age, ability to follow directions
   Physical findings, e.g., functional abilities/needs, neurodevelopmental and musculoskeletal impairments
   Family characteristics such as lifestyle, attitudes, and economic factors
   Environment, including geographic setting, climate, home/community
3. Gather information regarding orthosis options and support such as
   Materials, facilities, and team members' skills related to fabrication
   Costs, ranging from actual orthosis cost to travel for fittings
   Professional support for training in use, follow-up of program
4. Evaluation of the data by the team
5. Write a prescription
6. Fabricate the orthosis

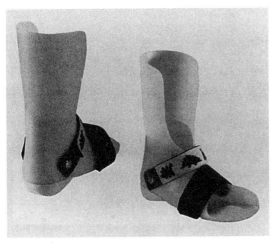

Figure 16-13. Solid or fixed AFO. (Reprinted with permission from Cascade Inc.)

lowing dorsiflexion. Additional clinical findings that indicate use of an AAFO or HAFO are

- Some or all voluntary control of dorsiflexion, but no plantarflexion control
- Limited voluntary control of *both* dorsiflexion and plantarflexion
- A need to use ankle motion in skill development

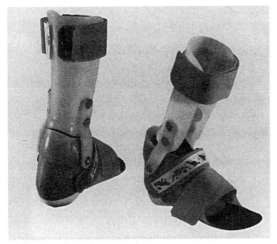

Figure 16-14. Articulated or hinged AFO (AAFO or HAFO). (Reprinted with permission from Cascade Inc.)

One clinical finding that contraindicates use of an AAFO or HAFO is a contracture of the ankle musculature. Interventions to minimize or eliminate the contracture must occur before the AFO is prescribed.

Dorsiflexion-Assist AFOs

There are a variety of dorsiflexion assists that may be used. These assists are typically used with AFOs. In a conventional orthosis, as discussed above, a posterior spring-loaded channel (known as Klenzak) is a dorsiflexion-assist device. A clinical finding that indicates use of a dorsiflexion-assist AFO is limited or no voluntary control of dorsiflexion and/or plantarflexion but an adequate range of passive motion.

Two different types of plastic orthoses are designed to assist with dorsiflexion. The first type is a spiral that coils around the shaft of the lower leg and supports the foot (Fig. 16-15). The second type is known as a posterior leaf

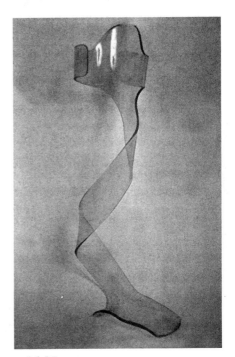

Figure 16-15. Spiral orthosis.

orthosis (PLO) or posterior leaf-spring orthosis (PLS) (Fig. 16-16). The PLS is designed for flexibility. The trim lines are posterior to the malleoli to allow both ankle dorsiflexion and plantarflexion to occur in gait. The PLS provides a spring-like dorsiflexion assist in terminal stance. The PLS may be custom molded to a particular client or custom fit as an-off-the shelf AFO. All of the AFOs (except the spiral) can limit mediolateral motion by extension of the plastic over the sides and top of the foot (also called extending the trim-lines). Motion may also be limited via ankle and foot straps.

Floor-Reaction or Ground-Reaction AFOs

A floor-reaction orthosis (FRO) or ground-reaction AFO (GRAFO) is molded to fit around the front of the leg (Fig. 16-17). The straps on the back of the leg hold the leg and heel in place. These straps and the anterior shell limit the forward movement of the tibia at initial contact and throughout the stance phase of gait. Therefore knee extension is promoted. The anterior shell may contain a patellar shelf to increase the size of the weight-bearing surface. By limiting dorsiflexion range,

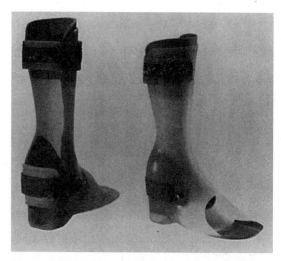

Figure 16-17. Floor reaction orthosis or ground reaction AFO (FRO or GRAFO). (Reprinted with permission from Cascade Inc.)

this orthosis may enable the wearer to assume a full upright posture. Additional clinical findings that indicate the need for a FRO or GRAFO are

- Excessive knee flexion in weight bearing
- Excessive ankle dorsiflexion in weight bearing

Clinical findings that contraindicate use of the FRO or GRAFO are a fixed knee and ankle flexion contracture.

Knee–Ankle–Foot Orthoses

A knee–ankle–foot orthosis (KAFO) controls and aligns the knee and ankle for weight bearing. Indications and contraindications for use of a KAFO are listed in Pros and Cons Box 16-2. The neurologic reasons for KAFO use are reviewed later in this chapter.

Common components of the KAFO include

- An AFO that usually has a limited motion stop or is fixed
- Two metal or plastic uprights running from the AFO to the thigh

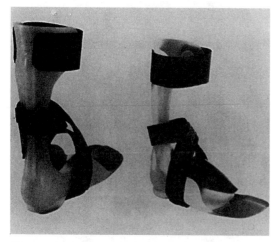

Figure 16-16. Posterior leaf spring orthosis (PLS). (Reprinted with permission from Cascade Inc.)

PROS & CONS BOX 16-2

General indications for use of a KAFO
- Little or no voluntary control at the knee and foot, with some or all voluntary control of the hip and trunk musculature
- Malalignment of the knee, such as genu valgus, genu varus, or knee flexion contracture

General contraindications for use of a KAFO
- Unable to meet energy demands
- Lack of adequate strength, especially in the trunk and upper extremities, to control standing balance or use assistive equipment
- Open wound in the area of the orthosis

- A hinged knee joint, with or without knee locks
- Patellar pad, straps, and thigh band (Fig. 16-18)

The patellar pad supports the anterior aspect of the knee, may help maintain extension during stance, but allows flexion in sitting. Straps may be added to the patellar pad to provide additional medial or lateral control.

Types of Knee Locks

Types of knee locks that may be used with a KAFO are as follows:

1. The drop lock is the most common lock used with KAFOs; it drops into place once the knee is extended. The client must possess the following abilities to unlock the knee so it may flex for sitting:

   Enough upper-extremity strength to raise the drop lock manually

   Enough finger dexterity to manipulate the lock

Enough standing balance, with or without an assistive device, to bend slightly forward, reach, and manipulate the lock

The client must possess one of the following abilities to lock the knee when coming to stand:

Enough strength to lift and extend the leg while still sitting so the locks drop into place. The ability to come to stand with legs extended is also needed.

Enough strength and balance to come to upright standing and have the locks drop into place. Standing may be accomplished by the use of an assistive device to support the body to get the weight line in front of the knee to extend the knee mechanically so the lock will drop into place.

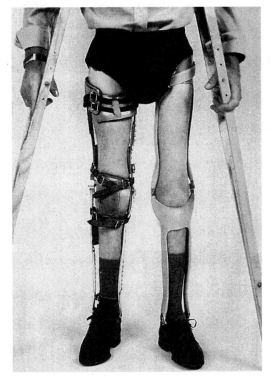

Figure 16-18. Comparison of a conventional KAFO on the *left* and a plastic KAFO on the *right*.

For patients with poor balance skills, the drop lock may be attached to a ring at midthigh level, and via a spring mechanism, the drop lock may be disengaged. The use of this spring mechanism enables the wearer to avoid having to bend to unlock the knee joint. Relocking the knees for standing would require the same characteristics as above. Individuals who are lighter weight and have more voluntary control and good balance may use one drop lock instead of two. This lock is then placed on the lateral upright. Drop locks are the most durable and have the lowest maintenance of those discussed here (Fig. 16-19).

2. The offset knee joint is placed posterior to the anatomic knee joint to increase the extension moment at the knee for increased stability in stance. An offset knee joint with a lock, the design in a reciprocal-gait orthosis (RGO), is used to assist upright standing posture and reduce the pressure on the

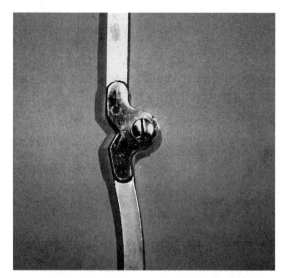

Figure 16-20. Offset knee joint with the mechanical axis posterior to the upright.

patellar pad to maintain knee extension (Fig. 16-20).

3. The bail lock is a horizontal semicircular lever placed behind the knee joint. When this lever is pulled up, the knee unlocks. The client may catch this lever on the seat of a chair to unlock the knee before sitting. To unlock the knee so it may flex for sitting, the client must have enough balance to back up to a chair. A strap attached to the bail lock is termed a *Swiss lock* (Fig. 16-21). The client must possess the same abilities to lock the knee as with the drop lock. Overall, the bail lock requires less effort and skill than the drop lock, therefore, it may be used by those with the use of only one hand such as a client with a cerebral vascular accident. One disadvantage of this lock is that it may disengage inadvertently when bumped.

Special KAFOs

Two special designs of KAFO are found in the literature; the Walkabout orthosis and Vannini-Rizzoli stabilizing orthosis. Even though they are KAFOs, they are designed for patients with

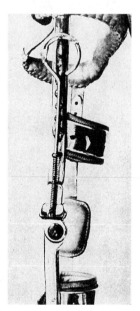

Figure 16-19. Spring-loaded pull rod attached to a drop lock.

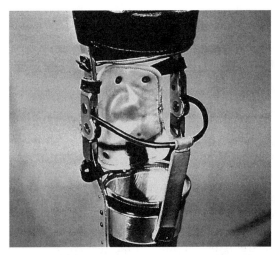

Figure 16-21. Swiss lock.

characteristics similar to those of a patient needing an HKAFO, which is discussed in the next section.

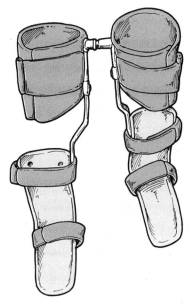

Figure 16-22. Walkabout orthosis. (Adapted from Burns. Y., & MacDonald, J. (1996). Physiotherapy and the growing child. Philadelphia: W. B. Saunders.)

Walkabout Orthosis

The Walkabout orthosis is a KAFO with a low-friction joint that attaches the legs at the knees (Fig. 16-22).[24] This joint spaces the legs at an appropriate width in standing and works to control abduction/adduction and/or rotation of the hips. With the use of assistive devices such as walkers, canes, or crutches, ambulation in the Walkabout occurs with a reciprocal pattern. Applying and removing the Walkabout requires the ability to balance in long and short sitting as well as upper-extremity strength and hand dexterity to lift the orthosis and manipulate the straps. A patient with limited hand function may require assistance.

Vannini-Rizzoli Stabilizing Orthosis

The Vannini-Rizzoli stabilizing orthosis or boot covers the foot and extends to the knee (Fig. 16-23).[25] This orthosis fixes the ankle and foot in 15° of plantarflexion to stabilize the knee when in the upright position. The patient achieves balance by tucking the chin,

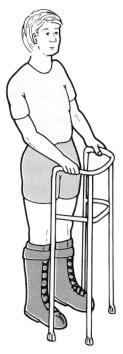

Figure 16-23. Vannini-Rizzoli stabilizing orthosis.

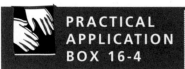

PRACTICAL APPLICATION BOX 16-4

The Impact of Orthoses on Selection of Clothing

Clothing selection may be more difficult because

- Repeated locking and unlocking of knees or hip joints may easily tear some clothing, thus limiting selection and possibly affecting the user economically
- If the orthosis is worn under clothing, larger sizes or certain styles may be needed, for example skirts instead of pants for girls; this is especially needed because of the large size of the bail lock
- If the orthosis is worn over clothing, size, shape, and textures may interfere with fit, thus limiting clothing selection; this limitation, as well as wearing the orthosis in full view, may be cosmetically unappealing to some individuals

hyperextending the back, and keeping hips and knees straight. Ambulation is achieved by shifting the upper body slightly right or left and progressing the leg forward by elevating the hip using trunk musculature. With the use of assistive devices, ambulation in the Vannini-Rizzoli stabilizing orthosis generally occurs with a reciprocal pattern. This orthosis was designed to eliminate the need for the more extensive stability and energy consumption of the HKAFOs. Applying and removing the Vannini-Rizzoli stabilizing orthosis is similar to putting on a boot. Contraindications for use of this orthosis are laxity of knee ligaments, unstable spine, and contractures of the hips and knees.

The effect of a KAFO or HKAFO on selection of clothing is described in Practical Application Box 16-4.

Hip–Knee–Ankle–Foot Orthoses

The most extensive lower-extremity orthosis is the HKAFO, which may be used with or without thoracic support. There are many different types of HKAFOs; some types provide support for standing only, while others also allow locomotion. Indications and contraindications for use of a HKAFO are listed in Pros and Cons Box 16-3. The neurologic reasons for use of a HKAFO are reviewed below in this chapter.

The basic components of the HKAFO include

1. An AFO that usually has a fixed joint
2. Two uprights (usually metal for added strength) running from the AFO to the pelvis or waist
3. Locking knee joints with patellar pads
4. Hip joints that may or may not be locking, with thigh bands
5. Pelvic or waist band that anchors the orthosis to the body

HKAFO variations are described below.

PROS & CONS BOX 16-3

General indications for use of a HKAFO

- Complete or partial loss of voluntary control of the trunk and lower extremities
- Need to stabilize the body in upright standing posture to provide the opportunity for different planes of movement to be experienced

General contraindications for use of an HKAFO

- Unable to meet high energy demands
- Inadequate neck and upper extremity strength and coordination
- Fixed hip flexion contracture, generally of more than 30°

HKAFOs That Enable Standing in Children

Standing orthoses offer a significant amount of stability and enable an upright posture. They can be used by the child who is nonambulatory but of the appropriate age to learn more about pulling to stand. They may also be used by a child just learning to walk. These orthoses are most often recommended for children with spina bifida but may also be suggested for early standing for children with cerebral palsy or developmental delay. These orthoses enable a child to weight bear and initially learn to develop body control. Upright posture may also foster cognitive, social, and emotional development. Since development of body control includes the function of the head, trunk, and extremities, a child must experience different postures that provide an environment for learning awareness and control of muscle function in different planes. An HKAFO provides an environment for learning that differs from weight bearing in prone, supine, or sitting. A more complete understanding of the interaction among motor learning, motor control, and motor development and their influence on intervention strategies and cognitive, social, and emotional development is beyond the scope of this book. The reader is directed to pediatric physical therapy texts for further information.[14,23,26]

There are generally two types of standing orthoses that fully support upright posture. These are the parapodium[27] (Fig. 16-24) and the standing shell[28] (Fig. 16-25).

Parapodium

The Parapodium is an HKAFO plus a thoracolumbar orthosis (TLO) that fully supports the trunk, hips, knees, and feet.[27] The TLO provides limited control of the trunk. The Parapodium is an adjustable orthosis with a wide base and hip and knee joints locks to allow sitting and hands-free standing. It is used to enable standing and ambulation. The Parapodium adjusts to allow for changes in height and width

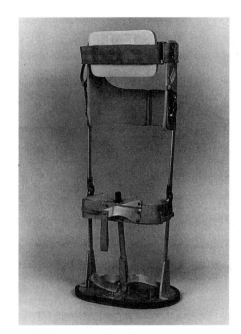

Figure 16-24. Parapodium.

and is most often used for a child. Due to its size, the Parapodium is heavy. Children can learn to apply and remove the Parapodium, as well as roll, come to stand from the floor, sit in and stand up from a chair, and locomote with

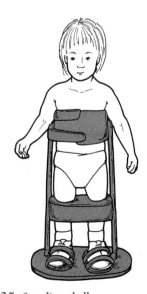

Figure 16-25. Standing shell.

and without assistive devices while wearing the Parapodium. However, all these activities require increased energy, strength, and coordination. The need for many children to be placed in the Parapodium by an adult is a limitation. The Parapodium as an ambulation device is discussed later in this chapter.

Standing Shell

A standing shell, or body-shaped orthosis,[28] reaches from the floor to the middle of the thorax, much like the Parapodium. However, the standing shell has a much smaller support surface that may allow a child to be placed into a mobility device such as a wheelchair and be easily transported. The standing shell has many of the same advantages and limitations as the Parapodium. However, the standing shell may tip more easily because of its small base of support.

HKAFOs That Enable Ambulation

HKAFOs developed to enhance the ability to ambulate include

1. Conventional HKAFO
2. Hip-guidance orthosis (HGO) or Parawalker
3. Parapodium
4. Orthotic Research and Locomotor Assessment Unit (ORLAU Swivel)
5. Reciprocating Gait Orthosis (RGO) with its various versions such as advanced RGO (ARGO), isocentric RGO, and hybrid RGO, or RGO II

Applying and removing any of the HKAFOs independently requires the following abilities:

- Enough neck, upper-extremity, and trunk strength to lift and position the orthosis
- Enough upper-extremity strength and balance control to lift and position oneself into or out of the orthosis
- Enough upper-extremity strength and hand dexterity to fasten and unfasten the straps of the orthosis

For many adults, walking with the assistance of the HKAFO is very seldom the primary means of mobility, since the HKAFO requires too much energy to be efficient. As a result, the HKAFO is primarily used for exercise and change of position. However, for children who are first learning to walk and in whom growth factors (contractures, deformities, and weight) have not interfered significantly with function, spending large portions of the day in an HKAFO for standing and walking may be their primary focus, with the secondary backup of a wheelchair.

Conventional HKAFOs

A conventional HKAFO may have locked or unlocked hips, depending upon the amount of hip control the client demonstrates (Fig. 16-26). A conventional HKAFO allows free range of hip flexion for sitting, but hip extension may be limited. A conventional HKAFO controls hip abduction/adduction and rotation. If the hips are locked, ambulation with crutches or a walker may be achieved by a swing-to or swing-through gait pattern. If the hips are unlocked, a reciprocal gait pattern is possible. As noted in the review of the literature section of this chap-

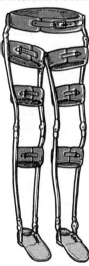

Figure 16-26. Conventional hip-knee-ankle-foot orthoses (HKAFO).

ter, the HKAFO requires the most effort to use for ambulation.

Hip Guidance Orthosis

The HGO or ParaWalker[29] is similar to the conventional HKAFO in having a hip joint that allows or limits the amount of hip flexion and extension and locks for the hip and knee joints. It differs from the conventional HKAFO in having a

- Close-fitting rigid body orthosis
- Special low-friction hip joint
- Fixed-ankle shoe plate with approximately 6° of dorsiflexion
- Rocker sole contouring on the underside of the shoe plate

This orthosis is designed to reduce energy expenditure in walking. The HGO functions as follows in gait: when an individual pushes on a crutch or walker to shift toward the stance leg, weight is shifted from the opposite leg for swing. The shape of the rocker sole allows an easy lateral shift on the stance leg and an easy anterior shift on the swing leg. The swing leg, slightly unweighted, clears the floor by pendulum action. This pendulum action is possible because the line of the center of mass falls behind the hip joint when it is in extension during stance and a hip flexor moment is initiated. Once the leg is slightly unloaded, the response to the flexor moment is flexion of the hip. The rocker sole makes the toes clear the floor easily for forward progression. Excessive flexion is limited by stops at the hip joint. This cycle is then repeated, allowing forward progression. The HGO is easier to progress forward in a reciprocal pattern than a conventional HKAFO, but has the same limitations for applying and removing.

Parapodium and ORLAU Swivel Walker

The Parapodium may be used either as a standing device or to allow ambulation. While wearing the Parapodium and using crutches, walker, or canes, a young child can learn to ambulate with a swing-to or a swing-through gait. Without the use of an assistive device, a child may also be able to progress forward by pivoting in the Parapodium. The major limitations on use of the Parapodium are the lack of a reciprocal gait pattern and the high energy demand for locomotion. The section on research discusses the energy differences of the Parapodium and other HKAFOs.

The orthotic research and locomotor assessment unit (ORLAU) swivel walker has components similar to those of the Parapodium, with the exception of the base plate, which is mounted on swiveling ball-bearing footplates.[30,31] The ORLAU is designed so that the line of gravity falls just ahead of the footplate center. When weight is shifted from side to side, the ORLAU swivels automatically on one footplate as the other footplate clears the ground.[30] Thus, movement in any direction without an assistive device is possible. The amount of effort needed to move when wearing a conventional HKAFO, a Parapodium, swivel walker, or the HGO sparked development of the RGO, which is described below.

Reciprocal-Gait Orthosis

The RGO[32,33] includes some of the same components as a conventional HKAFO such as AFOs, knee joints, uprights, knee pads, thigh bands, and pelvic bands (Fig. 16-27). Unique aspects of the RGO include

- Knee joints that are offset posteriorly with lateral ring locks
- Rigid pelvis band covering the gluteal and sacral areas
- One or two cables connected to each hip joint

In addition, a plastic molded thoracolumbosacral orthosis (TLSO) with a chest strap may be attached to further support the trunk. The RGO provides support to the trunk, pelvis, and lower extremities, while allowing ambulation with the use of assistive devices such as a

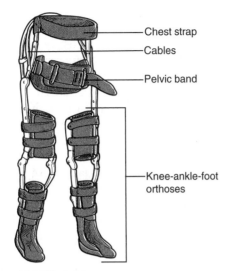

Chest strap
Cables
Pelvic band
Knee-ankle-foot orthoses

Figure 16-27. RGO.

walker, quad canes, or crutches in a reciprocal pattern. The cable system enables a coupling mechanism of the hips. While one leg is in stance, the cable provides stability of that hip through the tension created by the opposite advancing leg. As the advancing leg begins stance, the tension created at the opposite limb assists in unweighting, and a forward movement occurs. This cycle of tension and release is created over and over, enabling ambulation. In individuals with symmetric activity of the hip flexors, the cable system enhances the leg motion. In individuals without active hip musculature, a lateral, diagonal weight shift and leaning back with the upper body are needed to begin the process of creating tension on one side to initiate motion.[32,33]

The Advanced RGO (ARGO), in an attempt to reduce friction, replaced the two cables with one and modified the hip joints.[34] The isocentric RGO has the same components as the regular RGO. However, in this instance, the cables have been replaced by a central pivoting bar and tie-rod arrangement. These adaptations appear to have less breakage and reduce physiologic cost.[34] The hybrid RGO, or RGO II, is a combination of the RGO and functional electrical stimulation

(FES) that is designed to reduce the stress on the upper extremities and reduce energy expenditure.[35] Surface electrodes or electrodes incorporated into the plastic cuff stimulate hip and knee muscles to enhance ambulation. The hybrid RGO design is still experimental and currently the cost prohibits wide-spread use.

Orthosis-Wearing Schedule

Adjustment to wearing an orthosis is psychologic as well as physical, especially for children. The level of assistance that may be needed to apply and remove the orthosis, especially if the orthosis must be removed for toileting, needs to be considered. Time to apply and remove the orthosis needs to be factored into the wearing schedule. A client who wears a new orthosis may adopt the following schedule:

Days 1 and 2	Wear the orthosis for approximately 30–60 minutes per day. This time may best be broken up into AM and PM times. After applying the orthosis, check fit, making sure there is no pinching and that straps and locks work correctly. Allow some standing or ambulation as tolerated. When the orthosis is removed, check for redness, irritations, breakdown, or blistering of the skin. Any redness or irritation should disappear 15–20 minutes after removing the orthosis. If redness persists or blistering or skin breakdown develops, stop wearing the orthosis immediately until it can be rechecked by the therapist or orthotist.
Days 3 and 4	Increase AM and PM wearing time to approximately 1 hour each, or 2 hours total, per day. Check skin. Standing and walking should be done as tolerated.
Days 5–10	Increase AM and PM wearing time to approximately 2 hours each, or

4 hours total, per day. Check skin. Standing and walking should be done as tolerated.

Days 11–14   Apply the orthosis first thing in AM, remove, and check the skin before lunch. The orthosis can be put on again and checked after school or at dinner time. It may be applied a third time and worn until bedtime. Standing and walking should be done as tolerated throughout the day.

After Day 14   If no problems exist up to this point, the orthosis can be worn on a full-time basis as tolerated. The fit of the orthosis and skin should be checked at least once a day.[36] Standing and walking should be done as tolerated.

Skin and Orthosis Care

Clients wearing orthoses should be told to notify the orthotist or other health-care provider if any of the following problems are noticed:

- The orthosis rubs, causing skin discoloration that does not disappear in 15–20 minutes
- After removal of the orthosis, blistering or skin breakdown is evident
- The orthosis is cracked, broken, loose, or missing parts
- The orthosis is uncomfortably tight
- Excessive swelling develops within or around the trim lines of the orthosis
- Pain becomes a symptom or there is a change in character and intensity of pain
- The toes become discolored or difficult to move
- Odor or exudate develops from preexisting sores under the orthosis

Caring for the orthosis is a simple procedure. The orthosis should be cleaned regularly, using a cloth with mild soap and water. The orthosis should not be soaked in water, dried with a blow dryer, or placed near a heater. Heat may cause the orthosis to become misshapen. The orthosis should be towel dried or left at room temperature. A little talcum powder will help prevent odors.

There are two options for applying the plastic orthosis:
1. The orthosis is applied first, then the foot is slid into the footwear (shoe or sneakers), preferably with a shoehorn.
2. The orthosis is slid into the footwear first and then the foot is slid in, using the orthosis as a shoehorn.

Socks or stockings should be worn under the orthosis to reduce friction and protect the skin from perspiration. Socks composed of natural fibers such as cotton are best because they allow better air circulation and perspiration absorption. Seams of the sock should be kept away from bony areas such as dorsal toe surfaces, and socks should be smooth as possible against the skin. Any wrinkle or fold in the sock can create an area of irritation or increased pressure. Separate thigh socks can be worn for KAFOs or cotton tights for HKAFOs. Footwear with lace or Velcro closure allow a snug but not tight fit. Sandals, high heels, loafers, or other slip-on shoes should generally not be worn with the orthosis. Most sneakers have removable inserts and a wide last, which work well with orthoses. Extra-depth shoes are a good alternative when a dressier shoe is desired. The same heel height should be maintained when changing shoes. Changing to a different heel size may alter the GRF line and thus change the functions of the orthosis or create knee instability or back pain.[36]

Examination (Checkout) of an Orthosis

The checkout determines whether the orthosis is suitable for the client. A checkout procedure serves as a systematic method of examining the orthosis and the wearer and determines whether accepted standards of orthosis fabrication and fit have been met and, if not, possible corrective actions. During the checkout procedure, the therapist should consider the following:

- Comfort and fit
- Stability
- Alignment
- Appearance
- Workmanship

Specific checkouts may be done as follows:

- The orthosis should be easily applied. In most instances the wearer should be able to apply the orthosis with no assistance. However, children and patients who need HKAFOs may need help, and a goal to apply and remove the orthosis independently can be established. To facilitate application, the use of elastic or Velcro may be necessary to secure the orthosis around the limb.
- The sole and heel of the shoe should be flat on the floor and the wearer should feel stable. If the wearer feels that he or she is being forced forward or backward, the shoe may not be in even contact with the floor or the setting of the anterior or posterior stops may be incorrect. In addition, the knee joint of the orthosis may cause instability if it is placed too far forward or if the stops do not permit extension to 0°.
- There should be minimal rocking between the orthosis and the shoe. If the insert does not fit the contour of the insole of the shoe, the insole could move and produce instability.
- The wearer should sit comfortably with the knee flexed approximately 105°. If the client feels any discomfort, the shape or tilt of the calf band or placement of the mechanical ankle joint may be the cause.
- The wearer's skin should be free from signs of irritation after the orthosis is removed. If reddening disappears within 10 minutes and the client has no complaint of pressure or discomfort, there is probably no cause for concern.
- The uprights or plastic shells of the orthosis should conform to the contours of the leg and thigh. This contouring provides uniform pressure, reduces unnecessary bulk, and improves the appearance of the orthosis.[37]

Gait Analysis of the Client with an Orthosis

The following common gait deviations may be caused by either the orthosis or the wearer. One must determine the origin of the problem so that appropriate changes to the orthosis can be made as necessary. Some gait deviations may be normal, such as lateral trunk bending when using an RGO to assist with unweighting for forward progression.

Orthosis	Gait Deviation	Orthosis Causes	Wearer Causes
FO, AFO, KAFO, HKAFO	Excessive medial or lateral foot contact	Transverse plane malalignment at foot and/or knee	Weak ankle invertors or evertors Pes or genu valgus or varus
AFO	Hip hiking Circumduction Vaulting	Inadequate plantarflexion stop or dorsiflexion assist	Weak hip abduction Abduction contracture Increased tone in knee extensors Weak dorsiflexors Instability, fear, or habit
AFO	Knee instability	Inadequate dorsiflexion stop	Weak quadriceps Knee flexion contracture
	Knee recurvatum	Inadequate plantarflexion stop Ankle set in too much plantarflexion Uncontrolled pes equinus	Lax knee ligaments

Orthosis	Gait Deviation	Orthosis Causes	Wearer Causes
AFO	Inadequate dorsiflexion control	Inadequate plantarflexion or dorsiflexion assist	Weak dorsiflexors Increased tone of ankle musculature
KAFO	Abducted gait	Medial upright too high or too tight	Abduction contracture
	Circumduction	A locked knee	Weak hip abductors and adductors Instability
	Lateral trunk bend	Short leg requiring shoe lift Medial upright too high	Hip pain Habit
KAFO	Knee instability	Inadequate knee lock	Weak quadriceps
KAFO	Anterior trunk bend	Inadequate knee control	Weak quadriceps Weak hamstrings Hip flexion contracture
HKAFO	Any of the above deviations	Causes as noted above	Weak trunk muscles Causes as noted above

Review of the Literature

The rest of this chapter describes the use of orthoses in the care of clients with one of four different medical conditions: cerebral palsy, spina bifida, spinal cord injury, and cerebral vascular accident.

Orthoses and the Child with Cerebral Palsy (CP)

This section describes impairments, functional limitations, disabilities, the role of orthoses, and outcomes associated with the child with CP.

Impairments, Functional Limitations, and Disabilities

CP is a symptom complex caused by a nonprogressive lesion of the developing brain with a resultant movement disorder that may change presentation as the individual grows and develops.[38] This movement disorder is traditionally classified by the number of limbs impaired—diplegia (both legs), hemiplegia (arm and leg on the same side of the body), and quadriple-

gia (both arms and legs)—and by symptoms of *spasticity* (muscles perceived as excessively stiff and taut), **dyskinesia** (intermittent muscular tension and involuntary, uncontrolled, and purposeless movement), and *ataxia* (instability of movement).[38] Any of the above manifestations can vary from mild or moderate to severe. CP has multiple causes resulting in cerebral lesions. However, the extent of the cerebral lesions does not always relate to the extent of the disability, functional limitation, or impairment.[4]

Individuals with CP demonstrate neuromuscular and musculoskeletal system impairments either primary to pathophysiology or secondary to consequences over time.[26] These impairments may include malalignments, contractures, deformities, insufficient force generation, abnormal muscle tone, abnormal tissue extensibility, exaggerated or hyperactive reflexes, poor selective control and regulation of activity in muscle groups, abnormal timing, and decreased ability to learn unique movements.[26] Functional limitations of the child with CP are often noted in mobility, balance, and delays in acquiring motor milestones. Disabilities can be manifest in the amount of time and assistance the child and adult need in completing basic life functions. This increased time and assistance may limit their ability to engage in life and social roles. The examination and intervention for the scope of impairments alone does not provide an accurate appraisal of the extent of functional limitations or disabilities in these children.

The Role of Orthoses

For children with CP, one traditional intervention has been wearing orthoses.[12,19,20,23,26,39-43] Suggested applications of orthoses for the individual with CP include

- Preventing malalignments and contractures or correcting deformity, such as supporting joint alignment and mechanics, providing variable range of motion as needed, and protecting weak muscles
- Improving function; for example, promoting or facilitating training of skills via the opportunity to change positions (increased stability); providing appropriate biomechanical alignment for practice of a skill, especially gait; and providing a stable base of support for standing.[12,19-21,23,39,41,43]

To use an orthosis effectively, one must determine which of the above applications are being addressed and how the intervention may be affecting the child's development. At times, the function of an orthosis may interfere with the functional development of the child. For example, an AFO with the ankle set at 90° of dorsiflexion to control equinus in walking and maintenance of gastroc-soleus muscle extensibility may interfere with movement needed to come to standing from sitting in a chair.

Most children with CP who wear orthoses use an AFO. An SMO or FO may also be used. The HKAFO and KAFO are almost never used for the child with CP because of their weight and the effort needed to control balance and move about.[42] Most of the literature is dedicated to the various types of AFO and is reviewed on the basis of the expected outcomes identified.

Most of the children who serve as subjects in these studies have mild or moderate, spastic, diplegic or hemiplegic classifications and are ambulatory with or without an assistive device.

Outcomes: Prevention and Correction of Impairments

A primary outcome for intervention with children with CP is to prevent the impairments of malalignments, contractures, and deformities. One means of prevention is to respond to the consequences of abnormally high muscle tone, abnormal muscle extensibility, insufficient force production, and overactivity of muscles in children with CP. One consequence of these combined factors is increased muscle stiffness and reduced muscle lengthening. Prevention of malalignment, contracture, and deformity is aimed at the impairments of increased muscle stiffness and reduced muscle lengthening, both of which lead to shortened soft tissue (lessening range of motion) with limited ability to adapt movements.

Secondary deformities of the musculoskeletal system can be produced through the limited tissue adaptation coupled with a disproportionate bone-to-muscle growth and alterations in the direction and strength of muscle pull.[19] Secondary deformities need to be prevented because they may lead to functional limitations and disability. Common primary malalignments that can lead to fixed deformities of the lower extremities of children with spastic CP include internal rotation and adduction of the hips, genu valgus, hyperextension of the knees, equinus, and pronation of the foot.[20,22,26,44,45] Common deformities are hip flexion and adduction contractures, knee flexion, and ankle plantarflexion contractures. An orthosis that applies low pressure over time may alter the degree of deformity.[18]

Prevention of Impairments

There is scant research related to primary prevention of impairment in children with CP. Three group studies used repeated measures of passive range of motion of the ankle, hip, and knee to assess the usefulness of an AFO in preventing development of contracture and deformity.[46–48] In two studies, 41 children (1 to 7 years old) were the subjects. They were diagnosed with spastic hemiplegia or diplegia, were independent ambulators, and wore FAFOs or AAFOs. In the third study, 1200 circumferential FAFOs were prescribed and worn by children with CP from ages 3 to individual bony maturity. The evidence suggests that wearing any well-fitted AFO designed to maintain neutral or better ankle dorsiflexion affords some control toward preventing static equinus, especially for children with spastic hemiplegia or diplegia who begin wear at an early age. Prevention of static equinus may limit the need for surgery. One restriction to this recommendation is that the initial limitation at the ankle must be due to muscle imbalance, such as overactivity of certain muscles and insufficient force production, and not disproportionate muscle-to-bone growth.[49,50] Determining cause requires careful examination and evaluation of impairments. There is little or no evidence indicating that an AFO prevents knee and hip deformities.

Guidelines for AFO use are presented in Practical Application Box 16-5.

Correction of Impairments

Correction and prevention of the impairments of malalignments and deformities occur concurrently. Initially, the consequence of overactive or underactive muscles, insufficient force production, abnormal extensibility, and abnormal muscle tone may result in passively correctable postural malalignments or deformities. How these factors contribute to the development of dynamic deformity must be briefly considered.

Overactivity of spastic muscles, often described as *hypertonicity,* may limit the function or activity in antagonistic muscle groups. This limitation may be due to the biomechanical disadvantage of the antagonist that is placed in

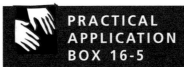

PRACTICAL APPLICATION BOX 16-5

Guidelines for AFO Use

For maximal effect in maintaining range of ankle motion, an AFO should have at least a 90° angle at the ankle. It should be worn throughout the child's growth years. It should be worn for an average of 6–7 hours of stretching per day, either day or night hours.[50] If surgery is performed, use of an AFO is recommended as a follow-up during either day or night hours to help prevent recurrence of contracture and deformity.[22] The AFO must be checked on a regular schedule for appropriate fit, otherwise its usefulness is diminished.

an overlengthened position. For example, the overactivity of the gastroc-soleus group holding the foot in equinus limits the activity of the anterior tibialis. Underactivity of muscles, often described as *hypotonicity,* may limit the function or activity in the agonist, antagonist, or both. These limitations may also be due to the biomechanical disadvantage (overlengthened or shortened range) based, for example, on the effects of gravity and consistently low electromyographic activity in affected muscle groups.[26]

When agonistic and antagonistic muscle groups do not act in concert, an imbalance of muscle power may result. This imbalance of muscle power can set the stage for developing joint hypomobility or hypermobility and malalignment. For example, a response to limited force production (e.g., weakness of the quadriceps) may be to hyperextend the knee to maintain upright posture, which keeps the line of gravity in front of the knee joint. The cycle of hyperextension of the knee, malalignment of the joint, and further distortion of alignment continues to affect force production.

This imbalance of power may also influence how sensory input to and from muscles is modulated, interpreted, and used for development and correction of movement. Inadequate sensory input (e.g., too much input to one set of muscles and too little to another) may enhance the retention of primitive patterns of movement (including dominating primitive reflexes such as plantar grasp), stimulate the development of malalignment (e.g., overactivity of the gastroc-soleus muscles pulling the foot and ankle into equinus), and influence the selection of muscle activity (e.g., contracting the plantar flexors rather than dorsiflexors at initial contact in gait).[20,41]

An orthosis may address these limitations. For example, wearing an orthosis, especially one with a contoured footplate, may provide constant pressure and protection to the sole of the foot, thus helping to decrease the sensory input that boosts overactivity. An orthosis may also affect the level of muscle activity by altering biomechanical alignment and forces. For example, fixing the foot in slight dorsiflexion limits the plantarflexion response that can occur at initial contact in gait. Attention to structural alignment should promote improved balance of muscle activity. Specifically, it should promote improved balance of muscle power. If muscle power is balanced, overactivity of certain muscle groups may be avoided, which should reduce the need to seek stability via compensatory balancing mechanisms. For example, the lower extremities may no longer internally rotate and adduct in an effort to seek stability. Increased internal rotation and adduction of the lower extremities in an effort to seek stability further limits reciprocal movement in gait. If muscle activity is balanced, the performance of certain underactive muscle groups may also be enhanced. For example, the knee may no longer need to hyperextend to maintain upright in response to quadriceps weakness. In addition, an orthosis can be designed to provide constant pressure and pro-

tection to the sole of the foot, which may help control the sensory input that boosts overactivity.

Consideration of these factors has influenced the design elements of orthoses: location of trim lines, addition of joints, and contours of footplates. Based on the concepts of structural alignment and the influence of sensory input on muscle activity, the contoured footplate for molding of a plaster cast has been developed. The footplate is designed to improve alignment and reduce sensory input to reflex areas of the foot. Depressions are made under the metatarsal heads and in the center of the distal end of the footplate to hold the calcaneus in place. A buildup of plaster is provided to support extension of the toes, the cuboid notch, medial and sometimes lateral longitudinal arch, and the calcaneus. Additionally, the first or fifth metatarsal head is supported as necessary. This design allows appropriate sensation of weight distribution of the foot and is the hallmark of the DAFO.[20]

The literature relating to the correction of deformity contains two distinct, but overlapping, factors:

1. The impact of orthoses on maintaining or altering alignment
2. The impact of orthoses on the distribution of the balance of muscle tone

Nine recent studies (seven group and two single-subject studies that compare multiple conditions of orthosis wear) address the influence of an AFO or SMO on alignment and function in gait.[52-60] The common, multiple variables of measurement used in these studies include gait analysis and force vector analysis. In the nine studies, a total of 130 children with the following characteristics were the subjects: age range (2.5 to 20 years old), diagnosis (spastic, hemiplegic or diplegic), functional status (independent ambulators with or without assistive devices), and range of motion (at least neutral passive dorsiflexion and no fixed ankle contractures). The results from these studies for each joint—ankle, knee, and hip and pelvis—are reviewed below, with suggestions for application.

Alignment

One major conclusion to be drawn from research studies on the effect of orthoses on alignment is that an AFO can influence alignment in children (2–20 years of age) with CP, with each joint affected differently.[52–60] The impact on malalignment is seen only while the orthosis is worn. The outcome of the AFO is most often control of malalignment or dynamic deformity rather than its correction. Correction of static deformity is not reported.

Ankle Alignment

The results of these studies support the use of any AFO (FAFO, AAFO, DAFO, or PLS) that limits plantarflexion (set at least at 90° of dorsiflexion) because it controls or prevents dynamic equinus better than no orthosis use during gait analysis.[52–60] The AFO must limit plantarflexion (set at least at 90° of dorsiflexion) to be effective. The implications of these results are tempered, however, because none of the orthosis styles significantly affect plantarflexion power generation at preswing[53,55,57] or appear to affect timing of ankle musculature activity in gait.[52,56] Burtner, Woolcott, and Qualls also found that neither a spiral DAFO nor a FAFO assisted in better organization of muscle recruitment during attempts to maintain upright balance by four children with spastic diplegic CP (3.6–15 years of age) who were independent ambulators and had no fixed contractures or past surgeries.[61] The spiral DAFO supports the foot while allowing dynamic activity at the ankle. However, from a functional viewpoint, when balance was challenged via a moveable platform, the spiral DAFO increased the probability of using an ankle strategy, improved upright posture (more knee extension), and increased the frequency of remaining in standing, compared with no AFO or FAFO use.[61]

Wilson et al. also evaluated a functional task to determine the role of orthosis type on control of equinus and task performance. Sit-to-stand behavior was compared in 15 children with spastic diplegia (2–5 years of age) while wearing an AAFO or an FAFO or going barefoot.[62] The children were able to sit on a bench unsupported, stand from the bench independently with or without use of a pole, had less than 20° of hip flexion contracture, and had 5° or more of passive dorsiflexion with dynamic equinus during weight bearing. The children fell into two groups. The first group could not actively control dynamic equinus and performed more slowly than typically developing children. However, they did significantly better (improved speed in achieving stable standing) when wearing AAFOs. The second group could actively control dynamic equinus and performed more like their typically developing peers. They slowed significantly in their task behavior when wearing either the AAFO or FAFO. The authors concluded that dynamic equinus interferes with the sit-to-stand task, but if the child can control the equinus, an orthosis is not needed to master this task. If the child needed help in controlling equinus, an AAFO aided the ability to come to stand. This finding was also supported by Baker et al., who noted that while wearing a FAFO, children 3–8 years of age with spastic CP were significantly better in forward trunk lean in the sit-to-stand task than they were while wearing AAFOs or shoes.[63] In conclusion, even though an AFO can help to control equinus, before a final prescription is written, one must consider the effect on ankle function for multiple tasks and the child's own ability to control the equinus.

Knee Alignment

Based upon the results from most of the studies, wearing an AFO has little or no effect on knee alignment[52–57] or timing of knee musculature activity[56] during gait in children with CP. There are three notable exceptions, however. Two studies concern the effect of the AFO on genu recurvatum,[59,64] and the third considers the effect of an SMO in controlling excessive knee flexion.[60] Butler, Thompson, and Major found that children with genu recurvatum could learn to reduce the knee-extending moment in gait and control hyperextension through the use of an FAFO coupled with physical therapy aimed at gaining control of the knee in static and dynamic balance.[59] Rosenthal et al. also found that an FAFO set in 5° of dorsiflexion, limiting knee extension, helped 12 ambulatory children (2–11 years of age) with spastic CP control genu recurvatum.[64] The genu recurvatum was attributed to knee flexor weakness secondary to overlengthening of the hamstrings, ankle plantarflexor weakness secondary to overlengthening, and hypertonicity of the lower extremities. There was an immediate 5° to 20° reduction of the genu recurvatum in all children. Over time (follow-up to 26 months), one child completely corrected 10° of recurvatum, eliminating the need for the orthosis. Three other children showed a tendency toward permanent correction at the second measurement. In summary, an orthosis set in at least 5° of dorsiflexion aids in control and possible correction of hyperextension of the knee during gait. The other exception to change in knee alignment involved one child who received neurodevelopmental treatment coupled with the use of an SMO to stabilize the foot. This child learned to control excessive knee flexion in gait.[60]

Even though the literature shows little or no effect of AFO use on knee alignment or timing of knee musculature activity, no studies were found that included the use of the FRO designed specifically to assist knee alignment. In conclusion, since an AFO has little effect on knee alignment, it may need to be addressed through other interventions such as strengthening and training in task. The reader is encouraged to review the literature related to strength training in children with CP.[65]

Hip and Pelvis Alignment

The results of these studies are conflicting about the effect of AFOs on hip and pelvic alignment. Two studies found no differences in hip and pelvic alignment, and one study found no effect on timing of hip musculature activity.[55,56] However, four studies noted hip and pelvic alignment changes. Through the use of an FAFO, Abel et al.[53] found increased hip and pelvic excursion, Butler et al.[59] noted reduced hyperflexion of the hip and compensatory lordosis used to hyperextend the knee, and Brunner, Meier, and Ruepp[54] reported increased abduction and symmetry of the hips. Brunner et al.[54] also noted that wearing the spring-type orthosis increased pelvic tilt appropriately. Carmick's[58] single-case photographs showed an immediate reduction of internal rotation of the hip when the child wore an AAFO rather than the FAFO.

In summary, a review of literature

- Supports the use of an AFO (fixed, articulated, dynamic, or spiral) to control the dynamic deformity of equinus. The final choice may be dictated by the additional active movement that the child needs to perform and the amount of support needed if other malalignment of the foot exists.
- Demonstrates the reduction of dynamic genu recurvatum through the use of a FAFO or a AAFO (with a plantarflexion stop) set in slight dorsiflexion.
- Demonstrates significant improvement in upright posture and the availability of an ankle strategy in static standing when wearing a spiral DAFO.
- Suggests improvement in symmetry and excursion of motion of the hip and pelvis through the use of an FAFO, AAFO, and spiral AFO, compared with no orthosis use.

Abnormal Muscle Tone

Control of malalignment at the foot and ankle does not appear to be due to changes in bony alignment, at least in the short term. Ricks and Eilert examined 27 children (2–16 years of age) with hyperreflexia and dynamic foot and ankle deformities (ankle plantarflexion, calcaneal valgus, forefoot pronation, and toe clawing).[66] All of the children had a diagnosis of either CP ($n = 20$) or head injury ($n = 7$).

Twenty children could ambulate independently with or without an assistive device, and the remaining seven could stand independently. Each child received two standing lateral x-rays while in and out of a FAFO, an AAFO or inhibitory casts. Each device was constructed when the foot was in 90° of dorsiflexion, subtalar joint and midtarsal joints neutral, and slight extension of the phalanges. The devices were worn from 1 to 3 weeks, with the casts worn 24 hours a day. With the exception of a significant difference in the calcaneal inclination while wearing the AAFO, x-rays showed no significant difference in the bony alignment of the foot and ankle during weight bearing among the three groups. The authors suggested that this study was limited because it did not include either immediate changes at initial fitting, changes over an extended period of time, or dynamic changes. They concluded that the effectiveness of orthoses to control and prevent deformity may not be due to the pressure concentration over certain bones but to the effect on distribution of muscle tone.

The basis for making tone-reducing orthoses, as noted above, was inhibitive casting with the distinctive footplate. Initial research in this area centered upon the effect of tone-reducing or inhibitive casts. Effectiveness of either casts or orthoses has been measured directly through the use of the Ashworth Scale and torque or indirectly through clinical observations.[3] The changes in clinical observations were assumed to be due to changes in tone. There are problems with these methods of measurement for tone because of the variability and confusion in the definition of tone. The Ashworth Scale and torque seek to measure spasticity or velocity-dependent hyperreflexia. The clinical observations include such activity as decreased toe clawing or increased time in unassisted static standing. Seven recent studies considered the effect of inhibitive casting or inhibitive orthoses on measures of tone.[67–73] Seventy-five children (age range, 18 months to 6.3 years) were subjects of these studies. Most

of these children, diagnosed with spastic diplegia, hemiplegia, or quadriplegia, were ambulatory with and without assistive devices. They wore inhibitive walking casts or FAFOs (set at least at neutral dorsiflexion). There were some reported changes in resistance to passive stretch (Ashworth scale measure), manifestation of primitive reflexive patterns (decreased toe clawing), and balance posture (increased time in static stand). These changes may be due to the lengthenings and adaptations of the muscle units rather than changes in the neurologic excitability of muscles.[26] Despite the suggestion that the effectiveness of orthoses in controlling and preventing deformity may be due to the effect on muscle tone, the direct evidence for any specific tone-reducing or tone-inhibiting effect of orthoses is inconclusive.[19] A more promising intervention to affect hyperreflexia may be the use of botulinus toxin, and the reader is encouraged to review this literature.[70]

Motor Function

Functional improvement can be judged in many ways. Usually in children with CP functional improvement means the acquisition of biomechanical alignment and retention of gait. Improvement may also mean that upright skills such as standing and sit-to-stand are acquired. Achievement of gait and upright skill acquisition are reviewed below through the research on functional outcomes and the effect of orthoses.

Gait

Gait is affected significantly by CP and is the functional outcome most often studied in relation to the intervention of orthoses. Gaits of children with CP differ from those of age-matched, typically developing peers.[74] For example, children with CP on average have the following significant differences from their peers:

- Later first-walking age
- Shorter stride lengths

- Longer time in double support; shorter time in single support
- Greater (1.5 to 3 times) energy demands for walking[74,75]
- Slower walking speeds that become increasingly slower with age[76]

Gage advocates eliminating impairments to improve the function of gait: specifically, reducing hyperreflexia, restoring stance-phase hip and knee stability (malalignment correction), and eliminating foot drag (correction of dynamic equinus deformity).[75]

The studies cited above report the results of orthosis use on the temporal–distance parameters of gait in children with CP.[52-60] Most of the gait improvements seen in the kinematic parameters did not translate into changes in temporal-distance parameters. In six group studies that used self-selected walking speed, velocity did not change significantly among conditions that included comparison of FAFOs, AAFOs, DAFOs, PLSs, shoes, and bare feet, with one exception.[52-57,59] The only significant increase in speed occurred with the spring-type AFO.[54] Cadence decreased[54,56] or remained the same[52,53] as long as an AFO was worn. Cadence was significantly better than that in bare feet. Stride length was generally significantly better while wearing any AFO than when wearing shoes or with bare feet, most often with a concurrent velocity increase or cadence decrease.[53,54,56] Double-support time was usually significantly better when wearing any AFO than when wearing shoes.[52,54]

Two conclusions may be drawn from these studies. First, reduction in impairments does not automatically lead to changes in function such as gait. Secondly, the final orthosis prescription must take into account all expected outcomes, weighing the importance of each outcome (e.g., need for speed vs. the increased stability of double-support time) as well as the individual's biomechanical limitations and needs. Orthoses do establish a better weight-bearing surface during stance, especially com-

pared with bare feet. Speed may be significantly enhanced through the use of a spring-type AFO, but use of the spring-type AFO may be limited if equinus is difficult to control. These studies lack the effect on function in environments other than the gait-analysis laboratory and the possible long-term effects on physiologic (e.g., cardiac) and psychologic (e.g., feeling of comfort and safety) function.

Functional Tests

Like the findings related to change in the functional aspects of gait, the following studies generally do not support the effectiveness of orthoses on various measures of function. Evans et al. compared scores on the standardized functional tests (Gross Motor Function Measure and Gross Motor Performance Measure) for 34 children (age range, 3–16 years) with severe to mild CP (spastic, ataxic, and dyskinesia). Seventeen children received weekly physical therapy and wore orthoses and 17 received weekly therapy only.[77] The children were tested before and after 4 months of intervention. No significant difference in status between the two groups was found. Held and Kott, in a preliminary study of 19 children (age range, 4–19 years) diagnosed with mild-to-moderate CP (ataxic, spastic, and dyskinetic) and independent ambulators without assistive devices, using standardized measures of function (examining time to complete tasks, loss of balance while moving around and carrying objects, standing, stooping, reaching, and turning within a set environment), found no significant difference in performances with and without orthoses.[78] Two case reports offer mixed results regarding the effect on balance when children used FAFOs.[72,73] One child demonstrated increased duration of static independent standing and ease of maintaining and regaining balance when wearing orthoses. The second child had no change in standing balance time, but shoulders were not elevated, abducted, and externally rotated when orthoses were worn. Finally, Mossberg, Linton, and Friske studied 18 children (3–14 years of age) with spastic diplegia CP who were independent ambulators. They found that 72% of the children (13 of 18) expended significantly less energy ambulating at a self-selected walking speed while wearing orthoses than when wearing no orthoses.[79] Mossberg et al. note, however, that because of individual differences, the decision about wearing an orthosis should be made on a case-by-case basis.[79]

In summary, a review of literature

- Offers mixed results on the impact of orthoses on the child's performance of temporal parameters of gait and other functional skills, especially for children with mild-to-moderate CP
- Demonstrates that an AFO will control ankle and foot positions and genu recurvatum that are dynamic and not fixed, thus improving the kinetics of gait
- Lacks evidence for a long-term effect of orthoses as a variable that affords the best biomechanical environment for motor learning in children with CP[59]
- Reveals an interesting psychologic effect when performing functional skills, a reported feeling of increased security and comfort while wearing orthoses;[78] the impact of this effect upon retention of long-term functional gait needs further exploration
- Suggests that there is no one right orthosis for all children with CP

Therefore, an orthosis as an adjunct intervention, must be prescribed on an individual basis after consideration of the examination findings and expected outcomes.

Orthoses for the Child with Myelodysplasia

This section describes the impairments, functional limitations, and disabilities associated with the disorder myelodysplasia. The role of orthoses and expected outcomes, based upon current literature, are also included.

Impairments, Functional Limitations, and Disabilities

Myelodysplasia is defined as a developmental defect of any part of the spinal cord. *Spina bifida* is the commonly used term to refer to the various forms of myelodysplasia. This defect occurs in utero with varying degrees of severity. These defects cause spinal cord lesions that are open or hidden, with the degree of motor and sensory loss ranging from none to severe impairment.[80] At birth, when the lesion is open, an external sac is present on the infant's back. In the worst case, this sac contains meninges, cerebrospinal fluid, and the spinal cord (a meningomyelocele, or MM), which interrupts the functioning of the motor and sensory connections at the level of the lesion. Because of these deficits in motor and sensory functions, individuals with MM exhibit paralysis from the level of the lesion down. Commonly, these lesions are located in the lumbar region, but they may be at any level of the spinal cord.

The major impairment of muscle paralysis can be the direct cause or a contributor to the musculoskeletal deformities seen in individuals with MM, such as joint contracture, asymmetric alignment, and postural deviations. Lack of muscle control and the presence or progression of deformities can affect positioning, weight bearing, and energy expenditure. Postural deformities, which vary by level of the lesion, typically include (a) hip and knee flexion contractures and (b) knee, ankle, and foot deformities. Hip and knee contractures are usually severe to moderate in children with high-level (thoracic to L2) and mid- to low lumbar (L3–L5) lesions but are generally mild in children with sacral level lesions. Plantarflexion contractures are frequently seen in children with high-level lesions. Children with mid- to low lumbar lesions may have genu and calcaneal valgus malalignment with pronated feet when weight bearing. Children with sacral level lesions can have either ankle and/or foot varus or valgus deformities combined with forefoot pronation or supination.[80,81]

Myelodysplasia, a developmental disorder, can have far-reaching effects on total development. The musculoskeletal deformities, motor and sensory deficits, and additional concerns related to hydrocephalus and cognitive dysfunction affect the functional limitations of balance and mobility noted throughout life. The extent of all the impairments associated with MM is beyond the scope of this text; the reader is encouraged to review pediatric physical therapy texts for further information.[80,81] Disability in social roles can be related to lack of independent mobility, limitations with activities of daily living such as personal hygiene, play and recreation, and prolonged periods of bed rest related to secondary complications.[81]

The Role of Orthoses

For children with MM, the need for orthoses is clearly defined. The major objective of a lower-extremity orthosis is to compensate for lack of muscle control by supporting joint alignment and mechanics. The purposes of supporting joint alignment and mechanics are to

- Prevent deformities[12,80,81]
- Facilitate function[12,80,81]
- Help decrease or prevent pain (especially of the knee in mid- to low lumbar and sacral level lesions)[82–86]

General guidelines for use of orthoses for children with MM include[12,80,81]

- Positioning and early support for all infants to help maintain adequate extension of the hip and knee and plantigrade position of the ankle for later weight bearing
- Stabilizing the trunk and pelvis while achieving lower-extremity alignment (use of a thoracolumbar orthosis as needed)
- Holding a limb in a corrected position after surgery
- Supporting an upright posture in preambulatory individuals

- Using the level of the lesion as the initial guide for choosing an orthosis for the individual who is ambulatory or is being taught to ambulate. Remember that all aspects of physical examination, including sensation, active movement, malalignment, cognitive status, respiratory status, and expected outcomes must be considered to choose the correct orthosis.

The following are orthosis types and suggested uses related to level of the lesion[12,80,81]

- An HKAFO with thoracic support, such as the Parapodium, standing shell, or swivel walker, is suggested for initial practice with upright positioning and learning to walk by children with higher-level lesions (thoracic and high to midlumbar (L3)). It may also be used for children with lower-level lesions (L4–L5) with decreased trunk control who need more extensive support to begin to stand. This type of orthosis would be prescribed about the time a typically aged peer would pull to stand. It may also be used for children with higher-level lesions when walking is an exercise and progression to household or community ambulation is not an expected outcome.
- An HKAFO, such as the RGO, is suggested for children who are younger (approximately 2–10 years) and lighter weight with thoracic, high and midlumbar lesions (L1–L3), to improve ambulation ability.
- An HKAFO with hip-guidance system is suggested for older (approximately 7 years and up) children with high to midlumbar lesions (L1–L3), to offer increased stability in standing.
- A KAFO is suggested for children with mid- to low lumbar lesions (L3–L4) to support weak knee musculature and provide medial and lateral stability of the knee in gait.
- An AFO or GRAFO is suggested for children with low lumbar–high sacral lesions (L4–S1) to support weak or absent ankle musculature, help toe clearance, provide

medial and lateral stability for the knee or ankle, and/or assist inadequate knee extensors.

- An SMO or FO is suggested for children with sacral-level lesions with no loss of motor function i.e., normal strength of all lower limb muscle groups with a grade of 4 in one or two groups and no loss of bowel or bladder function. The SMO or FO may assist with weight distribution in the foot and alignment of the subtalar joint and/or provide medial and lateral stability as needed.

Key features of these orthoses include

- Achievement of mediolateral stability through the use of subtalar-neutral trim lines and posting[80]
- Correction of flexible deformities of the feet, such as valgus or varus or accommodating the fixed foot with posting to achieve a plantigrade foot[21]
- Correction of knee extension moment with a rigid dorsiflexion stop set in 5° of plantarflexion; if there is a foot-clearance problem, the ankle can be set at less than 5°, but no more than neutral[87]
- Decreased energy expenditure with use[12,80]

Motor Function

Research on the use of specific orthoses by children or adults with MM is limited. Much of the research focuses upon orthosis use and long-term retention of ambulation, especially for individuals with higher-level lesions.[82,83,88–93] Ambulation is viewed as the highest level of independent mobility, with assumed benefits from upright posture; therefore, it is given a high priority during periods of intervention. Descriptive studies from the 1970s through the present day indicate that many individuals, especially those with high-thoracic and upper-lumbar lesions, may abandon walking for the wheelchair or deteriorate in their ability to walk as they move from childhood into adolescence.[12,82,89–92,94–96] Cur-

rent literature also reports that the gait of individuals with sacral-level lesions tends to deteriorate over time. These individuals report activity-related knee pain, feelings of increased instability, development of knee deformities, increased use of an orthosis, and a possible change of ambulation status from community to household ambulator.[82–86] Since better orthosis design was suggested as a possible solution to the loss of ambulation function, much of the research is related to developing an orthosis that is effective; comfortable; light weight; durable; easy to maintain, apply, and remove; adjustable for growth; and not a prohibition to any activities of daily living.[97] Outcomes to consider, besides ambulatory status, may be the benefits of upright posture and ambulation during the growing years and the reasons for deterioration of ambulatory function. These outcomes are reviewed as follows.

Wheelchair Use Compared with Walking

Despite the benefits of upright posture and ambulation, there remains a question about the long-term benefits versus the cost in time, energy, and finances of stressing ambulation in the young child with high-level lesions. This question is especially important in light of multiple studies that point to loss of ambulation skills in adolescents. One major study compares the benefits of early ambulation with early and continuous wheelchair use in individuals with high-level lesions.[96] This study was possible because of philosophical differences in two major centers regarding wheelchair versus walking for mobility. Thirty-six matched clients in each center were compared. The results considered the functional benefits derived from early walking. The children who walked early had better transfer skills. These transfer skills were retained even if ambulation was not the major form of mobility. The children who walked early and the children who did not walk had equal skill levels in activities of daily living. It was mistakenly hypothesized that activities of daily living would be compromised because too much time was spent learning to walk. The children who walked from an early age also had major physiologic benefits. The physiologic benefits of walking are discussed below.

In a single-subject design study over 15 days, three children (9, 10, and 15 years of age, with lumbar-level lesions) were compared by a physiologic cost index in wheelchair use and walking while in school. These authors found that the energy consumption for walking was significantly higher than that for wheelchair use and immediately after ambulating throughout the school, all the children had significantly lower visual–motor accuracy during fine motor tasks.[98]

Use of the RGO was compared with use of a conventional HKAFO and wheelchair for speed and energy expenditure in eight children with thoracic to low-lumbar-level MM (4–19 years of age).[99] The children had significantly higher heart rates and oxygen consumption using the HKAFO (with a swing-through gait pattern) than with wheelchair use. The heart rate and oxygen consumption values associated with use of the RGO (reciprocal gait pattern) did not differ significantly from those with wheelchair use. These authors concluded that the RGO did not put a significant metabolic burden on the individual, compared with wheelchair use.

Gait

Research on gait has focused on the development of better orthoses that decrease the energy needed to ambulate.[97] Most of the studies concerning the use of HKAFOs (with or without thoracic support) for children with high and midlevel MM have measured energy expenditure and speed (velocity) as the key dependent variables. Even though Vo_2max is the most widely used criterion for measuring cardiorespiratory endurance, the use of heart rate and velocity has been demonstrated to be a reliable and valid means of determining energy

expenditure.[29,95] The following studies compare these variables progressing through the various HKAFO designs.

Lough and Nielsen compared heart rate and velocity in 10 children (4–9 years of age) with T7–L2 lesions, during walking when wearing the Parapodium and the swivel walker.[100] When walking in the swivel walker at self-selected and maximal walking speed, the children required significantly less energy and had a significantly lower metabolic cost than with the Parapodium. When walking in the Parapodium, the children had a significantly higher velocity because the mechanism of the swivel walker did not allow a significant difference in self-selected and maximal walking speeds. Overall, the average speed was significantly slower (5–10 times) than that of typically developing peers, but energy cost was approximately the same. The reason that the energy cost did not differ significantly from that of peers may be that individuals naturally select a walking speed that corresponds to their level of energy expenditure.

Rose, Stallard, and Sankarankutty studied 27 children (age range, 5.8–15.7 years) with low thoracic–high lumbar lesions. Each child replaced previous systems of mobility—for example, wheelchair (3 children), swivel walker (17 children), conventional HKAFO (5 children), and KAFO (2 children)—with an HGO.[101] The HGO was designed to allow reciprocal gait. The children's initial mode of ambulation (reciprocal, drag-to, and swing-through) and ambulation status (community: independent indoors and outdoors on all surfaces; household: independent mainly indoors and some outdoors if flat, smooth surfaces; and therapeutic: indoors under assistance or supervision or chair bound) were recorded. Heart rate and speed were measured while walking 20-foot lengths, first wearing the original orthosis and then wearing the HGO at follow-up (at least 6 months later). Fourteen children completed both sets of measures. Thirteen children improved their ambulation classification by at least one level, for example, moving from a household to community ambulator. Two children improved from standing only to therapeutic status. Significant mean changes in speed were found. The children's mode of ambulation was reciprocal, which all parents preferred. This study concluded that the HGO could improve ambulation status in children with thoracic to high-lumbar-level lesions. Despite these changes, most of these children walked more slowly than their peers and required more energy expenditure. Other limitations of this study included the need for assistive devices (crutches, rollator, walkers) when wearing the HGO if the child had previously used a swivel walker and the need for larger spaces to maneuver in the HGO. Most of the children had difficulty applying and removing the HGO independently. This was an activity that most of the children could do with the swivel walker or KAFO. Also, only 50% of the children returned for reevaluation, and after the trial period, two children reverted back to their use of swivel walkers.

The introduction of the RGO allowed new comparisons to be made to determine efficiency and effectiveness of different orthoses on gait, especially for children with higher-level lesions. Two studies compared the RGO with and without the mechanism functioning (simulating a conventional HKAFO), with hips locked and unlocked, in 58 children (age range, 1–15 years) with thoracic-to-high-lumbar- (70%) and low-lumber-to-sacral- (30%) level lesions[102,103] The children had lower pulse rates (approximately 15%) and higher velocities when the reciprocal mechanism was functioning. In both studies, the gait with the mechanism working was described as smooth, compared with the abrupt swing-through or short-stepped pivot patterns with the hips locked. When the hips were unlocked, three children could not ambulate at all. Most of the children preferred the reciprocal pattern. Of the 41 children in the second study, 78% achieved community or household ambulation

status. In addition, hip flexion contractures up to 30° and knee flexion contractures up to 20° did not negate use of the RGO, and shorter, lighter-weight children did best.[103]

Eight children (2.2–11.9 years) with thoracic- or high-lumbar-level lesions participated in a crossover study to compare the light-weight HKAFO with the RGO (isocentric mechanism).[104] Each child received, and was trained to use, the HKAFO first. Measures of heart rate, oxygen consumption, and self-selected velocity were taken after 3–46 months (average, 26 months) of use. After initial data collection, the RGO pelvic section was fitted to the existing KAFO segments and gait training occurred. The second data collection occurred 4–17 weeks (average, 7 weeks) after receiving the RGO. There was a significantly higher oxygen cost during ambulation in the HKAFO for the children with thoracic- level lesions. Overall, the metabolic cost of walking in the RGO was twice that of typically developing peers, and when walking in the HKAFO, it was six times that of typically developing peers. The velocity achieved during ambulation was greater in the RGO, especially for the children with thoracic-level lesions. For the children with lumbar-level lesions, the differences between the two orthoses were not significant. The authors concluded that for individuals with thoracic-level lesions, the RGO can provide a faster, more-energy efficient gait, especially if hip flexion contractures are less than 30°.

Gerritsma-Bleeker et al. found that the presence of hip flexion contracture (up to 20°) and knee flexion contractures (up to 30°) as well as scoliosis of 90° did not stop use of the RGO in 7 children with low-lumbar-level lesions. The authors also stated that extensive surgery to permit fitting of the orthosis to change outcome is not often justified.[93]

Recent data identify characteristics of the child that may influence prescription and use of the RGO or HGO. Phillips and colleagues reviewed 21 children (age range at first fitting, 1.5–9.5 years) with T10–L4 lesions.[105] After use of the RGO for a mean period of 2.6 years, 12 children continued to use the RGO, 7 children used an HGO, 1 child progressed to a KAFO, and 1 child died. The authors concluded the following:

- It is easier to teach initial ambulation in the RGO, especially to a lightweight, young child without spinal deformity.
- It is easier for children to use the RGO when they have good upper body strength and coordination.
- It is easier to provide more stability in upright posture with less effort and more feelings of security in a HGO.
- An HGO is preferred by older, larger children.
- Body shape (height, weight, girth) was more important in selecting orthoses than the level of the lesion.
- No active hip flexion is needed to ambulate with the RGO, so children with higher thoracic lesions should have a prescription for the RGO.

In summary, from the literature review

- To date, the RGO is the most energy-efficient orthosis for children with thoracic-level lesions; however, the energy and time costs should be weighed against the energy and time costs of wheelchair use.
- Children with thoracic-level lesions, even those with hip and knee flexion contractures of 30° or less, can be fitted and can learn to ambulate with an RGO.
- Children do best learning and maintaining the ability to ambulate in the RGO if they have good upper body strength and coordination.
- Children with a high lumbar lesion may learn the reciprocal motion of ambulation more easily in the RGO, but it may not offer the best speed or energy efficiency, compared with those of an HGO or lightweight HKAFO
- As children get heavier and taller, the HKAFO or HGO may offer more stability

and maintenance of standing and walking skills.
- Use of an HKAFO requires a greater metabolic burden than use of the wheelchair.

Lacking from these studies are the use of these orthoses in environments outside the laboratory settings. A final determination to use any of the orthoses for ambulation must also consider the monetary costs; the need for extensive time for training; the possibility for independent use, including independence in putting on and taking off the orthosis; and any additional benefits of use.

Physiologic Function

The suggested physiologic benefits of upright posture and ambulation for children with MM include improved circulation, kidney and bowel function, respiratory status, and bone mass and density (with a concurrent decrease in deformities and fractures), normal joint development and the prevention of weight gain and pressure sores. Few studies support these benefits in children with MM. Decreased bone density is often noted in nonambulatory children with disabilities.[106–108] Rosenstein et al. evaluated the bone density in ambulatory and nonambulatory individuals with MM.[109] The density in the tibia and metatarsals correlated more strongly with neurologic levels than with ambulatory status. They concluded that weight-bearing status and neurologic status (ability to contract muscles) were both important factors in maintaining bone density. Upright posture must be as close to vertical as possible for there to be increased weight bearing on the legs.[110,111]

In the study by Mazur and associates, physiologic measures, including the number of fractures, number of pressure sores, and frequency and severity of obesity, were compared in 72 children with high-level lesions.[96] Greater physiologic benefits were found for the 36 children who were ambulatory from an early age (even if they stopped walking in their teens). In particular, the children who had ambulated had significantly fewer fractures and pressure sores. However, there were no differences in obesity between the two groups.

In conclusion, there must be additional study of the physiologic effects of ambulation and upright posture to support an educated decision about orthosis use.

Psychologic Function

Few or no studies to date have compared the psychologic growth or current well-being of ambulators and nonambulators. Gerritsma-Bleeker et al. reported that children 2–9 years of age using the Parapodium and RGO enjoyed achieving upright position and an increased level of independence.[93] Katz et al. stated that subjects, 2–11 years old, preferred the variability in gait pattern that an RGO offers.[104]

Since psychologic well-being is important throughout life, there is a great need for research on interrelated and interdependent factors, especially as they may benefit physical well-being. These studies are missing from research related to the achievement and maintenance of movement through the use of orthoses.

Prevention of Impairments

As stated above, prevention of fractures was noted as a benefit of early ambulation, compared with wheelchair use, in individuals with higher-level lesions.[96] Prevention of pain in the individual with a sacral-level lesion may also be a goal of orthosis use. Despite the ability to ambulate, individuals with sacral-level lesions tend to have a gait that slows and becomes more unsteady over time. In addition, these individuals often report increased knee pain over time.[83–86] Research on the use of the solid AFO set in slight plantarflexion suggests that its use may reduce the activity of the quadriceps (particularly the rectus femoris), which is hypothesized to be a major cause of knee pain.[86] In contrast, however, Thomson et al. suggest that the solid AFO, while helping to reduce the quadriceps activity and excessive knee flexion

in stance, was most beneficial to individuals with L4–L5 lesions and detrimental to the knee in individuals with S1–S2 lesions. The solid AFO reduced the power-generating capabilities at the ankle and increased transverse-plane rotation on the knee.[85] Prevention is an area that needs further research.

In conclusion, the unique characteristics of individuals with congenital lesions of the spinal cord make it important to consider all factors when prescribing an orthosis system. Research has focused on compensation for the impairments of paralysis, stressing the functional limitation of ambulation. Researchers have primarily studied the impact of different orthosis types on energy expenditure in gait. While there seems to be some physiologic benefit from early upright standing and walking, little is known about psychologic limitations or benefits or the prevention of impairments in individuals with MM. Further research needs to determine the long-term effects of the efforts to ambulate in settings other than a laboratory and the effects of perceived disability and functional limitation other than ambulation.

Orthoses for Adults with Spinal Cord Injury

This section describes impairments, functional limitations, and disabilities associated with spinal cord injury in adults. It includes the role of orthoses and outcomes expected based upon current literature.

Impairments, Functional Limitations, and Disability

Spinal cord injuries (SCIs) may occur from many causes (e.g., gunshot wounds, stabbings, motor vehicle accidents, falls, vascular malfunction, and vertebral subluxations). The causes are different, and therefore, the severity, level, and extent of the lesion varies from patient to patient. The average client with SCI is male (4:1 ratio to females), between the ages of

16 and 30. The estimated incidence each year is approximately 10,000 new cases. In 1998, it was estimated that the number of individuals with SCI in the United States was between 183,000 and 203,000.[112]

Generally, there are two categories of SCI according to the American Spinal Cord Injury Association (ASIA) system:

- *Tetraplegia* is partial or complete paralysis of muscles of the trunk and all four extremities resulting from lesions in the cervical cord.
- *Paraplegia* is partial or complete paralysis of some or all of the muscles of the trunk and the lower extremities from lesion in the thoracic or lumbar spinal cord or sacral roots.[112]

The extent of complete or partial impairment is specified by the ASIA Impairment Scale and designated by the letters A, B, C, D, and E. The letter A designates complete loss of motor and sensory function including the sacral segments S4 to S5. The letters B, C, and D designate sacral sparing plus variations of sensory preservation and increasing motor function. The letter E designates normal motor and sensory function. The impairments of individuals with a spinal cord lesion are similar to those of children with MM; there is incomplete or complete loss of motor and or sensory function. The motor impairment is classified by the neurologic level. For example, an individual with an intact C7 nerve root segment (no sensory or motor function below C7 nerve root with no sacral sparing) would be classified as having a C7 complete tetraplegia. Functional use of muscles above the C7 level is assumed. Actions such as facial expression, breathing, elbow flexion, and wrist extension would be functioning. A major difference to consider between the individual with a congenital lesion and one with an acquired SCI is the assumption of intact systems and development to the time of injury. Individuals with SCI, unless they have other preexisting conditions, do not have initial bony deformity or malformations. Additional complications may develop from lack of movement and possible muscle imbalances, including the development of contractures, spasticity, deep venous thrombosis, osteoporosis, renal calculi, and physical deconditioning. Maintaining preexisting range of motion becomes a major area of preventive care for individuals with SCIs.

For most individuals and in the eyes of society, the inability to walk is considered a major disability.[34] However, lack of movement can create other functional limitations of mobility, self-care, respiration, and continence. In addition, the inability to carry on with expected life roles such as working, child rearing, and leisure activities may also be significant disabilities for individuals with SCI. The incidence of SCI may be relatively low compared with that of other disabilities, but it extracts a high cost in the limitation of independence and financial burdens placed on the individuals, their families, and society as well.

The Role of Orthoses

Since SCI involves a complete or partial loss of motor function below the level of the lesion, the primary purposes of orthoses are to

- Provide support and stability for upright activities such as standing or activities of daily living
- Prevent or correct deformities
- Assist with mobility and control[34]

Orthoses may play an additional role in prevention of some complications of loss of motor function. Historically and physiologically, individuals with SCI benefit from upright posture, weight bearing, and walking.[34] However, clinicians often differ in deciding which clients are suitable for orthoses and what factors need to be considered in making that decision. As with the child with MM, the level of the lesion helps predict which type of orthosis may be suggested initially for standing and ambulation. Examples include HKAFOs, KAFOs, and AFOs. Whether an individual with an SCI achieves functional ambulation is closely related to the level of the lesion but is also influenced by additional factors such as motivation, physical condition, and the presence of spasticity, decubitus ulcers, weight, spinal and limb deformities, renal function, coordination, cognition, and psychosocial support.[34] Taken together these factors may reduce the likelihood of achieving functional ambulation. The following evidence for orthosis use is reviewed in relation to standing, walking, and prevention outcomes.

Standing and Ambulation

Standing and ambulating have a high psychologic priority after an SCI and have long-term physiologic benefits for individuals with SCIs. To achieve these objectives, the goal of standing and ambulating is considered therapeutic and essential if the individual is to achieve any degree of functional ambulation.

The extent to which walking will be a practical method of mobility is difficult to predict.[113] For the patient with an SCI there is a direct relationship between muscle power, reciprocal gait, and walking ability. Most patients who do walk in the community must have at least grade 3 hip flexor strength, some pelvic control, and at least one knee with grade 3 extensor strength. These individuals can use a reciprocal pattern.[114] Changes in orthosis design (as in the RGO) help patients who cannot maintain knee and ankle stability and hip flexion to achieve a reciprocal pattern of gait. Despite progress in orthosis design, most individuals with complete spinal cord injury do not achieve functional ambulation.[115–117] However in the future, with the combination of orthoses and FES, it may be possible for all clients, despite the level of SCI, to walk functionally. The research in this area is reviewed below.

The typical individual with complete paraplegia (T10 and below) or an incomplete lesion can usually achieve functional ambulation with unilateral or bilateral KAFOs and AFOs. The gait pattern most often used when wearing bilateral KAFOs is crutch-assisted swing-through. This individual will have a greater chance at successful ambulation with bilateral KAFOs with grade 4 or better for muscles controlling the trunk, grade 3 or better for muscles controlling pelvic movement, adequate arm strength to lift and swing the body forward, and no cardiorespiratory comorbidity. While walking, patients who use bilateral KAFOs may need to consume oxygen at a rate 160% above normal.[114]

Clients with complete lesions above T10 have traditionally not been considered appropriate for ambulation training and have often not been fitted with an orthosis. Wheelchair mobility is often emphasized in therapy for these individuals. This has been especially true in light of the high energy cost of ambulation.[114] However, newer evidence of recovery from SCI suggests that facilitation of weight bearing and locomotion through partial-body-support gait training may have benefits in inducing neuroplasticity and motor recovery—a more proactive approach than conventional compensatory strategies.[118] The following studies consider the merits of using HKAFO systems such as the Parawalker or HGO, RGO and its variations, KAFOs and medially linked KAFOs known as the Walkabout for individuals with high level, complete paraplegia and complete and incomplete tetraplegia.

In 1983, through the use of an RGO (Louisiana State University–RGO), a 30-year-old male with a complete T9 neurologic level SCI was reported to have achieved independent standing and walking with a rollator.[32] More recent studies report patients learning to stand and walk, generally for therapeutic purposes. These studies document the success of 85 adults with complete SCI from C6 to T12 while using either the RGO or ARGO.[119–121] Seventy-five adults, most with complete SCI from C2 to L1, also learned to stand and walk with the use of FES in combination with an RGO or KAFO.[122–127]

Yarkony et al. reported that six individuals with complete and incomplete SCIs (T4–T6) learned to stand at home unassisted by another person using FES plus KAFOs and the aid of a standing frame. Fifteen others with complete and incomplete SCIs (C7–T11) stood in the lab only. The average standing time was 5 to 15 minutes several times per day, two to five days per week.[122] Phillips et al. describe two individuals with SCI (incomplete C7 and complete T9) who learned to safely ambulate in the laboratory setting on level ground with FES plus a RGO. The patient with the incomplete tetraplegia learned to put on and take off the system, making this functionally most feasible.[123] Thoumie et al. summarized data from 26 individuals with complete SCI lesions (C8–T11 levels) using an FES plus a RGO. After 8–12 weeks of training over two sessions, 19 subjects were able to stand alone. At a follow-up 2 months after training, 15 subjects used the system at home. Four were only able to use the system during therapy because of later complications. The authors concluded that initial patient fitness was the most important factor in performance.[124]

Solomonow et al. reported on 70 individuals with complete C6/7–T11/12 levels of SCI who were fitted with an FES plus a RGO or a RGO alone. Forty-one of these individuals learned to stand and demonstrated limited walking, which included continuous walking without assistance; 77% of these individuals achieved independent walking on grass, ramps, and curbs and 21% were able to walk on flat, smooth surfaces only. One individual would walk on grass, curbs, and ramps only with assistance. There was a significant relationship between level of the injury, motivation, and successful completion of the training. These authors concluded that individuals with injuries at levels from T3 to T12 with good motivation do best with a FES plus the RGO system.[125]

Two studies demonstrated that nine individuals with complete SCI from T4 to L1 level of injury could learn to ambulate with the HGO or Parawalker. However, it is not clear whether these individuals continued to walk.[119,128] Three studies demonstrated the effectiveness of learning to stand and walk with the Walka-

bout system for 35 individuals with SCIs from C5 to T12 levels.[24,120,128–129] Middleton et al. however, reported that the level of independence is greater with the Walkabout than with a RGO or HGO. Activities such as transfers, toileting, and household chores including food preparation were achieved because the Walkabout allowed easier leg positioning.[24] There are, however, discrepancies in study results. Harvey et al. reported that subjects did not perceive a difference between use of the Walkabout or the isocentric RGO.[120] Kent reported the use of the Vannini-Rizzoli stabilizing orthosis or boot by 29 individuals with complete SCI (C5–L1) lesions with a 90% success rate for learning to walk safely.[25] However, a significant limitation to use of the boot is that trunk hyperextension is needed so that the line of gravity remains behind the hips.

In summary, the literature shows that for individuals with levels of injury above T10

- An orthosis may aid in standing and walking
- Orthoses may include a RGO, a ARGO or KAFO with FES, a boot, or a Walkabout device
- Standing and walking will most likely be at a therapeutic or household mobility level
- Long-term use has not been well documented

In the final analysis, for prescribing an orthosis for individuals with any level SCI, a complete examination and evaluation includes energy costs and other physiologic functioning, psychologic status, the cost of training, the patient's cognitive ability, possible connection to the FES system, the cost of the equipment, the system reliability, and cosmesis. All of these factors must be weighed against the expected outcome.[34]

Prevention of Impairments

Prevention for the adult with a SCI has a different emphasis than prevention in the child with MM or even a SCI. Factors of prevention in children relate more to the physical aspects of growth and development. In the adult, prevention could include lessening or elimination of psychologic and physiologic complications that result from lack of movement and walking combined with normal changes of aging and overuse. The psychologic benefits include

- Increasing and or maintaining self-esteem
- Preventing or reducing depression
- Increasing or maintaining a sense of independence

The physical benefits include

- Preventing osteoporosis, pressure sores, and contractures
- Reducing the incidence of fractures, urinary calcinosis, spasticity, and heterotropic ossification
- Reducing muscle soreness or injury from overuse
- Enhancing respiratory function
- Aiding digestion[34,117]

To enhance physiologic benefits, individuals with an SCI must maintain the ability to stand. The following section on prevention reports physiologic and psychologic outcomes as they relate to the client with a SCI.

Psychologic Effects

A few recent studies consider the psychologic effect of orthosis use. Regardless of the orthosis used (HKFO, FES with RGO, ARGO, Walkabout) or the level of the injury (C5–L5), positive psychologic effects have been noted.[24,115,116,121,125] Middleton et al. reported on data collection from 25 participants evaluated for use with the Walkabout. Upon initial receipt of the orthosis, 16 participants reported improved self-image with standing, because they could talk with others at the same level and were happy to be back on their feet.[24] Jaspers et al. documented the psychologic advantages of standing upright in 14 participants using an ARGO.[121] Coughlan et al. reported an increased overall sense of independence, such as ability to change position or work in standing, in six users of HKAFOs,[115] and Ferguson et al. described one subject's subjective measure of increased independence with the FES plus a

RGO, compared with the RGO alone.[127] Solomonow et al. reported that the use of an FES plus a RGO seemed to have significant importance in the psychologic well-being of 33 of 70 individuals who completed training.[125] Heinemann et al. analyzed 147 surveys and compared attitudes regarding wheelchair use compared with use of a KAFO.[116] The wheelchair was rated more positively and used more often to increase activity such as moving around and outside the home, going to work, and taking care of household chores. However, these participants still expressed a desire for a more adequate means of mobility. Lacking from all these studies are data that relate orthosis use to measures of depression.

In summary, no matter what type of orthosis is used, some individuals report psychologic benefits. However, for most individuals, the physiologic costs and increased time for use appear to far outweigh any positive psychologic effects.[115–117] More precise psychologic examination is needed to ascertain the benefits of continued orthosis use and to determine the psychologic profile of individuals who continue with orthosis use.[125]

Physiologic Effects

Despite the number of physiologic impairments assumed to be prevented by upright posture and ambulation by the client with a SCI, very few studies measure these impairments.[115,130–133] The variables measured in these studies include the effects of the use of HKAFOs on factors such as blood pressure, heart rate, vital capacity, bone density, bowel and bladder functions, spasticity, and skin integrity. In addition, the effect of specific HKAFO designs on the reduction of energy while standing and ambulating has been studied.

Strachan et al. examined the effect of upright posture with clients wearing a full-body orthosis termed a *pneumatic suit*.[132] The suit provided support throughout the trunk and lower extremities for standing and walking. In a study of eight adults with complete SCI (T3–T9), the authors noted mixed results related to muscle spasms but significant reduction in symptoms of postural hypotension, improved forced expiratory volume in upright posture, and improved total body calcium. They concluded that early standing in a full-body support is warranted because of the compression forces it exerts to the lower extremities and trunk.

Other studies have investigated various types of HKAFOs. One study showed no effect on blood flow measured after ambulation or after sitting by transcutaneous blood gas partial pressures of O_2 and CO_2 in the lower extremities of individuals with paraplegia.[134] Similarly, Ogilvie et al. documented little effect of orthosis use on objective measures of respiratory mechanics. In addition, subjective reports of reduction in urinary tract infection with no concurrent change in bacteria level were found in individuals with paraplegia. This study also found a slight improvement in bone density 18–30 months after beginning a program of walking.[130] Thoumie et al. summarized data from 20 individuals with complete SCI levels (C8–T12) before and immediately after completion of a training session in the use of FES plus an RGO. This group did not find significant changes in spasticity or improvement in bone mineral density, but did find significant cardiovascular changes and right colonic function.[133] Waters and Mulroy also reported conditioning effects in patients with SCI who continued to walk 1 year after discharge from rehabilitation.[114]

Solomonow's group conducted a comprehensive evaluation of physiologic factors.[131] Seventy adults with complete SCI (C6/7–T11/12) lesions were fitted and trained to use FES plus RGO or an ARGO alone (T11/12 level). Results from this study included reduction in spasticity, particularly for individuals with lesions above T10 who were able to combine the electrical stimulation with the RGO, and reduction in cholesterol levels, with a trend toward improved bone metabolism, vital capacity, and cardiac output.

The differences in study results may be due to a number of factors. The different reports of

the effect on spasticity in two studies by Solomonow et al. and Thoumie et al.[131,133] may be related to the measures of spasticity used by the authors. Solomonow et al. had each client complete a questionnaire, describing any possible changes in spasticity since entering the program.[131] No predetermined categories of spasticity were developed as a measure. Thoumie et al. used client self-report of spasticity, but each documented self-report had to fall into one of four levels derived from a modification these authors made to the Ashworth Scale.[133] Skold et al. reviewed documentation from 354 individuals with SCI to assess spasticity and its relationship to common SCI complications. Spasticity was measured by a physical examination scored through the Modified Ashworth Scale and self-reported symptoms. There was a significant association found between reduced range of motion and the increased presence of spasticity.[135] One implication of this finding is that use of an orthosis results in a prolonged stretch increasing or maintaining range of motion. Therefore, spasticity is reduced.

Finally, Coughlan and colleagues documented a statistically significant reduction of pressure sores in functional walkers who used HKAFOs daily for mobility, compared with occasional walkers, exercise walkers, standers, or nonusers of orthoses.[115]

The following studies address another physiologic effect, the differences in energy expenditure with the use of various orthoses. Overall, energy costs (energy requirements per unit of distance measured) in relation to speed of locomotion is correlated with the level of the SCI. A higher level of lesion results in increased energy costs and lower speeds.[34] All patients with SCI require more energy than their able-bodied peer to stand and ambulate.[114] Merkel et al. studied energy efficiency in nine patients with complete low-, mid-, or high-thoracic SCI while standing and walking with a walker and wearing a KAFO. Energy efficiency was measured by comparing oxygen consumed per kilogram of body weight per meter walked. The individuals with high-thoracic SCI levels used 25 times more energy than normal, and individuals with low and mid thoracic SCI levels used 7 to 9 times more energy. In relation to velocity, individuals with high thoracic SCI levels were approximately 25% slower than the other subjects.[136] These results imply that SCI patients who cannot improve oxygen consumption rates, such as patients with coexisting cardiopulmonary disease, may not be candidates for ambulation training.

Compared with bilateral KAFOs, the HGO, Walkabout, and RGO (and its variations) all have significantly lower energy requirements (measured by changes in heart rate, vital capacity, and oxygen consumption) at self-selected walking speeds.[34,129,131,137–139] In particular, use of a RGO was reported to lower energy cost by 16% compared with use of a KAFO.[34] Use of FES plus a RGO yielded significantly lower heart rates than the RGO, a HGO and conventional HKAFO.[125] Sykes, however, found no significant difference in terms of energy expenditure between the RGO and FES plus RGO if the systems were used for 5 minutes of continuous walking.[126] While heart rates and energy demands change with systems, individuals generally matched the energy costs and speed to decrease energy consumption.[124] Even with use of FES plus an RGO, average speed remains slow compared with that of able-bodied peers.[126,131]

In summary, the literature indicates that

- Standing and walking requirements (e.g., energy, strength, time to put on and take off) increase with higher levels of SCI. A careful look at all patient characteristics such as the ability to learn, perform safe mobility, fitness level, and cardiopulmonary functioning will assist in decision making regarding use of an orthosis.
- Many different orthosis systems have demonstrated effectiveness in helping individuals with SCI achieve standing and therapeutic walking with use of walking aids such as a walker and crutches.

- Some positive physiologic effects are reported for standing and short-distance walking or other activities of daily living and generally vary little from one orthosis system to another.
- Psychologic benefits need to be more closely measured.

Orthoses for Adults after a Cerebrovascular Accident

This section describes impairments, functional limitations, and disabilities associated with a cerebrovascular accident in an adult. It includes the role of orthoses and outcomes expected on the basis of current literature.

Impairments, Functional Limitations, and Disabilities

A *cerebrovascular accident* (CVA) is an abnormality in the cerebral circulation that results in a stroke or an acute onset of neurologic dysfunction. The symptoms of a CVA can be caused by ischemic or hemorrhagic lesions, most typically on one side of the brain. Severity and extent of impairment vary, since the lesions can occur in different locations within the brain, affect different-sized areas, and are influenced by the availability of collateral blood flow. A stroke may cause death or leave an individual with an array of short- or long-term impairments, functional limitations, and disabilities. These may range from complete recovery of function to dependence upon a wheelchair and the need for total care in all activities of daily living.[140] Although a stroke can occur at any age, the incidence increases with age. According to the American Heart Association's 1998 statistics, in the United States, approximately 600,000 individuals per year suffer strokes, and the current estimated number of survivors is 4,500,000.[141]

Impairments may include sensory, motor, cognitive, and perceptual deficits. Descriptions of the multiple impairments that can occur are beyond the scope of this book, and the reader is encouraged to review texts in physical rehabilitation.[140,142] The reader is also reminded that a detailed examination is necessary to determine a patient's capabilities, limitations, and expected outcomes as they relate to successful orthosis use.

Motor impairments include paralysis (hemiplegia) or weakness (hemiparesis) on one side of the body, opposite the site of the lesion. This may be manifested in such deficits as delays in onset of motor activity, abnormal timing and sequencing of muscle activity, and inappropriate coactivation of the agonist and antagonists. Initially the client may experience flaccidity of the muscles with no voluntary movement. From the early flaccid state, the muscles may develop hypertonicity, hyperreflexia, and overactivity. With recovery, the extent of return of voluntary movement varies and is often seen as overactivity in synergistic mass patterns of movement. These occur in both the lower and upper extremities. These mass patterns include flexion or extension components. For example, in the lower extremity, attempts to perform hip flexion are accompanied by hip abduction and external rotation, knee flexion, ankle dorsiflexion and inversion, and toe flexion. The extension synergy in the lower extremity includes hip extension, adduction, and internal rotation; knee extension; ankle plantarflexion and inversion; and toe plantarflexion. These mass patterns commonly seen in the execution of gait have a strong association with muscle weakness and altered muscle activation.[143,144] For example, weakness in the ankle dorsiflexors and premature firing of the triceps surae both contribute to the equinovarus position of the foot and ankle when loading the leg in gait.[144] If recovery continues, the severity of the mass patterns of movements, hyperreflexia, and hypertonicity may lessen. Recovery from stroke and decreasing the risk of complications are also impaired by coexistent diagnoses such as hypertension, coronary heart disease, congestive heart disease, and diabetes in many patients.[140]

The combination of the motor and other impairments may cause functional limitations in postural control and balance for sitting, standing, and walking. Asymmetry and unsteadiness are commonly seen, with slow speed a primary functional limitation of gait.[114] Most (70–80%) individuals do recover the ability to walk (with or without an assistive device). These patients may be limited in their independence beyond household ambulation because of the slow speed of walking or the extent of impairments and functional limitations such as cognitive and sensory processing and cardiopulmonary functions.[114,140,143,145]

The Role of Orthoses

A major focus for use of an orthosis for individuals with CVA is to prevent persistent problems that limit safe ambulation. Because of the effect of the CVA on one side of the body, only one orthosis is commonly prescribed. The primary purposes of an orthosis for a patient after a CVA are to

- Stabilize and support the ankle, foot, and knee (as necessary) for standing and walking
- Assist with the efficiency and control of gait
- Prevent or correct deformity[146-149]

The AFO is most commonly used to control problems of the knee and ankle/foot. The KAFO is rarely if ever used or successful because of the added weight and restriction on function and because the knee can often be controlled by positioning of the ankle in the AFO.[148-149] The major outcome focused upon in the literature has been the effect of the AFO on control or enhancement of gait through changes in alignment, temporal parameters, and energy consumption. The following review considers these topics.

Gait

Gait of the patient with hemiplegia is best described as asymmetric and interrupted, compared with that of able-bodied peers with equal weight bearing on both lower limbs and equal time in single support.[145,150] Commonly seen deviations in gait are persistent equinus or equinovarus, ankle mediolateral instability, clonic response to quick stretch of the gastro-soleus group, and knee hyperextension at stance, all affecting the efficiency of the gait. After a stroke, individuals often rely on the mass pattern of extension or flexion during the phases of gait because of impaired selective control and weak flexor muscles.[144,150]

Activation of extensor muscles in the beginning of stance is characterized normal timing and use of the hip and knee muscles. However, mass pattern of extension may limit the ability to achieve dorsiflexion by premature activation of the ankle plantar flexors as the limb is loaded.[144,146–147] This premature use of the plantar flexors in terminal swing also ultimately affects the timing of terminal stance and limits preswing on the affected side.[144,150] This mass pattern of extension may have elements of weakness, such as the knee extensors that compensate by hyperextending during weight bearing.

Common gait characteristics of the typical patient with CVA include

- Reduced walking speed
- Decreased step and stride length on the affected side
- Increased double-stance and decreased single-stance time on the affected side
- Higher rate of oxygen consumption than able-bodied peers walking at the same speed
- Abnormal affected-side lower extremity deviations, e.g., circumduction, external rotation/adduction of the hip, and backward leaning of the trunk.

Alignment During Gait

Like the child with CP, the individual with hemiplegia from a CVA often presents with equinus or equinovarus in gait. An orthosis may help decrease the plantigrade position of the foot during stance and clear the toes during swing. Malalignment at the knee can include too much flexion or hyperextension in the stance phase of gait. Genu recurvatum may be seen in the effort to place the foot flat on the floor from a variety of causes. These include the equinus or equinovarus position of the foot to compensate for weak knee muscles, the lack of dorsiflexion range, or impaired proprioception at the knee. Increased knee flexion is often seen in response to weak knee extensors, ankle dorsiflexion range past neutral, and impaired proprioception at the knee. The following studies review the changes to ankle and knee alignment with the aid of an AFO.[146,151–154]

Ankle Alignment

Lehmann et al. studied six individuals with hemiplegia who had strong mass patterns of extension. Each patient wore plastic FAFOs fixed in slight dorsiflexion and trim lines set at five different positions anterior and posterior to the malleoli. The authors found that the AFO with trim lines anterior to the malleoli provided the best control for ankle alignment.[151] Likewise, Ohsawa et al., in a study of individuals with strong mass extensor pattern, determined that anterior trim line positioning offered the best control.[152]

Hesse et al. further supported the use of an AFO to control the flexible equinovarus deformity. Twenty-one adults with hemiplegia used a rigid AFO that consisted of a metal caliper with an ankle set at 90° of plantarflexion and spring assist dorsiflexion. Compared with a barefoot condition, these individuals demonstrated better clearance of the foot at swing and increasing dorsiflexion appropriately at stance. However, a negative effect of AFO use was decreased activity of the tibialis anterior throughout gait. The authors concluded that a rigid AFO may lead to disuse atrophy of the tibialis anterior muscle and hence long-term dependency on the AFO.[153]

Burdett et al. compared no orthosis, an Air-stirrup, and two styles of AFO in 19 individuals with hemiplegia and excessive subtalar joint motion.[154] The AFO consisted of either metal double-action ankle joints with a 90° plantarflexion stop or a plastic FAFO set at neutral or 5° of dorsiflexion. The Air-stirrup only provided mediolateral stability but allowed both dorsiflexion and plantarflexion. Both the air-stirrup and AFOs decreased plantarflexion during midswing, compared with no orthosis use. The metal AFO significantly decreased plantarflexion at initial contact, compared with the other two conditions. The air-stirrup provided more calcaneal stability during stance than the no orthosis condition. The authors concluded that the air-stirrup is a viable substitution for the more expensive AFO if the client has only medial or lateral instabilities.

In summary, an AFO (metal or plastic) can correct dynamic ankle alignment during gait. The AFO, whether metal or plastic, is best if set at neutral or slight dorsiflexion (5° or less). For optimal benefit, the angle must be set very carefully to produce the best results for each individual client. In an attempt to control strong mass extension pattern, if a plastic AFO is used, the trim lines should be anterior to the malleoli to make it more rigid and most resistive to the pattern. One limitation to use of any AFO is causing decreased activity of the tibialis anterior. An air-stirrup may be warranted if short-term use of an assistive device is needed to position the foot for mediolateral stability and assistance is only needed to position the foot in dorsiflexion.

Knee Alignment

Lehmann et al. defined the adjustment to the AFO that is most effective in correcting knee position.[146] Seven individuals with hemiplegia walked without the orthosis or with a custom-fit metal single upright orthosis with double-action joints and rigid sole plate set at 5° of dorsiflexion or 5° of plantar flexion. Significant increases were noted in total knee flexion moments, and knee extension was assisted with the ankle in 5° of dorsiflexion.

Ohsawa et al., in a study of 23 patients with genu recurvatum due to severe mass extension pattern, were able to correct the genu recurvatum with trim lines anterior to the malleoli.[152] Hesse et al., in a study of 21 patients, found that activity of the quadriceps muscles increased appropriately in stance when a rigid-metal, double-upright, metal caliper set in slight dorsiflexion was used.[153]

In conclusion, knee alignment can be significantly changed through the use of an AFO (metal or plastic) that is set in slight dorsiflexion, which places the GRF line behind the knee during weight bearing.

Temporal Parameters of Gait

As noted above, temporal parameters of gait in individuals with CVA are altered significantly. In children with CP, change in alignment did not always change the functional parameters of gait significantly. However, in patients with impairments due to a CVA, changes in alignment of the knee, foot, and ankle do appear to have significant benefits on gait.

Lehman et al. found significant temporal parameter changes for patients wearing a AFO with the ankle set in slight dorsiflexion compared to plantar flexion or no orthosis use. These patients demonstrated increased walking speed, increased duration of time with the heel in contact with the floor at initial contact, and increased single-limb stance time on the affected limb.[146] Burdett et al. found an increased step length on the paretic side when patients were wearing AFO or air-stirrups.[154] Hesse et al. found significant differences in increased stride length and decreased cadence when nineteen patients with hemiplegia wore a metal AFO single medial upright with double-stop and spring assisted dorsiflexion compared to wearing firm shoes or no shoes.[155] In a subsequent study, Hesse et al. reported that the same metal caliper assisted individuals with hemiplegia to demonstrate better single-stance duration time on the paretic side and better swing symmetry.[153]

In another study, two single subjects also were found to have changes in temporal parameters of gait, specifically while wearing DAFOs.

Walking velocity and step length were significantly better wearing the DAFO than with the AFO or barefoot conditions.[156] In another study, one subject with hemiplegia who was an independent ambulator with a FAFO set at neutral dorsiflexion was fitted with a dynamic SMO. Total foot area contact and total force generated at single stance were significantly increased and total stance duration was significantly decreased when wearing the SMO.[157]

In summary, the literature indicates that compared with shoe or barefoot ambulation, use of any AFO during gait significantly improved

- Stride length and step length on both the paretic and the nonparetic side
- Single-limb stance time on the paretic limb
- Symmetry of motion, especially in swing
- Walking speed and cadence

Energy Consumption

Energy expenditure for individuals with hemiplegia varies. The extent of neurologic dysfunction and the coexistence of cardiopulmonary disease play a role. Because there is a marked reduction in walking speed, oxygen consumption is still higher than that of able-bodied peers walking at the same rate.[114] Corcoran et al., in a study of 13 individuals with hemiplegia who walked at self-selected walking speeds, found they had a 64% higher oxygen consumption than able-bodied peers.[158] This oxygen consumption was reduced significantly to 54% with a metal AFO and 51% with a plastic FAFO each set to control plantarflexion. The authors concluded that either orthosis was effective in significantly reducing oxygen consumption during walking.

In summary, an AFO is frequently prescribed for the individual with hemiplegia with walking difficulties. Clients with hemiplegia who used an AFO with 5° or less of dorsiflexion. showed the following benefits; a faster cadence with longer strides and steps, a decreased plantarflexion position of the foot helping to clear the floor during swing, con-trolled genu recurvatum with a possible increase in activity of the quadriceps, and lower oxygen consumption. One limitation to the use of an AFO was a significant decrease in the activity of the tibialis anterior muscle.

Chapter Summary

The purpose of this chapter is to provide the reader with an overview of the components and applications of shoes and orthoses for patients with neurologic disorders. Shoes and orthoses are only one aspect of intervention for these individuals, and they should be prescribed only after consideration of each individual patient's needs, expressed outcomes, identified impairments, functional limitations, and disabilities. Awareness of the biomechanics of the shoe or orthosis and outcomes identified from research will aid clinical decision making.

CRITICAL THINKING QUESTIONS

1. Compare and contrast the orthosis prescription for a child with CP spastic hemiplegia and an adult with a CVA.

2. Discuss the rationale for prescribing an orthosis for a toddler with MM.

3. Identify orthosis options and appropriate components for a patient with complete T9 paraplegia. Explain the expected outcomes from use of the orthosis.

4. Discuss the key principles for orthosis prescription for a child with high-thoracic-level MM and an adult with high- thoracic-level SCI.

5. Develop a clinical decision making model for the problem of equinus in a child with CP. The model should be the thinking process leading to either prescription or no prescription. It should include the identified problem, components of examination of disability, functional limitations, and impairments related to the problem, key aspects of evaluation, and expected outcomes.

6. Identify the purpose of shoes for the patient with an insensitive foot.

7. Develop an program of instruction for a patient who has received a new orthosis.

REFERENCES

1. American Physical Therapy Association. (2001). A guide to physical therapist practice. *Physical Therapy, 81.*

2. Palisano, R. L., Campbell, S. K., & Harris, S. R. (2000). Decision making in pediatric physical therapy. In S. K. Campbell, D. W. Van der Linden, & R. J. Palisano (Eds.), *Physical therapy for children* (2nd ed., pp. 198–224). Philadelphia: W. B. Saunders.

3. Boyd R. (2000, February 1). *Conservative and surgical options in the management of the motor problems in children with cerebral palsy: An evidenced based medicine approach.* Paper presented at the American Physical Therapy Association combined sections meeting. New Orleans, Louisiana.

4. Sackett, D. L. (1986). Rules of evidence and clinical recommendations on the use of antithrombotic agents. *Chest, 39,* 25–35.

5. Stuberg, W. (1994). The aims of lower limb orthotic management of cerebral palsy: A critical review of the literature. Report of a consensus conference on the lower limb orthotic management of cerebral palsy. *International Society of Prosthetics and Orthotics (ISPO),* 27–34.

6. Frey, C., Thompson, F., Smith, J., Sanders, M., & Horstman, H. (1993). American Orthopaedic Foot and Ankle Society Women's Shoe Survey. *Foot and Ankle, 14,* 78–81.

7. Redford, J. B. (1986). *Orthotics etcetera* (3rd ed.) Baltimore: Williams & Wilkins.

8. Redford, J. B., Basmajian, J. V., & Trautman, P. (1995). *Orthotics: Clinical practice and rehabilitation technology.* New York: Churchill Livingstone.

9. Weber, G., & Cardile, M. A. (1993). Neurologic manifestations in the lower extremity in the elderly person. *Clinics in Podiatric Medicine and Surgery, 10,* 161–178.

10. Frantz, S., Lawton, R., Schmagel, C., & Zimmerman, C. (1987). The physical therapist's role in the treatment of diabetes. *Clinical Management, 7,* 30–31.

11. Wernick, J. (1997). Treating the diabetic foot. *Rehabilitation Management, 10,* 50.

12. Knutson, L., & Clark, D. (1991). Orthotic devices for ambulation in children with cerebral palsy and myelomeningocele. *Physical Therapy, 71(12),* 947–960.

13. Meyer, P. (1974). Lower limb orthotics. *Clinical Orthopaedics and Related Research, 102,* 58–71.

14. Larin, H. (2000). Motor learning: Theories and strategies for the practitioner. In S. K. Campbell, D. W. Van der Linden, & R. J. Palisano (Eds.), *Physical therapy for children* (2nd ed., pp. 170–197). Philadelphia: W. B. Saunders.

15. McCollough, N. C. (1974). Rationale for orthotic prescription in the lower extremity. *Clinical Orthopaedics and Related Research, 102,* 32–45.

16. Norkin, C. C., & Levangie, P. K. (1992). *Joint structure and function.* (2nd ed.) Philadelphia: F. A. Davis.

17. Butler, P., & Nene, A. (1991). The biomechanics of fixed ankle foot orthoses and their potential in the management of cerebral palsied children. *Physiotherapy, 77,* 81–88.

18. Michael, J. (1990). Pediatric prosthetics and orthotics. *Physical and Occupational Therapy in Pediatrics, 10,* 123–146.

19. Walker, J., & Stanger, M. (1998). Orthotic management. In J. Dormans, & L. Pellegrino (Eds.), *Caring for children with cerebral palsy: A team approach* (pp. 391–426). Baltimore: Paul H. Brooks.

20. Cusick, B. (1990). *Progressive casting and splinting for lower extremity deformities in children with neuromotor dysfunction.* Tucson, AZ: Therapy Skill Builders.

21. Doxey, G. E. (1985). Clinical use and fabrication of molded thermoplastic foot orthotic devices. *Physical Therapy, 65,* 1679–1682.

22. Hylton, N. M. (1989). Postural and functional impact of dynamic AFOs and FOs in a pediatric population. *Journal of Prosthetics and Orthotics, 2,* 40–53.

23. Styer-Acevedo, J. (1999). Physical therapy for the child with cerebral palsy. In J. S. Tecklin (Ed.), *Pediatric physical therapy* (3rd ed., pp. 107–162). Philadelphia: Lippincott Williams & Wilkins.

24. Middleton, J., Yeo, J. D., Blanch L, Vare V, Perterson K, & Brigden K. (1997). Clinical evaluation of a new orthosis, the Walkabout, for restoration of functional standing and short distance mobility in spinal paralysed individuals. *Spinal Cord, 35,* 574–579.

25. Kent, H. O. (1992). Vannini-Rizzoli stabilizing orthosis (boot): Preliminary report on a new ambulatory aid for spinal cord injury. *Archives Physical Medicine Rehabilitation, 73*, 302–307.

26. Olney, S., & Wright, M. J. (2000). Cerebral palsy. In S. K. Campbell, D. W. Van der Linden, & R. J. Palisano (Eds.), *Physical therapy for children* (2nd ed., pp. 533–570). Philadelphia: W. B. Saunders.

27. Motloch, W. (1971). The Parapodium: An orthotic device for neuromuscular disorders. *Artificial Limbs, 15*, 36–47.

28. Brogren, E. (1995). Use of a standing shell in Swedish habilitation. *Pediatric Physical Therapy, 7*, 145–147.

29. Butler, P., & Major, R. (1987). The ParaWalker, a rational approach to the provision of reciprocal ambulation for paraplegic clients. *Physiotherapy, 73*, 393–397.

30. Stallard, J., Rose, G. K., & Farmer, I. (1978). The Orlau swivel walker. *Prosthetics and Orthotics International, 2*, 35–42.

31. Butler, P., Farmer, I., Poiner, R., Patrick J. (1983). Use of the Orlau swivel walker. *Physiotherapy, 68*, 324–326.

32. Douglas, R., Larson, P. F., D'Ambrosia, R., McCall, R. E. (1983). The LSU reciprocation-gait orthosis. *Orthopedics, 6*, 834–839.

33. Kahn, D., Angelo, L. (1989). The reciprocal-gait orthosis for children with myelodysplasia. *Physical and Occupational Therapy in Pediatrics, 9*, 107–117.

34. Nene, A. V., Hermens, H. J., Zilvoid, G. (1996). Paraplegic locomotion: A review. *Spinal Cord, 34*, 501–524.

35. Solomonow, M., Baratta, R. V., Hirokawa, S., Rightor, N., Walker, W., Beaudette, P., Shoji, H., D'Ambrosia, R. (1989). The RGO Generation II: Muscle stimulation powered orthoses as a practical walking system for thoracic paraplegics. *Orthopedics, 12*, 1309–1315.

36. Marshall Labs LTD. *Care and use guidelines for AFOs and KAFOs.* 131 Intrepid Lane Syracuse, New York.

37. *Lower limb orthotics* (1986). New York: Prosthetic-Orthotic Publications.

38. Albright, A. L. (1996). Spasticity and movement disorders in cerebral palsy. *Journal of Child Neurology, 11*, (Suppl. 1), S1–S4.

39. Barry, M. (1996). Physical therapy interventions for clients with movement disorders due to cerebral palsy. *Journal of Child Neurology, 11* (Suppl. 1), S51–S59.

40. Binder, H., & Eng, G. (1989). Rehabilitation management of children with spastic diplegic cerebral palsy. *Archives of Physical Medicine Rehabilitation, 70*, 481–489.

41. Cusick, B., & Sussman, M. (1982). Short leg casts: Their role in the management of cerebral palsy. *Physical and Occupational Therapy in Pediatrics, 2*, 93–110.

42. Jones, E. T., & Knapp, R. (1987). Assessment and management of the lower extremity in cerebral palsy. *Orthopedic Clinics of North America, 18*, 725–738.

43. Kurtz, L. A., & Scull, S. (1993). Rehabilitation for developmental disabilities. *Pediatric Clinics of North America, 40*, 629–643.

44. Bleck, E. E. (1987). *Orthopedic management in cerebral palsy.* Philadelphia: J. B. Lippincott.

45. Bleck, E. E. (1984). Forefoot problems in cerebral palsy—diagnosis and management. *Foot and Ankle, 4*, 188–194.

46. Baumann, J., & Zumstein, M. (1985). Experience with a plastic ankle-foot orthosis for prevention of muscle contracture. *Developmental Medicine and Child Neurology, 27*, 83. (Abstract)

47. Sankey, R. J., Anderson, D. M., & Young, J. A. (1989). Characteristics of ankle-foot orthoses for management of the spastic lower limb. *Developmental Medicine and Child Neurology, 31*, 466–470.

48. Hainsworth, F., Harrison, M. J., Sheldon, T. A., & Roussounis, S. H. (1997). A preliminary evaluation of ankle orthoses in the management of children with cerebral palsy. *Developmental Medicine and Child Neurology, 39*, 243–247.

49. Tardieu, C., Huet de laTour, E., Bret, M. D., & Tardieu, G. (1982). Muscle hypoextensibility in children with cerebral palsy: I. Clinical and experimental observations. *Archives of Physical Medicine and Rehabilitation, 63*, 97–102.

50. Tardieu, G., Tardieu, C., Cobeau-Justin, P., & Lespargot, A. (1982). Muscle hypoextensibility in children with cerebral palsy: II Therapeutic implications. *Archives of Physical Medicine and Rehabilitation, 63*, 103–107.

51. Tardieu, C., Lespargot, A., Tabary, C., & Bret, M. D. (1988). For how long must the soleus muscle be stretched each day to prevent contracture? *Developmental Medicine and Child Neurology, 30*, 3–10.

52. Rethlefsen, S., Kay, R., Dennis, S., Forstein, M., & Tolo, V. (1999). the effects of fixed and articulated ankle-foot orthoses on gait patterns in subjects with cerebral palsy. *Journal of Pediatric Orthopedics, 19*, 470–474.

53. Abel, M., Juhl, G., Vaughan, C., & Damiano, D. (1998). Gait assessment of fixed ankle-foot orthoses in children with spastic diplegia. *Archives of Physical Medicine and Rehabilitation, 79,* 126–133.

54. Brunner, R., Meier, G., & Ruepp, T. (1998). Comparison of a stiff and a spring-type ankle-foot orthosis to improve gait in spastic hemiplegic children. *Journal of Pediatric Orthopedics, 18,* 719–726.

55. Carlson, W., Vaughan, C., Damiano, D., & Abel, M. (1997). Orthotic management of gait in spastic diplegia. *American Journal of Physical Medicine Rehabilitation, 76,* 219–225.

56. Radtka, S., Skinner, S. R., Dixon, D. M., & Johanson, M. E. (1997). A comparison of gait with solid, dynamic, and no ankle-foot orthoses in children with spastic cerebral palsy. *Physical Therapy, 77,* 395–409.

57. Ounpuu, S., Bell, K., Davis, R., & DeLuca, P. (1996). An evaluation of the posterior leaf spring orthosis using joint kinematics and kinetics. *Journal of Pediatric Orthopedics, 16,* 378–384.

58. Carmick, J. (1995). Managing equinus in a child with cerebral palsy: merits of hinged ankle-foot orthoses. *Developmental Medicine and Child Neurology, 37,* 1006–1110.

59. Butler, P., Thompson, N., & Major, R. (1992). Improvement in walking performance of children with cerebral palsy: Preliminary results. *Developmental Medicine and Child Neurology, 34,* 567–576.

60. Embrey, D. G., Yates, L., & Mott, D. H. (1990). Effects of neuro-developmental treatment and orthoses on knee flexion during gait: A single-subject design. *Physical Therapy, 70,* 626–637.

61. Burtner, P., Woollacott, M., & Qualls, C. (1999). Stance balance control with orthoses in a group of children with spastic cerebral palsy. *Developmental Medicine and Child Neurology, 41,* 748–757.

62. Wilson, H., Haideri, N., Song, K., & Telford, D. (1997). Ankle-foot orthoses for preambulatory children with spastic diplegia. *Journal of Pediatric Orthopedics, 17,* 370–376.

63. Baker, M. J., Guiliani, A., Sparling, J., & Schenkmann, M. L. (1993). Effects of ankle foot orthoses on sit-to-stand task in children with cerebral palsy. *Pediatric Physical Therapy, 5,* 193. (Abstract)

64. Rosenthal, R. K., Deutsch, S. D., Miller, W., Schumann, W., & Hall, J. (1975). A fixed-ankle, below the knee orthosis for the management of genu recurvatum in spastic cerebral palsy. *Journal of Bone and Joint Surgery (Am), 57,* 545–547.

65. Damiano, D., & Abel, M. (1998). Functional outcomes of strength training in spastic cerebral palsy. *Archives of Physical Medicine and Rehabilitation, 79,* 119–125.

66. Ricks, N., & Eilert, R. (1993). Effects of inhibitory casts and orthoses on bony alignment of foot and ankle during weight bearing in children with spasticity. *Developmental Medicine and Child Neurology, 35,* 11–16.

67. Bertoti, D. B. (1986). Effect of short leg casting on ambulation in children with cerebral palsy. *Physical Therapy, 66,* 1522–1529.

68. Otis, J. C., Root, L., & Kroll, M. (1985). Measurement of plantar flexor spasticity during treatment with tone-reducing casts. *Journal of Pediatric Orthopedics, 5,* 682–686.

69. Watt, J., Sims, D., Harckham, F., Schmidt, L., McMillan, A., & Hamilton, J. (1986). A prospective study of inhibitive casting as an adjunct to physiotherapy for cerebral-palsied children. *Developmental Medicine and Child Neurology, 28,* 480–488.

70. Corry, I. S., Cosgrove, A. P., Duffy, C. M., McNeill, S., Taylor, T. C., & Graham, H. K. (1998). Botulinum toxin A compared with stretching casts in the treatment of spastic equinus: A randomised prospective trial. *Journal of Pediatric Orthopedics, 18,* 304–311.

71. Burroughs, J. (1982). Modified ankle-foot orthoses for a child with mild spastic diplegia: A case report. *Physical and Occupational Therapy in Pediatrics, 2,* 111–115.

72. Taylor, C. L., & Harris, S. R. (1986). Effects of ankle-foot orthoses on functional motor performance in a child with spastic diplegia. *American Journal of Occupational Therapy, 40,* 492–494.

73. Harris, S. R., & Riffle, K. (1986). Effects of inhibitive ankle-foot orthoses on standing balance in a child with cerebral palsy. *Physical Therapy, 66,* 663–667.

74. Norlin, R., & Odernick, P. (1986). Development of gait in spastic children with cerebral palsy. *Journal of Pediatric Orthopedics, 6,* 674–680.

75. Gage, J. (1993). Gait analysis an essential tool in the treatment of cerebral palsy. *Clinical Orthopaedics and Related Research, 288,* 126–134.

76. Johnson, D., Damiano, D., & Abel, M. (1997). The evolution of gait in childhood and adolescent cerebral palsy. *Journal of Pediatric Orthopedics, 17,* 392–396.

77. Evans, C., Gowland, C., Rosenbaum, P., William, A., Russell, D., Weber, D., & Plews, N. (1994). The effectiveness of orthoses for children with cerebral palsy. *Developmental Medicine and Child Neurology, 70,* (Suppl.), 26–27.

78. Held, S., & Kott, K. (1999). Effects of orthotics on upright functional skills of individuals with cerebral palsy [Abstract]. *Pediatric Physical Therapy, 11,* 217.

79. Mossberg, K., Linton, K. A., & Friske, K. (1990). Ankle-foot orthoses: Effect of energy expenditure of gait in spastic diplegic children. *Archives of Physical Medicine and Rehabilitation, 71,* 490–494.

80. Hinderer, K., Hinderer, S., & Shurtleff, D. (2000). Myelodysplasia. In S. K. Campbell, D. W. Van der Linden, & R. J. Palisano (Eds.), *Physical therapy for children* (2nd ed., pp. 621–670). Philadelphia: W. B. Saunders.

81. Tappit-Emas, E. (1999). Spina bifida. In J. S. Tecklin (Ed.), *Pediatric physical therapy* (3rd ed., pp. 163–222). Philadelphia: Lippincott Williams & Wilkins.

82. Bartonek, A., Saraste, H., Samuelsson, L., & Skoog, M. (1999). Ambulation in clients with myelomeningocele: A 12-year follow up. *Journal of Pediatric Orthopedics, 19,* 202–206.

83. Brinker, M. R., Rosenfeld, S. R., Feiwell, E., Granger, S. P., Mitchell, D. C., & Rice, J. C. (1994). Myelomeningocele at the sacral level. Long-term outcomes in adults. *Journal of Bone and Joint Surgery (Am), 76,* 1293–1300.

84. Park, B. K., Song, H. R., Vankoski, S. J., Moore, C. A., & Dias, L. S. (1997). Gait electromyography in children with myelomeningocele at the sacral level. *Archives of Physical Medicine and Rehabilitation, 78,* 471–475.

85. Thomson, J. D., Ounpuu, S., Davis, R. B., & DeLuca, P. A. (1999). The effects of ankle-foot orthoses on the ankle and knee in person with myelomeningocele: An evaluation using three-dimensional gait analysis. *Journal of Pediatric Orthopedics, 19,* 27–33.

86. Williams, J. J., Graham, G. P., Dunne, K. B., & Menelaus, M. B. (1993). Late knee problems in myelomeningocele. *Journal of Pediatric Orthopedics, 13,* 701–703.

87. Lehmann, J., Condon, S., deLateur, B., & Smith, C. (1985). Ankle foot orthoses: Effect on gait abnormalities in tibial nerve paralysis. *Archives of Physical Medicine and Rehabilitation, 66,* 212–218.

88. Richings, J. C., & Eckstein, H. B. (1970). Locomotor and educational achievements of children with myelomeningocele. *Annals of Physical Medicine, 10,* 291–298.

89. Hoffer, M., Feiwell, E., Perry, R., Perry, J., & Bonnett, C. (1973). Functional ambulation in clients with myelomeningocele. *Journal of Bone and Joint Surgery (Am), 55(8),* 137–148.

90. Barden, G. A., Meyer, L. C., & Stelling, F. H. (1975). Myelodysplastics: Fate of those followed for twenty years or more. *Journal of Bone and Joint Surgery (Am), 57,* 643–647.

91. DeSouza, L. J., & Carroll, N. (1976). Ambulation of the braced myelomeningocele client. *Journal of Bone and Joint Surgery (Am), 58,* 1112–1118.

92. Samuelsson, L., & Skoog, M. (1988). Ambulation in patients with myelomeningocele: A multivariate statistical analysis. *Journal of Pediatric Orthopedics, 8,* 569–575.

93. Gerristma-Bleeker, C. L. E., Heeg, M., & Vos-Niel, H. (1991). Ambulating with the reciprocating-gait orthosis. *Acta Orthopaedica Scandinavica, 68,* 470–473.

94. Selber, P., & Dias, L. (1998). Sacral-level myelomeningocele: Long-term outcome in adults. *Journal of Pediatric Orthopedics, 18,* 423–427.

95. Findley, T. W., & Agre, J. C. (1988). Ambulation in the adolescent with spina bifida. II. Oxygen cost of mobility. *Archives of Physical Medicine and Rehabilitation, 69,* 855–861.

96. Mazur, J. M., Shurtleff, D., Menelaus, M., & Colliver, J. (1989). Orthopedic management of high-level spina bifida. *Journal of Bone and Joint Surgery (Am), 71,* 56–61.

97. Carroll, N. C. (1974). The orthotic management of the spina bifida child. *Clinical Orthopaedics and Related Research, 102,* 108–114.

98. Franks, C. A., Palisano, R. J., & Darbee, J. C. (1989). The effects of walking with an assistive device and using a wheelchair on school performance in students with myelomeningocele. *Physical Therapy, 71,* 570–578.

99. Flandry, F., Burke, S., Robert, J. M., Hall, S., Drouilhet, A., Davis, G., & Cook, S. (1986). Functional ambulation in myelodysplasia: the effect of orthotic selection on physical and physiologic performance. *Journal of Pediatric Orthopedics, 6,* 661–665.

100. Lough, L., & Nielsen, D. (1986). Ambulation of children with myelomeningocele: Parapodium versus Parapodium with ORLAU swivel modification. *Developmental Medicine and Child Neurology, 28,* 489–497.

101. Rose, G. K., Stallard, J., & Sankarankutty, M. (1981). Clinical evaluation of spina bifida clients using hip guidance orthosis. *Developmental Medicine and Child Neurology, 23,* 30–40.

102. McCall, R. E., & Schmidt, W. T. (1986). Clinical experience with the reciprocal gait orthosis in myelodysplasia. *Journal of Pediatric Orthopedics, 6,* 157–161.

103. Yngve, D. A., Douglas, R., & Robert, J. M. (1984). The reciprocating gait orthosis in myelomeningocele. *Journal of Pediatric Orthopedics, 4,* 304–310.

104. Katz, D. E., Haideri, N., Song, K., & Wyrick, P. (1997). Comparative study of conventional hip-knee-ankle-foot orthoses versus reciprocating-gait orthoses for children with high-level paraparesis. *Journal of Pediatric Orthopedics, 17,* 377–386.

105. Phillips, D. L., Field, R. E., Broughton, N. S., & Menelaus, M. B. (1995). Reciprocating orthoses for children with myelomeningocele. *Journal of Bone and Joint Surgery (Br), 77,* 110–113.

106. Jeffries, L. M., McEwen, I. R., Venkataram, P. S., et al. (1994). Relations among age, weight, bone mineral content, and bone mineral density in children with spastic cerebral palsy and children without disabilities. *Pediatric Physical Therapy, 6,* 210. (Abstract)

107. Lock, T. R., & Aronson, D. D. (1989). Fractures in patients with myelomeningocele. *Journal of Bone and Joint Surgery (Am), 71,* 1153–1157.

108. Stuberg, W. (1992). Considerations related to weight-bearing programs in children with developmental disabilities. *Physical Therapy, 72,* 35–40.

109. Rosenstein, B. D., Greene, W. B., Herrington, R. T., & Blum, A. (1987). Bone density in myelomeningocele: The effects of ambulatory status and other factors. *Developmental Medicine and Child Neurology, 29,* 486–494.

110. Cunningham, E., McCulloch, P., & Schenkman, M. (1992). The evaluation of weight bearing in children with cerebral palsy on prone, supine, and upright standers. *Pediatric Physical Therapy, 4,* 193. (Abstract)

111. Miedaner, J. (1990). An evaluation of weight bearing forces at various standing angles for children with cerebral palsy. *Pediatric Physical Therapy, 2,* 215. (Abstract)

112. Schmitz, T. J. (2001). Traumatic spinal cord injury. In S. B. O'Sullivan, & T. J. Schmitz (Eds.), *Physical rehabilitation assessment and treatment* (4th ed., pp. 873–923). Philadelphia: F. A. Davis.

113. Waters, R., Yakura, J., & Adkins, R. (1993). Gait performance after spinal cord injury. *Clinical Orthopaedics and Related Research, 288,* 87–96.

114. Waters, R., & Mulroy, S. (1999). The energy expenditure of normal and pathological gait. *Gait and Posture, 9,* 201–231.

115. Coughlan, J. K., Robinson, C. E., Newmarch, B., & Jackson, G. (1980). Lower extremity bracing in paraplegia—a follow-up study. *Paraplegia, 18,* 25–32.

116. Heinemann, A. W., Magiera-Planey, R., Schiro-Geist, C., & Gimines, G. (1987). Mobility for persons with spinal cord injury: An evaluation of two systems. *Archives of Physical Medicine and Rehabilitation, 68,* 90–93.

117. Mikelberg, R., & Reid, S. (1981). Spinal cord lesions and lower extremity bracing: An overview and follow-up study. *Paraplegia, 19,* 379–385.

118. Basso, D. M. (2000). Neuroanatomical substrates of functional recovery after experimental spinal cord injury: Implications of basic science research for human spinal cord injury. *Physical Therapy, 80,* 808–817.

119. Franceschini, M., Baratta, S., Zampolini, M., Loria, D., & Lotta, S (1997). Reciprocating gait orthoses: A multicenter study of their use by spinal cord injured clients. *Archives of Physical Medicine and Rehabilitation, 78,* 582–586.

120. Harvey, L., Newton-John, T., Davis, G. M., Smith, M. B., & Engel, S. (1997). A comparison of the attitude of paraplegic individuals to the walkabout orthosis and the isocentric reciprocal gait orthosis. *Spinal Cord, 35,* 580–584.

121. Jasper, P., Peeraer, L., Van Petegem, W., & Van der Perre, G. (1997). The use of an advanced reciprocating gait orthosis by paraplegic individuals: a follow-up study. *Spinal Cord, 35,* 585–589.

122. Yarkony, G. M., Jaeger, R., Roth, E., Kralj, A., & Quintern, J. (1990). Functional neuromuscular stimulation for standing after spinal cord injury. *Archives of Physical Medicine and Rehabilitation, 71,* 201–206.

123. Phillips, C. A., & Hendershot, D. M. (1991). A systems approach to medically prescribed functional electrical stimulation. Ambulation after spinal cord injury. *Paraplegia, 29,* 505–513.

124. Thoumie, P., Perrouin-Verbe, B., LeClaire, G., Bedoiseau, M., Busnel, M., Cormerais, A., Courtillon A., Mathe, J. F., Moutet, F., Nadeau, G., Tanguy, E., Beillot, J., Dassonville, J., & Bussel, B. (1995). Restoration of functional gait in paraplegic clients with the RGO-II hybrid orthosis. A multicentre controlled study. I. Clinical evaluation. *Paraplegia, 33,* 647–653.

125. Solomonow, M., Aguilar, E., Reisin, E., Baratta, R. V., Best, R., Coetzee, T., & D'Ambrosia, R. (1997). Reciprocating gait orthosis powered with electrical muscle stimulation (RGO II). Part I: Performance evaluation of 70 paraplegic clients. *Orthopedics, 20,* 315–324.

126. Sykes, L., Campbell, I. G., Powell, E. S., Ross, E. R. S., & Edwards, J. (1996). Energy expenditure of walking for adult clients with spinal cord lesions using reciprocating gait orthosis and functional electrical stimulation. *Spinal Cord, 34,* 659–665.

127. Ferguson, K. A., Polando, G., Kobetic, R., Triolo, R. J., & Marsolais, E. B. (1999). Walking with a hybrid orthosis system. *Spinal Cord, 37,* 800–804.

128. Saitoh, E., Suzuki, T., Sonoda, S., Fujitani, J., Tomita, Y., & Chino, N. (1996). Clinical experience with a new hip-knee-ankle-foot orthotic system using a medial single hip joint for paraplegic standing and walking. *American Journal of Physical Medicine and Rehabilitation, 75,* 198–203.

129. Middleton, J., Sinclair, P. J., Smith, R. M., & Davis, G. (1999). Postural control during stance in paraplegia: effects of medically linked versus unlinked knee-ankle-foot orthoses. *Archives of Physical Medicine and Rehabilitation, 80,* 1558–1565.

130. Ogilvie, C., Bowker, P., & Rowley, D. I. (1993). The physiological benefits of paraplegic orthotically aided walking. *Paraplegia, 31,* 111–115.

131. Solomonow, M., Reisin, E., Aguilar, E., Baratta, R. V., Best, R., & D'Ambrosia, R. (1997). Reciprocating gait orthosis powered with electrical muscle stimulation (RGO II). Part II: Medical evaluation of 70 paraplegic clients. *Orthopedics., 20,* 411–418.

132. Strachan, R., Cook, J., Wilkie, W., & Kennedy, N. (1985). An evaluation of pneumatic orthoses in thoracic paraplegia. *Paraplegia, 23,* 295–305.

133. Thoumie, P., LeClaire, G., Beillot, J., Dassonville, J., Chevalier, T., Perrouin-Verbe, B., Bedoiseau, M., Busnel, M., Cormerais, A., Courtillon, A., Mathe, J. F., Moutet, F., Nadeau, G., & Tanguy, E. (1995). Restoration of functional gait in paraplegic clients with the RGO-II hybrid orthosis. A multicentre controlled study. II. Physiological evaluation. *Paraplegia, 33,* 654–659.

134. Messenger, N., Rithalia, S., Bowker, P., & Ogilvie, C. (1989). Effects of ambulation on the blood flow in paralysed limbs. *Journal of Biomedical Engineering, 11,* 249–252.

135. Skold, C., Levi, R., & Seiger, A. (1999). Spasticity after traumatic spinal cord injury: Nature, severity, and location. *Archives of Physical Medicine and Rehabilitation, 80,* 1548–1557.

136. Merkel, K. D., Miller, N. E., & Merritt, J. L. (1985). Energy expenditure in clients with low-, mid-, or high- thoracic paraplegia using Scott-Craig knee-ankle-foot orthoses. *Mayo Clinics Proceedings, 60,* 165–168.

137. Merritt, J. L., Miller, N. E., & Hanson, T. J. (1983). Preliminary studies of energy expenditures in paraplegics using swing through and reciprocating gait patterns. *Archives of Physical Medicine and Rehabilitation, 64,* 510.

138. Isakov, E., Douglas, R., & Berns, P. (1992). Ambulation using the reciprocating gait orthosis and functional electrical stimulation. *Paraplegia, 30,* 239–245.

139. Nene, A. V., & Patrick, J. H. (1989). Energy cost of paraplegic locomotion with the Orlau Parawalker. *Paraplegia, 27,* 5–18.

140. O'Sullivan, S. B. (2001). Stroke. In S. B. O'Sullivan, & T. J. Schmitz (Eds.), *Physical rehabilitation assessment and treatment* (4th ed., pp. 519–581). Philadelphia: F. A. Davis.

141. Stroke Statistics. Available at: http://www. Americanheart.org. Accessed June 30, 2001.

142. Ryerson, S. (2001). Hemiplegia. In D. Umphred (Ed.). *Neurological rehabilitation* (4th ed., pp. 741–786). Philadelphia: Mosby.

143. Kramers deQuervain, I., Simon, S., Leurgans, S., Pease, W., & McAllister, D. (1996). Gait pattern in the early recovery period after stroke. *Journal of Bone and Joint Surgery (Am), 78,* 1506–1514.

144. Yelnick, A., Albwet, T., Bonan, I., & Laffont, I. (1999). A clinical guide to asses the role of lower limb extensor overactivity in hemiplegic gait disorders. *Stroke, 30,* 580–585.

145. Roth, E., Merbitz, C., Mzoczek, K., Dugan, S., & Suh, W. (1997). Hemiplegic gait relationships between walking speed and other temporal parameters. *American Journal Physical Medicine and Rehabilitation, 76,* 128–133.

146. Lehmann, J., Condon, S., Price, R., & deLateur, B. (1987). Gait abnormalities in hemiplegia: Their correction by ankle-foot orthoses. *Archives of Physical Medicine and Rehabilitation, 68,* 763–771.

147. Lehmann, J. (1993). Push-off and propulsion of the body in normal and abnormal gait: Correction by ankle-foot orthoses. *Clinical Orthopaedics and Related Research, 288,* 97–108.

148. Ofir, R., & Sell, H. (1980). Orthoses and ambulation in hemiplegia: A ten year retrospective study. *Archives of Physical Medicine and Rehabilitation, 61,* 216–220.

149. Waters, R., & Montegomery, J. (1974). Lower extremity management of hemiparesis. *Clinical Orthopaedics and Related Research, 102,* 133–143.

150. Perry J. (1993). Determinants of muscle function in the spastic lower extremity. *Clinical Orthopaedics and Related Research, 288,* 10–26.

151. Lehmann, J., Esselman, P., Ko, M., Smith, J., deLateur, B., & Dralle, A. (1983). Plastic ankle-foot orthoses: Evaluation of function. *Archives of Physical Medicine and Rehabilitation, 64,* 402–407.

152. Ohsawa, S., Ikeda, S., Tanaka, S., Takahashi, T., Takeuchi, T., Utsunomiya, M., Ueno, R., Ohkura, M., Ito, Y., Katagi, Y., Ueta, M., & Hirano, T. (1992). A new model of plastic ankle foot orthosis (FAFO(II)) against spastic foot and genu recurvatum. *Prosthetics and Orthotics International, 16,* 104–108.

153. Hesse, S., Werner, C., Matthias, K., Stephen, K., & Berteanu, M. (1999). Non-velocity related effects of rigid double-stopped ankle-foot orthosis on gait and lower limb muscle activity of hemiparetic subjects with equinovarus deformity. *Stroke, 9,* 1855–1861.

154. Burdett, R., Borello-France, D., Blatchly, C., & Potter, C. (1988). Gait comparison of subjects with hemiplegia walking unbraced, with ankle-foot orthosis, and with air-stirrup brace. *Physical Therapy, 68,* 1197–1203.

155. Hesse, S., Luecke ,D., Jahnke, M., & Mauritz, K. (1996). Gait function in spastic hemiplegic patients walk. *International Journal of Rehabilitation Research, 19,* 133–141.

156. Diamond, M., & Ottenbacher, K. (1990). Effect of a tone-inhibiting dynamic ankle-foot orthosis on stride characteristics of an adult with hemiparesis. *Physical Therapy, 70,* 423–430.

157. Mueller, K., Cornwall, M., McPhoil, T., Mueller, D., & Barnwell, J. (1992). Effect of a tone-inhibiting dynamic ankle-foot orthosis on the foot-loading pattern of a hemiplegic adult: A preliminary study. *Journal of Prosthetics and Orthotics, 4,* 86–92.

158. Corcoran, P., Jebsen, R., Brengelmann, G., & Simons, B. (1970). Effects of plastic and metal leg braces on speed and energy cost of hemiparetic ambulation. *Archives of Physical Medicine and Rehabilitation, 51,* 69–77.

Chapter 17

ORTHOSES FOR SPINAL CONDITIONS—CLINICAL DECISION MAKING

Objectives

1. Describe the beneficial and negative effects of a spinal orthosis
2. Differentiate the indications, advantages, and disadvantages of the orthoses used for scoliosis
3. Describe the indications for spinal orthoses
4. Differentiate orthoses used for thoracic and lumbar injuries
5. Given a particular patient with a cervical spine injury, provide a rationale for recommending a specific cervical orthosis

This chapter is divided into the following sections:

Spinal orthoses have a long history as devices used to correct or protect a musculoskeletal condition. Early spinal orthoses consisted of tree bark that was cut circumferentially and placed around the patient. In 1582, Ambroise Paré developed a metal device padded with rags that was applied to the torso of a patient with scoliosis. Nicholas Andry described corsets to assist in spinal support in 1741. Lorenz Heister (1683–1758) introduced a spinal orthosis consisting of shoulder and abdominal straps that helped to support the head.[1]

The Committee on Prosthetics–Orthotics Education (CPOE) developed a systematic nomenclature to clarify orthosis terminology.[2] Common acronyms used to describe spinal orthoses are as follows:

SIO, sacroiliac orthosis
LSO, lumbosacral orthosis
TLSO, thoracolumbosacral orthosis
CO, cervical orthosis
HCTO, head–cervical–thoracic orthosis

There are two types of spinal orthoses; prefabricated and custom. Most patients are fitted with prefabricated or "off-the-shelf" orthoses ordered according to measurements. However, difficulty in ensuring a proper, patient-specific fit with prefabricated orthoses may occur. Custom-made orthoses that are molded to the patient are often considered preferable.[3]

An estimated 1,856,000 people used spinal orthoses in 1994, making them the most popular anatomic assistive device used.[4] Spinal orthoses apply forces to the trunk. The location, direction, and magnitude of these forces vary with the design of the orthosis, the tightness with which it is worn, and the patient's attempts to move against it. Many spinal orthoses often use a three-point force distribution system in which one directional force is balanced by two others that are above and below. The three-point force distribution is illustrated in Figure 5-20.

◆◆◆

Effects of Spinal Orthoses

There are beneficial and negative effects of a spinal orthosis. These are outlined as follows.

Beneficial Effects

1. Trunk support

Trunk support is accomplished by two mechanisms: a three-point pressure system and an abdominal corset. The abdominal corset increases the effectiveness of the abdominal muscles in elevating intracavitary pressure. An example of this beneficial effect is the use of a thoracolumbar anterior control or hyperextension orthosis (Fig. 17-1).

2. Motion restriction

Motion restriction may help to reduce pain and provide stability while fractures and inflamed soft tissues heal. A spinal orthosis is often worn for 6–12 weeks to allow fracture heal-

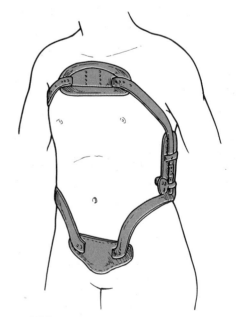

Figure 17-1. Thoracolumbar anterior control or hyperextension orthosis.

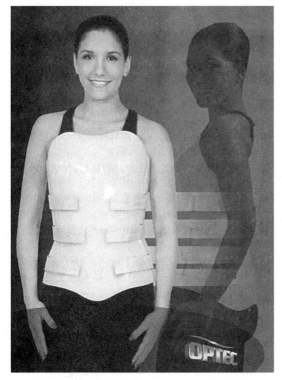

Figure 17-2. OPTEC TLSO. (Reprinted with permission from OPTEC Inc.)

ing.[3] An example of this beneficial effect is the use of a TLSO. (Fig. 17-2).

3. Modification of skeletal alignment

Modification of skeletal alignment is seen with an orthosis used in the intervention for a spinal deformity such as scoliosis or kyphosis. A Boston Brace is an example of this beneficial effect (Fig. 17-3).

Negative Effects

- Muscle atrophy and possible weakness
- Joint contracture after a period of immobilization
- Psychologic dependence or emotional disorders such as those associated with correction or maintenance of scoliosis

- Hypermobility in areas above or below the immobilized areas
- Respiratory difficulties due to compression
- Discomfort
- Poor cosmetic appearance

The Role of Orthoses in Intervention for Scoliosis

Six of every 1000 children, 3 to 5 years of age, develop spinal curves that are considered large enough to need interventions. In 80–85% of those with scoliosis, the cause is idiopathic, or unknown.[5] Some authors are skeptical about the efficacy of orthosis wear for idiopathic scoliosis.[6] However, the use of orthoses is the only nonoperative modality consistently shown to alter the natural progression of scoliosis curvatures.[7] Exercise has not been proved beneficial in reducing or altering the progression of curvature.[8] Electrical stimulation to strengthen the muscles on the convex side has also proved ineffective.[9] A multicenter, multinational prospective study sponsored by the Scoliosis Research Society evaluated the effectiveness of the care of ado-

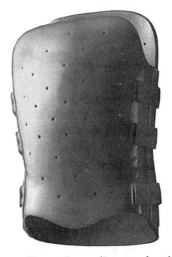

Figure 17-3. Boston Brace. (Reprinted with permission from Boston Brace International Inc.)

lescent idiopathic scoliosis. This care included observation, electrical stimulation, and TLSO wear. Results of this study showed no difference between electrical stimulation and observation. However, a statistically significant difference was seen between observation and wearing a TLSO.[10] Likewise, two other studies found no benefit from use of electrical stimulation in the intervention for scoliosis. One study found that use of surface electrical stimulation was significantly less effective than orthosis use in preventing progression of scoliosis.[11] Another study of 62 subjects with scoliosis found that electrical stimulation was unsuccessful in altering the natural history of idiopathic scoliosis.[12]

Some investigators believe that many patients with scoliosis wear orthoses needlessly, since curve progression continues, and surgical stabilization is eventually necessary. Others believe that while substantial improvement of the scoliosis curves is evident while a spinal orthosis is worn, long-term follow-up indicates that the orthosis prevents the curve from increasing beyond its original contour.[13] Scoliosis curvature progression may be limited, but not corrected, by the use of spinal orthoses. The degree of deformity seen at the start of orthosis wear is about the same as the final outcome after completion of wearing the orthosis. Therefore, orthosis wear should begin before the scoliosis curvature reaches an unacceptable magnitude.[6]

Radiographs taken while the patient is wearing the orthosis are the best way to assess the effect of the orthosis. Every 3–4 months, the orthosis can be checked for proper fit and a posteroanterior radiograph can be taken of the patient in the orthosis. Comparisons can be made with previous radiographs to determine the effect of the orthosis. Cessation of growth curvature may be determined by serial measurements. Since some curve progression frequently occurs with orthosis discontinuance, a gradual weaning process is recommended.[3]

Determining Scoliosis Curvature

There are three widely used methods of determining scoliosis curvature; The Cobb method, The Risser-Ferguson method, and the Scoliometer.

1. The Cobb method is shown in Figure 17-4.[14]
2. The Risser-Ferguson method is shown in Figure 17-5.[13]
3. The Scoliometer is a fluid-filled inclinometer that shows angles of trunk rotation on a scale with 1° increments from 0 to 30°. A study of 105 patients with trunk asymmetry in a scoliosis clinic compared the Scoliometer with the Cobb method. Interexaminer agreement was excellent in the thoracic spine but problematic in the lumbar spine. The investigators in this study concluded

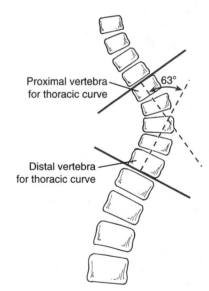

Figure 17-4. Cobb method of determining scoliosis. A line is drawn perpendicular to the margin of the upper vertebra that inclines most toward the concavity. Another line is drawn on the inferior border of the lower vertebra with the greatest inclination toward the concavity. A supplemental or identical angle is constructed by drawing lines perpendicular to the end vertebral lines. The angle formed by these intersecting lines is the degree of curvature.

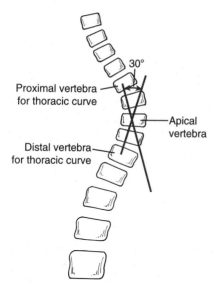

Figure 17-5. The Risser-Ferguson method of determining scoliosis uses lines drawn from the centers of the bodies of the highest (proximal) and lowest (distal) vertebrae of the curve to the center of the body of the middle vertebra of the curve. The proximal vertebra is the highest vertebra whose superior surface tilts to the concavity of the curve. The distal vertebra is the lowest vertebra whose inferior surface tilts to the concavity of the curve. The apical vertebra is parallel to the transverse plane of the body and is between the proximal and distal vertebrae. The angle formed by the two lines that intersect the apex from the proximal and distal midpoints is the degree of curvature.

that the Scoliometer has a high level of interexaminer measurement error that limits its use as an outcome instrument.[15] Classifications of scoliosis have been advocated by the Scoliosis Research Society as illustrated in Table 17-1.[14] Other classifications of scoliosis are as follows:

- Congenital—due to birth defects such as a hemivertebra, in which one side of the vertebra fails to develop normally
- Neuromuscular—due to loss of control of muscles or nerves that support the spine; this is seen in conditions such as cerebral palsy and muscular dystrophy

- Degenerative—may be caused by disk degeneration or arthritis
- Nonstructural (functional)—a structurally normal spine appears curved; this is often caused by conditions such as leg length discrepancy, muscle spasms, or inflammatory states
- Structural (fixed)—may result from congenital, neuromuscular, degenerative, or idiopathic causes[7]

A "C" curve is called right or left, depending on the convexity, e.g., a right curve has right convexity. An "S" curve is a compensation for the "C" curve. For example, Figure 17-5 shows an "S" right thoracic and left lumbar scoliosis curve. A high shoulder, rib hump, and low hip are on the convex side of the curve.

Indications for Orthosis Intervention for Scoliosis

Indications for orthosis intervention in cases of scoliosis are as follows:

10–20° curves are generally only observed.
20–30° curves are observed initially; if the curvature increases by more than 5° in a skeletally immature patient, the use of an orthosis is indicated
30–40° curves require the prompt use of orthoses; these patients are at high risk of progression of curvature and may rapidly

Table 17-1. Classification of Scoliosis

Group	Curve
1	0–20°
2	21–30°
3	31–50°
4	51–75°
5	76–100°
6	101–125°
7	126° and above

progress beyond the ability of the orthosis to be of assistance

40–50° curves usually require surgical intervention; however, if the patient has a well-balanced spine and the curvature is flexible, there may be some benefit to the use of an orthosis rather than surgery. In very young patients, orthoses may retard progression long enough to allow further trunk growth before the inevitable fusion[6]

Skeletal maturity is often determined by using a Risser sign, which quantifies the degree of iliac crest ossification from grades 0 (absence of ossification) to 5 (cessation of increase in height).

Objectives of Using an Orthosis

Objectives of using an orthosis for intervention of scoliosis include

1. Stopping the progression of scoliotic curvature and preventing the curve from increasing; an increase might mandate surgical stabilization
2. Gaining permanent correction in anticipation of skeletal maturity
3. Allowing for continued growth of the spine during adolescence; ideally a fusion should not be performed in the juvenile years because of the possibility of limiting trunk growth[2]

Types of Orthoses Used in the Intervention for Scoliosis

Which orthosis to prescribe depends on the patient, initial curve, progression of the curve, relevant research, and preference of the orthotic team. Regional differences may also affect the selection of a particular orthosis. There are several orthoses used in the intervention of scoliosis, the Milwaukee CTLSO and several types of TLSOs. Each of these is described as follows.

Milwaukee CTLSO

The Milwaukee CTLSO was first used in 1945 and was a crude orthosis with turnbuckles on the sides and a rigid screw fixation of the thoracic pad. In the 1950s, the turnbuckles were abandoned and replaced by three extensible uprights, one anteriorly and two posteriorly. Distraction of the thoracic spine is possible with a flat, firm chin pad and a notched occipital support mounted on a neck ring.[3] As the patient's head rocks back against the occipital pads of the neck ring, the resulting axial traction acts to further straighten the upper thoracic and cervical spine. Various pads may be attached to the posterior uprights. A pad is necessary for every major curve present.[3] The rib pad is the most commonly used and is placed over the rib convexity. An active element is incorporated because of the discomfort of the pads, with the patient actively moving away from the pads (Fig. 17-6).[3]

Longitudinal studies on the effectiveness of the Milwaukee CTLSO have yielded varied results. One investigator stated that the Milwaukee CTLSO is still the orthosis of choice for any major thoracic curvature with the apex above the T7 level and for cervicothoracic curves.[6] TLSOs have been recommended for thoracic curves with the apex below T7.[3,6] In an investigation of 95 children with thoracic curves between 30 and 39°, the Milwaukee CTLSO was effective in limiting progression of the curve in 84% of cases. Patients who complied with wearing the Milwaukee CTLSO had statistically much better results than noncompliant patients.[17]

Components of the Milwaukee CTLSO

The components of the Milwaukee CTLSO are

- A contoured girdle that grasps the pelvis firmly. Hinges permit the pelvic girdle to open for application and removal. The pelvic section may be custom molded from a positive mold of the patient's torso or prefabricated. Prefabricated girdles can be

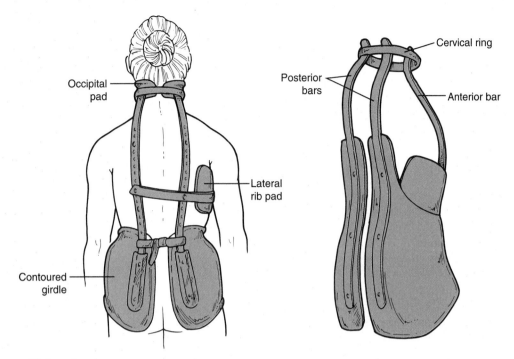

Figure 17-6. Milwaukee CTLSO.

applied more rapidly and fit 90% of patients[18]
- One anterior bar and two posterior bars that extend from pelvic girdle to cervical ring
- A cervical ring that unlocks to permit application and removal
- An occipital pad that is notched to avoid pressure on the occipital protuberance
- A chin pad
- Lateral pads that may be placed over the rib hump. The lateral pads push in and rotate toward the curve concavity

Advantages of the Milwaukee CTLSO

- It may be removed for activities of daily living.
- Because of its open design, there is minimal restriction of respiration.
- It allows good air circulation to minimize skin problems.
- It is adjustable to growth and curve changes.

- Physical activities are permitted when wearing this orthosis, except gymnastics. During gymnastics, the neck ring may create potential hazards.

Disadvantages of the Milwaukee CTLSO

- It must be worn for most of the day and night (typically over 20 hours) until the patient is mature as shown by closure of the vertebral epiphyses. Time out of the orthosis is allowed for bathing, swimming, and sporting activities.[19]
- It is noncosmetic, since the occipital and chin pads extend above the clothing.
- Fabrication is more difficult and time consuming than that of other orthoses.
- Little correction can be expected if the curves are major. However, use of the Milwaukee CTLSO does prevent further progression of the curve.

Thoracolumbosacral Orthoses

In the 1970s, several TLSOs were developed for patients with scoliosis or kyphosis.[2] They extend from the thorax to the sacrum and are often called *low-profile TLSOs*. These TLSOs are more cosmetic than the Milwaukee CTLSO since they do not have a neck ring and can be hidden easily under clothing. They are often named for the town or area where they were designed, such as Boston, Wilmington, and Charleston. Using thermoplastic materials, these orthoses have been effective in treating scoliosis with greater patient acceptance due to increased cosmesis and comfort.[6] While the Milwaukee CTLSO depends on longitudinal traction, these underarm TLSOs are passive devices, depending on fit and appropriate padding for control. They are primarily effective in patients with thoracic curvature with the apex of the curve below T7.[3,6] All TLSOs have either a three-point or four-point corrective system. The three-point system is used for single curves, as illustrated in Figure 17-7.

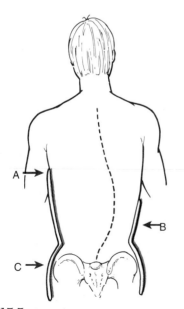

Figure 17-7. Three-point pressure of a TLSO for scoliosis. Forces applied to the lower thoracic curve (B) are balanced by high thoracic (A) and pelvic forces (C).

Boston Brace

The Boston Brace was developed in 1972, at Children's Hospital in Boston, Massachusetts. The Boston Brace is a prefabricated orthosis available in six sizes, which comes as a mass-produced polypropylene module that the orthotist alters to meet the needs of the individual patient. This orthosis is often used for curves between 20 and 45°. The Boston Brace opens posteriorly and is primarily designed for a lower scoliosis condition, below T8 (Fig. 17-3). The effectiveness of the Boston Brace has been reported in several studies. A study of 295 patients who wore a Boston Brace found that 39% achieved a correction of 5–15°, and 4% achieved more than 15° correction compared with preorthosis curves. Young age at the initiation of orthosis wear and greater preorthosis curvature increased the incidence of surgery.[20] A study of 21 children with myelomeningocele found no further progression of scoliosis 2 years after Boston Brace discontinuance. The average time of use of the Boston Brace was 2.5 years.[21] In a study of 40 adolescents, the Boston Brace reduced Cobb angles of the thoracic spine by 19–27%.[22]

In contrast, several studies showed little benefit and serious complications of Boston Brace wear. One study showed that use of the Boston Brace had a negative effect on pulmonary conditions. A study of 15 adolescents (mean age, 14.1 years) with scoliosis found that use of a Boston Brace resulted in an immediate, predictable, uniform reduction in lung volume and pulmonary compliance.[23] A study of 25 patients that investigated the long-term effect of the Boston Brace, at a mean follow-up of 8.5 years, found that the Boston Brace did not improve scoliosis curvature, but did prevent progression of vertebral rotation, translation, rib hump, and Cobb angle in idiopathic scoliosis. Investigators could not determine if the results reflected prevention of progressive deformity or merely the natural history of idiopathic scoliosis.[24] Another study found no statistically significant difference in scoliosis curve progression between 32 adolescents wearing the Boston Brace and 32 adolescents that were untreated.[25] In one study of 60 patients, despite use of the Boston Brace, a significantly greater average progression rate of the scoliotic curve was seen. The investigators in this study felt that the Boston Brace had little effect during a period of moderate to rapid skeletal growth.[26]

Wilmington Orthosis

The Wilmington orthosis is a custom-molded TLSO that is fabricated in one piece from thermoplastic material such as Orthoplast. Construction begins with a negative mold formed from the trunk. The Wilmington orthosis is then built around a positive mold. In a study of 71 patients, the Wilmington orthosis showed an average improvement of 1.4 cm in thoracic and thoracolumbar curves and 1.5 cm in double structural curves. Thirty-one percent of the subjects with thoracic curves had an improvement of 5° or more, while 33% were unchanged. These investigators concluded that the Wilmington orthosis was successful in treating scoliosis (Fig. 17-8).[27]

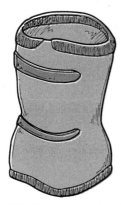

Figure 17-8. Wilmington orthosis. (Figure adapted from Bassett, G. S., & Bunnell, W. P. (1987). Influence of the Wilmington orthosis on spinal decompensation in adolescent idiopathic scoliosis. *Clinical Orthopaedics and Related Research, 223,* 164–169.)

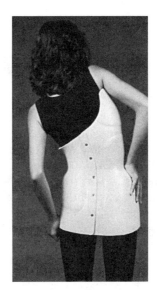

Figure 17-9. Charleston Bending Brace. (Reprinted with permission from SeaFab.)

Charleston Bending Brace

The Charleston Bending Brace, developed in 1978 in Charleston, South Carolina, is a nighttime bending orthosis that holds the patient in reversed position from the scoliotic curvature. This orthosis is molded in maximal reverse bending so that the curvature is forcibly straightened to the greatest degree allowed.[6] One long-term study of 149 patients with structural scoliosis curves showed less than 5° change in curvature. Preliminary results of the use of this orthosis have shown that 83% of skeletally immature patients have had satisfactory control of curvature. In this study, the investigators advocated continued use of the Charleston Bending Brace (Fig. 17-9).[28]

Advantages of TLSOs for Scoliosis

Two advantages of TLSOs, such as the Boston, Wilmington, and Charleston, in the intervention of scoliosis are

- TLSOs, in contrast to the Milwaukee CTLSO, are low profile and can be worn under clothing.[3]

- TLSO fabrication is quicker than Milwaukee CTLSO fabrication.

Disadvantages of TLSOs for Scoliosis

Disadvantages of TLSOs are

- The solid design of the TLSO limits adjustments for vertical growth. A new TLSO must be fabricated when the patient outgrows the TLSO.
- Heat retention can lead to possible skin problems because of the closed design of the TLSO.
- Respiration is restricted because of thoracic compression of the TLSO
- Because of its low profile, thoracic curves with an apex above T8 cannot be treated.

Research Studies

Which orthosis to use in an intervention for scoliosis may be confusing. One study of 244 female subjects with adolescent idiopathic scoliosis found that the Milwaukee CTLSO had a five times greater risk of failure than the Boston Brace. Investigators concluded that the Boston Brace was more successful than the Milwaukee CTLSO irrespective of initial curve magnitude and skeletal maturity.[29] Follow-up after 1 year of Milwaukee CTLSO use, showed an average curve correction of 18–29%, slightly less for high left thoracic curves and slightly more for lumbar curves.[3] However, at follow-ups more than 5 years after orthosis discontinuance, the final scoliosis curve was close to the initial preorthosis curve.[30] Therefore, use of the Milwaukee CTLSO resulted in scoliotic curve stabilization but not correction.[31] Either a Milwaukee CTLSO or a low-profile TLSO is recommended with a single lumbar or thoracolumbar curve. The choice of orthosis often depends on the philosophy of the orthotic team and what the skeletally immature patient is willing to wear.[3]

One common criticism of the Milwaukee CTLSO is its poor cosmesis. However, one study comparing the Milwaukee CTLSO with other TLSOs found no difference in wearing compliance among orthoses.[18] In addition, another study of the psychosocial characteristics of 95 female patients who wore a Milwaukee CTLSO for idiopathic scoliosis found, at an average follow-up of 7 years, no differences in depression or health locus of control.[32] Likewise, a study in Sweden found no statistically significant differences in body self-image of 54 adolescents with scoliosis and a normative group. No statistically significant differences were found between those preorthosis wear and at follow-up interviews an average of 1.7 years later.[33]

Several studies have compared the effectiveness of different TLSOs. One study compared the use of a TLSO a Charleston orthosis, and a Milwaukee orthosis by 177 patients. Results showed the TLSO superior at preventing curve progression in adolescent idiopathic scoliosis.[34] Another study found the Boston Brace more effective in preventing curve progression and in avoiding the need for surgery than the Charleston Bending Brace.[35] In a meta-analysis of 13 orthosis studies, the use of orthoses was significantly more successful than both electrical stimulation and observation in the treatment of idiopathic scoliosis. The weighted mean proportions of success were 0.99 for the Milwaukee Brace, 0.60 for the Charleston Brace, and 0.90 for all other types of orthoses. This study found the Milwaukee CTLSO significantly more successful than all other types of orthoses, and the Charleston Brace was significantly less successful than the Milwaukee CTLSO.[36] In summary, further investigations are needed to determine the most effective orthosis in scoliosis intervention.

Wearing Instructions

The amount of time a patient should wear the orthosis is controversial. Initially, patients were often required to wear orthoses for most of the day to prevent the progression of scoliosis.[32] In a meta-analysis of 13 orthosis studies, orthoses that were worn 23 hours per day were significantly more successful than those worn 8–16 hours a day.[36] However, other studies have shown that patients who wear their orthoses part time have outcomes as satisfactory as those who wear their orthoses full time.[37,38] One study of 162 subjects with idiopathic scoliosis who wore the Boston Brace found no significant differences in curve progression between wearing the orthosis 12 hours a day or 23 hours a day.[35] Many physicians now recommend wearing the orthosis part time, usually in a 16 hour a day protocol.[6]

Weaning from the orthosis may begin when the child reaches skeletal maturity. Weaning usually begins by allowing the patient out of the orthosis for 4 hours in the afternoon or evening. Time out of the orthosis is increased by 4-hour increments at sequential physician visits 4 months apart. Even after the patient has reached the point when the orthosis is not worn during the day, the orthosis should be worn at night for an additional year. After that time, orthosis use is eliminated.[6]

Orthoses used in scoliosis intervention have the disadvantage of retaining body heat because of their polypropylene construction. As a result, an undershirt is usually worn under the orthosis for moisture absorption and skin protection.[3] A common problem initially in fitting is not maintaining a snug fit of the orthosis. The skin should be checked routinely for breakdown or dermatitis. The patient's weight and general conditioning should be assessed on a regular basis. Patients undergoing significant weight gain should be counseled about exercise and diet. Skin care instructions such as those in Resource Box 17-1 may be given to the patient who wears an orthosis for scoliosis.

Noncompliance is the primary cause of failure in orthosis intervention programs. The older the child at the beginning of intervention, the less likely the child is to comply with wearing the orthosis.[39] Education of the patient and family regarding the importance of ortho-

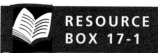

RESOURCE BOX 17-1

Skin Care Instructions for the Patient Who Wears an Orthosis for Scoliosis

1. Keep your skin as clean and dry as possible at all times. Bathe daily, and do not apply the orthosis until your skin is completely dry.
2. An undershirt should be worn under the orthosis and changed daily. The undershirt will absorb perspiration and protect your skin.
3. Avoid using lotion, talcum, or oils on the skin underneath the orthosis. These may soften the skin and cause areas of pressure. Additionally, they may soil the orthosis.
4. Inspect your skin whenever the orthosis is off for areas of pressure. If a pressure sore or a discolored area develops call your physician or orthotist immediately.

sis wear is critical to its acceptance. Peer support groups established through a scoliosis clinic may help adolescent patients deal with the potential social stigma of orthosis wear and can provide positive role models to assist with intervention compliance.[6]

Resources

Organizations that provide information on scoliosis are listed in Practical Application Box 17-1

Other Spinal Orthoses

Orthoses that are often used for lower thoracic or high lumbar fractures are described as follows.

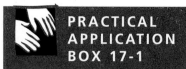

Resources for Scoliosis Information

National Scoliosis Foundation
  5 Cabot Place
  Stoughton, MA 02072
  (617)-341-8333
  http://www.scoliosis.com
The Scoliosis Research Society
  6300 North River Road
  Suite 727
  Rosemont, IL 60018
  (847)-698-1627
  http://srs.org
The Scoliosis Association Inc.
  P.O. Box 811705
  Boca Raton, FL 33481
  (800)-800-0669

Thoracolumbar Anterior Control or Hyperextension Orthosis

There are two types of thoracolumbar anterior control or hyperextension orthoses: the Jewett and the Cruciform Anterior Spinal Hyperextension (CASH) orthosis. The Jewett orthosis consists of an aluminum frame, sternal pad, suprapubic pad, and posterior thoracolumbar pad. It provides a three-point pressure system consisting of posteriorly directed forces from the sternal and suprapubic pads and an anteriorly directed force from the thoracolumbar pad. This configuration encourages a hyperextended posture (Fig. 17-1). With the patient seated in a proper posture and the orthosis properly aligned, the sternal pad will have its superior border $\frac{1}{2}$ inch below the sternal notch and the suprapubic pad will be $\frac{1}{2}$ inch above the symphysis pubis. The Jewett orthosis is most effective in preventing flexion and exten-

sion between T6 and L1. Above T6, the sternal pad may act as a fulcrum and actually increase the amount of motion in the upper thoracic spine.[3] The CASH orthosis is in a cruciform shape. Both of these orthoses use a three-point contact system, as shown in Figure 5-20, to prevent forward flexion of the thoracic spine (Fig. 17-10).

Thoracolumbosacral Orthoses

A TLSO has efficacy in scoliosis intervention and may also be used to restrict motion with vertebral fracture or instability that may result in neurologic damage such as paraplegia. TLSOs are designed to restrict midthoracic, low-thoracic, and lumbosacral movement. Thoracic fractures from T2 to T9 are stabilized by the rib cage. Fractures below T9 often require internal (via surgery) and/or external (via an orthosis) immobilization.[3] TLSOs extend superiorly to the upper chest and may include axillary straps. Inferiorly, the TLSO extends to the lower buttock border and to the inguinal ligaments. As mentioned previously, polypropylene

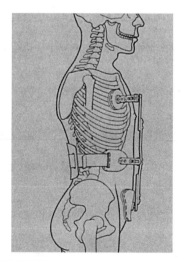

Figure 17-10. Cruciform anterior spinal hyperextension (CASH) orthosis. (Reprinted with permission from Ralph Storrs Inc.)

is often used in the construction of TLSOs and has the disadvantage of retaining body heat (Fig. 17-2).[3]

Lumbosacral Orthoses

LSOs may be divided into two categories, rigid and flexible.

Rigid LSOs

Rigid LSOs may be prefabricated or custom molded to the patient. Rigid LSOs may also include a corset with a rigid thermoplastic insert as well as a proximal leg extension. Each of these rigid LSOs is described as follows.

A prefabricated LSO is the lumbosacral anterior posterior lateral control (Knight) orthosis. This orthosis is often used in fractures of the lumbar spine. The prefabricated LSO is commonly constructed of aluminum and canvas (Fig. 17-11). The aluminum type consists of two lateral uprights, two posterior uprights, pelvic band, thoracic band, and abdominal support. This orthosis provides a

three-point pressure system consisting of posteriorly directed forces from the pelvic and thoracic straps and an anteriorly directed force from the posterior uprights in the lumbar area. This pressure system tends to limit lumbar flexion. A second three-point pressure system consisting of a posteriorly directed force from the abdominal support and anteriorly directed forces from the pelvic and thoracic bands, tends to limit trunk extension occurring in the lumbar spine, to reduce lordosis. Forces from the abdominal support assists in increasing intra-abdominal pressure. Lateral uprights may be added to this orthosis to prevent lateral flexion.[3] The polypropylene type may be prefabricated or custom molded to the patient. The polypropylene orthosis makes use of a circumferential force system (Fig. 17-12).[3]

Stable fractures of the lumbar spine may also be treated with a corset-type orthosis that has a rigid thermoplastic insert. This insert may be heated and molded to the lumbar spine, then put in a pocket of the corset LSO (Fig. 17-13).

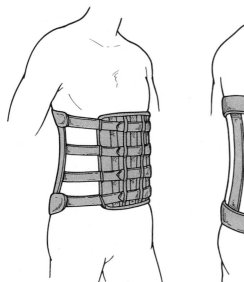
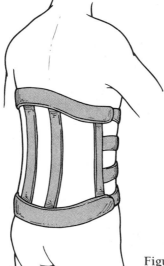

Figure 17-11. Lumbosacral orthosis anterior posterior lateral control (Knight).

Fractures at L5–S1 may need polypropylene rigid lumbar immobilization plus a proximal leg extension. This can be done with a single-leg spica that extends to the lumbar or the thoracic area (Fig. 17-14).

Flexible LSOs

The Flexible LSO, or lumbosacral corset, is a soft, flexible garment that wraps around the torso and hips. Straps suspend the belt like sus-

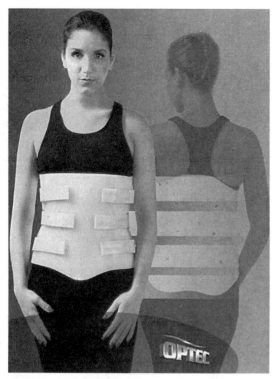

Figure 17-12. OPTEC polypropylene LSO. (Reprinted with permission from OPTEC Inc.)

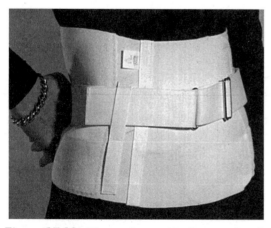

Figure 17-13. Thermoplastic LSO. (Reprinted with permission from Ortho Mold.)

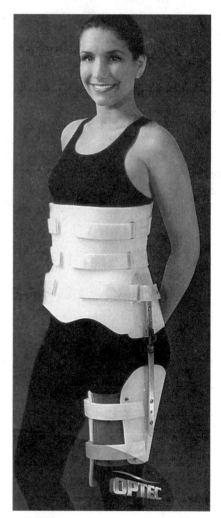

Figure 17-14. OPTEC LSO with hip spica. (Reprinted with permission from OPTEC Inc.)

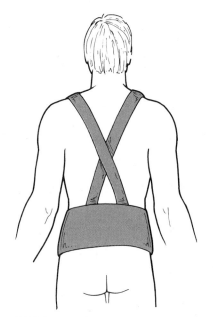

Figure 17-15. Flexible LSO.

penders, forming a "Y" in the back (Fig. 17-15). A flexible LSO may be used to restrict lumbar motion and help the abdominal musculature to elevate intracavity pressure. In the construction and retail occupations, the number of employees wearing these flexible LSOs has increased dramatically during the past several years.[37] Despite widespread use, these LSOs have little scientific support in preventing or reducing low back pain.[38–40] The usefulness of flexible LSOs in increasing intra-abdominal pressure to decrease intradiskal pressure has not been demonstrated conclusively.[41] However, one study done with a small sample of 10 volunteers found that wearing an abdominal belt increased lumbar spine stability. In this study, activities of the thoracic erector spinae in extension and the lumbar erector spinae muscles in flexion were decreased.[42] However, decreased muscle activity may have disadvantages. One study found that prolonged use of a flexible LSO was associated with trunk muscle weakness.[43] Because of these conflicting results, further research is needed to determine the efficacy of flexible LSOs.

Cervical Orthoses

There are three basic designs of cervical orthoses:

1. Orthopedic collars
2. Poster appliances
3. Custom-molded devices

Cervical orthoses, unlike TLSOs or LSOs, which are worn underneath clothing, are conspicuous. This visibility may affect compliance.

Orthopedic Collars

There are many different types of cervical orthopedic collars that may be used for post-trauma or postsurgical stabilization of the cervical spine. Two of the commonly used types of orthopedic collars are described as follows.

Soft Collar

The prefabricated, or off-the-shelf, soft collar is made of foam rubber and covered with cotton stockinette. It fits under the mandible and the occiput and provides minimal unweighting of the spine. The soft collar also serves as a reminder to guard against excessive motion. The soft collar frequently is used in whiplash injuries and minor muscular spasm associated with spondylosis or mild trauma. The collar may be worn in the conventional way with the closure posterior to put the cervical spine into slight flexion. Conversely, if the patient is more comfortable in slight extension, the soft collar may be reversed, with the closure in front. The soft collar should be adjusted to place the head and neck in the most comfortable position during an acute inflammatory phase (Fig. 17-16).

Plastazote Molded Soft Collar

The prefabricated Plastazote molded soft collar consists of molded chin and occipital supports extending down to the upper part of the thorax. This collar is reinforced on the anterior and posterior borders with longitudinal plastic

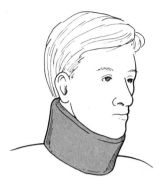

Figure 17-16. Soft cervical collar.

strips and is fastened by Velcro closures at the sides. It is often called a *Philadelphia collar*. It offers more stability than the soft collar; however its overall ability to limit motion is minimal. One study showed that the Plastazote molded soft collar allowed more motion in flexion and lateral bending than a plastic or polyethylene cervical collar. Skin breakdown over the chin has also been reported with this orthosis (Fig. 17-17).[44]

Poster Appliances

For patients who require more immobilization than that provided by an orthopedic collar, two types of poster appliances are commonly used.

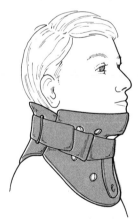

Figure 17-17. Plastazote molded soft collar.

Sternal Occipital Mandibular Immobilization (HCTO SOMI or Three-Poster)

This prefabricated orthosis consists of a rigid metal frame that rests on the front of the chest, with padded straps that pass over the shoulders, adjustable uprights that extend up to the mandibular and occipital supports, and a strap that goes around the trunk. The SOMI only has one anterior support. Since it does not have a back plate, the patient can often lie flat without discomfort (Fig. 17-18).

Cervical Anterior, Posterior, Lateral, and Rotary Control Orthosis (HCTO Four Poster)

This prefabricated orthosis applies forces under the chin and occiput to restrict flexion and extension of the head and the cervical spine. The Four Poster orthosis has mandible and occipital supports and two anterior and two posterior uprights. The front and back compo-

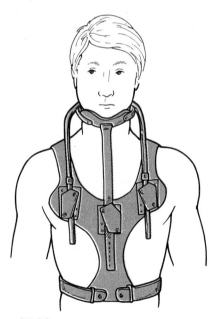

Figure 17-18. Sternal occipital mandibular immobilization (HCTO SOMI or Three Poster).

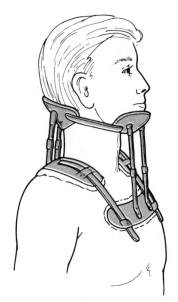

Figure 17-19. Cervical anterior, posterior, lateral, and rotary control orthosis (HCTO Four Poster).

nents are connected by straps around the head and over the shoulders.[45] The thoracic pad should be 1 inch below the inferior angle of the scapula, and the sternal plate should be 1 inch below the sternal notch. The HCTO Four Poster was found to be more effective in controlling midcervical than upper or lower cervical motion (Fig. 17-19).[46]

Custom-Molded Cervical Devices

The halo and the Minerva Body Jacket are two types of custom-molded cervical devices that are commonly used today.

Halo

Indications for the halo are a cervical or high thoracic spine instability or deformity. The halo is a metal ring secured to the periosteum of the skull with four pins. It is connected to the thorax by a prefabricated plastic body vest. The halo is rigidly connected to the body vest by metal uprights that allow adjustment. It controls motion better than any other cervical orthosis. The halo is particularly effective in limiting rotation, lateral bending, flexion, and extension in the upper cervical spine.[46] When precise limitation of upper cervical rotation and lateral flexion is necessary, the halo is the orthosis of choice. The halo may also provide longitudinal distraction of the middle and lower cervical spine. In one investigation, short-term placement of the halo stabilized the patient's neurologic status and facilitated the diagnosis and treatment of associated life-threatening injuries (Fig. 17-20).[47]

Surgical stabilization or internal fixation of the cervical spine may be done anteriorly, posteriorly, or in combination. The duration of immobilization depends on the healing time, the nature of the injury, and the type of surgical stabilization performed. At times, a surgeon may prefer to have the patient initially wear a halo postoperatively and then be weaned to a less restrictive orthosis such as a Plastazote molded soft collar.

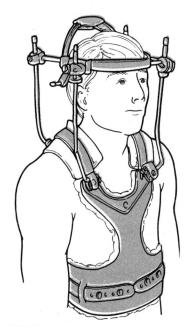

Figure 17-20. Halo Orthosis

While the halo does limit motion, it has not been shown to be effective in stopping cervical motion. A detailed analysis of the effect of the halo on overall cervical motion showed that 31% of motion was allowed.[48] The percentage of motion was greatest at C2/3 and least at C7/T1 (42 and 20%, respectively). One disadvantage of the halo device is pin site infection. Daily cleansing of pin sites minimizes skin and scalp infections. All sites should be swabbed with an antiseptic solution once or twice daily. Additionally, an antibiotic ointment may be applied.[3] Other disadvantages include pin slippage and supraorbital nerve problems. In addition the posts connecting the halo device to the body jacket often inhibit components of early rehabilitation such as rolling and prone activities.[49] One study of 179 patients found pin loosening in 36%, pin infections in 20%, skin problems in 11%, and serious complications such as dysphasia, nerve injury, and dural penetration in 1–2%.[50]

Wearers of a halo device are often more comfortable with a rolled-up towel placed in the cervical lordosis area when lying supine, or next to the cheek when side-lying. There are two excellent brochures concerning the care of a client wearing a halo vest. These are listed in Resource Box 17-2.

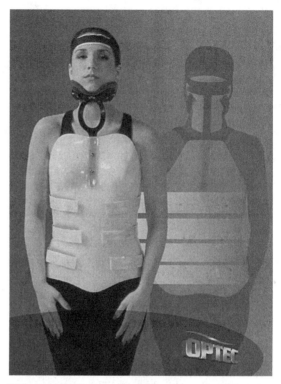

Figure 17-21. OPTEC Minerva CTO. (Reprinted with permission from OPTEC Inc.)

Minerva Cervicothoracic Orthosis (CTO)

The Minerva CTO is a thermoplastic custom-molded jacket that can be used instead of the halo. The Minerva CTO consists of two sections that immobilize the patient's thorax, mandible, and occiput to provide the necessary stabilization of the cervical spine. The bivalved nature of the thermoplastic jacket allows easy removal of either the posterior or anterior half while maintaining cervical alignment with the other half (Fig. 17-21).

Research Studies

There are multiple cervical orthoses available. Recommending a specific one may be confusing. A description of several research studies

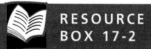

**RESOURCE
BOX 17-2**

Caring for the Client with a Halo Vest
   (caregiver version)
Your Guide to Wearing Your Halo Vest
   (wearer version)
Both are available from Bremer Medical
   4801 Dawin Road, Jacksonville, FL
   32207-9512. (800)-874-4256
Website information:
http://www.nbak.tierranet.com/halo.htm

may be helpful in deciding on a cervical orthosis for a particular patient.

A study comparing the effectiveness of five cervical orthoses found that the halo restricted flexion–extension the most between the occiput and T1. The Four Poster, SOMI, Plastazote molded soft collar, and finally the soft collar restricted motion in descending effectiveness. The soft collar was ineffective in controlling cervical flexion and extension. In addition to the halo, the SOMI was the most effective conventional orthosis in controlling flexion at C1–4. However, it was less effective than the Four Poster in controlling extension. This lack of extension control is because the SOMI's occipital support posterior upright is not rigid enough to restrict motion during voluntary neck extension. Although the SOMI restricts flexion better in the upper and middle cervical regions, the Four Poster is more effective in controlling extension.[46]

A study of 12 patients after surgical stabilization of the upper thoracic or cervical spine and the use of a combination halo–Milwaukee orthosis found that this orthosis was effective and versatile in the management of complex pediatric spinal deformities. This orthosis was well tolerated, allowed access to the posterior incision, and was easily converted to a standard Milwaukee CTLSO.[51]

One study using lateral cervical spine roentgenograms at extremes of flexion and extension found the Minerva CTO effective for limiting flexion and extension of C1–6.[49] Likewise, a study of 16 healthy male volunteers found that the Minerva CTO provided good control of the cervical spine below C1. However, occiput-to-C1 motion was poorly controlled.[52] A study comparing the Minerva and halo jackets found that the average movement from flexion to extension at each intervertebral level was significantly less in the Minerva jacket than with the Halo. This study concluded that the advantages of stability and comfort of the Minerva CTO makes it the orthosis of choice for ambulatory stabilization of most patients with an unstable posttraumatic cervical spine

injury.[53] Precautions with the use of the Minerva CTO are necessary however. One case report of an 83-year-old who wore a Minerva CTO following C1, odontoid, and C3 fractures reported dysphagia complications resulting in aspiration pneumonia. These conditions resolved when the Minerva CTO was replaced with a halo.[54] One investigator advocated use of the halo in immobilizing injuries above C2 and the Minerva for injuries below C2. However, both the halo and Minerva require considerable skill in application and maintenance.[55]

KEY POINTS

- The Committee on Prosthetics–Orthotics Education (CPOE) developed a systematic nomenclature to enhance communication in the area of orthoses.

- Most patients who need spinal orthoses are fitted with prefabricated, or off-the-shelf, orthoses ordered according to measurements. However, it may be difficult to ensure a proper, patient-specific fit with prefabricated orthoses. Custom-made orthoses that are molded to the patient are often considered preferable.

- Spinal orthoses have both beneficial and negative effects.

- The Milwaukee CTLSO and several types of TLSOs are used in the management of scoliosis.

- TLSOs and LSOs may also be used for vertebral fractures or postoperatively after spinal surgery.

- There are three basic designs of cervical orthoses: orthopedic collars, poster appliances, and custom-molded devices.

CRITICAL THINKING QUESTIONS

1. Describe the beneficial and negative effects of a spinal orthosis.

2. Summarize the research regarding different interventions in the care of scoliosis.

3. Compare and contrast the types of orthoses used in the care of the patient with scoliosis.

4. With a group of your classmates, decide what instructions you would give to a patient who wears an orthosis for scoliosis.

5. Describe conditions other than scoliosis in which a spinal orthosis would be indicated.

6. Differentiate the effectiveness of various orthoses in preventing cervical motion.

REFERENCES

1. Licht, S. H. (1966). *Orthotics Etcetera.* Baltimore: Waverly Press.
2. Harris, E. E. (1973). A new orthotics terminology—a guide to its use for prescription and fee schedules. *Orthotics Prosthetics, 27,* 6–19.
3. American Academy of Orthopaedic Surgeons Staff. (1996). *Atlas of orthotics. Biomechanical principles and application,* St. Louis: Mosby-YearBook.
4. Russell, J. N., Hendershot, G. E., LeClere, F., Howie, L. J., & Adler, M. (1994). Trends and differential use of assistive technology devices: United States 1994. *Advance Data, 292,* 3.
5. National Institute of Arthritis and Musculoskeletal Skin Diseases. (1998). *Questions & answers about scoliosis in children & adolescents.*
6. U.S. Preventive Services Task Force. (1993). Screening for adolescent idiopathic scoliosis: policy statement. *JAMA, 269,* 2664–2666.
7. McLain, R. F., & Karol, L. (1994). Conservative treatment of the scoliotic and kyphotic patient: Brace treatment and other modalities. *Archives of Pediatrics and Adolescent Medicine 1994, 148,* 646–651.
8. Tecklin, J. S. (1999). *Pediatric physical therapy* (3rd ed.). Philadelphia: Lippincott Williams & Wilkins.
9. Sullivan, J. A., Davidson, R., & Renshaw, T. S. (1986). Further evaluation of the Scolitron treatment of idiopathic scoliosis. *Spine, 11,* 903–906.
10. Nachemson, A. L., & Peterson, L. E. (1995). Effectiveness of treatment with a brace in girls who have adolescent idiopathic scoliosis. A prospective, controlled study based on data from the Brace Study of the Scoliosis Research Society. *Journal of Bone and Joint Surgery, 77A,* 815–822.
11. Durham, J. W., Moskowitz, A., & Whitney, J. (1989). Surface electrical stimulation versus brace in treatment of idiopathic scoliosis. *Spine, 15,* 888–892.
12. O'Donnell, C. S., Bunnell, W. P., Betz, R. R., Bowen, J. R., & Tipping, C. R. (1988). Electric stimulation in the treatment of idiopathic scoliosis. *Clinical Orthopaedics and Related Research, 229,* 107–113.
13. O'Sullivan, S. B., & Schmitz, T. J. (1988). *Physical rehabilitation: assessment and treatment* (3rd ed.). Philadelphia: F. A. Davis.
14. Rothstein, J. M., Roy, S. H., & Wolf, S. L. (1998). *The rehabilitation specialist's handbook* (2nd ed., pp. 208–209). Philadelphia: F. A. Davis.
15. Cote, P. (1998). A study of the diagnostic accuracy and reliability of the Scoliometer and Adam's forward bend test. *Spine, 23,* 796–803.
16. Keim, H. A. (1982). *The adolescent spine.* New York: Springer-Verlag.
17. Winter, R. B., Lonstein, J. E., Drogt, J., & Noren, C. A. (1986). The effectiveness of bracing in the nonoperative treatment of idiopathic scoliosis. *Spine, 11,* 790–791.
18. Watts, H. G., Hall, J. E., & Stanish, W. (1977). The Boston Brace System for the treatment of low thoracic and lumbar scoliosis by the use of a girdle without superstructure. *Clinical Orthopaedics and Related Research, 126,* 87.
19. Lonstein, J. E., & Winter, R. B. (1989). Milwaukee brace treatment of juvenile idiopathic scoliosis. *Orthopedic Transactions, 13,* 91.
20. Emans, J. B., Kaelin, A., Bancel, P., Hall, J. E., & Miller, M. E. (1986). The Boston Bracing system for idiopathic scoliosis. Follow-up results in 295 patients. *Spine, 11,* 792–801.
21. Muller, E. B., & Nordwall, A. (1994). Brace treatment of scoliosis in children with myelomeningocele. *Spine, 19,* 151–155.
22. Labelle, H., Dansereau, J., Bellefleur, C., & Poitras, B. (1996). Three-dimensional effect of the Boston Brace on the thoracic spine and rib. *Spine, 21,* 59–64.
23. Katsaris, G., Loukos, A., Valavanis, J., Vassiliou, M., & Behrakis, P. K. (1999). The immediate effect of a Boston orthosis on lung volumes and pulmonary compliance in mild adolescent idiopathic scoliosis. *European Spine Journal, 8,* 2–7.
24. Willers, U., Normelli, H., Aaro, S., Svensson, O., & Hedlund, R. (1993). Long term results of Boston Brace treatment on vertebral rotation in idiopathic scoliosis. *Spine, 18,* 432–435.

25. Goldberg, C. J., Dowling, F. E., Hall, J. E., & Emans, J. B. (1993). A statistical comparison between natural history of idiopathic scoliosis and brace treatment in skeletally immature adolescent girls. *Spine, 18,* 902–908.

26. Wever, D. J., Tonseth, K. A., Veldhuizen, A. G., Cool, J. C., & van Horn, J. R. (2000). Curve progression and spinal growth in brace treated idiopathic scoliosis. *Clinical Orthopaedics and Related Research, 377,* 169–179.

27. Bassett, G. S., & Bunnell, W. P. (1987). Influence of the Wilmington orthosis on spinal decompensation in adolescent idiopathic scoliosis. *Clinical Orthopaedics and Related Research, 223,* 164–169.

28. Price, C. T., Scott, D. S., Reed, F. E., Riddick, M. (1990). Night-time bracing for adolescent idiopathic scoliosis with the Charleston Bending Brace: Preliminary report. *Spine, 15,* 1294–1299.

29. Montgomery, F., & Willner, S. (1989). Prognosis of brace treated scoliosis. Comparison of the Boston and Milwaukee methods in 244 girls. *Acta Orthopaedica Scandinavica, 60,* 383–385.

30. Mellencamp, D. D., Blount, W. P., & Anderson, A. J. (1977). Milwaukee brace treatment of idiopathic scoliosis: Late results. *Clinical Orthopaedics and Related Research, 126,* 47–57.

31. Edmonson, A. S., & Smith, G. R. (1983). Long term follow-up study of Milwaukee brace treatment in patients with idiopathic scoliosis. *Orthopedic Transactions, 7,* 10

32. Noonan, K. J., Dolan, L. A., Jacobson, W. C., & Weinstein, S. L. (1997). Long-term psychosocial characteristics of patients treated for idiopathic scoliosis. *Journal of Pediatric Orthopedics, 17,* 712–717.

33. Olafsson, Y., Saraste, H., & Ahlgren, R. M. (1999). Does bracing affect self-image? A prospective study on 54 patients with adolescent idiopathic scoliosis. *European Spine Journal, 8,* 402–405.

34. Howard, A., Wright, J. G., & Hedden, D. (1998). A comparative study of TLSO, Charleston, and Milwaukee braces for idiopathic scoliosis. *Spine, 23,* 2404–2411.

35. Katz, D. E., Richards, B. S., Brone, R. H., & Herring, J. A. (1997). A comparison between the Boston Brace and the Charleston Bending Brace in adolescent idiopathic scoliosis. *Spine, 22,* 1302–1312.

36. Rowe, D. E., Bernstein, S. M., Riddick, M. F., Adler, F., Emans, J. B., & Gardner-Bonneau, D. (1997). A meta-analysis of the efficacy of non-operative treatments for idiopathic scoliosis. *Journal of Bone and Joint Surgery, 79A,* 664–674.

37. Redford, J. B. (1986). *Orthotics etcetera* (3rd ed.). Baltimore: Williams & Wilkins.

38. Green, N. E. (1986). Part time bracing of adolescent idiopathic scoliosis. *Journal of Bone and Joint Surgery, 68A,* 738–742.

39. Peltonen, J., Poussa, M., & Ylikoski, M. (1988). Three year results of bracing in scoliosis. *Acta Orthopaedica Scandinavica, 59,* 487–490.

40. Gurnham, R. B. (1983). Adolescent compliance with spinal brace wear. *Orthopedic Nursing, 2,* 13–17.

41. Minor, S. D. (1996). Use of back belts in occupational settings. *Physical Therapy, 76,* 403–408.

42. Cholewicki, J., Juluru, K., Radebold, A., Panjabi, M. M., & McGill, S. M. (1999). Lumbar spine stability can be augmented with an abdominal belt and/or increased intra-abdominal pressure. *European Spine Journal, 8,* 388–395.

43. Eisinger, D. B., Kumar, R., & Woodrow, R. (1996). Effect of lumbar orthotics on trunk muscle strength. *American Journal of Physical Medicine and Rehabilitation, 75,* 194–197.

44. McCabe, J. B., & Nolan, D. J. (1986). Comparison of the effectiveness of different cervical immobilization collars. *Annals of Emergency Medicine, 15,* 50–53.

45. Johnson, R. M., Owen, J. R., Hart, D. L., & Callahan, R. A. (1981). Cervical orthoses: A guide to their selection and use. *Clinical Orthopaedics and Related Research, 154,* 34–45.

46. Johnson, R. M., Hart, D. L., Simmons, E. F., Ramsby, G. R., & Southwick, W. O. (1977). Cervical orthoses. A study comparing their effectiveness in restricting cervical motion in normal subjects. *Journal of Bone and Joint Surgery, 59A,* 332–339.

47. Heary, R. F., Hunt, C. D., Krieger, A. J., Antonio, C., & Livingston, D. H. (1992). Acute stabilization of the cervical spine by halo/vest application facilitates evaluation and treatment of multiple trauma patients. *Journal of Trauma Injury Infection and Critical Care, 33,* 445–451.

48. Koch, R. A., & Nickel, V. L. (1978). The halo vest: An evaluation of motion and forces across the neck. *Spine, 3,* 103–107.

49. Millington, P. J., Ellingsen, J. M., Hauswirth, B. E., & Fabian, P. J. (1987). Thermoplastic Minerva Body Jacket—a practical alternative to current methods of cervical spine stabilization. *Physical Therapy, 67,* 223–225.

50. Garfin, S. R., Botte, M. J., Waters, R. L., & Nickel, V. L. (1986). Complications in the use of the Halo fixation device. *Journal of Bone and Joint Surgery, 68,* 320–325.

51. Godfried, D. H., Amory, D. W., & Lubicky, J. P. (1999). The Halo–Milwaukee brace. Case series of a revived technique. *Spine, 24,* 2273–2277.

52. Sharpe, K. P., Rao, S., & Ziogas, A. (1995). Evaluation of the effectiveness of the Minerva cervicothoracic orthosis. *Spine,* 20: 1475–1479.

53. Benzel, E. C., Hadden, T. A., & Saulsbery, C. M. (1989). A comparison of the Minerva and halo jackets for stabilization of the cervical spine. *Journal of Neurosurgery, 70,* 411–414.

54. Odderson, I. R., & Lietzow, D. (1997). Dysphagia complications of the Minerva Brace. *Archives of Physical Medicine and Rehabilitation, 78,* 1386–1388.

55. Pringle, R. G. (1990). Halo versus Minerva—which orthosis? *Paraplegia, 28,* 281–284.

Case Studies in *Guide to Physical Therapist Format*

APPENDIX

Case Studies

These three case studies present patient examples in a format used in the *Guide to Physical Therapist Practice*.[1] Each of these cases has examples of information taken from the history, systems review, tests, and measures, as well as outcome and procedural intervention examples. For more detailed information, the reader should refer to the chapters that pertain to each of these cases. Answers to the types of procedural interventions that should be designed for each of these cases are given at the end of all the case studies.

C A S E   1

PATIENT/CLIENT HISTORY

General Demographics

The patient, DM, is a 26-year-old, English-speaking male who had a left transtibial amputation 6 weeks ago secondary to infection. DM has poorly controlled type 1 diabetes.

History of Current Condition

DM has not been compliant with diet, exercise, or insulin regimens. He developed a left plantar surface foot infection that became gangrenous. A left transtibial amputation was done 3 weeks ago. He has been discharged from the hospital and is in a subacute rehabilitation unit affiliated with a large general hospital. Goals for this episode of care are completion of a preprosthetic training program and independence in all activities of daily living.

Social History

DM lives with his mother and 17-year-old sister. His father is absent. His mother works two jobs, one as a factory worker during the day, the other as an evening janitorial worker.

Occupation/Employment

DM has not worked for the past 2 years. He left school at age 16 because of multiple suspensions for disruptive behavior. He reads at a 7th grade level. He has rejected opportunities to obtain a high school equivalency diploma (GED).

Growth and Development

He is right handed. His foot dominance was not assessed.

Living Environment

He lives with his mother and sister in a three-bedroom mobile home. The home has two wooden steps leading to the back door and three concrete steps leading to the front door. No stair rails are present. The terrain from the carport to the mobile home is uneven. DM and his mother have a strained relationship because of DM's behavioral problems, including verbal abuse, inattention, and refusal to adhere to good health practices.

Functional Status and Activity Level

DM is independent in all activities of daily living with the exception of needing minimal assistance in wheelchair transfers to bed, commode, and shower chair. He is able to ambulate with minimal assist of one, using axillary crutches, non–weight bearing on left, for a distance of 30 feet. He fatigues quickly and must stop to rest for 5 minutes before continuing ambulation.

Medications

7.5/500 mg PRN Vicodin for pain
600 mg PRN Motrin for pain
100 mg PRN Colace for constipation
500 mg QID Keflex for infection
40 units Q AM 70/30 insulin for blood glucose level
25 units Q AM 70/30 insulin for blood glucose level

If blood sugar level exceeds 150, insulin is provided on a sliding scale, depending on the blood sugar level.

DM admits to daily marijuana use prior to the amputation and 1 pack/day cigarette use. Before this hospitalization, he drank two 40-oz bottles of beer per day. He denies use of other illicit drugs.

Other Tests and Measures

Laboratory Tests	DM Values	Normal Values[2]
WBC	12.8 mm³	5-10 mm³
RBC	4.0 million/mm³	4.8 million/mm³
HGB	11.0 g/dL	14–16.5 g/dL
HCT	34.0%	40–50%
Serum albumin	2.7 g/dL	3.5–5.0 g/dL
Calcium	8.0 mg/dL	8.5–10.5 mg/dL
Glucose	343 mg/dL, fasting	70–110 mg/dL, fasting

Laboratory values indicate a low-grade inflammatory response, resolving blood loss, and/or recovery from injury. His high glucose level shows poorly controlled diabetes.

Past History of Current Condition

Since his diagnosis of type 1 diabetes at age 12, DM has not been compliant with diet, exercise, or insulin regimens.

Past Medical/Surgical History

DM has had multiple sores on both feet, which have healed with topical antibiotic ointments. No known allergies.

Family History

DM's mother, maternal grandmother, and two maternal uncles have type 1 diabetes.

Health Status

Patient is overweight, sedentary, withdrawn, and often hostile.

Social Habits

DM has few friends, and he seldom interacts with other patients or staff on the subacute rehabilitation unit. His sister has been prohibited from bringing foods such as candy bars and potato chips into the subacute rehabilitation unit for DM.

TESTS AND MEASURES

These tests and measures have been put in the order of most importance.

Aerobic Capacity and Endurance

Respiratory rate, blood pressure, and heart rate are as follows at rest and after ambulating a distance of 30 feet using axillary crutches, non–weight bearing on the left.

Activity	Respiratory Rate	Blood Pressure	Heart Rate
Rest	24 breaths/min	138/88	90 bpm
After ambulation	28 breaths/min	160/90	115 bpm

Self-Care and Home Management

DM is independent in most activities of daily living. He needs minimal assistance in wheelchair transfers to bed, commode, and shower chair. He is anxious to return home to live with his mother and sister. His mother is supportive and willing to learn aspects of her son's care; however, she is distracted by financial concerns and the intermittent verbal abuse from her son.

Gait, Locomotion, and Balance

DM is able to ambulate with minimal assist of one, using axillary crutches, non–weight bearing on right for a distance of 30 feet. He quickly fatigues and must stop and rest for 5 minutes before continuing ambulation.

Integumentary Integrity

DM has a well-healed incision over the anterior distal surface approximately 23 cm (9 in.) below the inferior pole of the patella. There is edema present over the distal residual limb. The residual limb has a slightly bulbous appearance. Measurements are as follows:

Length from Inferior Pole of the Patella (cm)	Right Side (cm)	Left (Transtibial Residual Limb) Side (cm)
4	34	35
8	36	37
12	37	40
16	37	42
20	38	43

The skin is shiny and cool over the dorsum of the right foot. No hair is present on the dorsum of the toes or foot.

Pain

DM rates the pain in his left transtibial residual limb as 2/10 at rest; pain increases to 4/10 when the limb is in a dependent position and 6/10 when ambulating. He reports mild pain in his right foot when walking more than 200 feet.

Range of Motion

Range of motion is within normal limits except for left knee flexion, which is limited to 90°, and knee extension, which is lacking 10° from neutral. Right knee flexion is 125°, extension is 0°. Left ankle and foot measurements are not applicable.

Muscle Performance

Strength 5/5 overall except for left hip and knee strength, which is 4/5

Sensory Integrity

DM has decreased sensitivity to light touch and pinprick in the right (sound) foot. He cannot feel the touch of a 5.07 Semmes-Weinstein monofilament, indicating a loss of protective sensation. He is hypersensitive to light touch over the left residual limb.

Circulation

DM has an absence of the right dorsal pedis and posterior tibial pulses to palpation. An ankle brachial index (ABI) of 0.70 is present. An ABI between 0.50 and 0.75 indicates significant arterial symptomatology, including lower extremity pain with walking and rest pain.

Anthropometric Characteristics

Height 183 cm (6 ft. 0 in.); weight 102 kg (225 lb); BMI 29, indicating an overweight BMI

Arousal, Attention, and Cognition

Within normal limits

Assistive and Adaptive Devices

DM uses axillary crutches.

Work, Community, and Leisure Integration or Reintegration

DM has not worked for the past 2 years. He states he would like to resume playing basketball.

Environmental, Home, and Work Barriers

see "Living Environment" under "Patient/Client History" above.

Joint Integrity and Mobility

Within normal limits

Motor Function

Good coordination of the left residual limb in space

Orthotic, Protective, and Supportive Devices

DM wears a removable rigid dressing over the left transtibial residual limb. He has a wheelchair that belongs to the rehabilitation unit, with an elevating leg rest to assist in left knee extension.

Prosthetic Requirements

A transtibial prosthesis has been ordered consisting of patellar bearing (PTB) socket, sleeve suspension, and Carbon Copy II foot.

EVALUATION

DM is an overweight, deconditioned 26-year-old male with a variety of impairments. These include poor endurance, a slightly bulbous residual limb, weak left hip and knee strength, pain, limitation of right knee flexion, and dependence in transfers. Other problems include a history of poorly controlled blood glucose levels, lack of sensation and circulation in his sound foot including a low ABI, verbal abuse toward his mother, and problem drinking. He has a well-healed left transtibial residual limb.

DIAGNOSIS

The results of tests and measures show that DM's condition is consistent with a practice pattern of "Impaired Gait, Locomotion, and Balance and Impaired Motor Function Secondary to Lower Extremity Amputation" (4J). He has a left transtibial residual limb, with decreased sensation and circulation in his right foot.[1]

PROGNOSIS

The expected number of visits per episode of care according to practice pattern 4J ranges from 15 to 45. It is anticipated that 80% of the patients in this diagnostic group will achieve outcomes within 12 to 112 visits during a single continuous episode of care. It is estimated that DM will need 30 physical therapy visits. Even though DM is young, he may not be successful in achieving these outcomes because of his medical and behavioral problems.[1]

PROCEDURAL INTERVENTIONS

Manual Therapy Techniques

Mobilization techniques may be used on the left knee to increase knee flexion and extension.

Prescription, Application, and Fabrication of Devices and Equipment

DM may benefit from a soft vamp, high toe-box, and rocker bottom to avoid skin irritation for his right foot. Shoe modifications are reviewed in Chapter 16.

Primary Prevention/Risk Factor Reduction Strategies

DM is at risk for skin lesions or possible amputation of his right foot. He needs interventions by a diabetic educator, nutritionist, and physical therapist as described above in this case. In addition, a right shoe with modifications should be secured to prevent problems in an insensitive right foot.

Procedural Interventions

Questions

1a. Therapeutic exercise. What types of therapeutic exercise activities should be designed for DM? Refer to Chapter 7 for additional exercise suggestions.

1b. Functional training in self-care and home management. What arrangements need to be made in this area?

1c. Functional training in community and work integration or reintegration. What types of referrals to other health professionals are indicated?

1d. Goals/outcomes. Design short-term (2 weeks or less) and long-term (more than 2 weeks) impairment, functional, and disability goals for DM.

CASE 2

PATIENT/CLIENT HISTORY

General Demographics

The patient (WN) is an 87-year-old English-speaking male who was wounded in 1945 in World War II, resulting in a right transfemoral amputation.

History of Current Condition

WN is presently hospitalized in a Veterans Administration hospital. The hospitalization is due to a fall 2 weeks ago resulting in a left subcapital, impacted femoral fracture. A left total hip arthroplasty (THA) with an anterior lateral approach was done 10 days ago. The right transfemoral residual limb is abraded because of the fall, and the prosthesis was damaged. Goals for this episode of care in a general hospital setting include improvement in strength and functional activity independence. WN is scheduled to be discharged to a subacute rehabilitation facility in his hometown.

Social History

WN has been widowed for 13 years, has no children, lives alone, and relies on friends for transportation. His only surviving relatives include a 90-year-old sister who resides in a local nursing home and a grandniece who lives 2000 miles away. He is involved in Masonic Lodge activities and likes to play cards, read, collect coins, and watch television.

Occupation/Employment

WN has a high school education and is retired from his work as a cashier. Income per month is $730.00 from Social Security and $2112.00 from a service-connected disability.

Growth and Development

He is right handed. His foot dominance was not assessed.

Living Environment

WN lives in a split-level home; staircases have two railings. No elevator is available. His neighbor does not consider it safe for WN to live alone.

Functional Status and Activity Level

WN is able to feed himself; grooming, dressing, and toileting activities require verbal cues to minimal supervision. A lightweight, narrow wheelchair with removable armrests, elevating leg rests, antitipping devices, and seat belt has been ordered. A lightweight wheelchair is needed to facilitate propulsion and ease of transportation. He requires verbal cues to lock the wheelchair brakes, maneuver the leg rests, and propel the wheelchair 10 feet. WN needs moderate assistance with a transfer board to transfer from wheelchair to bed. He is not able to stand. The socket of his prosthesis is cracked because of the fall and needs to be replaced.

Medications

WN is currently taking the following medications:

650 mg PRN Tylenol for pain
0.4 mg PRN nitroglycerine for angina
25 mg QD atenolol for high blood pressure
100 mg PRN docusate for constipation
5 mg oxybutynin chloride (Ditropan) for prostate enlargement
Ensure Nutrition Supplement for weight gain

Other Tests and Measures

Laboratory values and normal values are as follows:

Laboratory Tests	WN Values	Normal Values[2]
WBC	13.2 mm³	5–10 mm³
RBC	3.72 million/mm³	4.8 million/mm³
HGB	10.8 g/dL	14–16.5 g/dL
HCT	32.1%	40–54%
Glucose	119 mg/dL	70–110 mg/dL, fasting
Creatinine	0.7 mg/dL	0.6–1.5 mg/dL
Urea nitrogen (BUN)	12 mg/dL	8–25 mg/dL
Serum albumin	2.7 g/dL	3.5–5.0 g/dL
K	4.4 mEq/L	3.5–5.0 mEq/L
Na	134 mEq/L	135–145 mEq/L
Chloride	100 mmol/L	100–108 mmol/L
Calcium	8.0 mg/dL	8.5–10.5 mg/dL

Laboratory values indicate a low-grade inflammatory response, resolving blood loss, and/or recovery from injury. Patient has a history of poor nutrition and hydration.

Past History of Current Condition

Patient had physical therapy after his right transfemoral amputation. He has had occasional visits to prosthetic facilities since 1945.

Past Medical/Surgical History

HN has a 20-year history of hypertension and angina
Moderate degenerative disk disease and osteophytes are scattered throughout the lumbar spine
Enlarged prostate that indents urinary flow
Heart slightly enlarged
Wears condom catheter
No known allergies

Family History

Mother and father died at ages 78 and 74 due to heart disease.

Health Status

Patient reports poor nutrition, decreased vision from cataracts, difficulty hearing, and pain in left hip from fracture and THA.

Social Habits

WN drinks occasionally, does not smoke or take recreational drugs.

TESTS AND MEASURES

These tests and measures have been put in the order of most importance.

Aerobic Capacity and Endurance

Respiratory rate, blood pressure, and heart rate are as follows at rest and after range-of-motion and strengthening activities:

Activity	Respiratory Rate	Blood Pressure	Heart Rate
Rest	26 breaths/min	130/84	92 bpm
After activity	30 breaths/min	164/92	118 bpm

Muscle Performance

Strength is as follows:

Movement	Right	Left
Hip flexion	4/5	3+/5
Hip extension	4/5	2/5
Hip abduction	4/5	2/5
Hip adduction	4/5	n/a[b]
Hip internal rotation	4/5	n/a[b]
Hip external rotation	4/5	n/a[b]
Knee flexion	n/a[a]	3+/5
Knee extension	n/a[a]	3+/5
Ankle dorsiflexion	n/a[a]	3/5
Ankle plantarflexion	n/a[a]	3/5

[a] Not applicable because of right transfemoral amputation.
[b] Not applicable because of THA precautions.

Integumentary Integrity

A 5-in. (11 cm) well-healing incision is present over the lateral aspect of the left proximal femur. A well-healing 3 by 3 in. (6.6 cm) abrasion is present over the distal anterior aspect of the right transfemoral limb. Both areas are covered with Curasol 4x4 dressings. A well-healed incision is present over the distal aspect of the right transfemoral residual limb. A 3 by 1 in. (6.6 by 2.2 cm) callus is present over the medial incision line.

Assistive and Adaptive Devices

WN is presently unable to stand or ambulate. Prior to his fall, he was ambulating independently with forearm crutches, with partial weight bearing on the right transfemoral prosthesis.

Gait, Locomotion, and Balance

WN can stand with moderate support of two and a walker. He can place his right transfemoral residual limb on a mat and partially weight bear on the left lower extremity. His right transfemoral prosthesis is being repaired.

Self-Care and Home Management

WN can feed himself. Grooming, dressing, and toileting activities require verbal cues to minimal supervision. He can propel a wheelchair 10 feet with verbal cues.

Sensory Integrity

WN has decreased response to light touch and pinprick on the calloused area over the medial incision line. Otherwise, sensation is intact.

Motor Function

Poor coordination of the right transfemoral residual limb

Prosthetic Requirements

WN has a transfemoral prosthesis with quadrilateral socket, pelvic band suspension, single-axis constant-friction knee, and SACH foot. The prosthetic socket is being repaired, and a manual-lock knee will be substituted for the single-axis constant-friction knee. The manual-lock knee will increase knee stability.

Range of Motion

Range of motion in all four extremities is within normal limits except for left hip, which was not assessed because of THA precautions.

Pain

Because of confusion, WN cannot rate the pain in his left hip and denies any phantom pain in the right transfemoral residual limb.

Anthropometric Characteristics

Height 175.3 cm (5 ft.9 in.); weight 66 kg (145 lbs); BMI 18.9 (5%) indicating a slightly underweight BMI

Arousal, Attention, and Cognition

WN is pleasant; he is confused at times to place and time. He denies depression, anxiety, or anger and has been referred to the Memory Disorders Clinic of the Veterans Administration hospital.

Environmental, Home, and Work Barriers

Not assessed, since WN will likely not be going home

Ergonomics and Body Mechanics

Not assessed, since WN is not independent in self-care or working

Circulation

Left dorsal pedis and posterior tibial pulses are present. ABI is 1.2, indicating normal blood flow.

EVALUATION

The patient is an 87-year-old male with a right transfemoral amputation and a left THA. He will benefit from intensive rehabilitation to enable functional activities with a minimum of supervision. Impairments include confusion to place and time, inability to stand independently or ambulate, decreased strength (left more affected than the right), and inability to transfer or perform activities of daily living. He has poor safety awareness, poor insights of impairments, poor awareness of THA precautions, and poor short-term memory.

DIAGNOSIS

The results of tests and measures show that WN's condition is consistent with two practice patterns: "Impaired Gait, Locomotion, and Balance and Impaired Motor Function Secondary to Lower Extremity Amputation" (4J) and "Impaired Integumentary Integrity Secondary to Skin Involvement Extending Into Fascia, Muscle, or Bone and Scar Formation" (7E). WN has impaired functional ability secondary to a right transfemoral amputation and left femoral fracture.[1]

PROGNOSIS

The expected range of number of visits per episode of care according to practice patterns 4J and 7E are 15 to 45 and 12 to 90, respectively. It is anticipated that 80% of the patients in this diagnostic group will achieve outcomes within 15 to 45 or 12 to 90 visits, respectively, during a single continuous episode of care. It is estimated that 70 physical therapy visits will be necessary. Because of WN's confusion to place and time and poor safety awareness, he may not be successful in achieving these outcomes in this time period.[1]

PRIMARY PREVENTION/RISK FACTOR REDUCTION STRATEGIES

Due to mental confusion, decreased vision, and pain in the left hip, WN is at risk for further falls. Presently, he cannot safely live alone and will need the care of a subacute rehabilitation facility. The Memory Disorders Clinic of the Veterans Administration hospital may assist in strategies to improve his mental capacities.

PROCEDURAL INTERVENTIONS

Prescription, Application, and Fabrication of Devices and Equipment

WN will need instruction in operation of a manual-lock prosthetic knee as well as retraining in application and removal of a transfemoral prosthesis.

Questions:

2a. Therapeutic exercise. What types of therapeutic exercise activities should be designed for WN? Refer to Chapter 7 for additional exercise suggestions.

2b. Functional training in self-care and home management. What types of functional training need to be done in this case?

2c. Goals/outcomes. Design short-term (2 weeks or less) and long-term (more than 2 weeks) impairment, functional, and disability goals for WN.

CASE 3

PATIENT/CLIENT HISTORY

General Demographics

The patient (LV) is an 7-year-old male who is bilingual in English and Spanish.

History of Current Condition

LV has a diagnosis of spastic diplegia cerebral palsy. LV has experienced hypertonus in both lower extremities and has received two separate botox injections in bilateral gastrocnemius muscles. He is being considered for a subcutaneous baclofen pump that is designed to decrease the spasticity in the lower extremities but will not affect the trunk or upper extremities. After insertion of a subcutaneous baclofen pump and strengthening, endurance, and motor-learning activities, goals of this episode of care in an outpatient setting include increasing selective muscle control and increasing gait parameters.

Social History

LV lives with his parents and 8-year-old brother who is developing typically. The patient plays modified baseball.

Occupation/Employment

The patient is in the regular second grade in a neighborhood public school. He uses a wheelchair to change classes but does ambulate using forearm crutches and bilateral DAFOs around the classroom.

Growth and Development

LV was born at 36 weeks gestation, with a birth weight of 5 lb. Development history was characterized by significant gross motor delay but no delay in verbal skills. He is right hand dominant. His foot dominance was not assessed.

Living Environment

LV lives in a single-level ranch home with two steps to get into the side door. His home is equipped with a ramp and is wheelchair accessible. He uses both his wheelchair and crutches around the house.

Functional Status and Activity Level

LV is independent in feeding, toileting, and most dressing activities. He needs moderate assistance to put on DAFOs and sneakers. LV requires moderate assistance of one to stand. He is independent in wheelchair-to-bed and wheelchair-to-commode transfers. LV requires the use of forearm crutches to walk around his house. He ambulates in the classroom but not in the community.

Medications

None

Other Tests and Measures

Gait analysis reports show greater than normal bilateral hip flexion, knee flexion, and ankle plantarflexion throughout most of stance and swing phases. Gait parameters of LV and typically developing individuals are shown below.

Gait Parameter	LV	Typically Developing[3]
Step length	31 cm	50 cm
Walking velocity	0.748 m/s	1.18 m/s
Cadence	136 steps/min	150 steps/min

In summary, LV walked with a shorter step length, lower walking velocity, lower cadence than to a typically developing 7-year-old.

Past History of Current Condition

LV receives physical and occupational therapy twice a week in 45-minute sessions while in school. Activities consist of flexibility, functional activities, and gait training.

Past Medical/Surgical History

Parents and LV have no history of toxic substance exposure or tranquilizer use. No known allergies.

Family History

No contributing factors

Health Status

Otherwise healthy

Social Habits

Enjoys playing modified baseball and watching major league baseball

TESTS AND MEASURES

These tests and measures have been put in the order of most importance.

Muscle Performance

Strength and endurance were examined through functional positions for the ability to hold and move through available ranges. Trunk flexion, hip flexion and knee flexion were tested by assuming and holding a "curled" position while supine. LV can partially lift his head and flex his hips and knees ($\frac{1}{2}$ range); holding, and repeating for a maximum of six times. Hip and knee extension were tested by assuming and holding a bridge position while in supine. LV could partially raise ($\frac{1}{2}$ range) hips and hold for a maximum of six repetitions. Knee extension was achieved through partial range in coming to stand for a maximum of three repetitions.

Neuromotor Development and Sensory Integration

Grading on a selectivity scale of voluntary movement of the lower extremities is as follows:

0–only patterned movement observed
1–partially isolated movement observed
2–complete isolated movement observed

Movement	Right	Left
Hip flexion	1	1
Hip extension	2	2
Hip abduction	2	2
Hip adduction	2	2
Knee flexion	1	1
Knee extension	2	2
Ankle dorsiflexion	1	1
Ankle plantarflexion	2	2
Ankle eversion	2	2
Ankle inversion	2	2

LV assumes a bilateral, crouched stance with excessive hip flexion, knee flexion, and ankle dorsiflexion while wearing DAFOs. LV cannot walk without DAFOs. LV initiates the walking sequence with the upper trunk and arms first, followed by the legs. More complete gait parameters are noted in the history.

LV demonstrates head and trunk righting, equilibrium reactions of protective extension of the upper extremities in long sitting and in standing with the use of crutches, and occasional stepping responses to challenges of balance in standing. Postural reactions in long sitting include the use of the upper extremities in a protective extension pattern forward and laterally with ease and backward with increased effort. In standing with crutches, the same patterns of protective extension emerge, with occasional forward stepping.

Orthotic, Protective, and Supportive Devices

LV can independently fasten and unfasten his wheelchair seat belt, lock brakes, remove leg rests, and maneuver through straight distances. He can put on hinged DAFOs with a 90° posterior or plantarflexion stop and sneakers with moderate assistance. He can fasten and unfasten straps and ties to remove the DAFOs and sneakers independently. LV needs minimal assistance to come to stand and secure forearm crutches. Once the forearm crutches are in place, he can ambulate independently.

Assistive and Adaptive Devices

See information under "Orthotics, Protective, and Supportive Devices."

Aerobic Capacity and Endurance

All values are age appropriate. Adequate expansion movement in the chest wall is noted.

Activity	Respiratory Rate	Blood Pressure	Heart Rate
At rest	22 breaths/min	100/70	125 bpm
After ambulation 153 m (500 feet)	33 breaths/min	110/74	130 bpm

Posture

LV has a slight thoracic kyphotic curve when in a short-sitting position. In standing, LV assumes a bilateral, crouched stance with excessive hip flexion, knee flexion, and ankle dorsiflexion.

Range of Motion

Range of motion is within normal limits except for bilateral ankle dorsiflexion, which is limited 15° from neutral in the knee-extended position. This indicates tightness in the gastrocnemius muscle. Bilateral dorsiflexion with the knee flexed is 0°, indicating less tightness in the soleus muscle than in the gastrocnemius. In addition, bilateral knee extension is limited 20° from neutral in a straight-leg (popliteal angle) position with the hip at 90° of flexion. In a Thomas test position, LV is missing 10° bilaterally from a neutral hip position, indicating tightness of the hip flexors.

Self-Care and Home Management

See "Orthotics, Protective, and Supportive Devices" under "Tests and Measures" above.

Gait, Locomotion, and Balance

LV can sit in the wheelchair and on a chair without arms, independently. Posture in sitting is slightly kyphotic, with head forward, but LV can assume full upright posture with verbal cues. He cannot come to stand without minimal assistance of his arms to initiate and cannot stand without support. He can stand and walk independently with support of forearm crutches while wearing DAFOs. LV walks with a reciprocal pattern on level ground, approximately 153 m (500 feet).

Reflex Integrity

Hyperreflexia is noted at the knees with a 3+ response (exaggerated response) and a 4+ (brisk response with intermittent clonus) at the ankles. Hypertonus is examined by changing the speed of the passive movements. With increased speed, hip flexors offer slight resistance. With increased speed, knee flexors and ankle dorsiflexors also offer greater resistance by catching or stopping the motion and then allowing the motion to continue. Developmental reflexive movement patterns such as an asymmetric tonic neck reflex (ATNR) can be elicited in the upper body and a flexor withdrawal in the lower body but are not obligatory.

Cranial and Peripheral Nerve Integrity

LV demonstrates appropriate response to visual tracking and auditory stimulus by locating sound. He is slow to respond to vestibular stimulus such as righting the body to tilting while sitting.

Anthropometric Characteristics

Height 122 cm (48 in.); weight 154 kg (70 lb)

Arousal, Attention, and Cognition

LV is alert and attentive during the examination. He can follow three-step verbal directions.

Work, Community, and Leisure Integration or Reintegration

Use of the School Function Assessment[4] allows description of LV's current performance of "travel" within the school environment. With a criterion score of 54 and a standard error of 2, LV is compared with the grade-level criterion of 100. Specifically, LV can partially or inconsistently perform "travel" via ambulation with forearm crutches in activities such as moving in line with classmates, moving in aisles, moving freely around the room, and keeping pace with peers as needed. He requires adaptations such as more time, supervision, and movement of obstacles in the environment by an adult to ambulate within the school environment.

Environmental, Home, and Work Barriers

Not tested; report of environment in history

Integumentary Integrity

No reddened areas noted on feet and legs after removing orthoses

Joint Integrity and Mobility

No joint hypermobility or hypomobility noted.

Pain

No complaints of pain

Sensory Integrity

Intact responses to superficial sensations of touch, temperature, and pressure. Intact responses to vision and hearing screening. Delays in response to vestibular stimulation equal in all directions.

EVALUATION

LV is a 7-year-old with a diagnosis of diplegia. LV and his parents' primary goal is to ambulate independently in school for longer distances to stay up with his peers. Achievement of improved ambulation, according to Gage,[5] includes the following:

1. Improvement in alignment to assist increased knee extension by allowing the ground reaction force (GRF) to move anterior to the knee
2. Improvement in foot clearance during swing
3. Reduction of spasticity surrounding the knee

LV's selective muscle control is unequal, resulting in better control of hip extension, abduction, and adduction; knee extension; and ankle plantarflexion. LV has limited strength and endurance in hip, knee, and ankle flexion and extension as well as hyperreflexia at the knees and ankles. Hamstring tightness affects alignment at the knees. His current DAFOs are not helping to limit crouch-knee posture. He is being evaluated for a subcutaneous baclofen pump. The pump will address the hyperreflexia noted in the lower extremities.

DIAGNOSIS

The results of tests and measures show that LV's condition is consistent with a practice pattern of "Impaired Motor Function and Sensory Integrity Associated With Congenital or Acquired Disorders of the Central Nervous System in Infancy, Childhood, and Adolescence" (5C). LV has impaired lower-extremity function regarding joint contractures, increased lower-extremity tone, and a crouched stance, resulting in functional limitations in ambulation.[1]

PROGNOSIS

The expected range of number of visits per episode of care according to practice pattern 5C is 6 to 90. It is anticipated that 80% of the patients in this diagnostic group will achieve outcomes within 6 to 90 visits during a single continuous episode of care. Considering LV's normal intelligence and supportive home environment, it is estimated that 10 physical therapy visits will be necessary. It is anticipated that after insertion of the baclofen pump, and strength, endurance, motor-learning training, LV will increase step length, walking velocity, and cadence to stay up with his peers in a school setting.[1]

PRIMARY PREVENTION/RISK FACTOR REDUCTION STRATEGIES

LV has a supportive home environment, normal intelligence, and appropriate equipment. After insertion of the baclofen pump, one hopes that he will show improvement in present impairment and functional abilities.

PROCEDURAL INTERVENTIONS

Questions:
3a. Therapeutic exercise/functional training. What types of therapeutic exercise/functional training activities should be designed for LV? Refer to Chapter 7 for additional exercise suggestions.
3b. Indirect interventions. What other interventions may be needed?
3c. Goals/outcomes. Design short-term (2 weeks or less) and long-term (more than 2 weeks) impairment, functional, and disability goals for LV.

Answers

C A S E   1

1a. Therapeutic exercise. Exercise should emphasize left hip and knee strengthening as well as increasing range of motion of the left knee. The following activities, such as those further described in Chapter 7, should be emphasized. Rotation exercises and ball throwing may increase trunk stability and coordination. Proprioceptive neuromuscular facilitation (PNF) exercises consisting of rhythmic stabilization and slow reversal may be used to strengthen the extremities, especially the weakened left hip and knee. Because of DM's sedentary lifestyle and underlying diabetes, cardiovascular activities are very important. Individuals with long transtibial residual limbs averaged a 10% higher energy expenditure and those with short residual limbs averaged a 40% higher energy expenditure than the able bodied.[3] Standing weight shift, progressing to weight shift on a compliant surface, to more challenging standing and ambulation activities should be done when the prosthesis is received. Upper-extremity strengthening will enable independent transfers. Desensitization exercises should be done to accustom the residual limb to weight bearing. Coordination exercises will facilitate controlled movement of the residual limb and, ultimately, the prosthesis.

1b. Functional training in self-care and home management. Arrangements need to be made for rails to be installed on the front and rear steps of the patient's home. Training in transfer techniques and independent ambulation with the left transtibial prosthesis on level and uneven surfaces should be done. A straight cane may be used initially, but DM should be able to ambulate independently more than 500 feet without an assistive device. Specific functional activities are further described in Chapter 7.

1c. Functional training in community and work integration or reintegration. Referral to a variety of health professionals is indicated. These include:

Vocational retraining for work-exploration activities
Nutrition regarding weight loss

Diabetic education for better blood glucose control, insulin monitoring, and education regarding care of his right foot
Psychology for counseling regarding his withdrawn personality and possible depression; in addition, interventions regarding family dynamics and problem drinking need to be explored
Support group for peer counseling; DM may benefit from interactions with an individual of the same age who has previously undergone an amputation
Social services to investigate family financial affairs

1d. Goals/outcomes

Short-term impairment goals. DM will
    Increase range of motion of the left knee to 125° of flexion and 0° of extension
    Increase strength in the left hip and knee to 5/5
    Decrease pain in the residual limb to a 0 level at rest, in a dependent position, and when ambulating
Short-term functional goals. DM will
    Transfer independently
    Independently apply and remove the prosthesis
Short-term disability goal. DM will
    Attend sessions with psychology, nutrition, diabetic education, and support groups
Long-term impairment goal. DM will
    Decrease respiration rates, pulse, and blood pressure to normal values
Long-term functional goal. DM will
    Ambulate independently in a normal cadence of 101-122 steps per minute for 5 minutes with the left transtibial prosthesis without an assistive device
Long-term disability goal. DM will
    Enroll in a job-retraining program and obtain a GED

C A S E   2

2a. Therapeutic exercise. Exercise should emphasize strengthening the left hip with the THA precautions of limiting hip flexion to 90° and adduction and external rotation to 0°. Strengthening and coordination activities of the right transfemoral extremity should also be emphasized to enable supervised ambulation with an assistive device.

2b. Functional training in self-care and home management. Training in wheelchair safety and mobility, transfer training, and activities of daily living such as dressing, grooming, and sit to stand should occur. Standing, progressing to weight shifting, and ambulation activities with an assistive device should be emphasized.

2c. Goals/outcomes

Short-term impairment goals. WN will
> Observe total hip precautions in limiting hip range of motion
> Complete healing of the incision over the left proximal femur and the abrasion over the right transfemoral residual limb

Short-term functional goals. WN will
> Propel wheelchair independently for functional distances on a level surface
> Independently lock wheelchair brakes and maneuver leg rests

Short-term disability goals. WN will
> Use a lightweight wheelchair to facilitate propulsion and attendance at hospital social functions
> Successfully arrange for repair of the transfemoral prosthesis and installation of a manual lock knee (with assistance from the rehabilitation team)

Long-term impairment goals. WN will
> Increase strength of left hip musculature to 4/5 to match that of the right hip
> Decrease respiration rate, pulse, and blood pressure to normal values

Long-term functional goals. WN will
> Independently apply and take off the prosthesis, including locking and unlocking the manual-lock knee
> Perform grooming, dressing, and toileting activities with only occasional verbal cues
> Transfer from bed to wheelchair with minimal assistance using a transfer board
> Ambulate 30 feet with minimal assistance using forearm crutches with partial weight bearing on the right transfemoral prosthesis

Long-term disability goal. WN will
> Successfully arrange for placement in a subacute rehabilitation facility in his hometown (with assistance from the rehabilitation team)

CASE 3

3a. Therapeutic exercise/functional training. Active and passive stretching activities should emphasize increasing length of the hip flexors, hamstrings, and plantarflexors. Functional motor activities should concentrate on strengthening, endurance, and selective control of hip flexion and extension, knee flexion and extension, and ankle dorsiflexion and plantarflexion to enable more-balanced control. Functional motor activities include ambulation as well as training in putting on and taking off DAFOs and sneakers.

3b. Indirect interventions

> Monitor crutches, DAFOs, and wheelchair for fit
> After insertion of the baclofen pump, assess the need for serial casting to gain ankle dorsiflexion
> After insertion of the baclofen pump, assess the need for a ground reaction orthosis rather than DAFOs to decrease crouched gait
> Communicate and document information provided to the school team regarding
>> Effects of baclofen
>> Goals of interventions
>> Strategies for carryover of motor learning into the school environment

3c. Goals/outcomes

Short-term impairment goals. LV will
> Increase range of motion by 10° in hip and knee extension and ankle dorsiflexion
> Perform isolated movements in bilateral hip flexion, knee flexion, and ankle dorsiflexion a minimum of 10 times

Short-term functional goal. LV will
> Require no assistance in putting on DAFOs and sneakers

Long-term functional goals. LV will
> Ambulate independently 100 feet in 2 minutes to stay up with his peers in school
> Perform isolated movement in bilateral hip flexion, knee flexion, and ankle dorsiflexion while ambulating 100 feet

References

1. American Physical Therapy Association. (2001). A guide to physical therapist practice. *Physical Therapy*, 81

2. Braunwald, E., Isselbacher, K. J., Petersdorf, R. G., Wilson, J. D., Martin, J. B., & Fauci, A. S. (2001). *Harrison's principles of internal medicine* (13th ed.). New York: McGraw Hill.

3. Sutherland, D. H., Olshen, R., Cooper, L., & Woo, S. Y. (1980) The development of mature gait. *Journal of Bone and Joint Surgery (Am)*, 62, 336–353.

4. Coster, W., Deeney, T., Haltiwangen, J., & Haley, S. *School function assessment (SFA): User's manual*. San Antonio, TX: Therapy School Builders, 1998.

5. Gage, J. (1993). Gait analysis. An essential tool in the treatment of cerebral palsy. *Clinical Orthopaedics and Related Research*, 288, 126–134.

GLOSSARY

Acquired amputation: not inherited, received after birth; most commonly due to trauma or disease.

Adductor roll: excess amount of soft tissue that forms high in the groin because of improper wrapping techniques.

Allograft: cadaver graft used to replace a portion of the shaft of bone.

Amelia: congenital absence of a limb.

Ankle rocker: refers to progression of the limb during gait at the time when the ankle serves as the pivot of motion.

Annular constricting band: ring of tissue that binds and squeezes; restricting further growth of parts of the developing fetus.

Arteriosclerosis: form of vascular disease characterized by loss of elasticity of arterial walls causing chronic ischemia of major organs and/or extremities.

Arthritis: inflammatory condition of joints, characterized by pain and effusion. Two common types are osteoarthritis, or degenerative joint disease (a slow, progressive process leading to breakdown of joint articular cartilage and subsequent pain and stiffness), and rheumatoid arthritis (a chronic, systemic inflammatory disorder usually involving numerous joints).

Arthrodesis: surgical fixation of a joint by fusion of the joint surfaces.

Arthroplasty: surgical procedure to fabricate an artificial joint.

Autograft: graft moved from one site to another in the same individual.

Bifid bones: cleft bones that are divided into two parts or branches.

BRIME: an isometric exercise regimen consisting of up to 20 maximum contractions, each held for 6 seconds, with a 20 second rest after each contraction.

Brittle: property of a material that shows little deformation under load, after the elastic limit is reached, before failure.

Bud: swelling on the trunk of the embryo that becomes a limb.

Cadence: the number of steps per unit time, often steps per minute.

Cerebral palsy (CP): a nonprogressive, nonhereditary involvement of the cerebral cortex that results in postural and motion disturbances.

Chopart amputation: amputation that occurs at the talonavicular and calcaneocuboid joints.

Chronic venous insufficiency (CVI): disorder characterized by decreased return of the venous blood from the legs to the trunk.

Complex regional pain syndrome (CRPS): another term for reflex sympathetic dystrophy (RSD). CRPS is chronic pain associated with abnormal sympathetic reflex response, severe pain, swelling, stiffness, and skin discoloration out of proportion to the injury.

Computer-aided design/computer-aided manufacturing system (CAD/CAM): a probe or digitizer that converts information from the negative impression of the residual limb into computer data, a software system, and a carver that makes a positive plaster mold.

Congenital: existing at, and usually before, birth; refers to conditions that are present at birth, regardless of the cause.

Contact dermatitis: inflammatory response to an irritant; may become a site for infection.

Contracture: fixed high resistance to passive stretch resulting from soft tissue or muscle shortening affecting joint position.

Creep: progressive deformation of a material caused by constant low loading over an extended period.

Definitive prosthesis: prescribed when the patient's residual limb no longer has marked edema. The patient may be ready for the definitive prosthesis 3–9 months after amputation.

Deformation: change in shape or volume in response to an applied force.

Degrees of freedom: the number of planes of motion a body (joint) can move through; one degree of freedom indicates that a segment can move through one plane of motion.

DeLorme technique: an isotonic regimen of exercise; also termed *progressive resistive exercise* (PRE).

Desensitization activities: activities such as massage or tapping to accustom the residual limb to weight bearing.

Diabetes mellitus: disorder characterized by hyperglycemia resulting from defects in insulin secretion, insulin action, or both.

Diagnosis: the process and the end result of evaluation information obtained from the examination.

Disability: the inability to engage in age- or gender-specific roles in a certain social context and physical environment.

Double stance: phase of the gait cycle when both feet are in contact with the ground.

Dressings: used after amputation to control edema and facilitate fitting of the prosthesis. Examples include

Air splint—plastic splint filled with air, which may allow partial weight bearing.

Removable rigid dressing (RRD)—dressing composed of a plaster shell, socks, a stockinet sleeve, and a thermoplastic supracondylar cuff; it allows easier visualization than the rigid dressing.

Rigid dressing—plaster cast that is very effective in controlling edema.

Semirigid dressing—dressing that uses an Unna paste bandage; it has better edema control than a soft dressing.

Soft dressing—dressing composed of gauze, cotton padding, and elastic bandages.

Ductile: describes a material that under load, exhibits considerable deformation before ultimate failure.

Duration: length of an exercise session.

Dynamic alignment: alignment of a prosthesis during weight bearing and/or walking.

Dynamic-response feet: feet that provide propulsion at terminal stance, enhancing the ability to walk long distances, run, and jump.

Dyskinesia: category of involuntary movements including ataxia, athetosis, or choreiform; difficulty in performing voluntary motion.

Elastic wraps: bandages that contain elastic, used to control residual limb edema.

Elasticity: property of material that returns to its original shape and size after being deformed.

Endoskeletal or modular prosthesis: soft covering over an inner tube; lightweight.

Epiphysis: end of a long bone, usually wider than the shaft, separated from the shaft by a cartilaginous disk.

Episode of care: all patient activities that are provided, directed, or supervised by the physical therapist from initial contact through discharge.

Equinovarus: plantarflexed and inverted foot position.

Equinus: lack of talocrural joint dorsiflexion, a plantarflexed foot.

Evaluation: dynamic process in which the therapist makes clinical judgments based on examination results.

Ewing's sarcoma: rapidly growing tumor that aggressively erodes the bone cortex to produce a tender, palpable mass.

Examination: the process of history taking, systems review, and selecting and administering specific tests and measures.

Examination (checkout) procedure: systematic method of examining a patient with an amputation and the prosthesis. The examination (checkout) procedure determines whether accepted standards of prosthesis fabrication and fit have been met and if not, a need for possible corrective actions.

Excessive heel rise: gait deviation characterized by increased knee flexion of the prosthesis compared with the sound side.

Exoskeletal prosthesis: prosthesis consisting of a hard outer cover made of plastic laminate; it is indicated when durability is important.

Flexibility or stretching exercises: exercises that increase range of motion to prevent muscle shortening and subsequent joint contractures.

Forefoot rocker: progression of the limb during gait when the forefoot serves as the pivot of motion.

Frequency: how often an exercise session is done; e.g., times per week.

Friction: tangential force resisting motion of one surface on another.

Functional limitations: restrictions in the ability to perform a physical action, activity, or task in an efficient manner.

Fusion: surgical procedure to join two bones together; an arthrodesis.

Gait cycle: the sequence of events that occur between two successive initial contacts of the same lower extremity.

Ground-reaction force: the force the ground exerts back on an object as a result of the weight of the object against the ground or surface on which it lies.

Ground reaction force vector: the graphic representation, including point of application, direction, and magnitude, of the ground-reaction force.

Heel rocker: progression of the limb during gait when the heel serves as the pivot of motion.

Hemimelia: developmental anomaly characterized by the absence of all or part of the distal half of a limb. A tibial hemimelia is the absence of the tibia, with the fibula intact.

Hemipelvectomy: loss of any part of the ilium, ischium, and pubis.

Hip disarticulation: loss of the complete femur.

Hip pointer: often caused by a blow to the inadequately protected iliac crest in an athlete. Pain is often caused by inflammation of muscles that attach to the iliac crest.

Hyperglycemia: elevated blood glucose level, primarily associated with diabetes mellitus.

Hypoplastic bones: defective or incompletely developed bones.

Hysteresis: energy loss exhibited by viscoelastic materials under loading; represented on a stress/strain curve as the area between the noncongruent curves of loading and unloading.

Ilizarov method: method of limb salvage using a distraction rate of 1 mm per day to facilitate bone formation.

Impairments: losses or abnormalities of physiologic, psychologic, or anatomic structure or function.

Impedance plethysmography: noninvasive blood flow assessment technique.

Inertia: tendency of an object at rest to stay at rest unless acted on by an outside force, and the tendency of an object in motion to stay in motion unless acted on by an outside force.

Intensity: difficulty of an exercise, often measured as a percentage of maximal heart rate.

Immediate postoperative prosthesis (IPOP): rigid dressing attached to a pylon and foot. The IPOP allows early ambulation after amputation.

Instant axis of rotation: the axis of motion at a given instant in time; as if it is a fixed or "pin" axis for that moment.

Intervention: purposeful, skilled interaction of the therapist with the patient to produce changes consistent with the diagnosis and prognosis.

Intermittent claudication: decrease in the arterial diameter resulting in insufficient blood flow, especially to the lower extremities.

Isokinetics: type of exercise in which movement occurs at a constant speed but a variable resistance.

Isometric: static form of exercise that occurs when a muscle contracts without an appreciable change in the length of the muscle or without visible joint motion.

Isotonics: type of exercise that is carried out against a constant or variable load as a muscle lengthens or shortens through the available range of motion.

Keel: hard inner part of the prosthetic foot, similar to the bones and ligaments of the anatomic foot. The keel is often surrounded by foam.

Kinematics: biomechanical term to describe motion without reference to mass or force.

Kinematic chain: in engineering, a series of links or segments interconnected by pin-centered joints.

Kinetics: biomechanical term to describe motion taking forces into account.

Knee disarticulation: an amputation through the knee joint.

Lateral whip: the heel moves laterally at toe-off.

Legg-Calvé-Perthes disease: flattening of the epiphysis of the femoral head; also called *coxa plana*. Avascular necrosis occurs because of a circulatory disturbance.

Liner: material placed between the residual limb and the hard socket to provide comfort and protection.

Lisfranc amputation: an amputation at the tarsometatarsal joint.

Longitudinal deficiency: total or partial absence of a segment; distally, beyond this deficient segment, normal skeletal structures may exist.

Meningocele: external protrusion of the meninges.

Mode: type of exercise that is most suited for the patient.

Moment arm: shortest distance from the action line to the axis of motion (a perpendicular from the axis to the action line); the longer the moment arm, the more torque can be created.

Myodesis: attachment of muscle to periosteal bone.

Myofascial flap: attachment of muscle to fascia.

Myelomeningocele: protrusion of the meninges and spinal cord.

Myoplasty: attachment of muscle to muscle.

Neuroma: collection of axons and fibrous tissue formed by the transected end of a peripheral nerve. Severe pain on weight bearing often results.

Neuropathy: inflammation of peripheral nerves characterized by weakness and pain; often seen in diabetes mellitus.

Orthotics: practice and manufacture of orthoses, or an example of a shoe insert.

Orthosis: device applied on the exterior of the body to restrict or enhance motion or reduce the load on a body segment.

Orthotist: person skilled in the profession of orthotics.

Osteomyelitis: infection resulting from penetrating trauma or a surgical procedure; commonly affects long bones such as the femur or tibia.

Osteosarcomas: tumors involving metaphyses of the long bones, particularly the lower end of the femur, upper end of the tibia, and upper end of the humerus.

Outcomes: results of patient management.

Oxford technique: isotonic regimen of exercise; the reverse of the DeLorme system.

Peripheral vascular disease (PVD): any abnormal condition that affects blood vessels peripheral to the heart.

Phantom limb sensation: perception of numbness, pressure, position, temperature, or "pins-and-needles" feeling in the amputated part.

Phantom pain: perception of pain in the absent distal extremity; described as shooting, burning, cramping, or crushing.

Phocomelia: absence of the proximal section of a limb(s).

Plantigrade: entire heel and sole of the foot is on the ground while walking.

Plasticity: property of material that does not return to its original shape with unloading; on the stress strain curve, plastic behavior occurs between the yield point and the failure point.

Positioning: placement or alignment performed to prevent soft tissue shortening and joint contractures.

Postoperative prosthesis: immediate postsurgical prosthesis (IPOP); usually used for younger patients with no vascular disease.

Prognosis: determination of the level of optimal improvement that may be attained and the amount of time to reach that level.

Proprioceptive neuromuscular facilitation (PNF): type of exercise that may improve strength and motor control of the trunk and limbs to enhance functional abilities such as bed mobility, transfers, and ambulation.

Proximal femoral focal deficiency (PFFD): underdeveloped or partial absence of the femur, especially the proximal third.

Pylon: metal tube that may extend between the rigid dressing and foot in an immediate postoperative prosthesis (IPOP).

Reflex sympathetic dystrophy (RSD): chronic pain associated with abnormal sympathetic reflex response; severe pain, swelling, stiffness, and skin discoloration out of proportion to the injury. Also called *complex regional pain syndrome* (CRPS).

Rhythmic stabilization: proprioceptive neuromuscular facilitation technique that involves isometric co-contraction of antagonists.

Rotationplasty: surgical procedure in which the ankle after rotation of 180° acts as the knee joint; commonly used in patients with tumor.

Shrinkers: customized elastic socks used to control edema; commonly used with patients with a transfemoral amputation.

Silicone liner: liner that may serve as a dressing to control edema as well as a prosthetic suspension; often used for patients with transtibial amputations.

Single stance: phase of the gait cycle when only one foot is in contact with the ground.

Slow reversal: proprioceptive neuromuscular facilitation technique that involves an isotonic contraction in one diagonal pattern with changes in direction performed alternately at the end of the range.

Soft bandage: bandage consisting of gauze, cotton padding, and elastic.

Speed: rate of position change over time; the magnitude portion of a velocity vector.

Spica: bandage that encircles the waist to secure a transfemoral wrap.

Spina bifida occulta: incomplete fusion of the vertebral lamina, often asymptomatic.

Static alignment: alignment of the prosthesis prior to wear; also referred to as *bench alignment*.

Step: part of the gait cycle that occurs between the initial contact of one foot and the initial contact of the opposite foot.

Stiffness: resistance to an external load as a material deforms; indicated by the slope of the stress/strain curve.

Stress: load per unit area.

Strain: deformation or change in dimension in response to a load.

Stride: part of the gait cycle that occurs between initial contact of one foot and the next initial contact of the same foot.

Supracondylar amputation: amputation at the distal femur in which the patella may be preserved.

Suspensions: elements that may be used to secure a prosthesis on the residual limb.

Syme amputation: ankle disarticulation in which the heel pad is maintained to cover the bottom of the limb for good weight bearing.

Synergy: specific movements of various joints occurring together as a result of a central nervous system defect.

Synostosis: union between two adjacent bones or parts.

Temporary prosthesis: unfinished prosthesis that allows early ambulation and residual limb shrinkage. These prostheses are usually used for 3–6 months following the amputation.

Terminal impact: gait deviation characterized by the prosthesis coming to an abrupt stop with visible and sometimes audible force as the knee extends fully.

TKA line: line used for static alignment of the transfemoral prosthesis in a lateral view.

Toe-out: angle formed by the line of progression (drawn by connecting the center of the heels for a stride) and a line drawn longitudinally in the foot from the center of the posterior heel to the second toe.

Torque: ability to rotate or turn a lever; equal to the force times the moment arm.

Trans: describes an amputation that extends across the axis of a long bone; e.g. transfemoral.

Translation: motion in which different regions of an object move the same distance in the same time frame.

Transverse deficiency: amputation that occurs across or at a right angle to the long axis of a bone. All structures distal to this level are absent.

Traumatic brain injury (TBI): head injury that may result in neurologic deficits.

Treatment: sum of all interventions provided by the physical therapist during an episode of care.

Unna paste bandage: bandage that consists of zinc oxide, gelatin, glycerin, and gauze, used in a semirigid dressing.

Vaulting: gait deviation characterized by excessive plantarflexion of the sound ankle and raising the entire body vertically, permitting the prosthesis to swing through.

Vector: quantity that includes a point of application, direction, and magnitude.

Velocity: speed and direction; the velocity of walking is the speed in a designated direction.

Vestigial phalanges: incomplete remnant with insufficient or no bony components.

Viscoelasticity: property combining some of the properties of viscosity and elasticity; shows varying degrees of stiffness depending on the rate of application and duration of the load.

Yield point: point on a load–deformation curve at which the material exhibits permanent deformation if loaded beyond that point; beginning of the plastic phase.

INDEX

Page numbers in italics followed by f denote figures; those followed by t denote tables.